Research of Pathogenesis and Novel Therapeutics in Arthritis 2.0

Research of Pathogenesis and Novel Therapeutics in Arthritis 2.0

Editor

Chih-Hsin Tang

MDPI • Basel • Beijing • Wuhan • Barcelona • Belgrade • Manchester • Tokyo • Cluj • Tianjin

Editor
Chih-Hsin Tang
China Medical University
Taiwan

Editorial Office
MDPI
St. Alban-Anlage 66
4052 Basel, Switzerland

This is a reprint of articles from the Special Issue published online in the open access journal *International Journal of Molecular Sciences* (ISSN 1422-0067) (available at: https://www.mdpi.com/journal/ijms/special_issues/arthritis2).

For citation purposes, cite each article independently as indicated on the article page online and as indicated below:

LastName, A.A.; LastName, B.B.; LastName, C.C. Article Title. *Journal Name* **Year**, *Volume Number*, Page Range.

ISBN 978-3-0365-7592-6 (Hbk)
ISBN 978-3-0365-7593-3 (PDF)

Contents

About the Editor

Chih-Hsin Tang

Chih-Hsin Tang (Professor): Chih-Hsin Tang is currently a professor at the Department of Pharmacology, China Medical University. He has served as the R&D Dean of the Research and Development Department since 2016 to present. His research mainly focuses on skeletal system diseases, including osteoporosis, arthritis, bone cancer, etc., to develop novel molecular targets and to find drugs with therapeutic potential. He has been listed in the "World's Top 2% Scientists 2020 (Scopus)", the "World's Top 2% Scientists 2021 (Scopus)", and the Best Scientists Ranking in the Medicine field in Taiwan (Research.com 2022).

International Journal of
Molecular Sciences

MDPI

Editorial

Research of Pathogenesis and Novel Therapeutics in Arthritis 2.0

Chih-Hsin Tang [1,2,3]

1 Department of Pharmacology, School of Medicine, China Medical University, Taichung 40001, Taiwan; chtang@mail.cmu.edu.tw; Tel.: +886-22052121 (ext. 7726)
2 Chinese Medicine Research Center, China Medical University, Taichung 40001, Taiwan
3 Department of Biotechnology, College of Health Science, Asia University, Taichung 41354, Taiwan

Received: 26 October 2020; Accepted: 28 October 2020; Published: 30 October 2020

Abstract: Arthritis has a high prevalence globally and includes over 100 types, the most common of which are rheumatoid arthritis, osteoarthritis, psoriatic arthritis, and inflammatory arthritis. All types of arthritis share common features of disease, including monocyte infiltration, inflammation, synovial swelling, pannus formation, stiffness in the joints and articular cartilage destruction. The exact etiology of arthritis remains unclear, and no cure exists as of yet. Anti-inflammatory drugs (NSAIDs and corticosteroids) are commonly used in the treatment of arthritis. However, these drugs are associated with significant side effects, such as gastric bleeding and an increased risk for heart attack and other cardiovascular problems. It is therefore crucial that we continue to research the pathogenesis of arthritis and seek to discover novel modes of therapy. This editorial summarizes and discusses the themes of the 27 articles published in our Special Issue "Research of Pathogenesis and Novel Therapeutics in Arthritis 2.0", a continuation of our 2019 Special Issue "Research of Pathogenesis and Novel Therapeutics in Arthritis". These Special Issues detail important novel research discoveries that contribute to our current understanding of arthritis.

Keywords: arthritis; treatment; molecular mechanisms; biomarkers; inflammatory cytokines; prevention

---

Arthritis has a high prevalence globally and includes over 100 types, the most common of which are rheumatoid arthritis (RA), osteoarthritis (OA), psoriatic arthritis (PsA) and inflammatory arthritis. All types of arthritis share common features of disease, including monocyte infiltration, inflammation, synovial swelling, pannus formation, stiffness in the joints and articular cartilage destruction. The exact etiology of arthritis remains unclear, and no cure exists as of yet. Anti-inflammatory drugs (NSAIDs and corticosteroids) are commonly used in the treatment of arthritis. However, these drugs are associated with significant side effects, such as gastric bleeding and an increased risk for heart attack and other cardiovascular problems. It is therefore crucial that we continue to research the pathogenesis of arthritis and seek to discover novel modes of therapy.

Our call for papers for this Special Issue—Research of Pathogenesis and Novel Therapeutics in Arthritis 2.0—Attracted a diverse collection of articles, which were closely examined by a panel of expert reviewers, who selected 27 (18 research papers and 9 reviews) for publication in this Special Issue. The majority of the research papers investigated the pathogenesis of arthritis and new biomarkers; three examined novel strategies in the treatment of arthritis. All of these papers are discussed below.

(i) The pathogenesis of arthritis. Research performed by Kmiolek and colleagues offers insights into how the interplay between transcriptional factors and microRNAs (miRNAs) contributes to RA pathogenesis [1]. Sanz and colleagues describe early immunomodulation in DMARD-naïve patients with new-onset RA and different patterns of CD4$^+$ modulation in methotrexate responders and nonresponders [2], while Lucchino and colleagues discuss their findings of early subclinical lung abnormalities in RA-associated autoimmunity, which may assist clinicians with the clinical management and therapeutic decisions in individual patients [3]. The preclinical research by Fujii and colleagues indicates that active exercise in established phase arthritis inhibits joint destruction and RA disease activity [4]. Upregulation of miR-941 in CD14$^+$ monocytes enhances osteoclast activation in patients with PsA, report Lin and colleagues [5], while other investigations reveal that age-related differences exist in knee joint transcriptome during the development of post-traumatic OA (PTOA) in mice, which may contribute to a severe PTOA phenotype in older individuals [6]. Akagi and colleagues offer novel insights into the pathophysiological function of angiotensin II (Ang II) in bone erosion and systemic bone loss in arthritis and they have found that excessive systemic activation of the renin–angiotensin system (RAS) is a risk factor for progressive joint destruction, which has important implications for the clinical use of RAS inhibitors in RA [7]. Teixeira and colleagues have addressed the interplay between inflammation and bone injury in collagen-induced arthritis (CIA) animal models of RA and confirm that such models are appropriate for investigating the mechanisms of bone repair/regeneration in chronic inflammatory conditions [8].

(ii) New biomarkers. Khanfar and colleagues describe preclinical findings showing that the transcription factor Nkx2-3 appears to regulate the development of autoimmune arthritis, probably via B cell signaling [9]. Li and Zheng have identified novel targets of knee OA shared by synovium and cartilage, which may help with the development of novel OA therapies [10]. Belluzzi and colleagues describe inflammatory and fibrotic changes in OA infrapatellar fat pad (IFP) characteristics, which suggests that targeting fibrosis could effectively counteract the disease progression and associated pain in patients with OA [11]. Groma and colleagues discuss their findings of persistent human herpesvirus 7 (HHV-7) infection in 81.5% of their study subjects with OA and reactivation in 20.5% of the subjects [12]. The study researchers discuss the significance of the immune system reaction to a foreign antigen and the impact on inflammatory cells in OA [12]. Chang and colleagues describe findings suggesting that electronegative low-density lipoprotein (LDL) may promote atherogenesis by augmenting macrophage foam cell formation, upregulating CD11c expression, and enhancing the expression levels of atherosclerosis-related mediators in RA [13]. In another study, Hähnlein and colleagues discuss evidence suggesting that human lymph node stromal cells (LNSCs) from RA patients regulate peripheral tolerance, making these cells a novel target to exploit in tolerance maintenance and induction [14]. Work by Yu and colleagues suggests that targeting peptidylarginine deiminase 2 (PADI2) may be a novel strategy for controlling inflammation caused by macrophages [15].

(iii) Novel strategies in the treatment of arthritis. Chou and colleagues discuss how the inhibition of discoidin domain receptors 1 (Ddr1) reduces chondrocyte apoptosis and promotes chondrocyte autophagy, leading to the attenuation of cartilage degradation, and so may therefore be a potential disease-modifying therapy for preventing OA progression [16]. Mendez and colleagues describe how chronic antibiotic treatment prior to the initial injury reduces inflammation and slows the development of PTOA in mice [17]. Hirata and colleagues detail promising findings showing that taurine inhibits mitochondrial dysfunction associated with glucocorticoid administration, preventing osteonecrosis in rabbits and cultured osteocytes [18].

Reviews. The nine reviews discuss recent findings on novel pathogenic aspects of inflammatory joint diseases and interesting investigations into treatment aspects of arthritis. Ailioaie and Litscher discuss the benefits of using photobiomodulation in juvenile idiopathic arthritis and adult RA [19], while Krajewska-Włodarczyk and colleagues focus on the immunopathogenic and therapeutic role of microparticles in chronic immune-mediated inflammatory joint diseases [20]. Tsukazaki and Kaito discuss the role of the interleukin (IL-23/IL-17) pathway in the pathogenesis of spondyloarthritis (SpA) and clinical evidence for biological agents that target IL-23 and IL-17 in the treatment of SpA [21]. Hong and colleagues discuss biological and molecular mechanisms that contribute to arthritis pain in animal models of RA and OA [22], while Kotyla and colleagues detail the activity of Janus kinase (JAK) inhibitors in the cardiovascular system of patients with RA, as well as the side effects of these medications [23]. Mikhaylenko and colleagues summarize genetic polymorphisms associated with the development of RA and they discuss how to apply the genetic variants in the selection of anti-RA medications [24]. MacDonald and colleagues describe the immunopathogenic characteristics of melatonin in RA disease [25], while Tanikella and colleagues discuss emerging genome-editing techniques against chronic degenerative joint conditions such as OA [26]. Finally, Cici and colleagues review the role of Wnt signaling in RA and SpA, focusing on the effect of biological therapy on this pathway and its possible clinical implications [27].

We hope that this Special Issue will provide new research insights and directions that ultimately inspire new arthritis prevention and treatment strategies.

Funding: This research received no external funding.

Conflicts of Interest: The author declares no conflict of interest.

References

1. Kmiolek, T.; Rzeszotarska, E.; Wajda, A.; Walczuk, E.; Kuca-Warnawin, E.; Romanowska-Prochnicka, K.; Stypinska, B.; Majewski, D.; Jagodzinski, P.P.; Pawlik, A.; et al. The interplay between transcriptional factors and micrornas as an important factor for th17/treg balance in ra patients. *Int. J. Mol. Sci.* **2020**, *21*, 7169. [CrossRef] [PubMed]
2. Monserrat Sanz, J.; Bohorquez, C.; Gomez, A.M.; Movasat, A.; Perez, A.; Ruiz, L.; Diaz, D.; Sanchez, A.I.; Albarran, F.; Sanz, I.; et al. Methrotexate treatment inmunomodulates abnormal cytokine expression by t cd4 lymphocytes present in dmard-naive rheumatoid arthritis patients. *Int. J. Mol. Sci.* **2020**, *21*, 6847. [CrossRef] [PubMed]
3. Lucchino, B.; Di Paolo, M.; Gioia, C.; Vomero, M.; Diacinti, D.; Mollica, C.; Alessandri, C.; Diacinti, D.; Palange, P.; Di Franco, M. Identification of subclinical lung involvement in acpa-positive subjects through functional assessment and serum biomarkers. *Int. J. Mol. Sci.* **2020**, *21*, 5162. [CrossRef] [PubMed]
4. Fujii, Y.; Inoue, H.; Arai, Y.; Shimomura, S.; Nakagawa, S.; Kishida, T.; Tsuchida, S.; Kamada, Y.; Kaihara, K.; Shirai, T.; et al. Treadmill running in established phase arthritis inhibits joint destruction in rat rheumatoid arthritis models. *Int. J. Mol. Sci.* **2019**, *20*, 5100. [CrossRef]
5. Lin, S.H.; Ho, J.C.; Li, S.C.; Cheng, Y.W.; Yang, Y.C.; Chen, J.F.; Hsu, C.Y.; Nakano, T.; Wang, F.S.; Yang, M.Y.; et al. Upregulation of mir-941 in circulating cd14+ monocytes enhances osteoclast activation via wnt16 inhibition in patients with psoriatic arthritis. *Int. J. Mol. Sci.* **2020**, *21*, 4301. [CrossRef]
6. Sebastian, A.; Murugesh, D.K.; Mendez, M.E.; Hum, N.R.; Rios-Arce, N.D.; McCool, J.L.; Christiansen, B.A.; Loots, G.G. Global gene expression analysis identifies age-related differences in knee joint transcriptome during the development of post-traumatic osteoarthritis in mice. *Int. J. Mol. Sci.* **2020**, *21*, 364. [CrossRef]
7. Akagi, T.; Mukai, T.; Mito, T.; Kawahara, K.; Tsuji, S.; Fujita, S.; Uchida, H.A.; Morita, Y. Effect of angiotensin ii on bone erosion and systemic bone loss in mice with tumor necrosis factor-mediated arthritis. *Int. J. Mol. Sci.* **2020**, *21*, 4145. [CrossRef]
8. Teixeira, J.H.; Silva, A.M.; Almeida, M.I.; Bessa-Goncalves, M.; Cunha, C.; Barbosa, M.A.; Santos, S.G. The systemic immune response to collagen-induced arthritis and the impact of bone injury in inflammatory conditions. *Int. J. Mol. Sci.* **2019**, *20*, 5436. [CrossRef]
9. Khanfar, E.; Olasz, K.; Gabris, F.; Gajdocsi, E.; Botz, B.; Kiss, T.; Kugyelka, R.; Berki, T.; Balogh, P.; Boldizsar, F. Ameliorated autoimmune arthritis and impaired b cell receptor-mediated ca(2+) influx in nkx2-3 knock-out mice. *Int. J. Mol. Sci.* **2020**, *21*, 6162. [CrossRef]
10. Li, C.; Zheng, Z. Identification of novel targets of knee osteoarthritis shared by cartilage and synovial tissue. *Int. J. Mol. Sci.* **2020**, *21*, 6033. [CrossRef]
11. Belluzzi, E.; Macchi, V.; Fontanella, C.G.; Carniel, E.L.; Olivotto, E.; Filardo, G.; Sarasin, G.; Porzionato, A.; Granzotto, M.; Pozzuoli, A.; et al. Infrapatellar fat pad gene expression and protein production in patients with and without osteoarthritis. *Int. J. Mol. Sci.* **2020**, *21*, 6016. [CrossRef] [PubMed]
12. Groma, V.; Tarasovs, M.; Skuja, S.; Semenistaja, S.; Nora-Krukle, Z.; Svirskis, S.; Murovska, M. Inflammatory cytokine-producing cells and inflammation markers in the synovium of osteoarthritis patients evidenced in human herpesvirus 7 infection. *Int. J. Mol. Sci.* **2020**, *21*, 6004. [CrossRef]

13. Chang, C.K.; Chen, P.K.; Lan, J.L.; Chang, S.H.; Hsieh, T.Y.; Liao, P.J.; Chen, C.H.; Chen, D.Y. Association of electronegative ldl with macrophage foam cell formation and cd11c expression in rheumatoid arthritis patients. *Int. J. Mol. Sci.* **2020**, *21*, 5883. [CrossRef] [PubMed]
14. Hahnlein, J.S.; Nadafi, R.; Jong, T.A.; Semmelink, J.F.; Remmerswaal, E.B.M.; Safy, M.; Lienden, K.P.V.; Maas, M.; Gerlag, D.M.; Tak, P.P.; et al. Human lymph node stromal cells have the machinery to regulate peripheral tolerance during health and rheumatoid arthritis. *Int. J. Mol. Sci.* **2020**, *21*, 5713. [CrossRef] [PubMed]
15. Yu, H.C.; Tung, C.H.; Huang, K.Y.; Huang, H.B.; Lu, M.C. The essential role of peptidylarginine deiminases 2 for cytokines secretion, apoptosis, and cell adhesion in macrophage. *Int. J. Mol. Sci.* **2020**, *21*, 5720. [CrossRef]
16. Chou, H.C.; Chen, C.H.; Chou, L.Y.; Cheng, T.L.; Kang, L.; Chuang, S.C.; Lin, Y.S.; Ho, M.L.; Wang, Y.H.; Lin, S.Y.; et al. Discoidin domain receptors 1 inhibition alleviates osteoarthritis via enhancing autophagy. *Int. J. Mol. Sci.* **2020**, *21*, 6991. [CrossRef]
17. Mendez, M.E.; Murugesh, D.K.; Sebastian, A.; Hum, N.R.; McCloy, S.A.; Kuhn, E.A.; Christiansen, B.A.; Loots, G.G. Antibiotic treatment prior to injury improves post-traumatic osteoarthritis outcomes in mice. *Int. J. Mol. Sci.* **2020**, *21*, 6424. [CrossRef]
18. Hirata, H.; Ueda, S.; Ichiseki, T.; Shimasaki, M.; Ueda, Y.; Kaneuji, A.; Kawahara, N. Taurine inhibits glucocorticoid-induced bone mitochondrial injury, preventing osteonecrosis in rabbits and cultured osteocytes. *Int. J. Mol. Sci.* **2020**, *21*, 6892. [CrossRef]
19. Ailioaie, L.M.; Litscher, G. Molecular and cellular mechanisms of arthritis in children and adults: New perspectives on applied photobiomodulation. *Int. J. Mol. Sci.* **2020**, *21*, 6565. [CrossRef] [PubMed]
20. Krajewska-Wlodarczyk, M.; Owczarczyk-Saczonek, A.; Zuber, Z.; Wojtkiewicz, M.; Wojtkiewicz, J. Role of microparticles in the pathogenesis of inflammatory joint diseases. *Int. J. Mol. Sci.* **2019**, *20*, 5453. [CrossRef]
21. Tsukazaki, H.; Kaito, T. The role of the il-23/il-17 pathway in the pathogenesis of spondyloarthritis. *Int. J. Mol. Sci.* **2020**, *21*, 6401. [CrossRef]
22. Hong, J.I.; Park, I.Y.; Kim, H.A. Understanding the molecular mechanisms underlying the pathogenesis of arthritis pain using animal models. *Int. J. Mol. Sci.* **2020**, *21*, 533. [CrossRef] [PubMed]
23. Kotyla, P.J.; Islam, M.A.; Engelmann, M. Clinical aspects of janus kinase (jak) inhibitors in the cardiovascular system in patients with rheumatoid arthritis. *Int. J. Mol. Sci.* **2020**, *21*, 7390. [CrossRef] [PubMed]
24. Mikhaylenko, D.S.; Nemtsova, M.V.; Bure, I.V.; Kuznetsova, E.B.; Alekseeva, E.A.; Tarasov, V.V.; Lukashev, A.N.; Beloukhova, M.I.; Deviatkin, A.A.; Zamyatnin, A.A., Jr. Genetic polymorphisms associated with rheumatoid arthritis development and antirheumatic therapy response. *Int. J. Mol. Sci.* **2020**, *21*, 4911. [CrossRef]
25. MacDonald, I.J.; Huang, C.C.; Liu, S.C.; Tang, C.H. Reconsidering the role of melatonin in rheumatoid arthritis. *Int. J. Mol. Sci.* **2020**, *21*, 2877. [CrossRef]
26. Tanikella, A.S.; Hardy, M.J.; Frahs, S.M.; Cormier, A.G.; Gibbons, K.D.; Fitzpatrick, C.K.; Oxford, J.T. Emerging gene-editing modalities for osteoarthritis. *Int. J. Mol. Sci.* **2020**, *21*, 6046. [CrossRef] [PubMed]
27. Cici, D.; Corrado, A.; Rotondo, C.; Cantatore, F.P. Wnt signaling and biological therapy in rheumatoid arthritis and spondyloarthritis. *Int. J. Mol. Sci.* **2019**, *20*, 5552. [CrossRef] [PubMed]

Publisher's Note: MDPI stays neutral with regard to jurisdictional claims in published maps and institutional affiliations.

International Journal of
Molecular Sciences

MDPI

Article

The Interplay between Transcriptional Factors and MicroRNAs as an Important Factor for Th17/Treg Balance in RA Patients

Tomasz Kmiołek [1], Ewa Rzeszotarska [1,*], Anna Wajda [1], Ewa Walczuk [1], Ewa Kuca-Warnawin [2], Katarzyna Romanowska-Próchnicka [3,4], Barbara Stypinska [1], Dominik Majewski [5], Pawel Piotr Jagodzinski [6], Andrzej Pawlik [7] and Agnieszka Paradowska-Gorycka [1]

1 Department of Molecular Biology, National Institute of Geriatrics, Rheumatology and Rehabilitation, 02-637 Warsaw, Poland; tomasz.kmiolek@spartanska.pl (T.K.); annawajda2046@gmail.com (A.W.); ewa.walczuk@spartanska.pl (E.W.); barbara.stypinska@wp.pl (B.S.); paradowska_aga@interia.pl (A.P.-G.)
2 Department of Pathophysiology and Immunology, National Institute of Geriatrics, Rheumatology and Rehabilitation, 02-637 Warsaw, Poland; ewa.kuca-warnawin@spartanska.pl
3 Department of Connective Tissue Diseases, National Institute of Geriatrics, Rheumatology and Rehabilitation, 02-637 Warsaw, Poland; katarzyna.prochnicka@gmail.com
4 Department of Pathophysiology, Warsaw Medical University, 02-091 Warsaw, Poland
5 Department of Rheumatology and Internal Medicine, Poznan University of Medical Science, 61-701 Poznan, Poland; dmajes@poczta.onet.pl
6 Department of Biochemistry and Molecular Biology, Poznan University of Medical Sciences, 61-701 Poznan, Poland; pjagodzi@ump.edu.pl
7 Department of Physiology, Pomeranian Medical University, 70-204 Szczecin, Poland; pawand@poczta.onet.pl
* Correspondence: ewa-rzeszotarska1@wp.pl

Received: 5 August 2020; Accepted: 25 September 2020; Published: 28 September 2020

Abstract: MicroRNAs regulate gene expression of transcriptional factors, which influence Th17/Treg (regulatory T cells) balance, establishing the molecular mechanism of genetic and epigenetic regulation of Treg and Th17 cells is crucial for understanding rheumatoid arthritis (RA) pathogenesis. The study goal was to understand the potential impact of the selected microRNAs expression profiles on Treg/Th17 cells frequency, RA phenotype, the expression profile of selected microRNAs, and their correlation with the expression profiles of selected transcriptional factors: SOCS1, SMAD3, SMAD4, STAT3, STAT5 in RA; we used osteoarthritis (OA) and healthy controls (HCs) as controls. The study was conducted on 14 RA and 11 OA patients, and 15 HCs. Treg/Th17 frequency was established by flow cytometry. Gene expression analysis was estimated by qPCR. We noticed correlations in RA Th17 cells between miR-26 and SMAD3, STAT3, SOCS1; and miR-155 and STAT3—and in RA Treg cells between miR-26 and SOCS1; miR-31, -155 and SMAD3; and miR-155 and SMAD4. In RA Tregs, we found a negative correlation between miR-26, -126 and STAT5a. The expression level of miR-31 in Th17 cells from RA patients with DAS28 $\leq$ 5.1 is higher and that for miR-24 is greater in Tregs from patients with DAS28 > 5.1. MiR-146a in Tregs is higher in rheumatoid factor (RF) positive RA patients.

Keywords: rheumatoid arthritis (RA); Treg; Th17; gene expression; microRNA; transcriptional factor

1. Introduction

Rheumatoid arthritis (RA) is one of the most widespread inflammatory diseases that affect the immune system. The most common symptoms are pain, joint swelling, and disability. In RA occurs proliferative synovitis leading to bone and cartilage destruction. The inflamed synovium contains synovial fibroblasts, macrophages, and T cells that secrete inflammatory cytokines. They activate osteoclasts, causing bone destruction. In RA occurs undue immune response of T cells. CD4+ T cells contain helper T cells (Th cells) and they stimulate the immune responses as well as regulatory T cells (Treg cells) that control these responses. Th cells include Th1, Th2, and Th17 cells subsets. RA is characterized by an imbalance in Th17/Treg, and Th17 is more activated than Treg [1].

In osteoarthritis (OA), disease joint surfaces are damaged, resulting in a lack of maintaining joint cartilage homeostasis. Damages are caused by excessive mechanical stress like tensile strains and compression forces, trauma, or inflammation. It results in structural damage and deformation [2].

In recent times, microRNAs are considered as an essential player connected with the onset as well as the progression of osteoarthritis [1,3,4]. MicroRNAs (miRNAs, miRs) are single-stranded, conserved, noncoding RNAs, which have approximately 22 nucleotides in length. There has been a lot of interest in miRNAs research in recent years, and more than two thousand microRNAs have been discovered so far. It is becoming increasingly clear that miRNAs contribute to the number of biological processes, e.g., apoptosis and cell proliferation. MicroRNAs regulate gene expression post-transcriptionally. About one-third of the genes in the human genome is under the control of the miRNAs [5]. Apart from the repression of translation, miRNAs moreover begin the affinity and enrollment of mRNA restriction factors, which leads to degradation of mRNA and disrupts gene expression. MicroRNAs regulate both acquired and innate immunity by their contribution to the cytogenesis and generation of immune cells (e.g., dendritic cells, T cells, B cells). Altered miRNAs stimulate the production of undue autoantibodies and inflammatory cytokines secretion. The abovementioned processes lead to an imbalance of the immune system. As a result, miRNAs are linked with various autoimmune diseases. MiRNAs have a crucial role in the pathogenesis of diseases like rheumatoid arthritis (RA), systemic lupus erythematosus (SLE), multiple sclerosis (MS), and primary biliary cholangitis (PBC) [4,5].

Yang et al. suggested that elevated miR-126 expression induces the hypomethylation of CD70 and CD11a genes, by the depression of DNMT1 protein, causing the onset and progression of RA [6]. Altered miR-24 occurs in RA and upregulation of this miRNA regulating the production of cytokines and causing deterioration of arthritis [7,8]. MiR-26a and miR-155 are linked to the immune responses and can suppress immune cell apoptosis; increase the activity of the immune system; and cause specific organ damage, including joint, skin, kidney, and lung [8]. Numerous microRNAs have been reported to be connected with synovial cell proliferation, osteoclast differentiation, and inflammatory cytokines and they have the potential to be used in the treatment of RA. MiR-155 and miR-146a are mentioned as representative miRNAs associated with the RA condition [2]. MiR-146a is critical for Treg cells suppressor function. The insufficiency of miR-146a in regulatory T cells caused a breach of immunological tolerance [9]. Suppressor of cytokine signaling 1 (SOCS1), the key negative controller of Janus kinase/Signal transducers and activators of transcription (JAK/STAT) signaling pathway [10], has been reported as the main target of miR-155 in peripheral blood mononuclear cells (PBMCs) of RA patients [2,11]. MiR-155 suppresses the expression of SOCS1 in activated CD4+ T cells and this leads to the stimulation of Interleukin-6/Signal transducer and activator of transcription 3 (IL-6/STAT3), and Interleukin-2/Signal transducer and activator of transcription 5 (IL-2/STAT5) signaling pathways, as well as the initiation of Treg/Th17 cells functions and differentiation [10].

Since microRNAs regulate gene expression of transcriptional factors, which impact Th17/Treg balance, assignment of the molecular mechanism of epigenetic as well as genetic regulation of Th17 and Treg cells is vital for comprehending RA etiology and pathogenesis. This study aimed to understand the potential influence of the selected microRNAs' expression profiles on the phenotype of RA. Moreover, we wanted to study and describe the regulation of five selected transcriptional factors, SOCS1, SMAD3, SMAD4, STAT3, and STAT5, by carefully chosen microRNAs in RA and control groups: OA and healthy control (HC). Moreover, we search for microRNAs that could be RA biomarkers.

2. Results

2.1. Increased Expression Levels of miR-146a and miR-155 in Treg Cells from RA and OA

Analysis of miRNAs expression levels in freshly isolated Th17 and Treg cells (Table S1) have shown that expression of miR-24 was 3 times higher in Th17 cells than in Treg cells from healthy subjects (p = 0.04). We did not see noticeable differences in OA and RA patients in the miR-24 expression level between Treg and Th17 cells (Figure 1A). We observed higher miR-26 expression levels in Treg cells from HCs than in RA Treg cells (p = 0.014). There were no differences in the miR-26 expression levels between Th17 cells and Treg cells in RA and OA patients (Figure 1B). We also observed that the miR-31 expression was 2 times higher in Th17 cells than in Treg cells from HCs (p = 0.0046, Figure 1C). For miR-146a, we noticed that its expression was 4 times higher in OA Treg cells than in OA Th17 cells (p = 0.008, Figure 1D), and 6 times higher in RA Treg cells than in RA Th17 cells (p = 0.0031, Figure 1D). MiR-155 expression was significantly higher in RA and OA Treg cells than in RA and OA Th17 cells (both p = 0.04, Figure 1E). In contrast, miR-155 expression was significantly higher in HC Th17 cells than in RA Th17 cells (p = 0.04, Figure 1E).

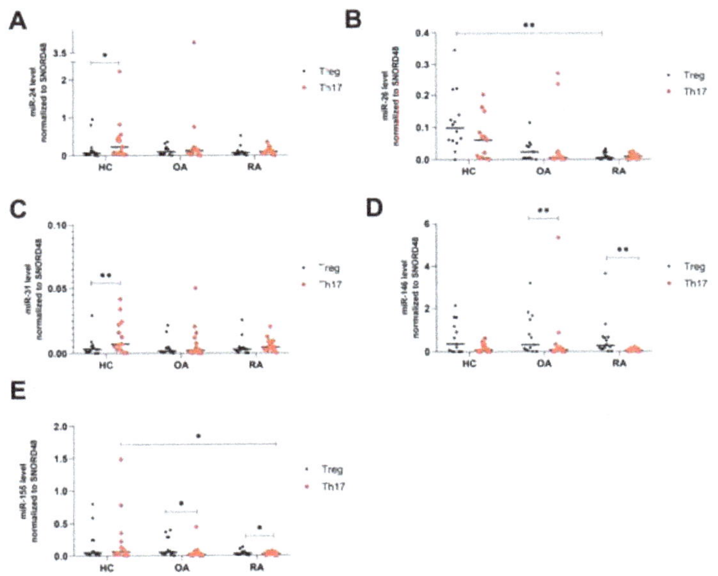

Figure 1. MicroRNA comparison in Treg and Th17 in healthy controls (HCs), osteoarthritis (OA), and rheumatoid arthritis (RA). MiR-24 level normalized to SNORD48 (**A**), miR-26 level normalized to SNORD48 (**B**), miR-31 level normalized to SNORD48 (**C**), miR-146a level normalized to SNORD48 (**D**), miR-155 level normalized to SNORD48 (**E**). Data are presented with the median as the scatterplot graph. Subtypes of Treg vs. Th17 cells within groups were analyzed by the Wilcoxon test. Multiple comparisons of HCs vs. RA vs. OA were conducted with the Kruskal–Wallis test with Dunn's post hoc. HC (n = 15), OA (n = 11), RA (n = 14). * $p < 0.05$, ** $p < 0.01$.

In the next step, we examined whether there exists a relationship between the mRNA expression and miRNAs expression. For this purpose, we analyzed correlations between examined miRNA and mRNA in the subpopulation of Th17 and Treg cells in RA patients. We found that the expression of miR-26 was positively correlated with SMAD3 (r = 0.78, p = 0.002), STAT3 (r = 0.63, p=0.02), and SOCS1 (r = 0.74, p = 0.005) expression, and expression of miR-155 was positively correlated with STAT3 expression (r = 0.67, p = 0.012) in Th17 cells from patients with RA (Figure 2).

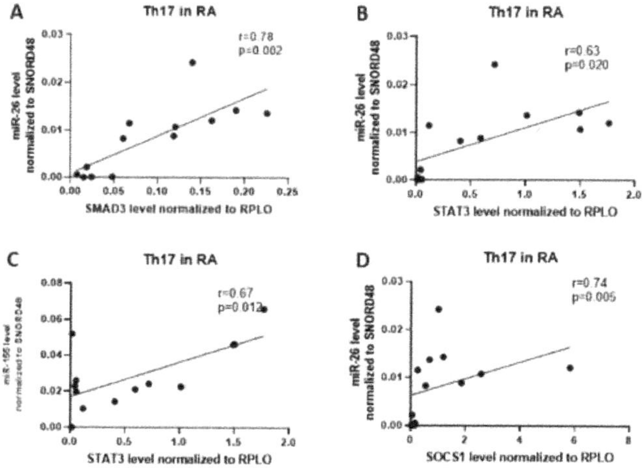

Figure 2. Correlation analysis of microRNA to SMAD3, STAT3, and SOCS1 in RA patients in Th17 cells. (**A**)- correlation between SMAD3 and miR-26; (**B**) correlation between STAT3 and miR-26; (**C**) correlation between STAT3 and miR-155; (**D**) correlation between SOCS1 and miR-26.

In contrast, in RA Treg cells, a strong positive correlation was observed between miR-26 and SOCS1 ($r = 0.68$, $p = 0.02$), between miR-31 and SMAD3 ($r = 0.66$, $p = 0.04$), and between miR-155 and SMAD3 ($r = 0.62$, $p = 0.06$) and SMAD4 ($r = 0.66$, $p = 0.04$). Furthermore, a significant, but negative correlation was observed between miR-26 and STAT5A ($r = -0.63$, $p = 0.04$) and between miR-126 and STAT5A ($r = -0.85$, $p = 0.0015$; Figure 3).

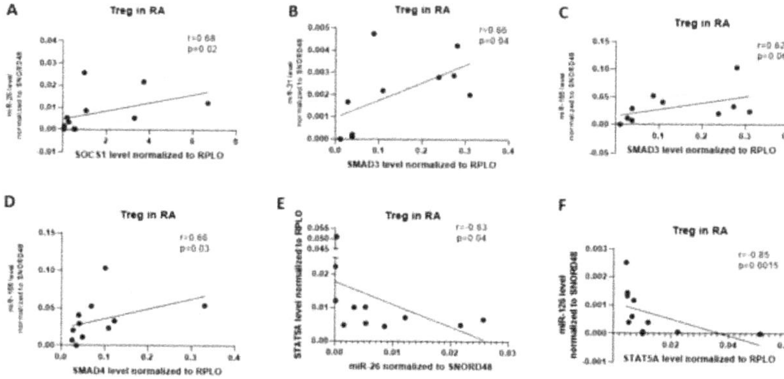

Figure 3. Correlation analysis of microRNAs to SMAD3, SMAD4, SOCS1, and STAT5A in RA patients in Treg cells. (**A**) correlation between SOCS1 and miR-26; (**B**) correlation between SMAD3 and miR-31; (**C**) correlation between SMAD3 and miR-155; (**D**) correlation between SMAD4 and miR-155; (**E**) correlation between miR-26 and STAT5a; (**F**) correlation between STAT5a and miR-126.

2.2. *Lack of Correlation between microRNA and mRNA in Th17 Cells in Control Groups: OA Patients and Healthy Subjects*

The aberrant expression of microRNAs through affecting the expression of target genes involved in Th17/Treg differentiation/function may contribute to the inflammatory responses in RA patients. To better understand the role of the examined miRNAs in Treg/Th17 cells balance, we conducted a correlation analysis between studied miRNA and expression of transcriptional factors playing a central role in the development of T cells. Data indicated that in OA Treg cells, a strong positive correlation was observed between miR-24 and SMAD3 (r = 0.66, p = 0.03), miR-31 and SMAD4 (r = 0.64, p = 0.037), miR-146a and SMAD3 (r = 0.62, p = 0.048), as well as between miR-155 and SOCS1 (r = 0.71, p = 0.02), STAT3 (r = 0.70, p = 0.02) and SMAD3 (r = 0.78, p = 0.006; Figure 4). In OA Th17 cells, we did not observe the correlation between examined miRNA and mRNA.

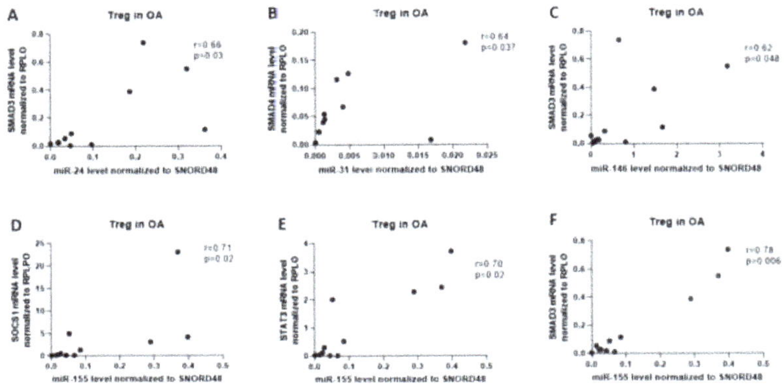

Figure 4. Correlation analysis of microRNAs to SMAD3, SMAD4, SOCS1, and STAT3 in OA patients in Treg cells. (**A**) correlation between miR-24 and SMAD3; (**B**) correlation between miR-31 and SMAD4; (**C**) correlation between miR-146a and SMAD3; (**D**) correlation between miR-155 and SOCS1; (**E**) correlation between miR-155 and STAT3; (**F**) correlation between miR-155 and SMAD3.

We found that the expression of miR-24 was positively correlated with SOCS1 (r = 0.73, p = 0.02), expression of miR-126 with SOCS1 (r = 0.77, p = 0.013), and expression of miR-155 with SOCS1 (r = 0.65, p = 0.049) in Treg cells from healthy subjects. In Treg cells from healthy subjects, we observed a high, negative correlation between miR-155 and SMAD3 (r = 0.70, p = 0.031) and STAT3 (r = 0.66, p = 0.044; Figure 5). In HCs' Th17 cells, we also did not observe the correlation between examined miRNA and mRNA.

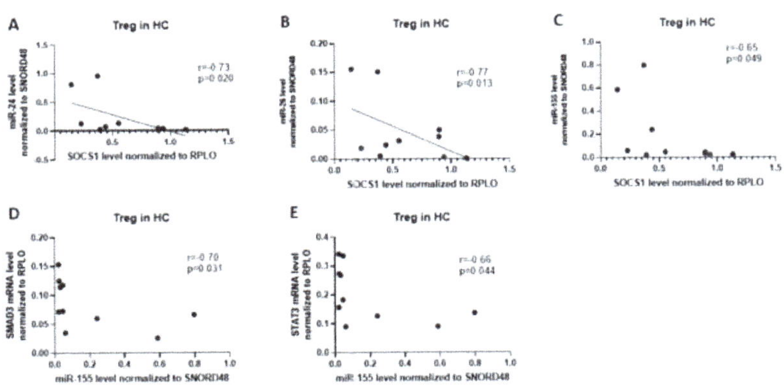

Figure 5. Correlation analysis of microRNAs to SMAD3, SOCS1, and STAT3 in HCs in Treg cells. (**A**) correlation between SOCS1 and miR-24; (**B**) correlation between SOCS1 and miR-26; (**C**) correlation between SOCS1 and miR-155; (**D**) correlation between miR-155 and SMAD3; (**E**) correlation between miR-155 and STAT3.

2.3. Correlation Analysis Of Related Target Genes Based on the mRNA–miRNA Interaction Network

Subsequently, we established miRNA–mRNA coexpression network analysis to identify the possible modulating mechanisms of the mRNAs. The miRNA–mRNA coexpression network analysis was constructed in Cytoscape software. This coexpression network analysis revealed that in RA Th17 cells, expression of miR-126 is correlated with expression of miR-26 and both may regulate expression of STAT3, SMAD3, and SOCS1 (Figure 6). In RA Treg cells, we did not observe this relationship.

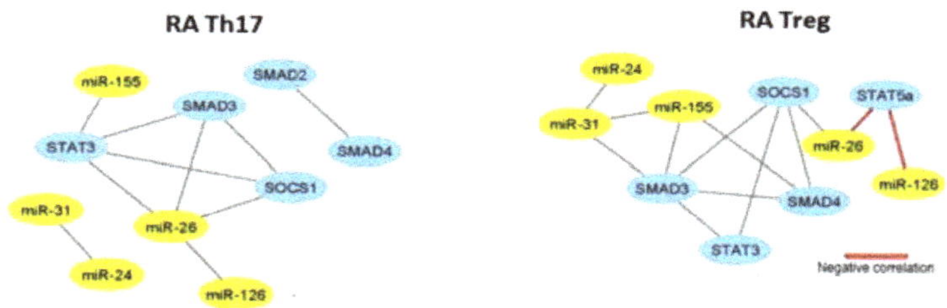

Figure 6. The network of high, significant correlation between selected microRNAs and transcriptional factors in RA patients (n = 14) in Th17 and Treg cells constructed in Cytoscape (coefficient of correlation higher than 0.6, significance < 0.05).

As it is shown in correlation networks (Figures 7 and 8), we did not find any correlation between miRNA and mRNA in Th17 cells from OA patients and healthy subjects. In OA Treg, we were able to observe correlation mostly between miR-155 and STAT3, SOCS1, and SMAD3. Moreover, SMAD3 was also correlated with miR-146a and miR-24. Additionally, we noticed a correlation between miR-31 and SMAD4.

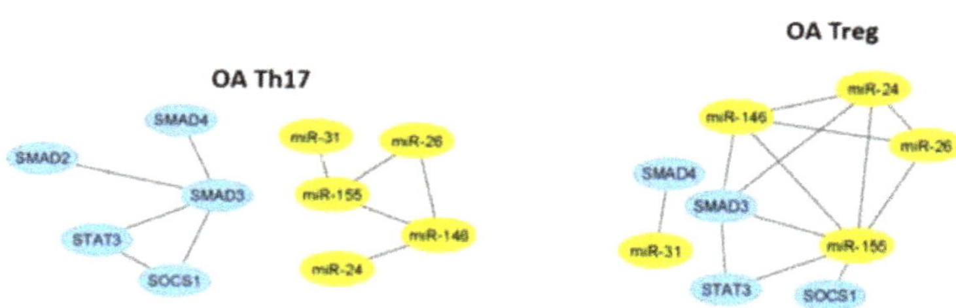

Figure 7. The network of high, significant correlation between selected microRNAs and transcriptional factors in OA patients (n = 11) in Th17 and Treg cells constructed in Cytoscape (coefficient of correlation higher than 0.6, significance < 0.05).

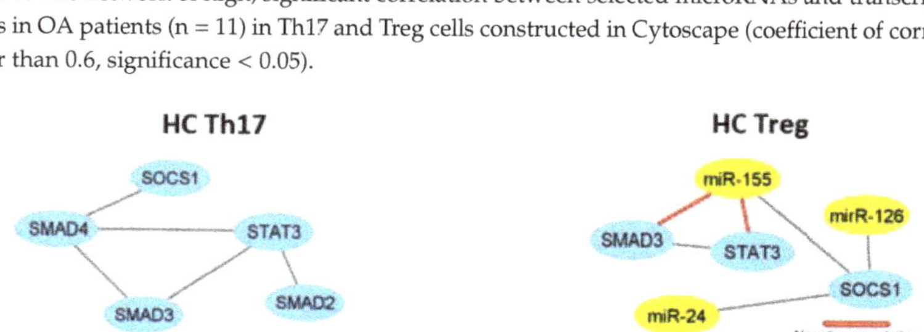

Figure 8. The network of high, significant correlation between selected microRNAs and transcriptional factors in HC (n = 15) in Th17 and Treg cells constructed in Cytoscape (coefficient of correlation higher than 0.6, significance < 0.05).

Similar to RA and OA patients, we prepared a correlation network to show how tested microRNAs may affect mRNAs in our healthy controls. We did not find any regulation of microRNA and mRNA in Th17 cells from healthy subjects. On the other hand, in Treg cells from healthy subjects, we observed that miR-126 and miR-24 were positively correlated with SOCS1 and that miR-155 was negatively correlated with SMAD3 and STAT3, but positively with SOCS1 (Figure 8).

2.4. MicroRNAs Are Significantly Correlated with Each Other in Th17 and Treg Cells in RA and OA Patients

Next, we investigated the correlation between examined miRNAs expression in Th17 and Treg cells isolated from RA and control groups: OA patients as well as from healthy subjects. We observed significant, positive correlations between miR-31 and miR-24 ($r = 0.73$, $p = 0.011$), between miR-31 and miR-155 ($r = 0.76$, $p = 0.006$) in Treg from RA, as well as between miR-126 and miR-26 ($r = 0.79$, $p = 0.003$) and between miR-24 and miR-31 ($r = 0.62$, $p = 0.0026$) in Th17 cells from RA patients (Figure 9).

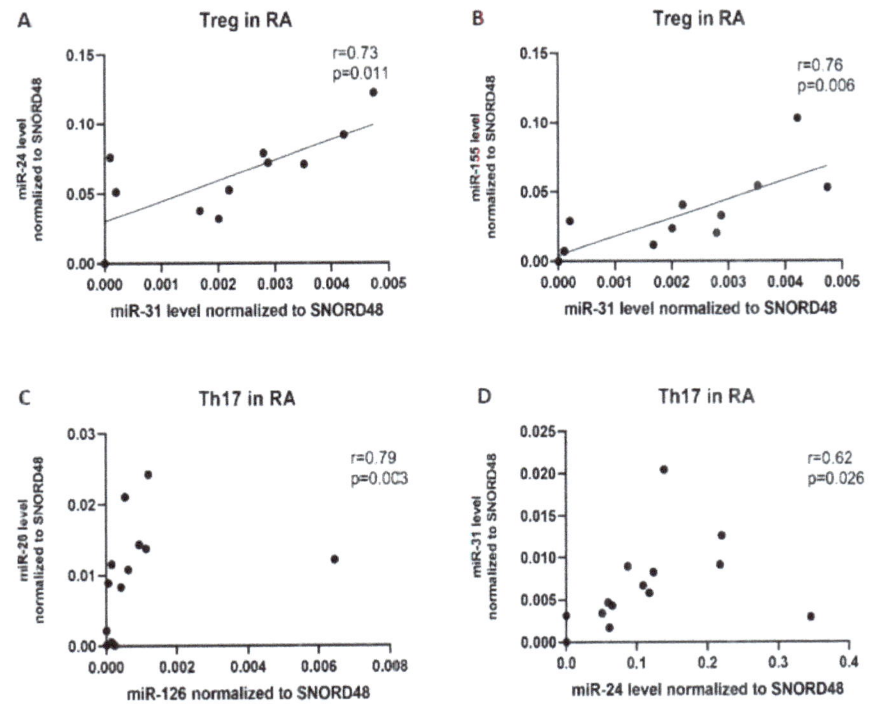

Figure 9. Correlation between microRNAs in Th17 and Treg cells in RA patients. (**A**) correlation between miR-31 and miR-24; (**B**) correlation between miR-31 and miR-155; (**C**) correlation between miR-126 and miR-26; (**D**) correlation between miR-24 and miR-31.

Figure S1 presents correlations between miRNAs in Treg cells from OA patients. We noticed a significant, positive correlations between miR-155 and miR-24 ($r = 0.81$, $p = 0.001$), between miR-155 and miR-26 ($r = 0.75$, $p = 0.004$), and between miR-26 and miR-24 ($r = 0.62$, $p = 0.02$).

Whereas in OA Th17 cells (Table S2), the highest correlation has been observed between expression of miR-24 and miR-146a ($r = 0.70$, $p = 0.0006$), expression of miR-26 and miR-146a ($r = 0.83$, $p < 0.0001$), expression of miR-26 and miR-155 ($r = 0.89$, $p < 0.0001$); and also between expression of miR-31 and miR-155 (r = 0.70, p = 0.007), and expression of miR-146a and miR-155 (r = 0.73, p = 0.004). In healthy controls, we have not noticed correlations between examined microRNAs in Th17 and Treg cells.

2.5. DAS-28, Anti-CCP and Rheumatoid Factor (RF) Parameters in Relation to miR-24, -26, -31, -146a, and -155 Expression Levels in Th17 and Treg Cells from RA Patients

To assess the contribution of the examined miRNAs in the RA phenotype, we stratified our patients based on the disease activity, anti-CCP presence, and RF presence. Based on disease activity, we divided RA patients into patients with active disease with DAS-28 > 5.1 (n = 6) and patients with moderate or low disease activity with DAS-28 ≤ 5.1 (n = 8).

MiR-31 expression was higher in RA patients with DAS-28 ≤5.1. We noticed significantly higher expression levels of miR-31 in Th17 cells from RA patients with DAS-28 ≤ 5.1 (p = 0.002). In Treg cells from RA patients with DAS28 > 5.1, miR-24 expression levels is twice higher than in those with DAS28 ≤ 5.1 (p = 0.048). Other outcomes were not statistically significant, however, it is interesting that in RA Treg cells with DAS28 > 5.1, we observed higher expression levels of miR-146a and miR-155 (Figure 10A,B). Moreover, we also found that miR-24, miR-26, miR-31, and miR-155 were downregulated, while miR-146a were upregulated in Th17 cells from RA patients with DAS28 ≤ 5.1.

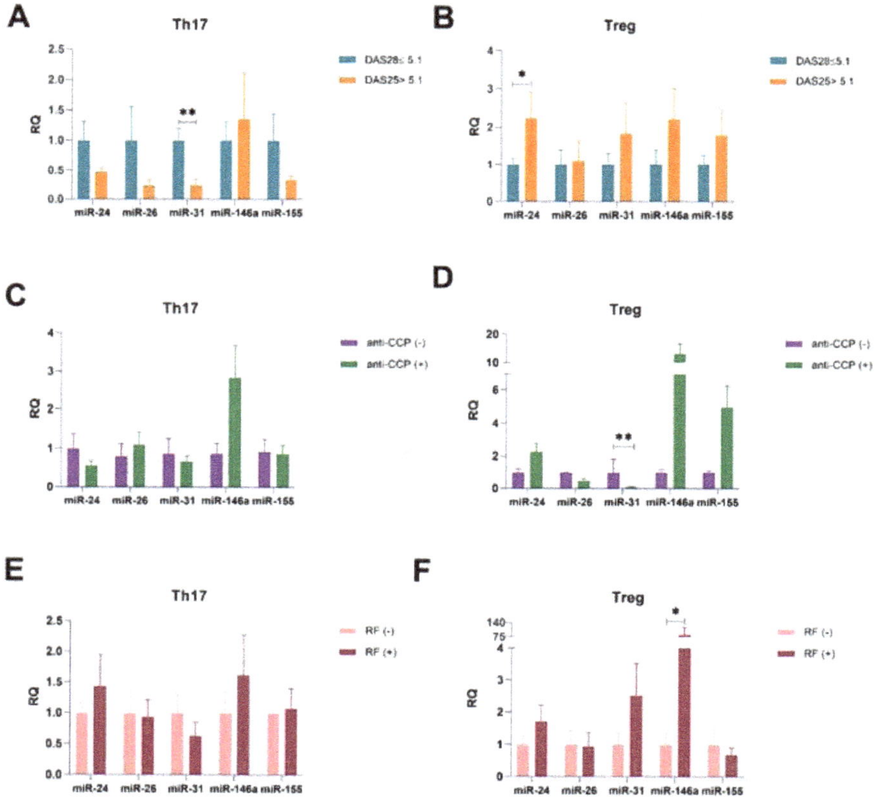

Figure 10. DAS-28 (**A**,**B**), anti-CCP (**C**,**D**), and rheumatoid factor (RF) (**E**,**F**) parameters in relation to miR-24, miR-26 miR-31, miR-146a, miR-155 expression levels in Th17 (**A**,**C**,**E**) and Treg (**B**,**D**,**F**) cells from RA patients. Data are presented as mean ± SEM. Expression of patients with DAS28 ≤5.1 (**A**,**B**), negative anti-CCP (**C**,**D**), and negative RF (**E**,**F**) was taken as 1. The Mann–Whitney test was used. * $p < 0.05$, ** $p < 0.01$.

Downregulation of miR-31 in Treg cells obtained from anti-CCP positive RA patients. Our results demonstrated that in Treg cells from anti-CCP positive RA patients, expression of miR-31 was significantly lower than in anti-CCP negative RA patients (p = 0.006; Figure 10D). In contrast, in Treg cells from anti-CCP positive RA patients, we noticed twice higher expression level for miR-24, 13 times higher for miR-146a, and 5 times higher for miR-155 than in anti-CCP negative RA patients; however, results were not significant. We also noticed that in Treg cells from anti-CCP negative RA patients, expression level of miR-26 is twice more than in anti-CCP positive patients; these outcomes were not significant. We also observed that in Th17 cells from anti-CCP positive RA patients, expression of miR-146a was higher and miR-24 and miR-31 were lower than in anti-CCP negative RA patients; these results were also not significant.

The higher expression level of miR-146a in RA patients with RF. In the present study, we reported almost twice higher miR-24, 2.5 times higher miR-31, and 82 times higher miR-146a (p = 0.02; Figure 10E,F) expression levels in Treg cells from RA patients with RF than in Treg cells from RA patients without RF. We also observed that expression levels of miR-155 were almost two times lower in Treg cells from RA patients with RF than in RA patients without RF, but this difference was not statistically significant. In contrast, expression levels of miR-126 were similar in both RF-positive and RF-negative RA patients. In RA patients with RF, we also observed the upregulation of miR-31 in Treg cells compared to Th17 cells.

MiR-26 and miR-155 May Be Good Potential Biomarkers for RA and OA. To estimate the further potential value of the examined miRNAs individually or as a panel as RA and/or OA biomarkers, receiver operating characteristic (ROC)–AUC (Area Under Curve) analyses were performed. The outcomes are presented in Table 1. MiR-26 after comparison of RA and HCs in Th17 (AUC = 0.75, p = 0.02) and Treg cells (AUC = 0.92, p = 0.0002) showed a prognostic value. We also revealed this potential for miR-26 in OA vs. HCs in Treg cells (AUC = 0.86, p = 0.0013). MiR-155 after comparison of RA and HCs in Th17 (AUC = 0.80, p = 0.006) and Treg cells (AUC = 0.73, p= 0.048) revealed a prognostic value. We also exposed this potential for miR-155 in OA vs. HCs in Th17 cells (AUC = 0.75, p = 0.03).

Table 1. Prognostic values of the relative expression level of the analyzed microRNAs in RA and OA patients as well as healthy subjects (HCs) based on the area under the curve receiver operating characteristic (ROC)–AUC (Area Under Curve).

microRNA	Group	AUC	Th17 *p*	Treg AUC	*p*
miR-26	HC RA	0.75	0.02	0.92	0.0002
	HC OA	0.66	0.16	0.86	0.0013
	RA OA	0.55	0.66	0.66	0.17
miR-155	HC RA	0.80	0.006	0.73	0.048
	HC OA	0.75	0.03	0.51	0.94
	RA OA	0.52	0.88	0.68	0.12

In the next step, we conducted the ROC curve analysis and estimated AUC to assess the diagnostic potential of candidate microRNAs that could distinguish RA and OA patients from healthy controls. Figure 11A–F shows the ROC curve analysis for miR-26 in Th17 and Treg cells in RA, OA, and HCs.

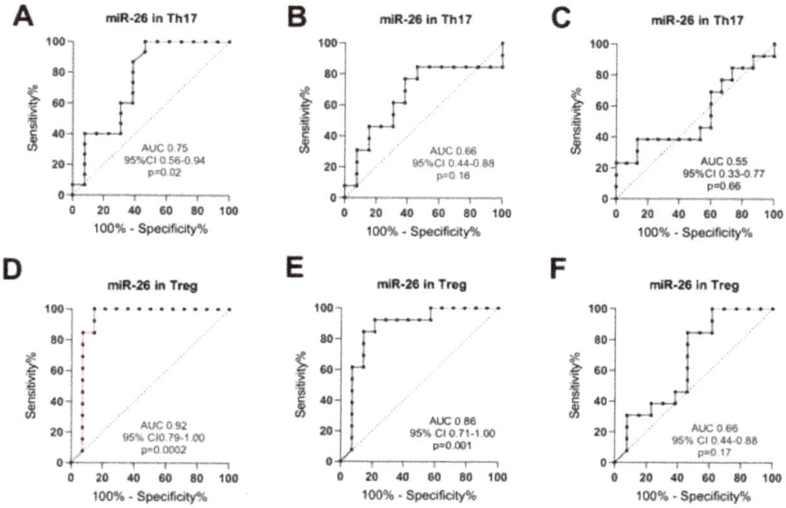

Figure 11. ROC curve analysis for miR-26. (**A**) RA vs. HC in Th17; (**B**) OA vs. HC in Th17; (**C**) RA vs. OA in Th17; (**D**) RA vs. HC in Treg; (**E**) OA vs. HC in Treg; (**F**) RA vs. OA in Treg.

The highest AUC value was obtained for miR-26 discriminating RA from healthy controls (AUC 0.92) and also differentiating OA from HCs (AUC 0.86) in Treg cells. The high AUC value was also obtained for miR-26 distinguishing RA from HCs (AUC 0.75) in Th17 cells.

Figure 12A–F shows the ROC curve analysis for miR-155 in Th17 and Treg cells in RA, OA, and HCs. The highest AUC value was obtained for miR-155 discriminating RA from healthy controls in Th17 cells (AUC 0.80) and Treg cells (AUC 0.73) and also differentiating OA from HCs in Th17 cells (AUC 0.75).

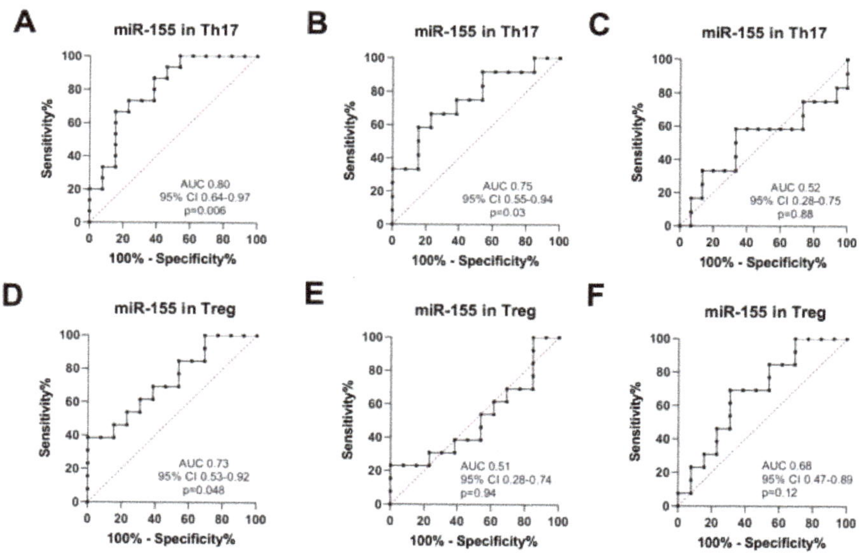

Figure 12. ROC curve analysis for miR-155. (**A**) RA vs. HC in Th17; (**B**) OA vs. HC in Th17; (**C**) RA vs. OA in Th17; (**D**) RA vs. HC in Treg; (E) OA vs. HC in Treg; (**F**) RA vs. OA in Treg.

Setting a cutoff value at the specific level permitted us to receive the maximum sensitivity and specificity values (Table S3). For miR-26 in RA vs. HC, we obtained 93.33% sensitivity and 53.85% specificity in Th17 (cutoff value = 0.022) and 84.62% sensitivity and 92.86% specificity in Treg cells (cutoff value = 0.025). In OA vs. HC, those values were 76.92% sensitivity and 61.54% specificity (cutoff value = 0.020) in Th17; and 84.62% sensitivity and 78.57% specificity (cutoff value = 0.051) in Treg cells. For miR-155 in RA vs. HC, we set a cutoff values at the levels 0.046 in Th17 (80% sensitivity, 61.54% specificity) and 0.118 in Treg cells (92.31% sensitivity, 30.77% specificity), respectively. For miR-155 in OA vs. HC, the cutoff values were 0.070 in Th17 (83.33% sensitivity, 46.16% specificity) and 0.075 in Treg cells (61.54% sensitivity, 30.77% specificity), respectively.

2.6. Multivariable Logistic Regression

Based on the results of the likelihood ratio test (LRT), multivariable logistic regression with a combination of miR-24, miR-26, miR-31, miR-146a, miR-155 as a predictor vector was used to assess their diagnostic accuracy for the possible diagnostic potential. Figure S2 presents ROC analysis for the combination of miR-26 and miR-155 in Th17 RA vs. HCs and miR-146a in Treg OA vs. HCs. Significant diagnostic potential in RA Th17 cells (AUC = 0.811) has only been demonstrated for the combination of miR-26 and miR-155. In Treg from OA patients, only miR-146a has been revealed as a significant estimator in the model (AUC = 0.4196).

3. Discussion

In the last years, we observe substantial progress in the field of miRNA-mediated regulation of immune function and T cell development. The clarification of miRNAs role in lymphocytes subtypes development/differentiation can be used to enhance our understanding of the molecular pathways that are involved in immune regulation. Currently, there is limited knowledge about the specific miRNAs participated in the regulation of immune-related molecular processes and to what extent their activity promotes rheumatoid arthritis pathogenesis. Rheumatoid arthritis is an autoimmune disease, which affects joints, and symptoms include pain and lead to disability through cartilage and bone destruction. This study confirmed the major imbalance between Th17 cells and Treg cells in patients with active RA, as was previously reported in the literature [12]. MicroRNAs play a multifaceted role in the development of RA and are part of the complex net of epigenetic interactions. Alternations to these interactions might be results of the disease or a contributing factor in RA pathogenesis [13]. Earlier studies on animal models have also confirmed the role of mir-155 as one of the factors contributing to arthritis development. Results of serum testing in arthritic rats showed an increased level of miR-155; on the other hand, mice lacking miR-155 were resistant to collagen-induced arthritis [14,15]. In the present study, we decided to focus on microRNAs since they are responsible for regulating gene expression of transcriptional factors that impact Th17/Treg balance [2,12]. Understanding the molecular pathway of genetic and epigenetic regulation of Treg and Th17 cells is critical to understand RA etiology and pathogenesis. We are the first, to our knowledge, who analyzed microRNAs from Th17 and Treg cells obtained from RA in comparison to control groups—OA patients also characterized among others by joint damage, but with different pathophysiology and without an autoimmune component and healthy subjects—and correlated them with some transcriptional factors important in Treg and Th17 cells differentiation.

The next focus of our study was to analyze the correlation between microRNAs and mRNAs in Treg and Th17 cells in tested groups used in this study: RA and controls; OA and HCs. In our study, we have shown a correlation between miR-155 and STAT3 as well as between miR-26 and STAT3, SMAD3, and SOCS1 in RA Th17 cells. Che et al. have shown that miR-155 shows the potential to be used as a biomarker [14]. For RA Treg cells, we found a correlation between miR-155 with SMAD3 and SMAD4, which again confirms the possibility to use miR-155 as a biomarker [16–19]. In the present paper, we have also shown a correlation between miR-31 and SMAD3 as well as between miR-26 and SOCS1; to our knowledge, our study is the first showing these correlations in RA patients.

However, the correlation between miR-31 and SMAD3 has already been reported by Hu et al. [20]. In Th17 cells from OA patients and healthy subjects, we did not found a correlation between analyzed microRNAs and mRNAs. On the other hand, our results confirmed earlier studies that in OA Treg cells, there exists/occurs/is a correlation between miR-24 with SMAD3; miR-31 with SMAD4; miR146a with SMAD3; and miR-155 with SOCS1, SMAD3, and STAT3 [17,18,21,22]. In accordance with an earlier study, in Treg cells from healthy subjects, we also found a few correlations between miR-24 and SOCS1, miR-126 and SOCS1, miR-155 and SOCS1; and two negative correlations between miR-155 and SMAD3 and STAT3 [18,19,21]. Both earlier studies and our present study indicate miR-155 as a potential diagnostic biomarker for RA/OA detection, because miR-155 has a negative correlation with SMAD3 and STAT3 in healthy subjects, but positive in RA patients and OA patients.

Analysis of selected microRNAs' expression in Treg and Th17 cells confirmed differences between Treg and Th17 cells, which is consistent with other studies [13,23]. We observed that the expression of miR-26 is significantly higher in healthy subjects than in RA patients. MiR-31, like miR-24, demonstrated a significant change in expression between Treg and Th17 cells within the HCs group. Our results for miR-146a and miR-155 confirmed the results of previous studies on the expression of microRNAs in RA [23]. We observed that miR-146a expression level in RA and OA Treg was significantly higher than in Th17 cells. The last studies demonstrated that miR-146a plays a considerable role in various aspects of immunopathogenesis. Our results emphasize the role of miR-146a as an anti-inflammatory agent. The downregulating miR-146a expression in Treg cells may promote their proliferation and alleviate the inflammation process. In comparison with the fact that miR-146a preferably reduces the proinflammatory immune response, miR-155 strengthens inflammation, which is consistent with our observations. In the present study, we observed that miR-155 expression in Th17 cells was higher in HCs than in RA patients and that miR-155 expression was higher in Treg cells from RA and OA patients than in Th17 cells. Treg cells from active RA patients with high disease activity (we have 42% RA patients with DAS-28 > 5.1) expressed elevated levels of SOCS1—a target of miR-155—which negatively regulates inflammatory processes. Moreover, our study confirms the value of miR-146a and miR-155 as an important factor in early detection of RA, but we were also able to show the potential use of miR-26 as a biomarker [17,23–25].

The present study revealed significant correlations between particular microRNAs. In RA Treg cells, we noticed the correlation between miR-31 and miR-24 as well as between miR-31 and miR-155 levels. In RA Th17 cells, correlations were between miR-126 and miR-26, miR-24, and miR-31 levels. OA Treg cells showed correlations between miR-155 and miR-24, miR-155 and miR-26, miR-26, and miR-24. In OA Th17 cells we saw significant correlations between miR-24 and miR-146a, miR-26 and miR-146a, miR-26 and miR-155, miR-31 and miR-155, and miR-146a and miR-155. In Bae et al. meta-analysis, levels of circulating miR-146a were significantly higher in RA patients than in controls. This study suggests the noteworthy role of miR-146a levels in RA proinflammatory processes [26].

Our study revealed some connections between microRNAs' expression levels and clinical parameters. We observed in RA patients with DAS28 ≤ 5.1 significantly higher miR-31 expression levels in Th17 cells and contrarily, in RA patients with DAS28 > 5.1 twice higher miR-24 in Treg cells. We also noticed in RA Treg cells upregulation of miR-155 and miR-146a, when DAS28 > 5.1. MiR-26 was at a similar level, independently of DAS score; however, these results were not statistically significant. Li et al. found that in PBMCs from active RA patients, miR-155 expression is positively correlated with DAS28 [11]. Moreover, miRNA-146a in RA patients was also positively correlated with DAS28 [27]. We did not notice significant differences in the anti-CCP level in RA patients, excluding that miR-31 in RA with positive anti-CCP was downregulated in comparison to the level observed in anti-CCP negative RA patients. Treg cells of RA patients with RF-positive results were characterized by a significantly higher level of miR-146a expression.

Our additional analysis revealed that the miR-26 and miR-155 reveal significant diagnostic potential for RA differentiation from healthy subjects. Moreover, high diagnostic potential has been revealed for the combination of miR-155 and miR-26 in RA Th17 cells. MiR-26a was reported as overexpressed in RA PBMCs and plasma in comparison to HC [7,19,28]. During interleukin (IL)-17 differentiation and T CD4+ cells generation, upregulation of miR-26a occurs. T CD4+ cells are crucial in RA pathology [27]. MiR-155 insufficiency reduces the number of Treg cells and downregulates IL-2 receptor (IL-2R) signaling and phosphorylation of STAT5, causing deficient SOCS1 suppression [29]. Yao et al. found that STAT3 and STAT5 phosphorylations are positively regulated by miR-155. That is probably due to miR-155 blocking the inhibitory effect on phosphorylations of STAT3 and STAT5 mediated by SOCS1 [10]. MiR-155 was assessed as a potential biomarker of response on methotrexate (MTX) in RA patients by AUC analysis by Singh et al. [30].

Our study has some limitations. The sample size should be enlarged. Further studies are necessary to elucidate the exact microRNAs influence on transcriptional factors as well as on Th17 and Treg cells in the etiology and pathogenesis of rheumatoid arthritis. Additional studies can identify and describe the microRNAs and their target genes signaling pathways, and interactions between them and Th17 and Treg cells included in the inflammatory processes, which may cause the development of new RA therapeutics.

4. Materials and Methods

4.1. Study Population

In this study, we used blood from 14 patients with RA and controls: 11 patients with OA and the group of 15 healthy controls (HCs), which were age and gender-matched to patients we used in this study. This study meets all criteria contained in the Declaration of Helsinki and was approved by the Ethics Committee of the National Institute of Geriatrics, Rheumatology, and Rehabilitation, Warsaw, Poland (approval protocol number 29 June 2016). All participants gave their written informed consent before enrollment. Patients with RA were recruited from the National Institute of Geriatrics, Rheumatology and Rehabilitation in Warsaw, Poland; and from the Poznan University of Medical Sciences, Poland. All RA patients fulfilled the American College of Rheumatology (ACR 2010) criteria for RA. Patients with OA were recruited from the National Institute of Geriatrics, Rheumatology and Rehabilitation in Warsaw, Poland. OA patients were diagnosed based on characteristic x-ray findings and the absence of features suggestive of inflammatory arthritis and must meet the ACR criteria for OA of the knee. RAand OA patients with an active infection, cancer, or other rheumatological diseases were excluded from the study. The HCs consisted of volunteers without clinical or laboratory signs of autoimmune diseases. The control group was chosen randomly between blood bank donors to match the age, gender, and ethnicity of patients with RA and OA. All participants who donated blood for this study had the same socioeconomic status and were from the same geographic region.

RA patients were qualified based on their physical examination and laboratory tests. The main factor based on which patients were qualified was age, gender, disease duration, swollen joints number, C-reactive protein (CRP), erythrocyte sedimentation ratio (ESR), platelets (PLT), and creatinine. Additionally, we evaluated them to study by presence of rheumatoid factor (RF $\geq$ 34 IU/mL), presence of anti-CCP antibodies (anticyclic citrullinated peptide autoantibodies, aCCP $\geq$ 17 IU/mL), disease activity score in 28 joints (DAS-28), visual analog scale (VAS, range 0–100), Larsen score, and information about the treatment were collected at the time of obtaining samples from patients. Demographic and clinical characteristics of subjects are summarized in Table 2 and detailed clinical characteristics of RA patients are summarized in Table 3.

Table 2. Demographic and clinical characteristics of the study population. ESR—erythrocyte sedimentation ratio; CRP—C-reactive protein

Parameter	RA n = 14	OA n = 11	HCs n = 15
Age	52 ± 19 64 (21–75)	70 ± 10 66.5 (56–85)	48 ± 6.6 45 (41–63)
Female/Male	13/1	7/4	9/6
ESR (mm/h)	14 (9–64)	15 (3–26)	
CRP (mg/L)	12.5 (5–73)	5 (5–10)	

Table 3. Detailed clinical characteristics of RA patients.

Clinical Characteristics of Patients with RA	
Disease duration (years)	6.5 (0.5–18)
DAS-28 > 5.1 n (%)	6 (42%)
Larsen 1–3 n (%)	9 (64%)
RF Positivity n (%)	5 (35%)
Anti-CCP Positivity n (%)	7 (50%)
Methotrexate (MTX) n (%)	9 (64%)
Somatostatin Analogue (SSA) n (%)	3 (21%)
Antimalarials Drug n (%)	7 (50%)
Glucocorticoids (GCs) n (%)	4 (28%)
IL-6 Inhibitor n (%)	1 (7.1%)
No Treatment n (%)	1 (7.1%)

4.2. *Detection of Th17 and Treg Cells Using Flow Cytometry.*

Using Ficoll-Paque (GE Healthcare Bio-Sciences, Uppsala, Sweden) and performing density gradient centrifugation, we were able to isolate PBMC. In the next step, cells were cultured in RPMI 1640 (Invitrogen, Paisley, UK), 10% heat-inactivated fetal bovine serum (FBS) (Gibco, Thermofisher, USA), 100 U/mL penicillin, and 100 ug/mL streptomycin (Sigma-Aldrich, Saint Louis, MO, USA) for 12 h. After that period, cells were harvested and stained for particular membrane antigens using anti-CD4 APC-Cy7, anti-CD25 PE, anti-CD127 FITC, anti-CCR6 APC, and anti-CXCr3 PE-Cy7 murine Abs. Cells were washed, then they were acquired, analyzed, and sorted using a FACSAria cell sorter/cytometer and Diva software. By using 7AAD staining, we were able to eliminate dead cells from analysis (Figure S3). All reagents used in the flow cytometry were purchased from Becton Dickinson (San Jose, CA, USA).

4.3. *Isolation of Total RNA from Th17 and Treg Cells*

Total RNA was isolated from earlier sorted Th17 and Treg cells using the miRNeasy Micro Kit (Qiagen, Germantown, MD, USA). The quantity and quality of isolated RNA were evaluated by the Quawell Q5000 spectrophotometer. Total RNA isolated during this procedure was used to perform the reverse transcription reaction using High-Capacity cDNA Reverse Transcription Kit (Applied Biosystems, Carlsbad, CA, USA). We stored synthesized cDNA at −20 °C for the next step. Preamplification of cDNA from this reverse transcription was performed using TaqMan® PreAmp Master Mix Kit (Applied Biosystem, Carlsbad, CA, USA) according to the manufacturer instructions. The rest of the isolated total RNA from Th17 and Treg cells were used to perform reverse transcription reaction using the miRCURY LNA RT kit (Qiagen) according to the manufacturer instructions. Both reverse transcriptions were conducted in a thermocycler (SensoQuest Labcycler 48 s, Göttingen, Germany).

4.4. *Quantitative Real-Time PCR*

We used following TaqMan primer and probes (Applied Biosystems, Foster City, CA, USA) SMAD3 (Hs00969210_m1), STAT3 (Hs00374280_m1), STAT5a (Hs00559647_m1), SOCS1 (Hs00705164_m1), GAPDH (Hs02786624_g1), and RPLO (Hs99999902_m1). The following assays were used in microRNA experiment: hsa-miR-24-3p (QG-339306_YP00204260), hsa-miR-26a-5p (QG-339306_YP00206023), hsa-miR-31-5p (QG-339306_YP00204236), hsa-miR-100-5p (QG-339306_YP00205689), hsa-miR-126-3p (QG-339306_YP00204227), hsa-miR-146a-5p (QG-339306_YP00204688), hsa-miR-155-5p (QG-339306_YP00204308), hsa-miR326 (QG-339306_YP00204512), SNORD48 (hsa) (QG-339306_YP00203903), and U6 snRNA (has, mmu) (QG-33906_YP00203907). To prepare quantitative Real-Time PCR, we used TaqMan Gene Expression Master Mix (Applied Biosystems); and for quantitative with microRNA, we used miRCURY SYBR Green PCR Kit (Qiagen). Quantitative Real-Time PCR was performed on real-time cycler (Quant Studio 5, Applied Biosystem, Foster City, CA, USA). Each sample was analyzed in duplicates. From that, we took the mean Ct value, and we used it in the next steps of the analysis. Ct values higher than 35 were taken out of analysis and considered below quantification. The housekeeping gene has been selected and relative expression was calculated by ΔΔCt method or ΔCt method normalized to RPLO; in the case of microRNA, SNORD48 was used as a reference.

4.5. Statistical Analysis

For microRNA, we used the Shapiro–Wilk test as a normality test. Analysis of statistical signification between Th17 cells and Treg cells was conducted with the Wilcoxon test. Statistical significance between two independent groups was determined by the nonparametric Mann–Whitney U test. As for the comparison between RA, OA, and HCs, we used independent tests—the Kruskal–Wallis test with Dunn's post hoc. Correlation analysis of the mRNA with microRNA in Th17 and Treg cells was conducted by the Spearman test. Data were analyzed using GraphPad Prism software version 8.2.1. and was presented as figures. In all tested values, $p < 0.05$ was considered significant. The receiver operating characteristic (ROC) curves analysis, an area under curves (AUC) likelihood ratio of chi-square, and p-value were obtained by multivariable logistic regression analysis and were calculated by the R program (R Development Core Team (2008) R: A language and environment for statistical computing. R Foundation for Statistical Computing, Vienna, Austria ISBN 3-900051-07-0, URL http://www.R-project.org.) with R:ggplot [31] and pROC [32] packages.

5. Conclusions

In conclusion, our association study revealed correlations of expression levels in Treg cells obtained from RA patients between miR-26 and SOCS1, miR-31 and SMAD3, miR-155 and SMAD3, SMAD4. Moreover, we also noticed correlations in Th17 cells from RA between miR-26 and SMAD3, STAT3, SOCS1, miR-155 and STAT3. The present study also showed that RA Treg cells have a negative correlation between STAT5a and miR-26 level as well as between miR-126 and STAT5a level. Our research established that miR-26 and miR-155 can be good possible biomarkers for rheumatoid arthritis and osteoarthritis. After analyzing gene expression in a tested group of patients, we assume that SMAD2 shows the most promise to be used in the future to allow for earlier recognition of RA Our study presented some interesting observations about connections between microRNAs' expression and the clinical characteristics of RA patients. The current study revealed that RA patients with DAS28 ≤ 5.1 have significantly higher miR-31 expression levels in Th17 cells and, on the contrary, the twice higher expression level of miR-24 in Treg cells from patients with DAS28 > 5.1. We also exposed that the expression level of miR-146a in Treg cells is much higher in RA patients with RF than those with RF-negative. Furthermore, our outcomes presented that anti-CCP positive RA patients have meaningfully lower miR-31 expression levels in Treg cells than anti-CCP negative RA patients.

We believe that our study may be useful in elucidating and describing the inflammatory processes leading to the RA development and RA course. There is a need for further studies with an enlarged sample size as well as the need for functional studies. Functional studies may provide insights into the effect of microRNAs on gene function. Further studies are essential to clarify the microRNAs' impact on Treg and Th17 cells, as well as transcriptional factors in the development and the course of rheumatoid arthritis. Moreover, we trust that this knowledge can lead to the development of new therapeutics for rheumatoid arthritis.

Supplementary Materials: The following are available online at http://www.mdpi.com/1422-0067/21/19/7169/s1

Author Contributions: T.K. and E.R. wrote and edited the original draft of the manuscript and performed experiments. E.W., A.W., B.S., E.K.-W. performed experiments. A.W. performed data analysis. K.R.-P., D.M. provided research material, developed clinical database. P.P.J. and A.P. reviewed the manuscript. A.P.-G. invented, designed, and supervised the experiment and reviewed the manuscript. All authors have read and agreed to the published version of the manuscript.

Funding: This research was funded by the Polish National Science Center, grant number 2015/19/B/NZ5/00247.

Acknowledgments: The technical assistance of Agnieszka Hertel and Wieslawa Frankowska is gratefully acknowledged. We are also thankful to all of the RA patients, OA patients and healthy subjects whose cooperation made this study possible.

Conflicts of Interest: The authors declare no conflict of interest.

Abbreviations

aCCP	Anti-cyclin citrullinated peptide autoantibodies
AUC	Area under curve
CD	Cluster of differentiation
CNS1	Conserved noncoding sequence 1
CRP	C-reactive protein
DAS	Disease activity score
DNMT 1	DNA methyltransferase 1
ESR	Erythrocyte sedimentation ratio
FBS	Fetal bovine serum
FOXP3	Forkhead box P3
GCs	Glucocorticoids
HCs	Healthy controls
IL-2	Interleukin-2
Il-6	Interleukin-6
JAK/STAT	Janus kinase/signal transducers and activators of transcription
miRNAs, miRs	MicroRNAs
MS	Multiple sclerosis
MTX	Methotrexate
OA	Osteoarthritis
PBC	Primary biliary cholangitis
PBMCs	Peripheral blood mononuclear cells
PLT	Platelets
pTreg	Peripherally derived Treg
RA	Rheumatoid arthritis
RF	Rheumatoid factor
ROC	Receiver operating characteristic
SLE	Systemic lupus erythematosus
SMAD2	SMAD family member 2
SMAD3	SMAD family member 3
SMAD4	SMAD family member 4
SOCS1	Suppressor of cytokine signaling 1
SSA	Somatostatin analogue
STAT3	Signal transducer and activator of transcription 3
STAT5	Signal transducer and activator of transcription 5
Th cells	T helper cells, helper T cells
Treg cells	T regulatory cells, regulatory T cells
VAS	Visual analog scale.

References

1. Tateiwa, D.; Yoshikawa, H.; Kaito, T. Cartilage and bone destruction in arthritis: Pathogenesis and treatment strategy: A literature review. *Cells* **2019**, *8*, 818. [CrossRef] [PubMed]
2. Glyn-Jones, S.; Palmer, A.J.R.; Agricola, R.; Price, A.J.; Vincent, T.L.; Weinans, H.; Carr, A.J. Osteoarthritis. *Lancet* **2015**, *386*, 376–387. [CrossRef]
3. Nugent, M. MicroRNAs: Exploring new horizons in osteoarthritis. *Osteoarthr. Cart.* **2016**, *24*, 573–580. [CrossRef] [PubMed]
4. Sondag, G.R.; Haqqi, T.M. The role of MicroRNAs and their targets in osteoarthritis. *Curr. Rheumatol. Rep.* **2016**, *18*, 1–23. [CrossRef] [PubMed]

5. Zhang, L.; Wu, H.; Zhao, M.; Chang, C.; Lu, Q. Clinical significance of MiRNAs in autoimmunity. *J. Autoimmun.* **2020**, *109*, 102438. [CrossRef]
6. Yang, G.; Wu, D.; Zeng, G.; Jiang, O.; Yuan, P.; Huang, S.; Zhu, J.; Tian, J.; Weng, Y.; Rao, Z. Correlation between MiR-126 expression and DNA hypomethylation of CD4+ T cells in rheumatoid arthritis patients. *Int. J. Clin. Exp. Pathol.* **2015**, *8*, 8929–8936.
7. Murata, K.; Furu, M.; Yoshitomi, H.; Ishikawa, M.; Shibuya, H.; Hashimoto, M.; Imura, Y.; Fujii, T.; Ito, H.; Mimori, T.; et al. Comprehensive MicroRNA analysis identifies MiR-24 and MiR-125a-5p as plasma biomarkers for rheumatoid arthritis. *PLoS ONE* **2013**, *8*, e69118. [CrossRef]
8. Zhang, L.; Wu, H.; Zhao, M.; Lu, Q. Identifying the differentially expressed MicroRNAs in autoimmunity: A systemic review and meta-analysis. *Autoimmunity* **2020**, *53*, 122–136. [CrossRef]
9. Lu, L.F.; Boldin, M.P.; Chaudhry, A.; Lin, L.L.; Taganov, K.D.; Hanada, T.; Yoshimura, A.; Baltimore, D.; Rudensky, A.Y. Function of MiR-146a in controlling treg cell-mediated regulation of Th1 responses. *Cell* **2010**, *142*, 914–929. [CrossRef]
10. Yao, R.; Ma, Y.; Liang, W.; Li, H.; Ma, Z.; Yu, X.; Liao, Y. MicroRNA-155 modulates treg and Th17 cells differentiation and Th17 cell function by targeting SOCS1. *PLoS ONE* **2012**, *7*, e46082. [CrossRef]
11. Li, X.; Tian, F.; Wang, F. Rheumatoid arthritis-associated microrna-155 targets Socs1 and upregulates TNF-α and IL-1β in PBMCs. *Int. J. Mol. Sci.* **2013**, *14*, 23910–23921. [CrossRef] [PubMed]
12. Samson, M.; Audia, S.; Janikashvili, N.; Ciudad, M.; Trad, M.; Fraszczak, J.; Ornetti, P.; Maillefert, J.F.; Miossec, P.; Bonnotte, B. Brief report: Inhibition of interleukin-6 function corrects Th17/Treg cell imbalance in patients with rheumatoid arthritis. *Arthritis Rheum.* **2012**, *64*, 2499–2503. [CrossRef] [PubMed]
13. Evangelatos, G.; Fragoulis, G.E.; Koulouri, V.; Lambrou, G.I. MicroRNAs in rheumatoid arthritis: From pathogenesis to clinical impact. *Autoimm. Rev.* **2019**, *18*, 102391. [CrossRef] [PubMed]
14. Dudics, S.; Venkatesha, S.H.; Moudgil, K.D. The Micro-RNA expression profiles of autoimmune arthritis reveal novel biomarkers of the disease and therapeutic response. *Int. J. Mol. Sci.* **2018**, 19. [CrossRef]
15. Kurowska-Stolarska, M.; Alivernini, S.; Ballantine, L.E.; Asquith, D.L.; Millar, N.L.; Gilchrist, D.S.; Reilly, J.; Ierna, M.; Fraser, A.R.; Stolarski, B.; et al. MicroRNA-155 as a proinflammatory regulator in clinical and experimental arthritis. *Proc. Natl. Acad. Sci. USA* **2011**, *108*, 11193–11198. [CrossRef]
16. Che, X.M.; Huang, Q.C.; Yang, S.L.; Chu, Y.L.; Yan, Y.H.; Han, L.; Huang, Y.; Huang, R.Y. Role of Micro RNAs in pathogenesis of rheumatoid arthritis. *Medicine* **2015**, *94*, e1326. [CrossRef]
17. Taganov, K.D.; Boldin, M.P.; Chang, K.J.; Baltimore, D. NF-kappaB-dependent induction of microRNA miR-146, an inhibitor targeted to signaling proteins of innate immune responses. *Proc. Natl. Acad. Sci. USA* **2006**, *103*, 12481–12486. [CrossRef]
18. Blüml, S.; Bonelli, M.; Niederreiter, B.; Puchner, A.; Mayr, G.; Hayer, S.; Koenders, M.I.; van den Berg, W.B.; Smolen, J.; Redlich, K. Essential role of microRNA-155 in the pathogenesis of autoimmune arthritis in mice. *Arthritis Rheum.* **2011**, *63*, 1281–1288. [CrossRef]
19. Churov, A.V.; Oleinik, E.K.; Knip, M. MicroRNAs in rheumatoid arthritis: Altered expression and diagnostic potential. *Autoimmun. Rev.* **2015**, *14*, 1029–1037. [CrossRef]
20. Hu, J.; Chen., C.; Liu, Q.; Liu, B.; Song, C.; Zhu, S.; Wu, C.; Liu, S.; Yu, H.; Yao, D.; et al. The role of the miR-31/FIH1 pathway in TGF-β-induced liver fibrosis. *Clin. Sci.* **2015**, *129*, 305–317. [CrossRef]
21. Monticelli, S.; Ansel, K.M.; Xiiia, C.; Socci, N.D.; Krichevsky, A.M.; Thai, T.; Rajewsky, N.; Marks, D.S.; Sander, C.; Rajewsky, K.; et al. MicroRNA profiling of the murine hematopoietic system. *Genome Biol.* **2005**, *6*, R71. [CrossRef] [PubMed]
22. Gao, J.; Kong, R.; Zhou, X.; Ji, L.; Zhang, J.; Zhao, D. MiRNA-126 expression inhibits IL-23R mediated TNF-α or IFN-γ production in fibroblast-like synoviocytes in a mice model of collagen-induced rheumatoid arthritis. *Apoptosis* **2018**, *23*, 607–615. [CrossRef] [PubMed]
23. Pesce, B.; Soto, L.; Sabugo, F.; Wurmann, P.; Cuchacivuch, M.; Lopez, M.N.; Sotelo, P.H.; Molina, M.C.; Aguillon, J.C.; Catalan, D. Effect of interleukin-6 receptor blockade on the balance between regulatory T cells and T helper type 17 cells in rheumatoid arthritis patients. *Clin. Exp. Immunol.* **2013**, *171*, 237–242. [CrossRef] [PubMed]
24. Niu, Q.; Cai, B.; Huand, Z.C.; Shi, Y.Y.; Wang, L.I. Disturbed Th17/Treg balance in patients with rheumatoid arthritis. *Rheumatol. Int.* **2012**, *32*, 2731–2736. [CrossRef] [PubMed]

25. Liu, J.; Hong, X.; Lin, D.; Luo, X.; Zhu, M.; Mo, H. Artesunate influences Th17/Treg lymphocyte balance by modulating Treg apoptosis and Th17 proliferation in a murine model of rheumatoid arthritis. *Exp. Ther. Med.* **2017**, *13*, 2267–2273. [CrossRef] [PubMed]
26. Bae, S.C.; Lee, Y.H. MiR-146a Levels in rheumatoid arthritis and their correlation with disease activity: A meta-analysis. *Int. J. Rheum. Dis.* **2018**, *21*, 1335–1342. [CrossRef] [PubMed]
27. Abou-Zeid, A.; Saad, M.; Soliman, E. MicroRNA 146a expression in rheumatoid arthritis: Association with tumor necrosis factor-alpha and disease activity. *Genet. Test. Mol. Biomarkers* **2011**, *15*, 807–812. [CrossRef]
28. Niimoto, T.; Nakasa, T.; Ishikawa, M.; Okuhara, A.; Izumi, B.; Deie, M.; Suzuki, O.; Adachi, N.; Ochi, M. MicroRNA-146a expresses in interleukin-17 producing T cells in rheumatoid arthritis patients. *BMC Musculoskelet. Disord.* **2010**, 11. [CrossRef]
29. Su, L.C.; Huang, A.F.; Jia, H.; Liu, Y.; Xu, W.D. Role of microRNA-155 in rheumatoid arthritis. *Int. J. Rheum. Dis.* **2017**, *20*, 1631–1637. [CrossRef]
30. Singh, A.; Patro, P.S.; Aggarwal, A. MicroRNA-132, miR-146a, and miR-155 as potential biomarkers of methotrexate response in patients with rheumatoid arthritis. *Clin. Rheumatol.* **2019**, *38*, 877–884. [CrossRef]
31. Wickham, H. *ggplot2: Elegant Graphics for Data Analysis*; Springer: New York, NY, USA, 2016.
32. Robin, X.; Turck, N.; Hainard, A.; Tiberti, N.; Frédérique, L.; Jean-Charles, S.; Markus, M. pROC: An open-source package for R and S+ to analyze and compare ROC curves. *BMC Bioinf.* **2011**, *12*, 77. [CrossRef] [PubMed]

International Journal of *Molecular Sciences*

MDPI

Article

Discoidin Domain Receptors 1 Inhibition Alleviates Osteoarthritis via Enhancing Autophagy

Hsin-Chaio Chou [1,2,3], Chung-Hwan Chen [2,3,4,5,6], Liang-Yin Chou [1,2,3], Tsung-Lin Cheng [2,3,7], Lin Kang [8], Shu-Chun Chuang [2,3], Yi-Shan Lin [2,3], Mei-Ling Ho [1,2,3,7,9,10], Yan-Hsiung Wang [2,3,11], Sung-Yen Lin [1,2,3,4,6,9,*] and Chau-Zen Wang [1,2,3,7,12,*]

1 Graduate Institute of Medicine, College of Medicine, Kaohsiung Medical University, Kaohsiung 80708, Taiwan; rna.studio2014@gmail.com (H.-C.C.); laining59@gmail.com (L.-Y.C.); homelin@kmu.edu.tw (M.-L.H.)
2 Orthopaedic Research Center, Kaohsiung Medical University, Kaohsiung 80708, Taiwan; hwan@kmu.edu.tw (C.-H.C.); junglecc@gmail.com (T.-L.C.); hawayana@gmail.com (S.-C.C.); 327lin@gmail.com (Y.-S.L.); yhwang@kmu.edu.tw (Y.-H.W.)
3 Regeneration Medicine and Cell Therapy Research Center, Kaohsiung Medical University, Kaohsiung 80708, Taiwan
4 Departments of Orthopedics, Kaohsiung Municipal Ta-Tung Hospital, Kaohsiung 80145, Taiwan
5 Institute of Medical Science and Technology, National Sun Yat-Sen University, Kaohsiung 80424, Taiwan
6 Division of Adult Reconstruction Surgery, Department of Orthopedics, Kaohsiung Medical University Hospital, Kaohsiung Medical University, Kaohsiung 80708, Taiwan
7 Department of Physiology, College of Medicine, Kaohsiung Medical University, Kaohsiung 80708, Taiwan
8 Department of Obstetrics and Gynecology, National Cheng Kung University Hospital, College of Medicine, National Cheng Kung University, Tainan 70101, Taiwan; kanglin@mail.ncku.edu.tw
9 Department of Orthopedics, College of Medicine, Kaohsiung Medical University, Kaohsiung 80708, Taiwan
10 Department of Marine Biotechnology and Resources, National Sun Yat-Sen University, Kaohsiung 80424, Taiwan
11 School of Dentistry, College of Dental Medicine Kaohsiung Medical University, Kaohsiung 80708, Taiwan
12 Department of Medical Research, Kaohsiung Medical University Hospital, Kaohsiung 80708, Taiwan
* Correspondence: tony8501031@gmail.com (S.-Y.L.); czwang@kmu.edu.tw (C.-Z.W.); Tel.: +88-6-7-3121101 (C.-Z.W.)

Received: 30 July 2020; Accepted: 16 September 2020; Published: 23 September 2020

Abstract: We recently reported that the chondrocyte-specific knockout of discoidin domain receptors 1 (Ddr1) delayed endochondral ossification (EO) in the growth plate by reducing the chondrocyte hypertrophic terminal differentiation, and apoptosis. The biologic and phenotypic changes in chondrocytes in the articular cartilage with osteoarthritis (OA) are similar to the phenomena observed in the process of EO. Additionally, autophagy can promote chondrocyte survival and prevent articular cartilage from degradation in OA. On this basis, we explored the effect of Ddr1 inhibition on OA prevention and further investigated the roles of autophagy in treating OA with a Ddr1 inhibitor (7 rh). The anterior cruciate ligament transection (ACLT)–OA model was used to investigate the role of 7 rh in vivo. Forty 8-week-old mice were randomly assigned to four groups, including the sham group, ACLT group, and two treated groups (ACLT with 7 rh 6.9 nM or 13.8 nM). According to the study design, normal saline or 7 rh were intra-articular (IA) injected into studied knees 3 times per week for 2 weeks and then once per week for 4 weeks. The results showed that 7 rh treatment significantly improved the functional performances (the weight-bearing ability and the running endurance), decreased cartilage degradation, and also reduced the terminal differentiation markers (collagen type X, Indian hedgehog, and matrix metalloproteinase 13). Moreover, 7 rh decreased chondrocyte apoptosis by regulating chondrocyte autophagy through reducing the expression of the mammalian target of rapamycin and enhancing the light chain 3 and beclin-1 expression. These results demonstrated that the IA injection of 7 rh could reduce the chondrocyte apoptosis and promote chondrocyte autophagy, leading to the attenuation of cartilage degradation. Our observations suggested that the IA injection of 7 rh could represent a potential disease-modifying therapy to prevention OA progression.

Keywords: discoidin domain receptors 1 (Ddr1); osteoarthritis (OA); autophagy; apoptosis; terminal differentiation

---

1. Introduction

Osteoarthritis (OA) is the most prevalent joint disease worldwide and also the leading cause of disability in aged patients. Because of aging and increasing obesity in the population, the prevalence of OA is rapidly increased. The current pharmacological therapy for OA was focused on symptomatic relief. Despite some promising disease-modifying therapy undergoing clinical trials, there is no currently effective therapy to prevent the progressive destruction of articular cartilage [1].

Chondrocyte death is the key pathogenesis of OA. The articular chondrocyte is the only resident cell in cartilage and is responsible for maintaining the equilibrium of the extracellular matrix. The compromising of chondrocyte survival leads to cartilage degradation; as a result, the prevention of chondrocyte death is an important research direction for OA prevention. The morphologic changes in chondrocytes in OA are resembling those happening in the growth plates, where the chondrocytes undergo hypertrophic terminal differentiation, featuring chondrocyte hypertrophic change, mineralization, and eventually apoptosis [2]. Recent research on parathyroid hormone 1-34 (PTH 1-34) in OA has indicated that the treatment can inhibit the apoptosis of chondrocytes in the growth plate, which can also be used to inhibit the apoptosis of chondrocyte in osteoarthritic articular cartilage, thereby reducing cartilage degradation [3–5].

Discoidin domain receptors (Ddr) are a group of the transmembrane receptors that triggers a ligand-induced kinase activation and receptor autophosphorylation after biding collagen and then to regulate cell migration, proliferation, differentiation, and cell survival [6]. Ddr1 and Ddr2 are two major types of Ddrs with similar amino acid sequences and both are expressed in the cartilage. The biological function of Ddrs has been widely investigated by gene knockout mice. Although the physiologic role of two Ddrs is different, the global Ddr1 or Ddr2 ablated mice all present with dwarfism [7]. The Ddr2 ablation reduces the chondrocyte proliferation and thus decreases bone growth; however, the reasons for dwarfism in Ddr1 ablation mice remain unclear. Our recent study using chondrocyte-specific Ddr1 knockout mice demonstrated that the Ddr1 ablation resulted in a decreased chondrocyte proliferation, terminal differentiation, and apoptosis in growth plates and caused a delayed EO [8]. Our findings indicated that Ddr1 is an imperative regulator of EO in the growth plate and maybe also a potential target for OA treatment.

Autophagy maintains the homeostatic equilibrium to cartilage following injury and is reported to be a cellular self-protection mechanism of normal cartilage. Previous researchers demonstrated that the deregulation of autophagy predisposed to the pathogenesis of OA and the activation of autophagy could protect articular cartilage from OA [9]. The mammalian target of rapamycin (mTOR) is a serine/threonine protein kinase regulating signal transduction during autophagy. A previous study showed that the cartilage-specific deletion of mTOR upregulated the autophagy signaling and reduced the articular degradation, chondrocyte apoptosis, and synovial fibrosis in surgical-induced OA mice [10]. Similarly, rapamycin (an inhibitor of mTOR) enhanced the activation of autophagy, maintained the cartilage cellularity, and reduced the severity of surgical-induced OA [11]. Although we do not fully understand the relationship between chondrocyte survival and autophagy, accumulating evidence suggests that the restoration autophagy of senescent chondrocyte can restore the reparative capacity and may be an effective therapeutic approach for OA [12].

While the inhibiting of Ddr1 can decrease chondrocyte apoptosis in the growth plate, it has yet to be demonstrated whether this phenomenon may occur in the articular cartilage and the inhibition expression of Ddr1 can protect against cartilage degradation in experimental-induced OA animal models. Ddr1 inhibition can reduce chondrocyte terminal differentiation and apoptosis in the growth plate, but whether autophagy contributes to the treatment of Ddr1 suppression on ameliorating OA progression remains unclear. The object of this study was to test the hypothesis that the inhibition of Ddr1 expression by intra-articular (IA) injection of Ddr1 inhibitor (7 rh) can reduce the OA progression in anterior cruciate ligament transection (ACLT)-induced OA mice. Specifically, we aimed to determine whether (1) IA of 7 rh can delay the articular cartilage degradation in histology and also improve knee function after OA induction; (2) IA of 7 rh can reduce the chondrocyte terminal differentiation and apoptosis; (3) the effects of 7 rh on prevention chondrocyte apoptosis are through the regulation of autophagy in chondrocytes.

2. Results

2.1. Low Cytotoxicity of 7 rh on Human Articular Chondrocytes Viability

A pilot study was conducted to choose the optimal concentrations of 7 rh for this experiment. The cytotoxicity of 7 rh on HAC was assessed by CCK8 assay. IC50 (6.9 nM) and IC100 (13.8 nM) of 7 rh were assessed to determine the cytotoxicity. Cell viability assay exhibited that the drug dosage in our study was low cell cytotoxicity to chondrocyte (Figure 1). Therefore, we selected the concentrations of 6.9 nM and 13.8 nM for the subsequent experiments. Additionally, the effects of 7 rh on IL-1β-stimulated HAC were assessed. As shown in Figure 1B, the results showed that the cell viability was suppressed after IL-1β stimulation and 7 rh could significantly prevent the inhibitory effects of IL-1β on cell viability at both selected concentrations ($p < 0.05$ in 6.9 nM and $p < 0.001$ in 13.8 nM).

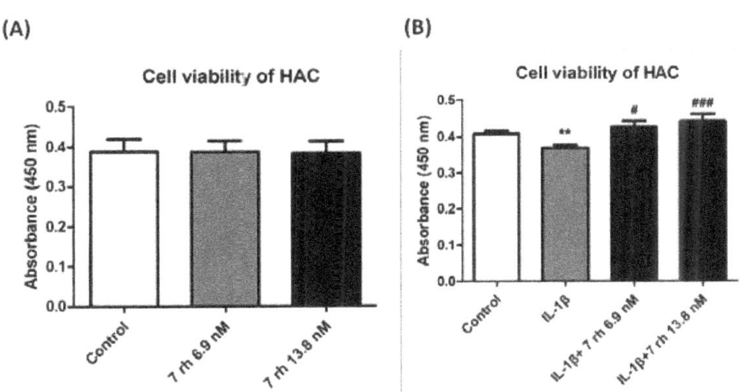

Figure 1. The cytotoxic effects of 7 rh on human articular chondrocytes (HAC). (**A**) The cell viability of HAC that was treated with 6.9 nM and 13.8 nM of 7 rh for 48 h was detected by CCK8 assay. (**B**) The chondrocytes were co-cultured with IL-1β and 7 rh (6.8 nM and 13.9 nM) for 48 h. The cell viability was measured by CCK8 assay. All experiments were performed in quadruplicate and repeated three times with similar results. (** $p < 0.01$ versus the control group; # $p < 0.05$, and ### $p < 0.001$ versus the IL-1β-treated group).

2.2. The IA Administration of 7 rh Improves the Weight Distribution Ability and Running Endurance after OA-Induction

The weight distribution test and running endurance assessment were used to evaluate the functional performance of knee joints after OA induction with or without 7 rh treatment. During the treatment course, we did not observe an apparent change in weight-bearing ability of the studied limb in both of the sham control groups (sham+ saline and sham+ 7 rh 13.8 nM), but a significantly reduced ability to bear weight in ACLT mice ($p < 0.001$ compared with the sham control groups). In contrast, the mice in 7 rh-treated groups could bear approximately 50% of their body weight since the third week, and the effects persisted to the residual treatment course (Figure 2A).

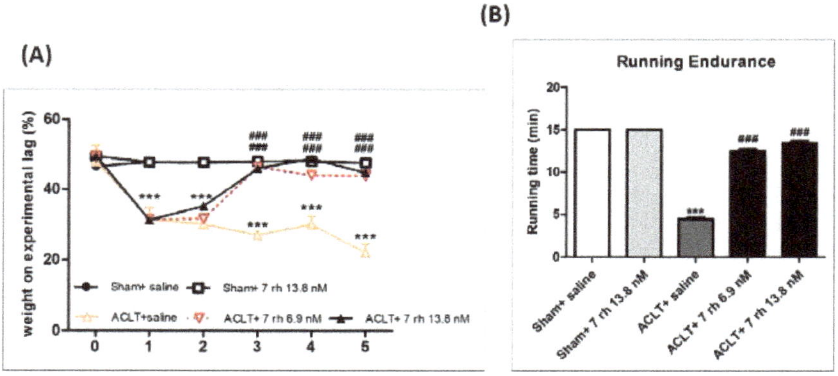

Figure 2. Treatment with 7 rh promoted knee function after anterior cruciate ligament transection (ACLT). (**A**) Weight-bearing test. There were no obvious influences in both of the sham control groups (sham+ saline and sham+ 7 rh 13.8 nM) during the treating courses. The weight-bearing ability of the studied limb was significantly reduced after osteoarthritis (OA) induction ($p < 0.001$). Mice in the OA + 7 rh group could bear significantly more weight since the third week ($p < 0.001$ at both concentrations) and thereafter until the end of the study (all $p < 0.001$). (**B**) Treadmill running test. The mice in the ACLT-OA group could endure less time in gait occurred than those in the sham control groups ($p < 0.001$) at 5 weeks. In both treating groups, the mice significantly increased their running endurance in the treadmill test (all $p < 0.001$) with no significant difference from mice in the sham control groups. (*** $p < 0.001$ versus the sham control groups; ### $p < 0.001$ versus the ACLT group).

The running endurance is an indicator of knee function improvement. As the results of the weight distribution test, the running endurance was significantly reduced after OA induction. The mice in both sham control groups could finish the 15 min running test, whereas the mice in the ACLT group could only endure 4.5 ± 0.8 min at 5 weeks. Notably, 7 rh significantly increased the mice' endurance levels to 12.5 ± 0.8 min in 6.9 nM 7 rh group and 13.5 ± 0.8 min in the 13.8 nM 7 rh group, respectively, at 5 weeks, which is not a significant difference compared to the sham control groups (Figure 2B).

2.3. The IA Administration of 7 rh Slows the Articular Cartilage Degradation

To evaluate the efficacy of 7 rh on ACLT-induced OA progression, the loss of GAG, and the structural integrity of the articular cartilage were examined by the Safranin O-Fast Green staining and OARSI histology grading scores. As shown in Figure 3A, there was no obvious structure destruction or GAG loss identified in the sham-operated knees that were treated either with normal saline or 7 rh 13.8 nM. In contrast, we observed apparent damages to articular cartilage with a marked loss of proteoglycans in the ACLT mice at 5 weeks, indicating the successful induction of OA. The IA injection of 7 rh (6.9 nM and 13.8 nM) attenuated the cartilage degeneration and reduced the GAG loss after ACLT compared with the sham-operated knees. These results were further confirmed by the OARSI scores. The articular cartilage in the sham-operated knees did not exhibit obvious OA pathological changes in the articular cartilage and had an average OARSI score of 3.2 ± 0.9 in saline group and 3.3 ±1.0 in 7 rh 13.8 nM group (Figure 3B). The cartilage in the ACLT-OA knees exhibited significant GAG loss, cartilage erosion, and chondrocyte clustering with a mean OARSI score 9.2 ± 0.9, which was significantly higher compared to the sham-operated knees ($p < 0.01$). In contrast, the cartilage in the 7 rh-treated mice revealed a less cartilage fibrillation and proteoglycans loss and the mean OARSI scores (4 ± 0.9 in 6.9 nM of 7 rh, and 2.8 ± 1 in 13.8 nM of 7 rh) were also significantly lower compared to ACLT-OA mice ($p < 0.01$ in both concentrations).

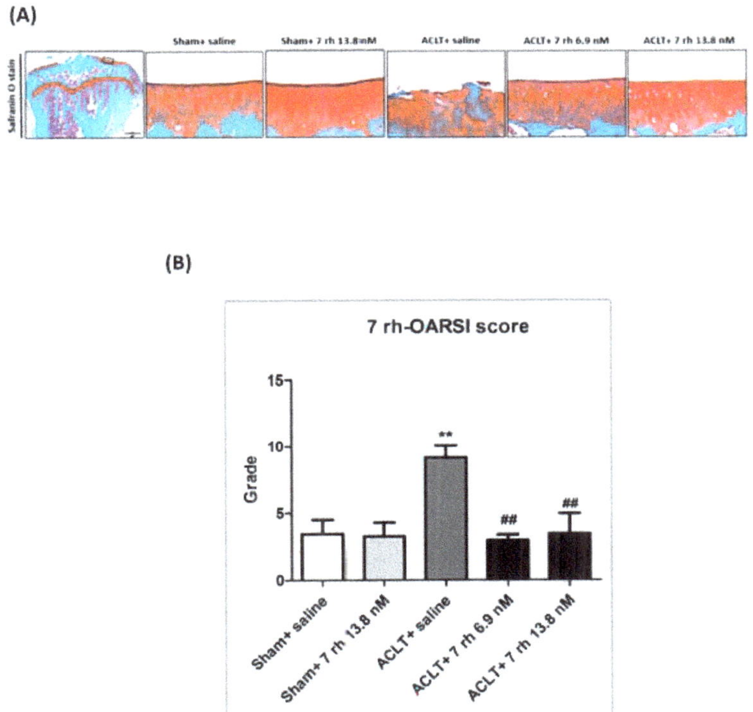

Figure 3. Intra-articular injection of 7 rh attenuated cartilage degradation in anterior cruciate ligament transection (ACLT)-induced osteoarthritis (OA). (**A**) The representative Safranin O-Fast Green stained articular cartilages micrographs of the proximal tibia from the right knee joints of mice in the sham control groups (sham+ saline and sham+ 7 rh 13.8 nM), ACLT, and two 7 rh treated groups. (**B**) Osteoarthritis Research Society International (OARSI) scores of articular cartilage at 5 weeks after ACLT surgery. (** $p < 0.01$ versus the sham control groups; ## $p < 0.01$ versus the ACLT group).

2.4. The IA Administration of 7 rh Decreases the Expression of Hypertrophic Markers (Col X, MMP13, and IHH) after OA Induction

IHC staining was performed to investigate whether 7 rh alleviated OA progression by reducing the chondrocyte hypertrophic differentiation. The representative images of IHC staining of chondrocyte hypertrophic markers, including Col X, IHH, and MMP13 at 5 weeks, are shown in Figure 4A–C and the results of the quantitative analysis are shown in Figure 4D–F. Col X, IHH, and MMP13 were well-established markers for detecting the chondrocyte during the hypertrophic differentiation. The ensity of immunolocalized Col X was significantly increased in the ACLT group, and the treatment of 7 rh (13.8 nM) in ACLT mice at 5 weeks significantly inhibited the expression of Col X (Figure 4A,D). As shown in Figure 4B,E, the levels of IHH expression also increased after OA induction and reduced significantly in the 7 rh-treated mice (13.8 nM group) compared to ACLT-OA mice at 5 weeks. As shown in Figure 4C,F, the immunolocalized MMP13 protein was predominantly found in the articular chondrocytes in the ACLT-OA mice and the expressions were decreased significantly after 7 rh treatment (13.8 nM group). These results revealed that chondrocytes undergo terminal differentiation after OA induction, but 7 rh (13.8 nM) can prevent chondrocytes from terminal differentiation.

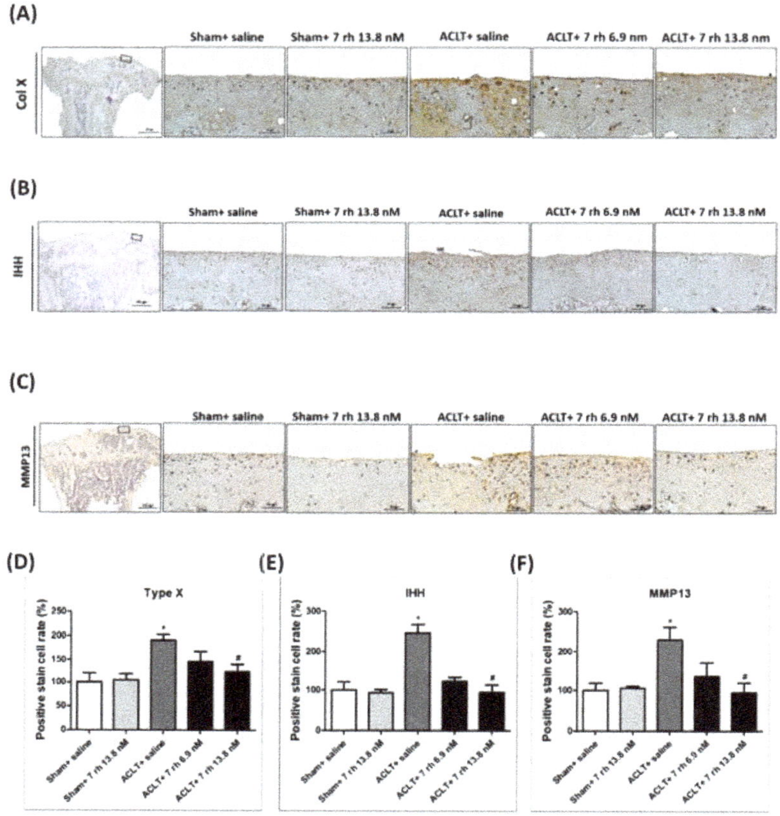

Figure 4. Intra-articular injections of 7 rh reduced the chondrocyte hypertrophic differentiation in anterior cruciate ligament transection (ACLT)-induced osteoarthritis (OA) cartilage. (**A**) The representative micrographs of immunolocalized type X collagen (Col X) in articular cartilage of the sham control groups (sham+ saline and sham+ 7 rh 13.8 nM), ACLT, and two 7 rh treating groups. (**B**) The representative micrographs of immunolocalized Indian hedgehog (IHH). (**C**) The representative micrographs of immunolocalized matrix metallopeptidase 13 (MMP13). (**D**) Quantitative analysis of the immunohistochemically (IHC) staining of Col X. (**E**) Quantitative analysis of the IHC staining of IHH. (**F**) Quantitative analysis of the immunohistochemical IHC of MMP13. In quantitative analysis, each bar represents the mean±SEM of 12 samples in each group. (* $p < 0.05$ versus the sham control groups; # $p < 0.05$ versus the ACLT group).

2.5. The IA Administration of 7 rh Decreases Chondrocyte Apoptosis

The results of TUNEL staining exhibited that 7 rh treatment prevented cell apoptosis in the ACLT-OA cartilage (Figure 5A). The apoptotic rate of chondrocytes in the articular cartilage of the ACLT-OA mice (22.4 ± 3.3%) was significantly more increased than in the sham + saline group (4.5 ± 0.7%, $p < 0.001$) and in the sham + 7 rh 13.8 nM group (1.0 ± 0.5%, $p < 0.001$). After 7 rh treatment at 5 weeks, the apoptotic rate of chondrocytes in the 7 rh-treated articular cartilage was significantly reduced to 7.6 ± 1.4% in the 7 rh 6.9 nM group and 5.8 ± 0.8% in the 7 rh 13.8 nM group, respectively (Figure 5C).

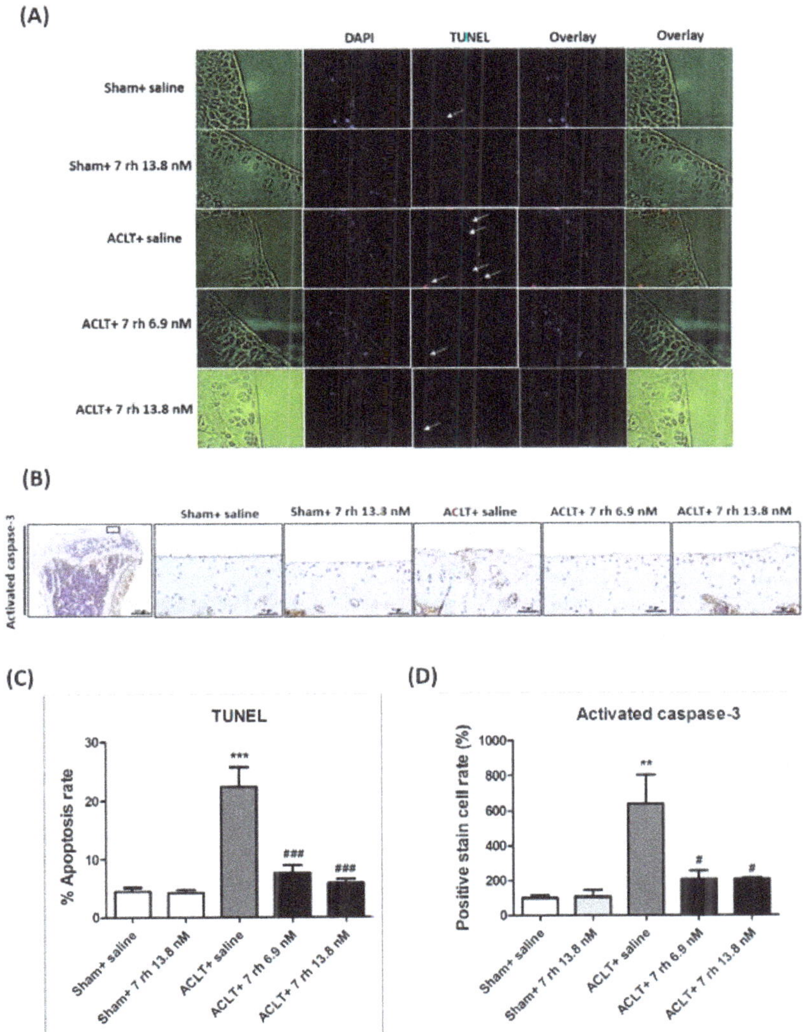

Figure 5. Effect of 7 rh on chondrocyte apoptosis in articular cartilage. (**A**) TUNEL staining in the articular cartilages of the sham control groups (sham+ saline and sham+ 7 rh 13.8 nM), ACLT, and two 7 rh treating groups. The arrows mean positive stain of TUNEL. (**B**) The representative micrographs of immunolocalized activated caspase 3. (**C**) Quantitative analysis of the apoptotic rate. (**D**) Quantitative analysis of the immunohistochemical staining of activated caspase 3. Each bar represents the mean±SEM of 12 samples in each group. (** $p < 0.01$ versus the sham control groups; *** $p < 0.001$ versus the sham control groups; $^{\#}$ $p < 0.05$ versus the ACLT group; $^{\#\#\#}$ $p < 0.001$ versus the ACLT group).

Caspase-3 is considered as the primary executioner for apoptosis; therefore, we used IHC staining of activated caspase-3 for the analysis of apoptosis activity. The results revealed that activated caspase-3 protein expression in the ACLT group was significantly increased compared with the sham control groups, but was significantly decreased in the OA-induced mice treated with 7 rh (both 6.9 nM and 13.8 nM) at 5 weeks (Figure 5B,D). These results showed that 7 rh significantly reduced chondrocyte apoptosis in ACLT mice.

2.6. The IA Administration of 7 rh Decreases mTOR Expression and Increases LC3 and Beclin 1 Expression

To clarify if 7 rh treatment can rescue the autophagy effect in the ACLT-OA model, we examined the expression of autophagy markers, including mTOR, LC3 and beclin-1 in the articular cartilage (Figure 6). The results of IHC staining showed that the autophagy dysfunction in response to ACLT-OA induction was rescued by 7 rh. The expression of phosphorylated mTOR in the 7 rh treated group was significantly lower than that in the ACLT group ($p < 0.05$ in 7 rh 6.9 nM group and $p < 0.01$ in 7 rh 13.8 nM group). Meanwhile, the density of LC3 and beclin 1 in the cartilage of the 7 rh treated group was significantly higher than that in the ACLT group at 5 weeks ($p < 0.05$ in LC3 and $p < 0.001$ in beclin 1).

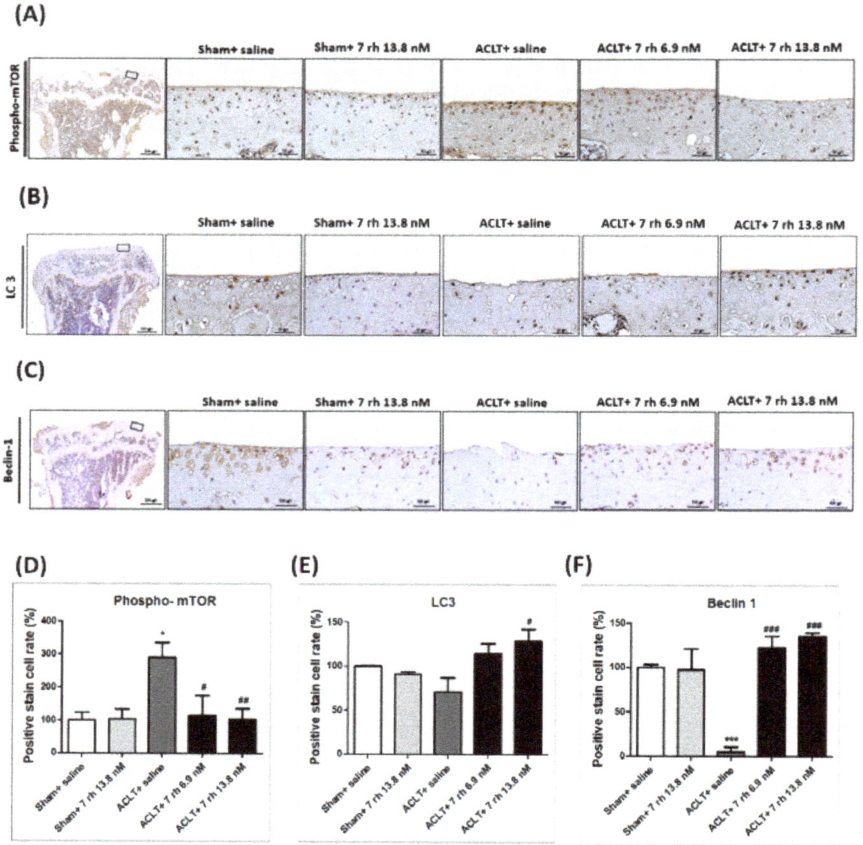

Figure 6. Effect of 7 rh mediated enhanced autophagy-related proteins in articular cartilage. (**A**) The representative micrographs of immunolocalized phosphorylation of mechanistic target of rapamycin (phospho-mTOR) in articular cartilage of the sham control groups (sham+ saline and sham+ 7 rh 13.8 nM), ACLT, and two 7 rh treated groups. (**B**) The representative micrographs of immunolocalized light chain 3 (LC3). (**C**) The representative micrographs of immunolocalized beclin-1. (**D**) Quantitative analysis of the immunohistochemical (IHC) staining of phospho-mTOR. (**E**) Quantitative analysis of the IHC staining of LC3. (**F**) Quantitative analysis of the IHC immunohistochemical staining of beclin-1. In quantitative analysis, each bar represents the mean±SE of 12 samples in each group. (* $p < 0.05$ versus the sham control groups; *** $p < 0.001$ versus the sham control groups; $^{\#}$ $p < 0.05$ versus the ACLT group; $^{\#\#}$ $p < 0.005$ versus the ACLT-OA group; $^{\#\#\#}$ $p < 0.001$ versus the ACLT group).

3. Discussion

The results of the current study are the first to show the central role of the Ddr1 inhibition in ameliorating OA progression in the ACLT induced OA model. By using a Ddr1 inhibitor (7 rh), we significantly slowed the articular cartilage degradation, improved the weight-bearing ability, and promoted the running endurance through treadmill tests at 5 weeks after ACLT. Histologically, the reduced expression of chondrocyte hypertrophic markers indicated the inhibition of chondrocyte terminal differentiation. Furthermore, 7 rh reduced the chondrocyte hypertrophic differentiation and apoptosis by enhancing autophagy.

Previous studies have indicated the similar biological behaviors of articular chondrocytes in OA progression with the chondrocytes of the growth plate in EO [2]. In the OA status, the articular chondrocytes become hypertrophic, with changes accompanied by the overexpression of the hypertrophic markers, including alkaline phosphatase, Col X, and MMP13 and subsequent chondrocyte mineralization and apoptosis, which is similar with the phenotype changes in EO [13]. It was already known that the chondrocyte differentiation and EO in the growth plate were regulated by the parathyroid hormone-related protein (PTHrP)-IHH feedback loop [14]. PTH 1–34, sharing the same receptors with PTHrP, was also reported to suppress the expression of Col X and IHH of hypertrophic chondrocyte in the fetal bovine growth plates [15]. In our previous study, we showed that IA injection of the PTH 1–34 at 3–5 weeks significantly attenuated the loss of proteoglycans and type II collagen, suppressed the expression of Col X, and reduced chondrocyte apoptosis in papain-induced OA in rats [3]. Similar results have also been reported in the systemic administration of PTH 1-34 [5] and in both surgical induced and spontaneous OA models [4]. These studies proved the concepts that treatments that can inhibit chondrocyte terminal differentiation in the growth plate and can also suppress chondrocyte apoptosis in articular cartilage and then inhibit the progression of OA.

Our recent research, investigating the role of Ddr1 in the regulation of EO, has indicated that the chondrocyte-specific Ddr1 knockout can delay the EO and accompany decreased chondrocyte proliferation, terminal differentiation, and apoptosis in growth plates of mice [8]. Accordingly, we hypothesized that the Ddr1 inhibitor (7 rh) may maintain the survival of articular chondrocytes and reduce the progression of OA. To test this hypothesis, we examined the efficacy of the IA injection of 7 rh on reducing the cartilage degeneration and inhibition of the chondrocyte apoptosis in the ACLT-induced OA model in mice. Our results indicated that the IA injection of 7 rh improved the function of the OA joint and reduced the OARSI score. We also found that 7 rh can decrease chondrocyte hypertrophic differentiation by inhibiting the expression of Col X, MMP13, and IHH. IHH signaling is not only essential for regulating normal chondrocyte proliferation and differentiation in the growth plate but also important in modulating chondrocyte terminal differentiation in OA cartilage. Lin A.C. et al. used genetically modified mice to exam the role of IHH signaling in OA chondrocytes and demonstrated that the expression of IHH was up-regulated by OA and was closely related to the severity of OA [13]. Moreover, the pharmacological inhibition of IHH signaling could decrease the hypertrophic differentiation of chondrocytes and ameliorate OA severity [13,14]. Accordingly, we reputed that the inhibition of the up-regulation of IHH signaling in OA plays a pivotal role in suppressing the degradation of cartilage.

The hypertrophy-like changes in chondrocytes secreted a number of proteins that are involved in tissue remodeling, and calcification has been associated with the early and late stage of OA [13]. The inhibition of chondrocyte hypertrophic differentiation was considered as a therapeutic target for OA progression. The Ddr2, a receptor tyrosine kinase, that can be activated by degrade type II collagen has been reported to play a role in chondrocyte differentiation in OA. The increased expression of Ddr2 was reported to be associated with OA progression and elevated MMP13 expression in the surgically induced OA in mice [14]. Moreover, Ddr2 modulated Runx2 activity and stimulated the expression of Col X in hypertrophic chondrocytes (ADTC5 cells) [15]. The role of Ddr1 in chondrocyte hypertrophic differentiation is still not clear. Col X and MMP13 were the mostly widely used markers for hypertrophic chondrocytes [13]. Apoptosis is also an important marker for detecting hypertrophic chondrocytes in late staged OA cartilage. The TUNEL staining of late-staged human OA cartilage showed that the chondrocytes in the upper zone of cartilage undergo terminal differentiation and eventually die by apoptosis [16]. In the current study, 7 rh treatment significantly decreased the expression of Col X and MMP13 and also reduced chondrocyte apoptosis by decreasing the expression of activated caspase 3 in OA cartilage. These findings suggested that the IA injection of 7 rh reduced chondrocyte hypertrophic differentiation and apoptosis in the OA cartilage, thereby reducing OA progression.

Autophagy is an essential process in maintaining cellular metabolism and homeostasis. Emerging evidence suggests that the deregulation of autophagy is a crucial factor in the pathogenesis of OA [17,18]. Caramés, B. et al. studied the expression of autophagy regulator and chondrocyte apoptosis in the articular cartilage of human OA and the experimental OA, and the authors demonstrated that the autophagy regulators were reduced in the human OA and the aging-related or surgically induced OA in mice accompanied by an increase in chondrocyte apoptosis [17]. Recently, the same researchers used green fluorescent protein–light chain transgenic mice to detect autophagy activation in normal and aging cartilage and indicated that the autophagy regulators were reduced before the onset of cartilage degradation and the decrease in chondrocyte cellularity [18]. The mTOR signaling pathway plays a central role in regulating the initiation, processing, and termination of autophagy. The cartilage-specific deletion of mTOR upregulated autophagy and protected mice from OA [10]. In addition, autophagy activated by rapamycin (an inhibitor of mTOR) reduced the severity of experimental OA [19]. Similar to previous studies, our results showed significantly increased mTOR expression after experimental OA induction, indicating that the reduction in the autophagy process leads to articular cartilage degeneration [11,19]. Furthermore, we also found that beclin1 and LC3, the major indicators for autophagosome formation, were expressed in normal cartilage, indicating a functional autophagy process. However, the expression of autophagy markers (beclin1 and LC3) was significantly suppressed after ACLT, implying insufficient autophagy in OA cartilage. These findings indicated that articular cartilage degradation after ACLT was related to autophagy dysfunction. In this study, our results showed that the IA of 7 rh significantly restored autophagy function and further reduced the progression of OA, as shown by the reduced immunostaining of activated mTOR, the increased immunostaining of beclin1 and LC3, and histologically lower GAG loss and a lower OARSI score. Based on these findings, we suggested that the reduction in chondrocyte apoptosis, mediated by the activation of autophagy, may be a part of the mechanism of action of 7 rh on preventing OA progression.

In conclusion, our results showed that the IA injection of 7 rh reduced cartilage degradation in ACLT-induced OA animals. The inhibition of Ddr1 can reduce chondrocyte hypertrophic differentiation and chondrocyte apoptosis in the OA cartilage, as well as recover the autophagy function that was impaired by OA. We demonstrated that the inhibition of Ddr1 in articular cartilage could modulate OA progression and prevent chondrocyte apoptosis by promoting autophagy in OA cartilage. These findings suggested that 7 rh may be a potential disease-modifying drug to prevention OA progression.

4. Materials and Methods

4.1. Human Articular Chondrocyte (HAC) Cultures

The human articular chondrocyte (HAC) cell line was purchased from Lonza Walkersville Inc. (8F3339, LONZA, MD, USA). The HAC cells were cultured in Dulbecco Modified Eagle Medium (DMEM) containing 10% fetal bovine serum (FBS), 100 IU/mL penicillin, and 100 μg/mL streptomycin at 37 °C in a humidified atmosphere of 5% CO_2.

4.2. Cell Viability Assay

Cell viability was measured using Counting Kit-8 (CCK-8 assay). A total of 10,000 HAC cells per well were cultured in 96-wells cell culture plate and then incubated for 48 h at 37 °C. After that, HAC cells were cultured in 200 μL culture medium with 7 rh (6.9 nM or 13.8 nM) or co-cultured with

7 rh and IL-1β (10 ng/mL) in 5% CO2 for 3h. Then, 10 μL of CCK-8 reagent (E-CK-A361, Elabscience, Houston, TX, USA) was added and the optical density at 450 nm was measured using a multifunction microplate reader (Synergy H1, BioTek, Winooski, VT, USA) after incubation for 2 h at 37 °C.

4.3. Animals Experiments

All animal experiments were performed following the approval of the Institutional Animal Care and Use Committee-IACUC from Kaohsiung Medical University (The project identification code and date: IACUC105127; 1 Aug 2017–31 July 2020). A total of 40 healthy male C57BL/6 mice (8-weeks-old) were obtained from the Jackson laboratory (National laboratory animal center, Taiwan), and were housed under the standard conditions in Animal Center of Kaohsiung Medical University (Kaohsiung, Taiwan). The animals were randomly assigned into four groups, including the sham group (sham operation treated by Normal saline, $n = 10$), ACLT group (OA induction treated by Normal saline, $n = 10$), ACLT plus 7 rh 6.9 nM ($n = 10$), and ACLT plus 7 rh 13.8 nM ($n = 10$). OA was surgically induced in 8-weeks-old C57BL/6 mice by ACLT in the right knee. According to study design, the mice either received IA injection with the same volume (10 μL) of Normal saline, 7 rh 6.8 nM, or 7 rh 13.8 nM three times per week from 7 to 9 weeks-old and then one dose per week until sacrifice at 13 weeks-old.

4.4. Weight Bearing Distribution Test

The weight-bearing ability after OA-induction was measured by Dual Channel Weight Averages (Singa Technology Corporation, Taiwan), which can analyze the weight-bearing of each hind paw. The changes in joint weight-bearing capacity represent the severity of the experimental joint symptoms. The weight-bearing test was performed at one week before ACLT and then every week until the mice were euthanized.

4.5. Running Endurance

Mice were subjected to run on a Columbus Instruments rodent treadmill (Columbus, OH, USA) once a week before and after OA-induction until the mice were euthanized. The running speed started from 8.5 m/min and lasted for 3 min. Thereafter, the treadmill speed increased by 2.5 m/min every 3 min with a treadmill angle of 5 degrees until the maximum running speed was 25 m/min. The limit of running endurance recording time was 15 min, and the experiment stopped after reaching the maximum duration. During the whole process, a mild electric shock caused an uncomfortable shock but not physical damage to the mice and was set according to the previous study [17].

4.6. Histopathological Assessments

The mice tibia samples were fixed in 10% buffered paraformaldehyde for 2 days and then decalcified with buffered ethylenediaminetetraacetic acid (0.5 M, pH 7.4). After dehydration and embedding in paraffin, the tissue blocks were cut in coronal with a thickness of 5 μm. Glycosaminoglycan (GAG) was stained by Safranin O-Fast Green (1% safranin O counterstained, 0.75% hematoxylin, and then 1% Fast Green; Sigma, St. Louis, MO, USA) and was used to evaluate the severity of OA. All of the histological results were assessed by two independent researchers blinded to any other information according to the histology grading system of Osteoarthritis Research Society International (OARSI) [18].

4.7. Immunohistochemistry (IHC) for Type X Collagen (Col X), Indian Hedgehog (IHH), Matrix Metalloproteinases 13 (MMP13), Caspase 3, mTOR, Light Chain 3 (LC3), Beclin-1

Tissue sections were deparaffinized, rehydrated and then blocked with 3% hydrogen peroxide. The samples were prepared for indirect immune detection by mouse- and rabbit-specific horseradish peroxidase/diaminobenzidine detection kit (ab64264, Abcam, Cambridge, MA, USA) following the manufacturer's instructions. The primary antibodies used in this study were rabbit polyclonal antibodies to Col X (ab58632, Abcam, Cambridge, MA, USA), IHH (ab52919, Abcam, Cambridge, MA, USA), MMP13 (ab39012, Abcam, Cambridge, MA, USA), activated caspase-3 (ab2302, Abcam,

Cambridge, MA, USA), phosphorylated-mTOR(Ser235/236)(4858s, Cell Signaling, Danvers, MA, USA), LC3 (14600-1-AP, Proteintech, Rosemont, IL, USA), and beclin 1 (11306-1-AP, Proteintech, Rosemont, IL, USA). The sections were counterstained with hematoxylin and the immunolocalized nuclei were stained in brown. For quantification, the sections of related target proteins staining were digitalized at 400 times magnification in a total of 2560 × 1920 pixel and 300 dpi digital images in JPG file format using TissueFAXS microscope (TissueGnostics GmbH, Vienna, Austria). The digital images were analyzed to quantify the total amount of related target proteins staining using HistoQuest (TissueGnostics, Los Angeles, CA, USA) analysis software. Total area of related target protein staining was detected after automatic color separation by HistoQuest. The staining intensity was measured as mean intensity of all pixels with an automatic background threshold range from 5 to 255. The results were given as percentage per mm^2 of total tissue area.

4.8. Terminal Deoxynucleotidyl Transferase dUTP Nick End Labeling (TUNEL) Assay

TUNEL assay was performed on proximal tibia tissue sections to detect chondrocyte apoptosis (12156792910, Roche, Branchburg, NJ, USA). The percentages of TUNEL-positive cells in chondrocytes relative to 4′,6-diamidino-2-phenylindole (DAPI)-stained cells were calculated and an analysis was conducted using a Leica immunofluorescence system (Leica MicroImaging). Photographs from three independent experiments were conducted and calculated for each experimental group.

4.9. Statistical Analysis

All data were presented as mean±SEM. The results were analyzed using one-way ANOVA, and multiple comparisons were conducted by Tukey's HSD using GraphPad Prism (version 5.0). The statistical significance was considered as $p < 0.05$.

Author Contributions: Conceptualization, H.-C.C., S.-Y.L., C.-H.C. and C.-Z.W.; methodology, H.-C.C.; software, H.-C.C., S.-C.C., L.-Y.C., Y.-S.L.; validation, Y.-S.L., L.-Y.C., S.-Y.L., M.-L.H., C.-Z.W. and C.-H.C.; formal analysis, H.-C.C., S.-Y.L., T.-L.C., L.K., Y.-H.W., C.-Z.W. and C.-H.C.; investigation, H.-C.C.; data curation, H.-C.C.; writing—original draft preparation, H.-C.C. and S.-Y.L.; writing—review and editing, S.-Y.L., C.-H.C. and C.-Z.W.; project administration, H.-C.C., S.-Y.L., C.-H.C. and C.-Z.W.; funding acquisition, S.-Y.L., C.-H.C. and C.-Z.W. All authors have read and agreed to the published version of the manuscript.

Funding: This study was supported in part by the Minister of Science and Technology of Taiwan (MOST 109-2314-B-037-026, MOST108-2320-B-037-008 and MOST109-2320-B-037-005), Kaohsiung Medical University Hospital (KMUH105-5M30), Kaohsiung Medical University (KMU-TP105B10 and KMU-DK105009), Kaohsiung Medical University (KMU-TC108A02-1). The funder had no conflicts of interest including in the study design, data collection, analysis, decision to publish, or preparation of the manuscript.

Acknowledgments: We appreciate the support from members of our orthopedic research center and Department of Physiology, Regeneration Medicine and Cell Therapy Research Center, Graduate Institute of Medicine, College of Medicine of Kaohsiung Medical University, Kaohsiung City, Taiwan.

Conflicts of Interest: The authors declare no conflict of interest. The funders had no role in the design of the study; in the collection, analyses, or interpretation of data; in the writing of the manuscript, or in the decision to publish the results.

References

1. Hunter, D.J.; Bierma-Zeinstra, S. Osteoarthritis. *Lancet* **2019**, *393*, 1745–1759. [CrossRef]
2. Blanco, F.J.; Guitian, R.; Vázquez-Martul, E.; de Toro, F.J.; Galdo, F. Osteoarthritis chondrocytes die by apoptosis. A possible pathway for osteoarthritis pathology. *Arthritis Rheum.* **1998**, *41*, 284–289. [CrossRef]
3. Chang, J.K.; Chang, L.H.; Hung, S.H.; Wu, S.C.; Lee, H.Y.; Lin, Y.S.; Chen, C.H.; Fu, Y.C.; Wang, G.J.; Ho, M.L. Parathyroid hormone 1-34 inhibits terminal differentiation of human articular chondrocytes and osteoarthritis progression in rats. *Arthritis Rheum.* **2009**, *60*, 3049–3060. [CrossRef] [PubMed]
4. Yan, J.Y.; Tian, F.M.; Wang, W.Y.; Cheng, Y.; Song, H.P.; Zhang, Y.Z.; Zhang, L. Parathyroid hormone (1-34) prevents cartilage degradation and preserves subchondral bone micro-architecture in guinea pigs with spontaneous osteoarthritis. *Osteoarthr. Cartil.* **2014**, *22*, 1869–1877. [CrossRef]

5. Sampson, E.R.; Hilton, M.J.; Tian, Y.; Chen, D.; Schwarz, E.M.; Mooney, R.A.; Bukata, S.V.; O'Keefe, R.J.; Awad, H.; Puzas, J.E.; et al. Teriparatide as a chondroregenerative therapy for injury-induced osteoarthritis. *Sci. Transl. Med.* **2011**, *3*, 101ra193. [CrossRef] [PubMed]
6. Leitinger, B. Molecular analysis of collagen binding by the human discoidin domain receptors, DDR1 and DDR2. Identification of collagen binding sites in DDR2. *J. Biol. Chem.* **2003**, *278*, 16761–16769. [CrossRef]
7. Vogel, W.F.; Aszódi, A.; Alves, F.; Pawson, T. Discoidin domain receptor 1 tyrosine kinase has an essential role in mammary gland development. *Mol. Cell. Biol.* **2001**, *21*, 2906–2917. [CrossRef] [PubMed]
8. Chou, L.Y.; Chen, C.H.; Lin, Y.H.; Chuang, S.C.; Chou, H.C.; Lin, S.Y.; Fu, Y.C.; Chang, J.K.; Ho, M.L.; Wang, C.Z. Discoidin domain receptor 1 regulates endochondral ossification through terminal differentiation of chondrocytes. *FASEB J.* **2020**, *34*, 5767–5781. [CrossRef] [PubMed]
9. Luo, P.; Gao, F.; Niu, D.; Sun, X.; Song, Q.; Guo, C.; Liang, Y.; Sun, W. The Role of Autophagy in Chondrocyte Metabolism and Osteoarthritis: A Comprehensive Research Review. *Biomed. Res. Int.* **2019**, *2019*, 5171602. [CrossRef] [PubMed]
10. Zhang, Y.; Vasheghani, F.; Li, Y.H.; Blati, M.; Simeone, K.; Fahmi, H.; Lussier, B.; Roughley, P.; Lagares, D.; Pelletier, J.P.; et al. Cartilage-specific deletion of mTOR upregulates autophagy and protects mice from osteoarthritis. *Ann. Rheum. Dis.* **2015**, *74*, 1432–1440. [CrossRef] [PubMed]
11. Caramés, B.; Hasegawa, A.; Taniguchi, N.; Miyaki, S.; Blanco, F.J.; Lotz, M. Autophagy activation by rapamycin reduces severity of experimental osteoarthritis. *Ann. Rheum. Dis.* **2012**, *71*, 575–581. [CrossRef] [PubMed]
12. Li, Y.S.; Zhang, F.J.; Zeng, C.; Luo, W.; Xiao, W.F.; Gao, S.G.; Lei, G.H. Autophagy in osteoarthritis. *Joint. Bone Spine* **2016**, *83*, 143–148. [CrossRef] [PubMed]
13. van der Kraan, P.M.; van den Berg, W.B. Chondrocyte hypertrophy and osteoarthritis: Role in initiation and progression of cartilage degeneration? *Osteoarthr. Cartil.* **2012**, *20*, 223–232. [CrossRef] [PubMed]
14. Xu, L.; Peng, H.; Glasson, S.; Lee, P.L.; Hu, K.; Ijiri, K.; Olsen, B.R.; Goldring, M.B.; Li, Y. Increased expression of the collagen receptor discoidin domain receptor 2 in articular cartilage as a key event in the pathogenesis of osteoarthritis. *Arthritis Rheum.* **2007**, *56*, 2663–2673. [CrossRef] [PubMed]
15. Zhang, Y.; Su, J.; Yu, J.; Bu, X.; Ren, T.; Liu, X.; Yao, L. An essential role of discoidin domain receptor 2 (DDR2) in osteoblast differentiation and chondrocyte maturation via modulation of Runx2 activation. *J. Bone Miner. Res.* **2011**, *26*, 604–617. [CrossRef] [PubMed]
16. Kirsch, T.; Swoboda, B.; Nah, H. Activation of annexin II and V expression, terminal differentiation, mineralization and apoptosis in human osteoarthritic cartilage. *Osteoarthr. Cartil.* **2000**, *8*, 294–302. [CrossRef] [PubMed]
17. Kim, B.J.; Kim, D.W.; Kim, S.H.; Cho, J.H.; Lee, H.J.; Park, D.Y.; Park, S.R.; Choi, B.H.; Min, B.H. Establishment of a reliable and reproducible murine osteoarthritis model. *Osteoarthr. Cartil.* **2013**, *21*, 2013–2020. [CrossRef] [PubMed]
18. Glasson, S.S.; Chambers, M.G.; Van Den Berg, W.B.; Little, C.B. The OARSI histopathology initiative—Recommendations for histological assessments of osteoarthritis in the mouse. *Osteoarthr. Cartil.* **2010**, *18* (Suppl. 3), S17–S23. [CrossRef] [PubMed]
19. Takayama, K.; Kawakami, Y.; Kobayashi, M.; Greco, N.; Cummins, J.H.; Matsushita, T.; Kuroda, R.; Kurosaka, M.; Fu, F.H.; Huard, J. Local intra-articular injection of rapamycin delays articular cartilage degeneration in a murine model of osteoarthritis. *Arthritis Res. Ther.* **2014**, *16*, 482. [CrossRef] [PubMed]

International Journal of
Molecular Sciences

MDPI

Article

Taurine Inhibits Glucocorticoid-Induced Bone Mitochondrial Injury, Preventing Osteonecrosis in Rabbits and Cultured Osteocytes

Hiroaki Hirata [1,†], Shusuke Ueda [1,†], Toru Ichiseki [1,*], Miyako Shimasaki [2], Yoshimichi Ueda [2], Ayumi Kaneuji [1] and Norio Kawahara [1]

1 Department of Orthopaedic Surgery, Kanazawa Medical University, Daigaku 1-1, Uchinada-machi, Kahoku-gun, Ishikawa 920-0293, Japan; hiro6246@kanazawa-med.ac.jp (H.H.); adeu221@kanazawa-med.ac.jp (S.U.); orthoped@kanazawa-med.ac.jp (A.K.); kawa@kanazawa-med.ac.jp (N.K.)

2 Department of Pathology 2, Kanazawa Medical University, Daigaku 1-1, Uchinada-machi, Kahoku-gun, Ishikawa 920-0293, Japan; miya0807@kanazawa-med.ac.jp (M.S.); z-ueda@kanazawa-med.ac.jp (Y.U.)

* Correspondence: tsy-ichi@kanazawa-med.ac.jp; Tel.: +81-76-286-2211 (ext. 3214); Fax: +81-76-286-4406

† These authors contributed equally to this work.

Received: 30 July 2020; Accepted: 16 September 2020; Published: 20 September 2020

Abstract: Mitochondrial injury has recently been implicated in the pathogenesis of glucocorticoid-induced osteonecrosis. Using cultured osteocytes and a rabbit model, we investigated the possibility that taurine (TAU), which is known to play a role in the preservation of mitochondrial function, might also prevent the development of osteonecrosis. To reduplicate the intraosseous environment seen in glucocorticoid-induced osteonecrosis, dexamethasone (Dex) was added to MLO-Y4 cultured in 1% hypoxia (H-D stress environment). An in vitro study was conducted in which changes in mitochondrial transcription factor A (TFAM), a marker of mitochondrial function, and ATP5A produced by mitochondria, induced by the presence/absence of taurine addition were measured. To confirm the effect of taurine in vivo, 15 Japanese White rabbits were administered methylprednisolone (MP) 20 mg/kg as a single injection into the gluteus muscle (MP+/TAU− group), while for 5 consecutive days from the day of MP administration, taurine 100 mg/kg was administered to 15 animals (MP+/TAU+ group). As a control 15 untreated rabbits were also studied. The rabbits in each of the groups were sacrificed on the 14th day after glucocorticoid administration, and the bilateral femora were harvested. Histopathologically, the incidence of osteonecrosis was quantified immunohistochemically by quantifying TFAM and ATP5A expression. In the rabbits exposed to an H-D stress environment and in MP+/TAU− group, TFAM and ATP5A expression markedly decreased. With addition of taurine in the in vitro and in vivo studies, the expression of TFAM and ATP5A was somewhat decreased as compared with Dex−/hypoxia− or MP−/TAU− group, while improvement was noted as compared with Dex+/hypoxia+ or MP+/TAU− group. In rabbits, the incidence of osteonecrosis was 80% in MP+/TAU− group, in contrast to 20% in the taurine administered group (MP+/TAU+), representing a significant decrease. Since taurine was documented to exert a protective effect on mitochondrial function by inhibiting the mitochondrial dysfunction associated with glucocorticoid administration, we speculated that it might also indirectly help to prevent the development of osteonecrosis in this context. Since taurine is already being used clinically, we considered that its clinical application would also likely be smooth.

Keywords: osteonecrosis; taurine; mitochondrial function; glucocorticoid

---

1. Introduction

Glucocorticoids are excellent therapeutic agents that are used effectively in diverse conditions, notably autoimmune disorders and asthma. The price for this, however, includes many well-known serious side effects including glucocorticoid-induced femoral head osteonecrosis. Glucocorticoid-induced femoral head osteonecrosis occurs at both young and elder ages, and is considered an intractable condition in which destruction of the hip joint markedly impairs quality of life (QOL) by causing pain and impaired ambulation. Once femoral head osteonecrosis is established, surgical intervention such as artificial joint implantation cannot be avoided in most cases. This situation makes the devising of optimal prophylactic countermeasures and greater elucidation of the underlying pathogenetic mechanisms of glucocorticoid-related injury very important so as to make glucocorticoid use safer.

However, despite the extensive research being focused on glucocorticoid-induced femoral head osteonecrosis, its causes and pathophysiology are still far from clear. Various studies using rabbit, rat, and other animal models have been conducted, with models of rabbit osteonecrosis induced by glucocorticoid administration being the most common [1]. Hitherto, various causative factors such as oxidative stress, vascular endothelium injury, coagulopathy, and dyslipidemia have been implicated, and much work has been devoted to their prevention and management [2–4]. Recently, attention has been turned to mitochondria because they are the site of oxidative stress development, and the involvement of mitochondrial injury in glucocorticoid-induced osteonecrosis is being recognized [5].

In general, cells of the mitochondrial electron transport system in vivo account for ≥90% of oxygen consumption, of which 1–5% is converted into reactive oxygen species, representing the major intracellular source of reactive oxygen species generation [6]. The acceleration of reactive oxygen species production induced by mitochondrial and mitochondrial DNA injury has been shown to be involved in the development of diverse pathological conditions. Moreover, it has been recognized that mitochondria exist in a state characterized by constant exposure to oxidative stress, with this having a considerable impact on disease development and progression. For this reason, the possibility has been raised that mitochondria may be an ideal target for both therapeutic trials and attempts at elucidating the underlying pathogenetic mechanisms of various disorders [7].

Taurine (TAU, 2-aminoethanesulfonic acid) has been attracting increasing attention as an easy to administer therapeutic agent with few side effects that can help to prevent mitochondrial injury. Taurine is made up of free amino acids present in large quantities in vivo, and has been proven to be effective in the therapy of mitochondrial cytopathies such as mitochondrial myopathy, encephalopathy, lactic acidosis, stroke-like episodes (MELAS) syndrome [8]. Taurine's anti-inflammatory and anti-oxidative actions have been exciting interest [9,10], while its impact on mitochondrial function including regenerative and prophylactic actions is also being reported [11,12].

These properties of taurine suggest to us the realistic possibility that it may also be effective in preserving mitochondrial function and thereby help to inhibit the development of glucocorticoid-induced osteonecrosis in which mitochondrial dysfunction has been implicated. In a recent study conducted under in vitro conditions, osteocytes exposed to a stress environment (H-D stress environment), namely a hypoxic environment to which dexamethasone (Dex) had been added, an intraosseous environment with successful reduplication of glucocorticoid-induced osteonecrosis has been described [13]. Here, in an in vitro study, we first sought to determine whether taurine exerts any inhibitory effect on osteocyte mitochondrial functional injury in this kind of H-D stress environment. Furthermore, to document any in vivo inhibitory effect of taurine on the development of glucocorticoid-induced osteonecrosis, we investigated the incidence of osteonecrosis and intraosseous mitochondrial function using a glucocorticoid-induced rabbit osteonecrosis model.

2. Results

2.1. TFAM and ATP5A Expression Due to Taurine Addition yo Cultured Osteocytes in an H-D Stress Environment

To confirm the functional preservation effect of mitochondria due to taurine, the expression of TFAM and ATP5A in osteocytes placed in an H-D stress environment was investigated. In the Dex+/hypoxia+ group, as compared with Dex−/hypoxia− group as a control, the expression of both TFAM and ATP5A decreased. In contrast, in the taurine addition group, the expression of both TFAM and ATP5A in Dex+/hypoxia+/taurine+ group as compared with Dex+/hypoxia+ group was markedly increased (Figure 1). In this way, it was confirmed that taurine preserved mitochondrial function in a stress environment.

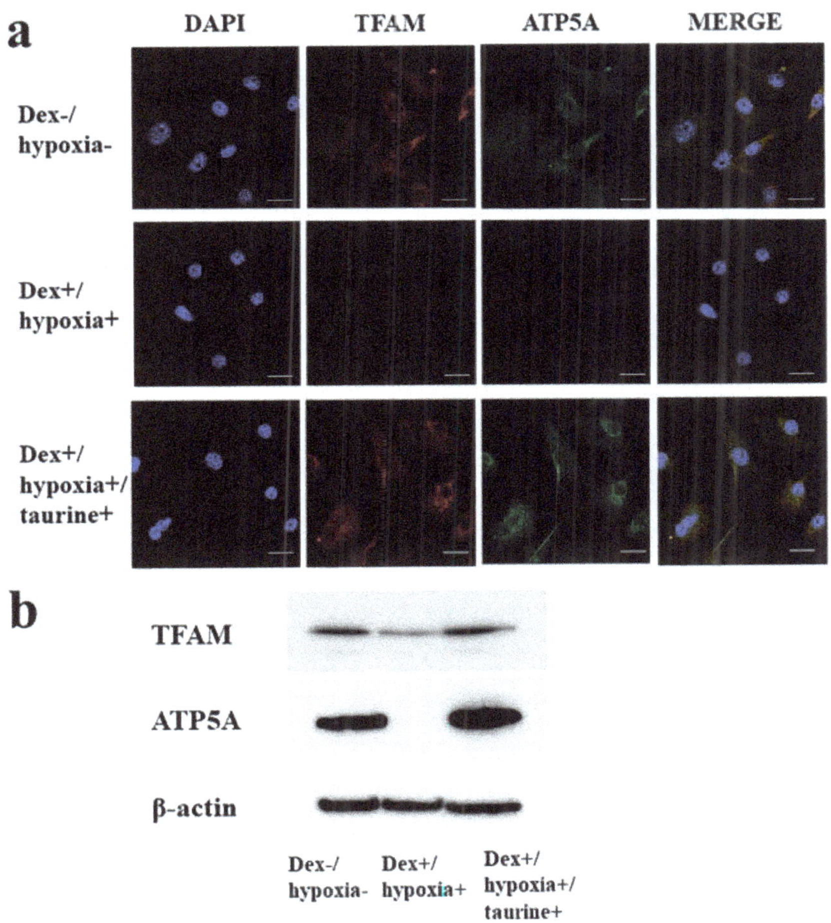

Figure 1. Mitochondrial transcription factor A (TFAM) and ATP5A expression in cultured osteocytes in an H-D stress environment. (**a**) Immunocytochemical study, (**b**) Western blot. TFAM (29 kDa), ATP5A (50–55 kDa), β-actin (42 kDa). In Dex+/hypoxia+ group as compared with Dex−/hypoxia− group, expression of TFAM and ATP5A levels was decreased. In Dex+/hypoxia+/taurine+ group with addition of taurine, as compared with Dex+/hypoxia+ group, levels of both TFAM and ATP5A expression were increased. Scale bar: 20 μm.

2.2. Prevention of Osteonecrosis by Taurine in a Glucocorticoid-Administered Rabbit Osteonecrosis Model

After preparing a glucocorticoid-administered rabbit osteonecrosis model, taurine was injected intravenously, and its inhibitory effect on osteonecrosis development was determined. In none of the animals in MP−/TAU− group, were there any sites showing necrosis of medullary haematopoietic cells or fat cells, and no empty lacunae or condensed nuclei in osteocytes were found. In 12 of 15 rabbits in the MP+/TAU− group, osteonecrosis was found. In 4 of 15 rabbits in the MP+/TAU+ group, necrosis of medullary haematopoietic cells or fat cells and empty lacunae or condensed nuclei in osteocytes were noted at some sites, and the osteonecrosis development rate was 20% ($p < 0.05$ vs. MP+/TAU−) (Figure 2). Since the decrease in the osteonecrosis development rate was significant, taurine was suggested to have inhibited osteonecrosis development in this experiment.

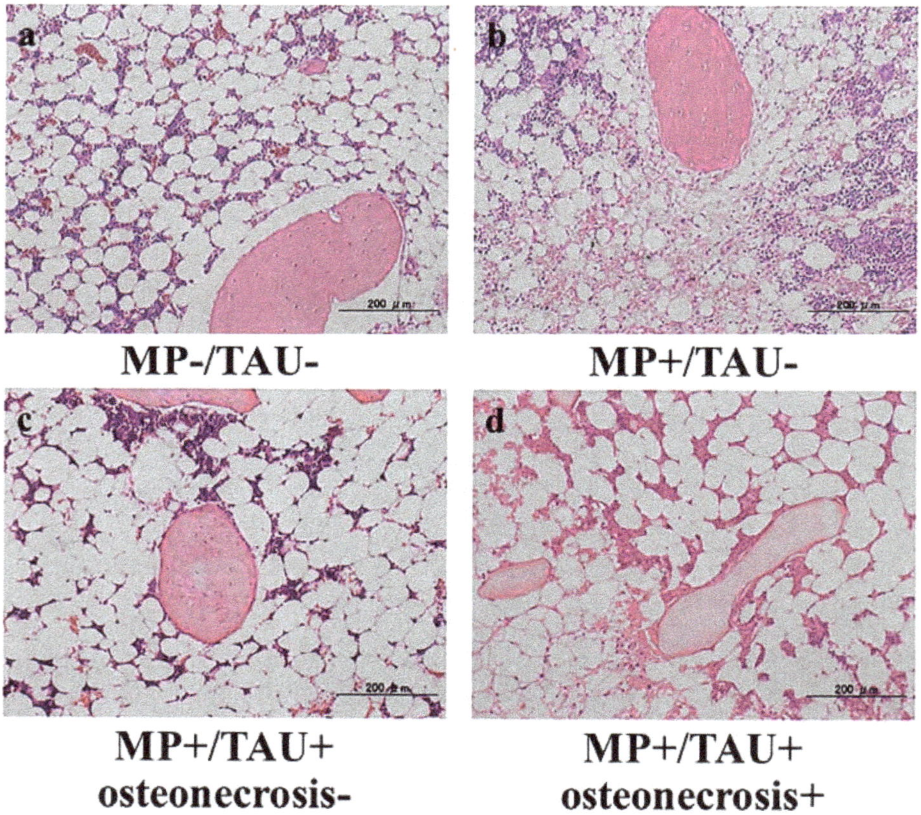

Figure 2. Osteonecrosis inhibition with intravenous administration of taurine in a glucocorticoid-induced rabbit osteonecrosis model. (**a**) MP−/TAU−, (**b**) MP+/TAU−, (**c**,**d**) MP+/TAU+. Osteonecrosis was found in 12 of 15 rabbits of MP+/TAU− group (**b**). In 4 of 15 rabbits of the MP+/TAU+ group, some portions showing necrosis of medullary haematopoietic cells or fat cells and empty lacunae or condensed nuclei in osteocytes were found (**d**). The osteonecrosis development rate was 20%, representing a significant inhibition of osteonecrosis as compared with the MP+/TAU− group ($p < 0.05$). Scale bar: 200 μm.

2.3. Inhibition of Mitochondrial Injury by Taurine in a Glucocorticoid-Administered Rabbit Osteonecrosis Model

To determine any mitochondrial protective effect of taurine in a glucocorticoid-administered rabbit osteonecrosis model, using the percentage of positive cells (%PC) in TFAM and ATP5A, the inhibitory effect of taurine on intraosseous mitochondria injury was investigated. In the MP−/TAU− group, TFAM was 73.95 ± 1.20% and ATP5A was 57.22 ± 2.23%. In the MP+/TAU− group, TFAM was 41.15 ± 2.93%, and ATP5A 31.85 ± 3.61% in contrast to MP+/TAU+ group in which TFAM was 67.19 ± 1.57%, and ATP5A 59.71 ± 2.01%, with increased expression found in this order (Figure 3). In this way, the preservation by taurine of mitochondrial function could be confirmed also in vivo.

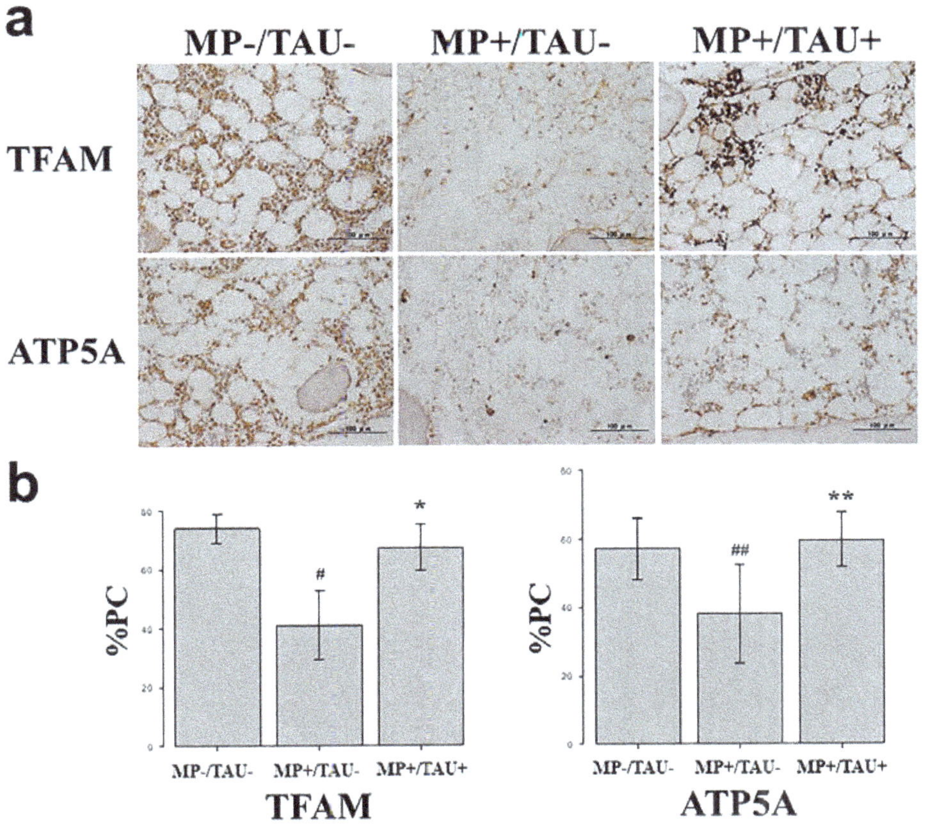

Figure 3. TFAM and ATP5A positive cell rate after taurine administration in a glucocorticoid-induced rabbit osteonecrosis model. (**a**) Immunohistochemical study of TFAM and ATP5A. Scale bar: 100 μm. (**b**) Graph indicates percentage of positive cells of TFAM and ATP5A in the indicated conditions. Columns and bars indicate means and S.E. As compared with MP−/TAU− group, in MP+/TAU− group the numbers of TFAM and ATP5A positive cells were significantly decreased ([#] $p < 0.0001$ vs. MP−/TAU−, [##] $p = 0.001$ vs. MP−/TAU−). In MP+/TAU+ group, TFAM and ATP5A levels were maintained as compared with MP−/TAU− group. (* $p < 0.0001$ vs. MP+/TAU−, ** $p < 0.001$ vs. MP+/TAU−).

3. Discussion

Recently, numerous studies have identified a role for oxidative stress in glucocorticoid-induced osteonecrosis [2,14,15]. Regarding mitochondria, which are the major site of oxidative stress generation, the intraosseous decrease of their TFAM levels induced by glucocorticoid administration has been implicated in osteonecrosis development, suggesting that mitochondrial stress plays a role in this process [5]. Accordingly, preservation of mitochondrial function may be an important factor helping to prevent osteonecrosis development [16].

The taurine used in this experiment has lately been recognized to be a useful therapeutic agent in various disorders, including cerebrovascular injury, cardiac disorders, and hepatic injury, by protecting cells from oxidative stress. Other beneficial effects lately emphasized include inhibition of cell injury and anti-ageing properties [9,12,17]. Taurine helps to keep Ca^{2+} concentrations in cardiomyocyte mitochondria normal, even when they are increased by H_2O_2-induced oxidative stress, and a possible action on the apoptosis pathway of mitochondria exposed to oxidative stress has been proposed [17]. Moreover, in mitochondrial cytopathies such as MELAS, taurine has attracted attention as a therapeutic agent that provides symptomatic improvement [8]. These findings allow hope that taurine may also help to inhibit mitochondrial injury, which is now thought to be an important step in the course of development of glucocorticoid-induced osteonecrosis.

In this study, to evaluate the efficacy of taurine against mitochondrial injury present in bone and osteocytes, TFAM, a factor strongly involved in mitochondrial function [5,16,18,19] and ATP5A, a marker of mitochondrial function produced by mitochondria, were used.

First, in vitro studies using cultured osteocytes were conducted. In these osteocytes exposed to a sufficiently stressful H-D environment so as to induce cell necrosis, both TFAM and ATP5A expression levels were markedly decreased, proving that mitochondrial functional injury had been engendered. On the other hand, with the addition of taurine under the same conditions, the decrease in TFAM and ATP5A levels was attenuated. These results show that taurine is firmly protective of mitochondrial function in vulnerable osteocytes exposed to a stressful environment.

In various glucocorticoid-induced osteonecrosis models, the occurrence of oxidative and mitochondrial injuries within 48–72 h after glucocorticoid administration is considered to be a contributing factor [2,5,15]. The period from injury to osteonecrosis development has been estimated to be approximately 72–120 h [15,20,21]. Referring to these estimates, in the present glucocorticoid-induced rabbit osteonecrosis model, taurine was administered for 5 consecutive days, and its dose was set to be consistent with that routinely used clinically, 100 mg/kg/day. With glucocorticoid-alone administration (MP+/TAU− group), the intraosseous expression of TFAM and ATP5A was significantly decreased as compared with the MP−/TAU− group. On the other hand, in the MP+/TAU+ group, similar to the in vitro results, TFAM and ATP5A showed improvement up to the levels seen in MP−/TAU− group, as well as a significant decrease in the incidence of osteonecrosis. In this way, together with the mitochondrial injury associated with glucocorticoid use leading to osteonecrosis development, it was considered that taurine protected or preserved mitochondrial function, thereby in turn, possibly helping to prevent the development of osteonecrosis.

For the purposes of the present work, the taurine dose was set to be comparable to that routinely used in daily clinical practice, but because side effects are few, in conditions such as MELAS even larger doses are being administered. In this study, although the osteonecrosis incidence was 20%, to be able to achieve an incidence approaching 0%, factors such as the administered dose of taurine, and its timing and duration will need to be determined. Since a significant decrease in the incidence of glucocorticoid-induced osteonecrosis was attained, considering the ease of taurine administration and the paucity of associated side effects, its clinical application in the near future can be anticipated.

In conclusion, preservation of intraosseous mitochondrial function is vital for the prevention of glucocorticoid-induced osteonecrosis. From the in vivo and in vitro results of taurine obtained here, preservation of mitochondrial function was demonstrated, and was in turn, considered to be related to the prevention of osteonecrosis.

4. Materials and Methods

4.1. Cell Culture

An established murine osteocytic cell line (MLO-Y4) (Kerafast, Boston, MA, USA) was maintained as a subconfluent monolayer culture in the alpha MEM medium (Gibco, Tokyo, Japan) supplemented with 10% fetal calf serum. When the culture reached 70% confluency being cultured at 37 °C under 20% O_2 and 5% CO_2, MLO-Y4 were treated with 1 μM dexamethasone (Dex, MSD, Tokyo, Japan) in 1% O_2 (hypoxia) for 24 h (Dex+/hypoxia+ group). A quantity of 0.8 μM taurine was added to the medium of Dex+/hypoxia+ group exposed to taurine-free medium (Dex+/hypoxia+/taurine+ group). As a control group, cells were cultured under 20% O_2 in the culture medium without either Dex or taurine (Dex-/hypoxia− group). Three independent experiments each were carried out.

4.2. Immunocytochemical Study

To determine the effect of taurine on cultured osteocytes in an H-D stress environment, an immunohistochemical study on TFAM which exerts a protective effect on mitochondria, and ATP5A which shows ATP production, which is the main function of mitochondria was conducted. Cells of each group were fixed in 4% paraformaldehyde, and permeabilized with 0.3% Triton X-100 in phosphate buffered saline (PBS). Blocking was then achieved with 10% bovine serum albumin (Dako Cytomation, Santa Clara, CA, USA) in PBS, and the primary antibody, anti-ATP synthase (ATP5A) (Proteintech, Rosemont, IL), and anti-TFAM (LSbio, Seattle, MA, USA) antibody each at 10.0 μg/mL were made to react at room temperature for 2 h. The secondary antibody, anti-mouse Alexa 488 (Thermo Fisher Scientific, Tokyo, Japan), and anti-rabbit Alexa 594 (Thermo Fisher Scientific) each at 10.0μg/mL were made to react while being shielded from light, and nucleus staining was done with DAPI. Then after washing in PBS, they were mounted using a prolong diamond antifade mountant (Thermo Fisher Scientific, Tokyo, Japan). Images were taken with a Zeiss-LSM710 camera (Zeiss, Baden-Württemberg, Germany). The taurine non-administered and administered groups were then compared.

4.3. Western Blot

For quantification, immunoblotting for TFAM and ATP5A was performed on MLO-Y4 cells. Protein was extracted using protein extraction solution (PRO-PREP, iNtRON Biotechnology, Kyungki-Do, Korea). The protein, 20 μg, was electrophoresed on a 10% polyacrylamide gel, and transferred to a nitrocellulose membrane (Atoh, Tokyo, Japan). The membranes were reacted overnight at 4 C with the primary antibodies. The Primary antibodies applied were anti-ATP5A (Proteintech) or anti-TFAM (Invitrogen, Waltham, MA, USA) antibody at a concentration of 0.5 μg/mL. After the incubation with peroxidase-labeled goat anti-mouse or anti-rabbit IgG antibody (Dako Cytomation, Santa Clara, CA, USA) at a concentration of 0.7 μg/mL each for 1 h at room temperature and vigorous washing, the nitrocellulose membrane was incubated with Chemiluminescence Luminol Reagent (Immuno Star LD, Wako, Tokyo, Japan) and photographed digitally using ImageQuant LAS 4000 mini (GE healthcare Japan Co, Tokyo, Japan). Immunoblot using anti-actin monoclonal antibody (Sigma Chemical Co. St. Louis, MO, USA) was used for standardization. Intensity was measured using the Multi Gauge v3.1 (Fujifilm, Tokyo, Japan). Experiments were repeated at least three times.

4.4. Animals

As the experimental animals, forty-five male Japanese White rabbits weighing about 3.5 kg each were used. As the glucocorticoid-induced rabbit osteonecrosis model [1], methylprednisolone (MP) 20 mg/kg was injected into a gluteus muscle only once in 15 rabbits of MP+/TAU− group. In 15 animals of MP+/TAU+ group, after MP injection into a gluteus muscle, taurine 100 mg/kg was injected via an auricular vein for 5 continuous days. A control group was also prepared in which physiological saline 3 mL was injected into a gluteus muscle in 15 rabbits (MP−/TAU− group). The animals in all of the groups were sacrificed 2 weeks later with thiopental sodium (NIPRO ES Pharma, Osaka, Japan) delivered by rapid injection via an auricular vein. The bilateral femora were then quickly resected. After fixation of the resected femurs in 10% neutral buffered formalin, decalcification was done with formic acid, and paraffin embedded specimens were cut into 4 μm thick sections with a microtome. This study was conducted in accordance with all guidelines of the Animal Research Committee of Kanazawa Medical University (#2018-13; approval date: 1 April 2020).

4.5. Histopathology

From the femoral sections of each group, sections thinly cut with a microtome from the femoral neck maximum cut surface of the forehead surface were used as hematoxylin and eosin (H&E)-stained specimens, and the presence/absence of osteonecrosis development was studied using a light microscope. Osteonecrosis was judged to be present when necrosis of medullary haematopoietic cells or fat cells or empty lacunae or condensed nuclei in osteocytes were noted [1]. Regarding the osteonecrosis development rate, all of the groups were compared with osteonecrosis considered to be present even if limited to a unilateral leg.

4.6. Immunohistochemical Study

To study the effect of taurine in a glucocorticoid-induced rabbit osteonecrosis model in vitro, an immunohistochemical study was performed using TFAM which has a mitochondria protective effect and ATP5A which shows ATP production. In all groups, femoral sections were prepared, and sections obtained from the femoral proximal medial diaphysis of each group were deparaffinized with xylene and ethanol, after which to activate antigen, protease K (Dako Cytomation, Santa Clara, CA, USA) was dribbled on tissue sections that were incubated at 37 °C for 40 min. Using 0.3% H_2O_2, endogenous peroxidase was eliminated, blocking was performed using mouse or goat normal serum, and the primary antibody was made to react. As the primary antibody, anti-TFAM rabbit polyclonal antibody (Invitrogen, Waltham, MA, USA) and anti-ATP5A goat polyclonal antibody (Lsbio, Seattle, MA, USA) were used at 0.1 μg/mL and 5.0 μg/mL, respectively. The reaction time was overnight at 4 °C in a cool dark room. After reacting the primary antibody, the secondary antibody (biotin), was reacted with an enzymatic agent (streptavidin), and after 5-minue immersion in DAB to allow for color development, the nuclei were stained and studied under a light microscope.

To quantify relative stainability, 3 fields were chosen at random from tissue adjacent to areas of osteonecrosis in the femoral proximal medial diaphysis, and the proportion of the positive cell count relative to that of the total cell number was calculated, and compared between each group as the percentage of positive cells (%PC).

4.7. Statistical Analysis

All quantified results were expressed as the mean ± SE. Significant differences in the osteonecrosis development rate in the H&E-stained specimens, were determined by Fisher's exact test. Statistical significance in the comparison of %PC of TFAM or ATP5A between the control and each of the experimental groups was analyzed with Dunnett's multiple comparison test. Significance was defined as $p < 0.05$. The statistical analysis was performed using Stat View J-5.0 software (SAS Institute, Cary, USA)

Author Contributions: All authors made a significant contribution to the study and are in agreement with the content of the manuscript H.H., T.I., M.S., S.U. and Y.U. conceived and designed the experiments; H.H., T.I., M.S. and S.U. performed the experiments; H.H., T.I., M.S. and S.U. analyzed the data; H.H., T.I., M.S., S.U., Y.U., A.K. and N.K. interpreted the data and drafted the manuscript. All authors have read and agreed to the published version of the manuscript.

Funding: This research received no external funding.

Conflicts of Interest: The authors declare no conflict of interest.

Abbreviations

H-D stress environment	dexamethasone was added to MLO-Y4 cultured in 1% hypoxia
TFAM	mitochondrial transcription factor A
Dex	dexamethasone
MP	methylprednisolone
TAU	taurine
QOL	quality of life
MELAS	mitochondrial myopathy, encephalopathy, lactic acidosis, stroke-like episodes
H&E-stain	hematoxylin and eosin-stain
%PC	percentage of positive cells

References

1. Yamamoto, T.; Irisa, T.; Sugioka, Y.; Sueishi, K. Effects of pulse methylprednisolone on bone and marrow tissues: Corticosteroid-induced osteonecrosis in rabbits. *Artritis Rheum.* **1997**, *40*, 2055–2064. [CrossRef] [PubMed]
2. Ichiseki, T.; Matsumoto, T.; Nishino, M.; Kaneuji, A.; Katsuda, S. Oxidative stress and vascular permeability in steroid-induced osteonecrosis model. *J. Orthop. Sci.* **2004**, *9*, 509–515. [CrossRef] [PubMed]
3. Kuroda, Y.; Akiyama, H.; Kawanabe, K.; Tabata, Y.; Nakamura, T. Treatment of experimental osteonecrosis of the hip in adult rabbits with a single local injection of recombinant human FGF-2 microspheres. *J. Bone Miner. Metab.* **2010**, *28*, 608–616. [CrossRef] [PubMed]
4. Motomura, G.; Yamamoto, T.; Miyanishi, K.; Jingushi, S.; Iwamoto, Y. Combined effects of an anticoagulant and a lipid-lowering agent on the prevention of steroid-induced osteonecrosis in rabbits. *Arthritis Rheum.* **2004**, *50*, 3387–3391. [CrossRef]
5. Tsuchiya, M.; Ichiseki, T.; Ueda, S.; Ueda, Y.; Shimazaki, M.; Kaneuji, A.; Kawahara, N. Mitochondrial stress and redox failure in steroid-associated osteonecrosis. *Int. J. Med. Sci.* **2018**, *15*, 205–209. [CrossRef]
6. Papa, S. Mitochondrial oxidative phosphorylation changes in the life span. Molecular aspects and physiopathological implications. *Biochim. Biophys. Acta.* **1996**, *1276*, 87–105. [CrossRef]
7. Oyewole, A.O.; Birch-Machin, M.A. Mitochondria-targeted antioxidants. *FASEB J.* **2015**, *29*, 4766–4771. [CrossRef]
8. Fakruddin, M.; Wei, F.Y.; Suzuki, T.; Asano, K.; Kaieda, T.; Omori, A.; Izumi, R.; Fujimura, A.; Kaitsuka, T.; Miyata, K.; et al. Defective Mitochondrial tRNA Taurine Modification Activates Global Proteostress and Leads to Mitochondrial Disease. *Cell. Rep.* **2018**, *22*, 482–496. [CrossRef]
9. Liu, Y.; Li, F.; Zhang, L.; Wu, J.; Wang, Y.; Yu, H. Taurine alleviates lipopolysaccharide-induced liver injury by anti-inflammation and antioxidants in rats. *Mol. Med. Rep.* **2017**, *16*, 6512–6517. [CrossRef]
10. Cheleschi, S.; De-Palma, A.; Pascarelli, N.A.; Giordano, N.; Galeazzi, M.; Tenti, S.; Fioravanti, A. Could Oxidative Stress Regulate the Expression of MicroRNA-146a and MicroRNA-34a in Human Osteoarthritic Chondrocyte Cultures? *Int. J. Mol. Sci.* **2017**, *18*, 2660. [CrossRef]
11. Ahmadi, N.; Ghanbarinejad, V.; Ommati, M.M.; Jamshidzadeh, A.; Heidari, R. Taurine prevents mitochondrial membrane permeabilization and swelling upon interaction with manganese: Implication in the treatment of cirrhosis-associated central nervous system complications. *J. Biochem. Mol. Toxicol.* **2018**, *32*, e22216. [CrossRef] [PubMed]
12. Wang, Q.; Fan, W.; Cai, Y.; Wu, Q.; Mo, L.; Huang, Z.; Huang, H. Protective effects of taurine n traumatic brain injury via mitochondria and cerebral blood flow. *Amino Acids* **2016**, *48*, 2169–2177. [CrossRef] [PubMed]
13. Ueda, S.; Ichiseki, T.; Yoshitomi, Y.; Yonekura, H.; Ueda, Y.; Kaneuji, A.; Matsumoto, T. Osteocytic cell necrosis is caused by a combination of glucocorticoid-induced Dickkopf-1 and hypoxia. *Med. Mol. Morphol.* **2015**, *48*, 69–75. [CrossRef] [PubMed]
14. Ichiseki, T.; Kaneuji, A.; Katsuda, S.; Ueda, Y.; Sugimori, T.; Matsumoto, T. DNA oxidation injury in bone early after steroid administration is involved in the pathogenesis of steroid-induced osteonecrosis. *Rheumatology (Oxford)* **2005**, *44*, 456–460. [CrossRef] [PubMed]
15. Ichiseki, T.; Kaneuji, A.; Ueda, Y.; Nakagawa, S.; Mikami, T.; Fukui, K.; Matsumoto, T. Osteonecrosis development in a novel rat model characterized by a single application of oxidative stress. *Arthritis Rheum.* **2011**, *63*, 2138–2141. [CrossRef] [PubMed]

16. Ueda, S.; Shimasaki, M.; Ichiseki, T.; Hirata, H.; Kawahara, N.; Ueda, Y. Mitochondrial Transcription Factor an Added to Osteocytes in a Stressed Environment Has a Cytoprotective Effect. *Int. J. Med. Sci.* **2020**, *17*, 1293–1299. [CrossRef]
17. Wang, J.; Qi, C.; Liu, L.; Zhao, L.; Cui, W.; Tian, Y.; Liu, B.; Li, J. Taurine Protects Primary Neonatal Cardiomyocytes Against Apoptosis Induced by Hydrogen Peroxide. *Int. Heart J.* **2018**, *59*, 190–196. [CrossRef]
18. Alam, T.I.; Kanki, T.; Muta, T.; Ukaji, K.; Abe, Y.; Nakayama, H.; Takio, K.; Hamasaki, N.; Kang, D. Human mitochondrial DNA is packaged with TFAM. *Nucleic Acids Res.* **2003**, *31*, 1640–1645. [CrossRef]
19. Kanki, T.; Ohgaki, K.; Gaspari, M.; Gustafsson, C.M.; Fukuoh, A.; Sasaki, N.; Hamasaki, N.; Kang, D. Architectural role of mitochondrial transcription factor A in maintenance of human mitochondrial DNA. *Mol. Cell Biol.* **2004**, *24*, 9823–9834. [CrossRef]
20. Sato, M.; Sugano, N.; Ohzono, K.; Nomura, S.; Kitamura, Y.; Tsukamoto, Y.; Ogawa, S. Apoptosis and expression of stress protein (ORP150, HO1) during development of ischaemic osteonecrosis in the rat. *J. Bone Joint Surg. Br.* **2001**, *83*, 751–759. [CrossRef]
21. Catto, M. A histological study of avascular necrosis of the femoral head after transcervical fracture. *J. Bone Joint Surg. Br.* **1965**, *47*, 749–776. [CrossRef] [PubMed]

International Journal of *Molecular Sciences*

MDPI

Article

Methrotexate Treatment Inmunomodulates Abnormal Cytokine Expression by T CD4 Lymphocytes Present in DMARD-Naïve Rheumatoid Arthritis Patients

Jorge Monserrat Sanz [1,2,*], Cristina Bohórquez [3], Ana Maria Gómez [1], Atusa Movasat [3], Ana Pérez [2,3], Lucía Ruíz [3], David Diaz [1,2], Ana Isabel Sánchez [3], Fernando Albarrán [3], Ignacio Sanz [4] and Melchor Álvarez-Mon [1,2,3,*]

1 Laboratory of Immune System Diseases, Department of Medicine, University Hospital "Príncipe de Asturias", University of Alcalá, Alcalá de Henares, 28871 Madrid, Spain; alahoz1199@gmail.com (A.M.G.); david.diaz@uah.es (D.D.)

2 IRYCIS Unit, Instituto Ramón y Cajal de Investigación Sanitaria, 28034 Madrid, Spain; aperezalcala@yahoo.es

3 Immune System Diseases-Rheumatology Service, Department of Medicine, University Hospital "Príncipe de Asturias", University of Alcalá, Alcalá de Henares, 28805 Madrid, Spain; crisbohorquez@yahoo.es (C.B.); atusa_m@yahoo.es (A.M.); luciaruiz83@gmail.com (L.R.); aisatrio@gmail.com (A.I.S.); falbarranhdez@gmail.com (F.A.)

4 Division of Immunology and Rheumatology, Department of Medicine, Emory University, Atlanta, GA 30322, USA; ignacio.sanz@emory.edu

* Correspondence: jorge.monserrat@uah.es (J.M.S.); mademons@gmail.com (M.Á.-M.); Tel.: +34-91-8854533 (J.M.S. & M.Á.-M.); Fax: +34-91-8854526 (J.M.S. & M.Á.-M.)

Received: 27 July 2020; Accepted: 14 September 2020; Published: 18 September 2020

Abstract: $CD4^+$T-lymphocytes are relevant in the pathogenesis of rheumatoid arthritis (RA), however, their potential involvement in early RA remains elusive. Methotrexate (MTX) is a commonly used disease-modifying antirheumatic drug (DMARD), but its mechanism has not been fully established. In 47 new-onset DMARD-naïve RA patients, we investigated the pattern of IFNγ, IL-4 and IL-17A expression by naïve (T_N), central (T_{CM}), effector memory (T_{EM}) and effector (T_E) $CD4^+$ subsets; their STAT-1, STAT-6 and STAT-3 transcription factors phosphorylation, and the circulating levels of IFNγ, IL-4 and IL-17. We also studied the RA patients after 3 and 6 months of MTX treatment and according their clinical response. $CD4^+$T-lymphocyte subsets and cytokine expression were measured using flow cytometry. New-onset DMARD-naïve RA patients showed a significant expansion of IL-17A^+, IFNγ^+ and IL-17A^+IFNγ^+ $CD4^+$T-lymphocyte subsets and increased intracellular STAT-1 and STAT-3 phosphorylation. Under basal conditions, nonresponder patients showed increased numbers of circulating IL-17A producing T_N and T_{MC} $CD4^+$T-lymphocytes and IFNγ producing T_N, T_{CM}, T_{EM} $CD4^+$T-lymphocytes with respect to responders. After 6 months, the numbers of $CD4^+$IL-17A^+T_N remained significantly increased in nonresponders. In conclusion, $CD4^+$T-lymphocytes in new-onset DMARD-naïve RA patients show IL-17A and IFNγ abnormalities in T_N, indicating their relevant role in early disease pathogenesis. Different patterns of $CD4^+$ modulation are identified in MTX responders and nonresponders.

Keywords: naïve rheumatoid arthritis; CD4+ T-lymphocytes; methotrexate response; IFNγ, IL-17A; STAT expression

1. Introduction

The immune system plays a relevant role in the pathogenesis of rheumatoid arthritis (RA) [1,2]. However, the involvement of $CD4^+$T-lymphocytes is only partially understood. $CD4^+$T-lymphocytes form a regulatory and functionally diverse population of the immune system. This cell heterogeneity includes different patterns of cytokine secretion and stages of differentiation/activation [3–6]. $CD4^+$T-lymphocytes subsets are characterized by their ability to produce cytokines such as IFNγ, IL-4 or IL-17A, and they are named Th1, Th2 and Th17, respectively [7,8]. Different signals are involved in promoting development, but the signal transducer and activator of transcription (STAT) family of proteins appears to be critical for the activation of the subset-characteristic transcription factors [9]. The binding of these STATs can activate lineage-specific enhancers associated with alternative cell fates [10]. STAT-1, STAT-6 and STAT-3 are recognized as essential for T-bet, Gata3 and RORc activation, which promote Th1, Th2 and Th17 cell differentiation, respectively.

Based on their distinctive functional and phenotype patterns, $CD4^+$T-lymphocytes are divided into $CD4^+$ naïve (T_N), central-memory (T_{CM}), effector-memory (T_{EM}) and effector (T_E) T subsets [11]. $CD4^+T_N$ exhibits noneffector functions, while $CD4^+T_{CM}$ can rapidly proliferate and express multiple different effector molecules such as cytokines after being stimulated by antigens, and exhibit diminished activation requirements [11–13]. $CD4^+T_{EM}$ produce effector cytokines but have limited proliferative capacity, and $CD4^+T_E$ are at a final differentiation stage and share high levels of cytokine production [14]. The requirements for the activation, proliferation and survival of these subsets are different, as well as their capacity to enter lymphoid and inflamed nonlymphoid tissues [15].

RA patients show several abnormalities in circulating $CD4^+$T-lymphocytes including an imbalance between circulating Th1, Th2 and Th17 subsets and abnormal serum levels of their hallmark IFNγ, IL-4 and IL-17A cytokines [16,17]. However, contradictory results have been published on the percentages of these T cell subsets and of the cytokine concentration in RA patients [18–23]. Several factors might be involved in this variability, including the clinical stage of the disease and the previous and active treatments. There is also evidence of an abnormal regulation of the expression and phosphorylation of the Th1, Th2 and Th17 inducers STAT-1, STAT-6 and STAT-3, respectively [24–26]. The treatment of RA has dramatically improved in recent decades by the introduction and use of methotrexate (MTX) [27]. MTX has become the most commonly used disease-modifying antirheumatic-drug (DMARD) in RA, but its mechanism of action remains elusive. Additionally, controversial effects have described the concerning results of MTX in the $CD4^+$T-lymphocytes distribution and activity of the Th1, Th2 and Th17 subsets [16,19,22,23]. Thus, the analysis of Th1, Th2 and Th17 subsets in new-onset DMARD-naïve RA patients may clarify the role of these cells in the pathogenesis of the disease and the study of the immunomodulatory and clinical effects of MTX treatment may favor the understanding of the heterogeneity in the response to this DMARD.

In this work, in a homogenous population of new-onset DMARD-naïve RA patients, we have investigated the pattern of IFNγ, IL-4 and IL-17A expression by T_N and T_{CM}, T_{EM} and T_E $CD4^+$T-lymphocytes. We have also studied the expression and phosphorylation of the Th1, Th2 and Th17 transcriptional factors, STAT-1, STAT-6 and STAT-3, as well as the circulating levels of IFNγ, IL-4 and IL-17A. Furthermore, we have followed the patients during the first six month of MTX treatment and stratified them according to the clinical response attained.

2. Results

2.1. Patient Demographic Characteristics

Table 1 shows the baseline characteristics of the 47 new-onset DMARD-naïve RA patients who eventually became responders (n = 31) or nonresponders (n = 16) after six months of MTX treatment. No significant differences were observed in terms of age, sex and clinical variables examined between both groups of patients. We analyzed the evolution of C-reactive protein (CRP), disease activity score of 28 (DAS28) and the Health Assessment Questionnaire (HAQ) in both groups of patients at a 6-month follow-up. After six months of MTX treatment, the responders, however, showed a significant reduction in CRP from 16.12 ± 6.39 to 4.90 ± 2.31 mg/dl, in DAS28 from 3.62 ± 0.49 to 2.23 ± 0.41, and in HAQ from 0.76 ± 0.56 to 0.47 ± 0.26. The nonresponders also showed a significant reduction in CRP, from 16.57 ± 5.33 to 9.09 ± 4.18 mg/dL. The reductions in DAS28 from 3.69 ± 0.46 to 3.61 ± 0.25 and in HAQ from 0.78 ± 0.79 to 0.72 ± 0.65 were not statistically significant.

Table 1. Patient demographics and clinical and biological characteristics at baseline.

	Healthy Controls (n = 29)	**Eventual Responders (n = 31)**	**Eventual Non-Responders (n = 16)**	
Variables	(mean ± SD)	(mean ± SD)	(mean ± SD)	p-value
Age (years)	48.70 ± 12.01	51.60 ± 10.01	52.02 ± 9.48	0.823
Gender (women)	72.10%	74.19%	75.00%	0.902
CRP (mg/L)	-	16.12 ± 6.39	16.57 ± 5.33	0.942
Rheumatoid factor (+)	-	225.34 ± 88.46	233 ± 91.18	0.907
Prevalence (+)		87.09%	87.50%	0.841
Anti-CCP (IU/mL)	-	435.72 ± 358.15	431.08 ± 276.10	0.965
Prevalence (+)		77.41%	81.25%	0.809
DAS28	-	3.62 ± 0.49	3.69 ± 0.46	0.689
Erosions (+)	-	27.01%	27.53%	0.759
HAQ	-	0.76 ± 0.56	0.78 ± 0.79	0.844

CRP, C-reactive protein; anti-CCP, anticyclic citrullinated peptide antibody; DAS28, Disease Activity Score 28; HAQ, Health Assessment Questionnaire.

2.2. New-Onset DMARD-Naïve RA Patients Show An Expansion of $CD4^+IL\text{-}17A^+$ and $CD4^+IFN\gamma^+$ T-Lymphocytes

We investigated IL-17A, IFNγ and IL-4 expression by circulating $CD4^+$T-lymphocyte subsets from 47 new-onset DMARD-naïve RA patients and 29 HCs (healthy controls) before starting MTX treatment and during the initial 6 months of treatment (Figure 1). There were no significant differences either in the number or in the percentage of circulating T-lymphocytes or $CD4^+$T-lymphocytes between RA patients and HCs at baseline (T-lymphocytes: 2801.99 ± 380.15 vs. 2002.15 ± 347.12 cells/μL and 49.47 ± 2.52 vs. 52.88 ± 5.95%; $CD4^+$ T-lymphocytes: 1131.60 ± 174.23 vs. 825.20 ± 79.84 cells/μL and 37.13 ± 2.17 vs. 40.29 ± 4.69%, respectively).

Next, we investigated the IL-17A, IFNγ and IL-4 expression by PMA (phorbol-12-myristate-13-acetate)-activated $CD4^+$T-lymphocytes from each individual. RA patients had significantly increased $CD4^+IL\text{-}17A^+$T-lymphocyte numbers with respect to HCs (Figure 1a, panel B). The percentage of $CD4^+IL\text{-}17A^+$ cells in the $CD4^+$T-lymphocyte population was also increased in patients (Figure 1a, panel E). This $CD4^+IL\text{-}17A^+$ lymphocyte expansion could mainly be explained by a significant broadening of the $CD4^+IL\text{-}17A^+T_N$ and $CD4^+IL\text{-}17A^+T_{CM}$ lymphocytes (Figure 1a, panel E).

RA patients also showed a significant increment in the numbers of $CD4^+IFN\gamma^+$ cells with an expansion of the $CD4^+IFN\gamma^+$ T_{EM} and $CD4^+IFN\gamma^+$ T_E lymphocytes (Figure 1a, panel A). However, there were no significant differences in the percentages of $IFN\gamma^+$-producing cells in the different $CD4^+$T-lymphocyte subsets between patients and HCs (Figure 1a, panel D). The numbers or percentages of $CD4^+IL\text{-}4^+$T-lymphocytes were similar in both groups of subjects (Figure 1a, panel C and F). A representative dot plot of IL-17A, IFNγ and IL-4 expression by $CD4^+$ T-lymphocytes is shown in Figure 1b.

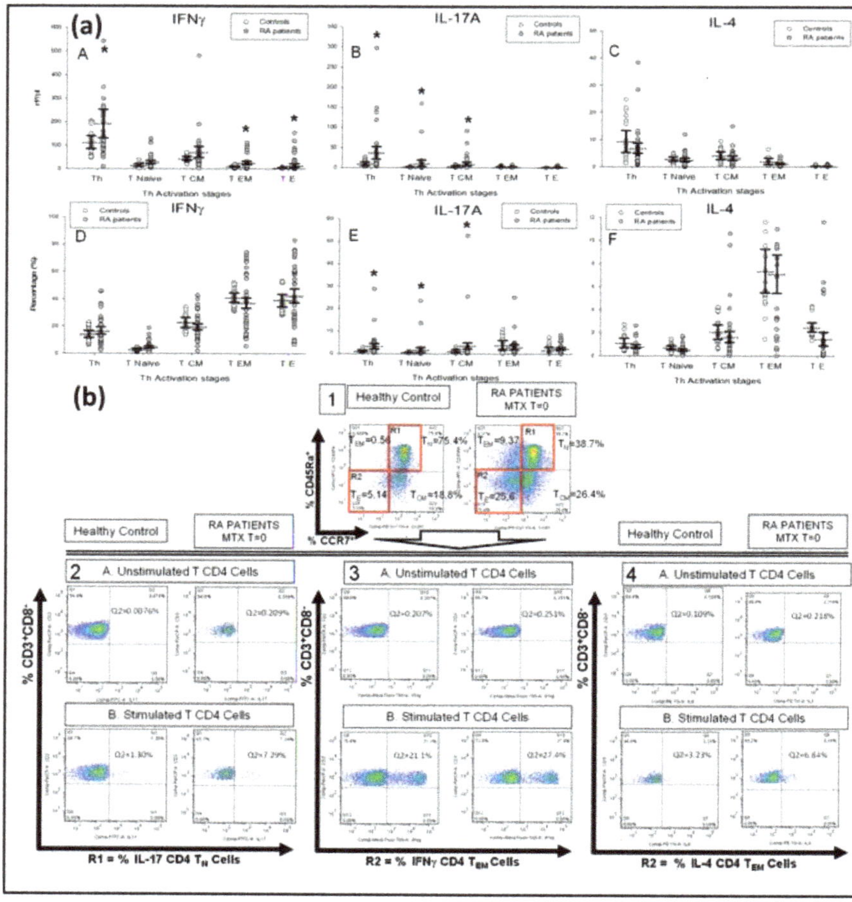

Figure 1. Intracellular IFNγ, IL-17A, IL-4 expression by the different activation/differentiation stages of T $CD4^+$ lymphocytes from rheumatoid arthritis (RA) patients. Note: (**a**) Data represent numbers (n°/γl) (A, B and C panels) and percentages (%) (D, E and F panels) of total $CD3^+CD4^+$ (Th), and the $T_{Naïve}$, T_{CM}, T_{EM} and T_E $CD4^+$ lymphocyte subsets that express intracellular IL-17A, IFNγ and IL-4 after in vitro phorbol-12-myristate-13-acetate (PMA) stimulation in disease-modifying antirheumatic drug (DMARD)-naïve RA patients (●) and healthy controls (○). % (percentages) refers to total population of the indicated lymphocytes. All values are expressed as the mean cell numbers ± S.E.M. *, $p < 0.05$ for RA patients vs. healthy controls. (**b**) Panel 1. The first dot plots represent the selected gates and percentages of T_N, T_{CM}, T_{EM} and T_E $CD4^+$ T-lymphocytes in two representative situations: a healthy control and RA patient at baseline before Methotrexate (MTX) treatment. Panel 2, 3 and 4. Dot plots represent the percentages of IL-17A, IFNγ and IL-4-producing $CD4^+$ T cells in the presence and absence of PMA stimulation in the two representative cases described in panel 1. R1 and R2 represents the regions that include the $T_{Naïve}$ and T_{EM} $CD4^+$ lymphocyte subsets, respectively.

Interestingly, the numbers of T_N and T_{MC} $CD4^+$T-lymphocytes expressing both IL-17A and IFNγ were significantly increased in patients compared with HCs (Figure 2a).

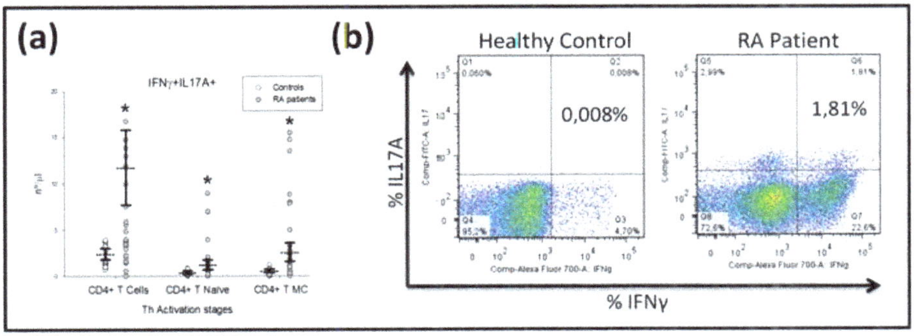

Figure 2. Intracellular $IFN\gamma^+IL\text{-}17A^+$ double-positive expression by $CD3^+$, T_N and T_{MC} $CD4^+$ lymphocytes in RA patients. Note: (**a**) Data represent numbers (n°/μL) of $CD4^+$, $T_{Naïve}$ and T_{CM} $CD4^+$ lymphocytes in (●) DMARD-naïve RA patients and (○) healthy controls. All values are expressed as the mean cell numbers ± S.E.M. *, $p < 0.05$ for RA patients vs. healthy controls. (**b**) Dot plots represent the percentages of $IFN\gamma^+IL\text{-}17A^+$ double-positive expression by $CD4^+$ T-lymphocytes after in vitro PMA stimulation in two representative situations: a healthy control and a RA patient at baseline before MTX treatment.

Next, we investigated the expression and phosphorylation of STAT-1, STAT-3 and STAT-6 transcription factors in $CD4^+$ T-lymphocytes from patients and HCs (Figure 3). Patients showed an increased percentage of phosphorylated STAT-1 and STAT-3 protein in the four different $CD4^+$T-lymphocyte subsets analyzed with respect to HCs. Simultaneously, each $CD4^+$T-lymphocyte subset from patients showed normal STAT-6 phosphorylation. Total STAT-3 protein was significantly increased in the four $CD4^+$T-lymphocyte subsets from patients with respect to the HCs, while total STAT-6 protein was significantly increased in the $CD4^+$ and T_N and T_{CM} subsets and total STAT-1 protein was normal.

Finally, we investigated the IL-17A, IFNγ and IL-4 serum levels from patients and HCs (Figure 4). We found that patients had significantly increased levels of IL-17A and IFNγ, but normal IL-4 concentrations.

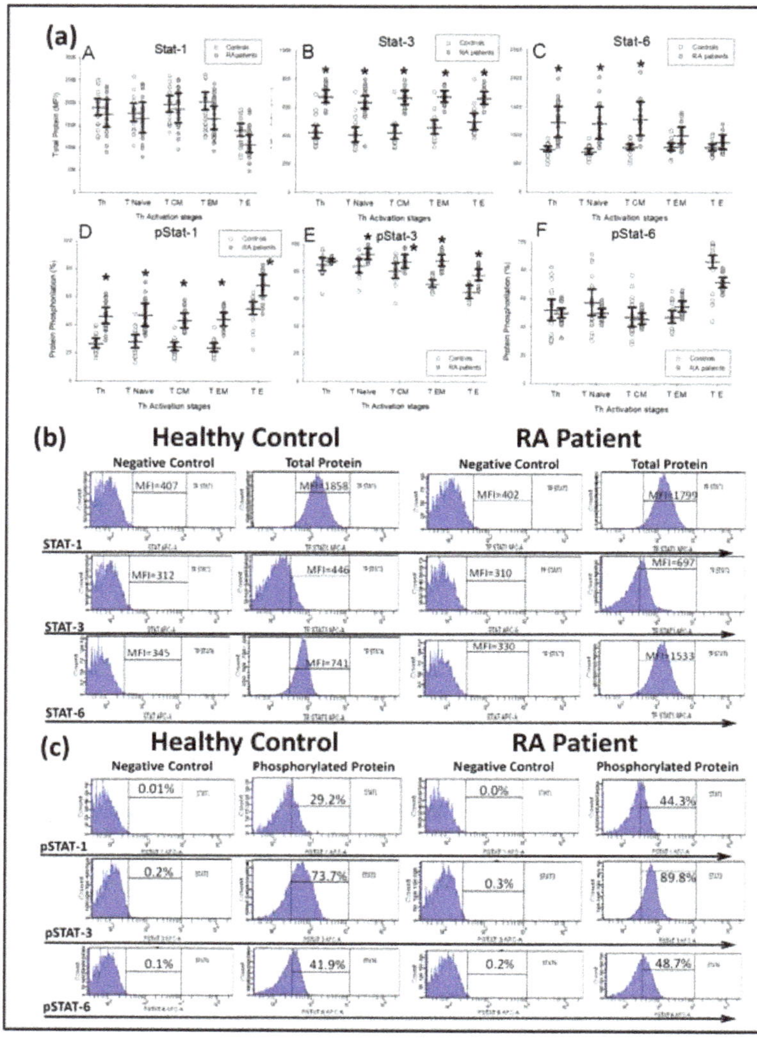

Figure 3. STAT-1, STAT-3 and STAT-6 phosphorylation and total protein expression by T CD4$^+$ lymphocyte subsets from new-onset DMARD-naïve RA patients. Note: (**a**) Data represent the mean florescence intensity (MFI) and percentage (%) of the total and phosphorylated proteins, respectively, in CD3$^+$CD4$^+$, $T_{Naïve}$, T_{EM}, T_E and T_{CM} CD4$^+$T-lymphocytes of (●) DMARD-naïve RA patients and (○) healthy controls. All values are expressed as the mean MFI or percentage ± S.E.M. *, $p < 0.05$ for RA patients vs. healthy controls. (**b**) Histograms represent the mean fluorescence intensity (MFI) of STAT-1, STAT-3 and STAT-6 total protein stimulated with IFNγ, IL-6 and IL-4, respectively, and their negative controls, in two representative cases: a healthy control and a RA patient at baseline before MTX treatment. (**c**) Histograms represent the percentages of STAT-1, STAT-3 and STAT-6 phosphorylation stimulated with IFNγ, IL-6 and IL-4, respectively, and their negative controls in two representative cases: a healthy control and an RA patient at baseline before MTX treatment.

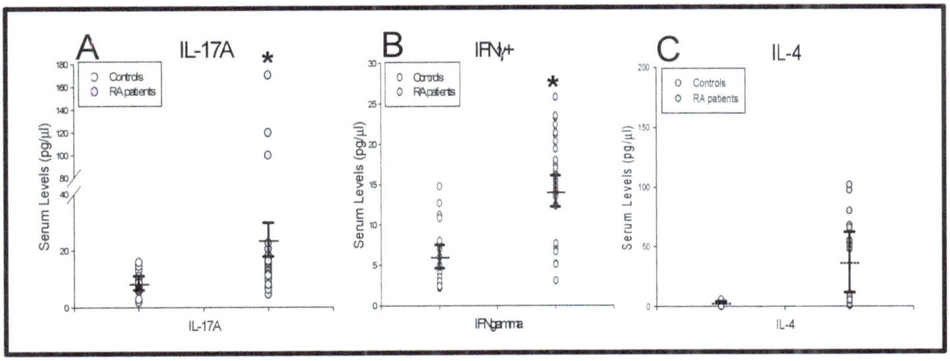

Figure 4. IL-17A, IFNγ and IL-4 serum levels in new-onset DMARD-naïve RA patients. Data represent the mean value serum levels of IL-17A, IFNγ and IL-4 in (●) RA patients and (○) as healthy controls (panels **A**, **B** and **C**). All values are expressed as the mean serum levels ± S.E.M. *, $p < 0.05$ for RA patients vs. healthy controls.

2.3. Different Patterns of Distribution Of IL-17A, IFNγ And IL-4 CD4⁺ T-Lymphocytes Are Observed in MTX Responder and Nonresponder Ra Patients

In new-onset DMARD-naïve patients, we investigated the expression of IL-17A, IFNγ and IL-4 by circulating $CD4^+$T-lymphocytes before and during the first 6 months of MTX treatment. We stratified the patients into two groups, which were defined according to the clinical response to MTX treatment attained after 6 months of treatment. There were 31 and 16 patients who met the criteria for responders and nonresponders to MTX, respectively. The patients were studied in parallel with 29 HCs. There were no significant differences in the number or frequency of circulating $CD4^+$T-lymphocytes between MTX nonresponder and MTX responder RA patients and HCs at baseline ($CD4^+$T cells: 821.99 ± 187.91 vs. 1101.54 ± 260.11 cells/µL and 33.07 ± 3.45 vs. 36.22 ± 2.73%, responder vs. nonresponder patients, respectively).

Under basal conditions, MTX nonresponder patients showed a significantly increased number of $CD4^+IL\text{-}17A^+$T-lymphocytes with respect to responder patients, which could be explained by an expansion of the $CD4^+IL\text{-}17A^+T_N$ and $CD4^+IL\text{-}17A^+T_{CM}$ subsets (Figure 5b). After 6 months of treatment, there were no differences in the numbers of $CD4^+IL\text{-}17A^+$T-lymphocytes between nonresponder and responder RA patients, but the numbers of $CD4^+IL\text{-}17A^+T_N$ remained significantly increased in nonresponders. During treatment, MTX responder patients did not show significant modifications in the number of $CD4^+IL\text{-}17A^+$T-lymphocytes.

Under basal conditions, the number of $CD4^+IFN\gamma^+$T-lymphocytes was significantly increased in MTX nonresponder patients with respect to responders, which was due to an increase in the $CD4^+IFN\gamma^+T_N$, $CD4^+IFN\gamma^+T_{CM}$ and $CD4^+IFN\gamma+T_{EM}$ subset numbers, which were significantly reduced after 6 months of MTX treatment. In MTX responder patients, there were no significant modifications of the $CD4^+IFN\gamma^+$T-lymphocytes numbers during the 6 months of treatment follow-up (Figure 5a).

There were no significant differences in $CD4^+IL\text{-}4^+$T-lymphocyte numbers between MTX responder and nonresponder patients under basal conditions. However, after 6 months of treatment, there was a significant increase in the number of $CD4^+IL\text{-}4^+$T-lymphocytes as well as in the $CD4^+IL\text{-}4^+T_{CM}$ and $CD4^+IL\text{-}4^+T_{EM}$ subsets in nonresponder patients. In contrast, MTX responder RA patients showed a significant reduction in numbers of $CD4^+IL\text{-}4^+$T-lymphocytes and $CD4^+IL\text{-}4^+T_{CM}$ subsets (Figure 5c).

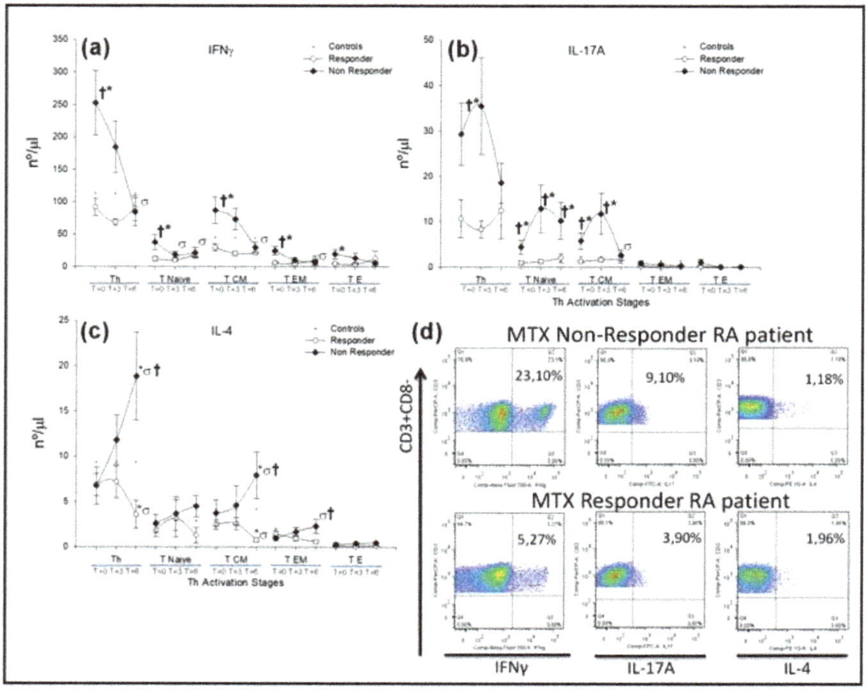

Figure 5. IFNγ, IL-4 and IL-17A-producing $CD3^+CD4^+$, $T_{naïve}$, T_{CM}, T_{EM} and T_E $CD4^+$ T-lymphocyte numbers in RA patients according to MTX response. Note: (**a–c**) Data represent numbers (n°/μL) of IFNγ, IL-4 and IL-17A-producing $CD3^+CD4^+$, $T_{Naïve}$, T_{CM}, T_{EM} and T_E $CD4^+$ T-lymphocytes according to the MTX response in (○) responder and (◆) nonresponder RA patients. The dotted line represents the mean value recorded in healthy controls (-◆-). All values are expressed as the mean cell numbers (n°/μL) ± S.E.M. *, $p < 0.05$ for responder or nonresponder RA patients vs. healthy controls; †, $p < 0.05$ for responders vs. nonresponders, σ $p < 0.05$ for 6 months of follow-up time vs. baseline. (**d**) Dot plots represent the percentages of $IFN\gamma^+$, $IL\text{-}17A^+$ and $IL\text{-}4^+$ expression by $CD4^+$ T-lymphocytes after in vitro PMA stimulation in two representative situations: a nonresponder and a responder RA patient at baseline before MTX treatment.

Next, we investigated the expression and phosphorylation of STAT-1, STAT-3 and STAT-6 transcription factors on $CD4^+$T-lymphocytes from MTX responder and nonresponder patients. Under basal conditions and at 3 and 6 months, there were no significant differences in either the percentage of phosphorylation or in the total protein in the different $CD4^+$T-lymphocytes between both groups of patients (Figure 6). However, there were significant differences in the total expression of STAT-1 and STAT-3 and STAT-6 phosphorylation by $CD4^+$T-lymphocytes from MTX nonresponder patients between basal conditions and after six months of treatment.

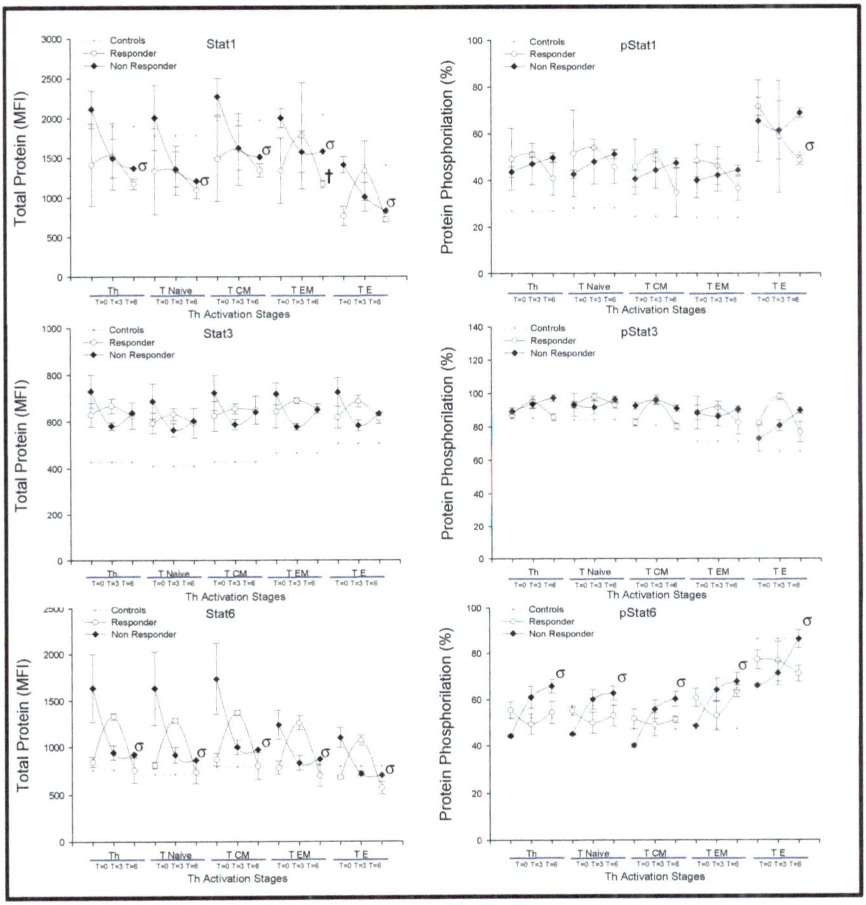

Figure 6. STAT-1, STAT-3 and STAT-6 phosphorylation in $CD4^+$ T-lymphocytes of RA patients according to MTX response. Note: Data represent the mean florescence intensity (MFI) and percentage (%) of total and phosphorylated proteins, respectively, on $CD3^+CD4^+$, $T_{Naïve}$, T_{CM}, T_{EM}, and T_E $CD4^+$ T-lymphocytes according to the MTX response in (○) responder and (◆) nonresponder RA patients. The dotted line represents the mean value recorded in healthy controls (-+-). All values are expressed as the mean cell numbers ± S.E.M. †, $p < 0.05$ for responders vs. nonresponders, σ $p < 0.05$ for 6 months of follow-up time vs. baseline.

Finally, we also investigated the serum levels of IL-17A, IFNγ and IL-4 in RA patients before and during the initial 6 months of treatment. Significantly increased levels of IL-17A were detected in MTX nonresponders with respect to responders under basal conditions and during the six months of treatment follow-up. Bot, MTX responder and nonresponder patients showed similar basal levels and significant reductions in IFNγ levels during the 6 months of MTX treatment. IL-4 serum levels were significantly increased in MTX nonresponders with respect to MTX responders before and during the 6 months of treatment (Figure 7).

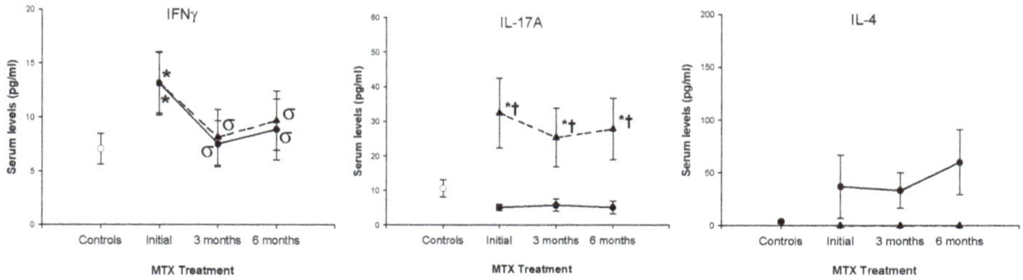

Figure 7. IFNγ, IL-4 and IL-17A serum levels in RA patients according to MTX response. Note: Data represent the mean value of serum levels of IFNγ, IL-4 and IL-17A in (▲) nonresponder, (●) responder RA patients and (○) healthy controls. All values are expressed as the mean serum levels ± S.E.M. *, $p < 0.05$ for responders or nonresponders vs. healthy controls; †, $p < 0.05$ for responders vs. nonresponders, σ $p < 0.05$ for 3 or 6 months of follow-up time vs. baseline.

3. Discussions

In this paper, we have shown that new-onset DMARD-naïve RA patients have abnormally functioning circulating $CD4^+$T-lymphocytes with an expansion of the $CD4^+IL\text{-}17A^+$, $CD4^+IFN\gamma^+$ and $CD4^+IL\text{-}17A^+IFN\gamma^+T$ subsets. This functional bias of the $CD4^+$ T cell population is associated with increased intracellular STAT-1 and STAT-3 stimulation and increased circulating levels of IFNγ and IL-17A. Furthermore, the pattern of $IL\text{-}17^+$, $IFN\gamma^+$ and $IL\text{-}4^+$ $CD4^+$T-lymphocytes production detected in new-onset DMARD-naïve RA patients could be modified by MTX treatment, and two different behaviors were identified in responders and nonresponders.

$CD4^+$T-lymphocytes play a critical role in the pathogenesis of RA [3–6,8,28]. Heterogeneous results, demonstrating increased, unchanged or reduced numbers and/or percentages of Th1, Th2 and Th17 $CD4^+$T-lymphocyte subsets in the circulation of RA patients have been reported [19–23,29–33]. This variability may be explained by different nonmutually exclusive mechanisms, including disease duration, previous and active DMARD and immunosuppressor treatments, concomitant diseases, the genetic and epidemiological backgrounds of the patients, cohort size, and the methodologies used to record different immune system variables. To minimize these potential interferences with the mechanisms directly associated with RA pathophysiology, we focused herein on a clinically homogeneous population of new-onset DMARD-naïve patients. Our data revealed increased numbers of circulating $CD4^+IFN\gamma^+$ and $CD4^+IL\text{-}17A^+$T-lymphocytes in new-onset DMARD-naïve RA patients, but normal $CD4^+IL\text{-}4^+$T-lymphocytes. The frequency of Th17 cells was also increased, but the percentages of Th1 and Th2 lymphocytes were similar to those found in HCs. The differences in the results obtained using both methods of quantification indicate that the analyses of these $CD4^+$T-lymphocytes subsets require the simultaneous study of numbers and percentages in RA patients. The numbers of circulating Th1, Th2 or Th17 cells appear to have special potential pathogenic relevance since they are a main source of IFNγ, IL-4 and IL-17A secretion [7,8]. In agreement with these cellular findings, the serum levels of IL-17A and IFNγ were increased, but those of IL-4 were normal in new-onset DMARD-naïve RA patients. Increased circulating IL-17A and IFNγ levels have been described in patients with early RA [34,35]. Interestingly, the numbers of circulating Th1, Th2 and Th17 cells showed differences under basal conditions and/or during MTX treatment between responder and nonresponder patients. Moreover, in agreement with a previous report, we found an expanded number of double $IL\text{-}17A^+IFN\gamma^+CD4+$T-lymphocytes in RA patients [23]. These different observations may contribute to understanding the established confusion concerning the normality or alteration of circulating Th1, Th2 and Th17 subsets in RA patients. Taken together, these findings improve knowledge of the involvement of $CD4^+$T-lymphocytes in the early clinical stages of RA patients. Furthermore, this $CD4^+$T-lymphocyte disturbance in RA patients cannot be ascribed to a single Th subset since both Th1 and Th17 were expanded with increased levels of circulating IFNγ and IL-17A cytokines.

In addition to the pattern of cytokine production, $CD4^{+}$T-lymphocytes are a heterogeneous population with different stages of differentiation/activation and patterns of circulation and tissue infiltration [11–15]. Interestingly, the number of $CD4^{+}T_{N}$ able to express IL-17A^{+} and IFNγ^{+}IL-17A^{+} was increased in new-onset DMARD-naïve RA patients. These data suggest an abnormal bias of nonantigen activated $CD4^{+}$T-lymphocytes from these patients toward IL-17A production, which is also observed in antigen-promoted T_{CM} $CD4^{+}$T-lymphocytes. The relevance of the predisposition and acquired activation of $CD4^{+}$T-lymphocytes to express cytokines is supported by the observation of the opposite results with respect to IFNγ production in naïve RA patients. The increasing numbers of IFNγ-producing $CD4^{+}$T-lymphocytes were mainly focused in the $CD4^{+}T_{EM}$ and $CD4^{+}T_{E}$ subsets in new-onset DMARD-naïve RA patients. Different mechanisms might be involved in these different functional findings, including the intrinsic/genetic characteristics of the patients, the activating microenvironment and preferential extra-vascular tissue migration, such as the inflamed joints in naïve RA patients. It has been proposed that the CD14^{+high}CD16^{+} monocyte subset participates in the expansion of Th17 T-lymphocytes in RA patients [36,37]. There is also evidence supporting the relevance of the cytokine microenvironment in the differentiation of naïve T-lymphocytes into Th1, Th2 and Th17 subsets [7]. Furthermore, precursors such as $CD4^{+}CD161^{+}$T-lymphocytes may differentiate into either Th1 or TH17 lymphocytes based on the presence of IL-1γ and IL-23 or TGFγ [7]. It is possible that this plasticity might be involved in the observed expansion of $CD4^{+}T_{N}$ able to express IL-17A^{+} and IFNγ^{+}IL-17A^{+} in new-onset DMARD-naïve patients with RA. In contrast, the selective overexpansion of IFNγ in $CD4^{+}T_{EM}$ and $CD4^{+}T_{E}$ lymphocytes suggests the occurrence of antigen stimulation in the IL-12 microenvironment.

The relevance of the different signals driving Th lymphocyte activation appears to be critical because the percentages of phosphorylation of the transcription factors STAT-1 and STAT-3 were increased in the four different CD4 differentiation/activation stages in the DMARD-naïve RA patients. It is possible to suggest that early RA is associated with an intrinsic $CD4^{+}$IL-17A$^{+}T_{N}$ differentiation. However, antigen pressure and cytokines favor Th1 differentiation with a predominance of $CD4^{+}T_{EM}$ and $CD4^{+}T_{E}$ lymphocyte activation. In addition, it has been proposed that Th17 cells are unstable and easily shift toward Th1 cells, named "non-classic Th1 cells", and they have been found in early RA with relevant pathogenic activity [34]. In cord blood or spondyloarthropathies, abnormal Th1 and Th17 differentiation have been postulated in response to IL-1β and IL-23 [38,39]. Our data showed the involvement of both Th1 and Th2 subsets in early RA patients; however, their pathogenic role remains to be elucidated.

Our data revealed a heterogeneous function of $CD4^{+}$T-lymphocytes in the early stages of RA. Analysis of the basal characteristics of new-onset DMARD-naïve patients who did not achieve a clinical response to MTX showed a significant expansion of $CD4^{+}$IFNγ^{+} and $CD4^{+}$IL-17A^{+} T_{N} and T_{CM} and $CD4^{+}$IFNγ^{+} T_{EM} and T_{E} lymphocytes with respect to those circulating in responders. Interestingly, during the 6 months of follow-up, MTX nonresponders maintained increased numbers of $CD4^{+}$IL-17A$^{+}T_{N}$ cells. Nevertheless, a normalization of $CD4^{+}$IFNγ^{+} cell subset numbers was observed with a concomitant increase in $CD4^{+}$IL-4$^{+}T_{CM}$ and $CD4^{+}$IL-4$^{+}T_{EM}$ cells. In addition, the significantly increased levels of circulating IL-17A persisted, but those of IFNγ were normalized, during the 6 months of MTX treatment in nonresponders. Thus, it is possible to suggest that the persistence of Th17 polarization during MTX treatment is associated with a defective response to treatment with this drug in early RA patients. The relevance of this Th17 differentiation is also supported by the normal numbers of $CD4^{+}$IFNγ^{+}, $CD4^{+}$IL-17A^{+} and $CD4^{+}$IL-4^{+} subsets in MTX responder patients. These results support the idea that these Th17 might be important in RA pathogenesis and in the response to immunomodulator treatments. There were no significant differences in the levels and phosphorylation of the STAT-1, STAT-3 and STAT-6 proteins in the different $CD4^{+}$T-lymphocytes between responders and nonresponders. Interestingly, the different behaviors of the CD4$^+$T-lymphocytes compartment in both groups of patients cannot be ascribed to different disease activities before starting MTX treatment.

The precise mechanism of action of MTX in RA patients remains obscure [40]. It may act by decreasing cell proliferation, enhancing the rate of apoptosis, increasing endogenous adenosine concentrations, or altering cytokine production [41,42]. However, MTX is not a general antiproliferative drug; indeed, it induces apoptosis only in highly activated immune system cells [42,43]. The present data indicate that MTX causes different regulatory effects on CD4$^+$T-lymphocytes in responders and nonresponders. This different CD4$^+$T-lymphocyte modulation cannot be ascribed to a differential effect on the levels and phosphorylation of STAT-1, STAT-3 and STAT-6 proteins. The absence of a clinical response to MTX does not, however, rule out a biological effect of the drug on patient CD4$^+$T-lymphocytes. Furthermore, the progression of uncontrolled diseases may be related to the expansion of CD4$^+$IL-17A$^+$T$_N$ lymphocytes. Determining whether this is the case is impossible since it would be unethical to maintain patients with active RA without treatment. These results support the knowledge of the relevance of an early immunomodulation in a subset of new-onset RA patients. Future works have to investigate the potential value of CD4$^+$T-lymphocytes parameters as biomarkers in new-onset DMARD-naïve RA patients.

4. Materials and Methods

4.1. Inclusion and Exclusion Criteria

The study subjects included 47 Caucasian patients with ACR/EULAR (American College of Rheumatology/The European League Against Rheumatism) 2010 classification criteria for RA [44]. Patients were studied in parallel with 29 healthy sex-, age-, ethnicity-matched controls. The patients were followed at the Rheumatology Service, Hospital Príncipe de Asturias, Alcala University, in Spain. All patients provided their informed consent to be included. The study was properly approved by the hospital's clinical/ethics committee: "Ethical committee for clinical research of the Hospital Principe de Asturias" (research proyect 1/2006, code P1-11-02433, committee approval date 26/1/2006).

Inclusion criteria:

Patients with new-onset RA (disease duration < 3-months), previously untreated with DMARDs and a disease activity score of 28 (DAS28) according to EULAR criteria, were evaluated for inclusion in the study [44].

Exclusion criteria:

To have (1) severe cardiovascular disease, (2) hypercholesterolemia or diabetes mellitus, hematopoietic, (3) lung, hepatic or renal disorders, (4) acute or chronic bacterial or viral infections, (5) other autoimmune diseases, (6) treatment with steroids, immunosuppressors or other drugs that would have interacted with the immune system in the previous 6 months, (7) possible pregnancy/lactation during the study period, and (8) simultaneous malignancy or congenital immunodeficiency.

4.2. Study Protocol

All patients were treated weekly for 6 months with 15 mg MTX (orally) plus 5 mg folic acid. The MTX dose was adjusted by increments of 5 to 25–30 mg weekly until the disease response criteria were met. Patients were advised to take 5 mg of Prednisone (orally) daily and a non-teroidal anti-inflammatory drug at fixed doses during the study. All patients were monitored monthly for clinical and analytical tolerance to MTX treatment and at 3 and 6 months to assess the clinical response and to undertake immunological studies. Disease activity was determined by the DAS28 score according to EULAR criteria and using a validated Spanish version of the Health Assessment Questionnaire (HAQ) [45]. The clinical response of the patients to MTX was defined according to EULAR criteria for RA [46], classifying patients as responders or nonresponders. The responder group included those patients with an actual DAS28 < 3.2 score, plus a DAS28 score decrease by at least 1.2 with respect to the initial value, after 6 months of MTX treatment.

Three peripheral blood samples were obtained from each patient by antecubital venipuncture at baseline (before starting MTX treatment) and at 3 and 6 months after starting MTX treatment.

4.3. Clinical Laboratory Assays

C-reactive prtein (CRP) y Rheumatoid factor (FR) was determined by an inmmunoturbidimetry assay in an Atellica Solution® CH (Siemens Healthineers, Erlangen, Germany), with 0–5 mg/L being the normal range for CRP and 3.5–90 IU/mL for RF. Anti-CCP was determined by a fluoroenzimo-immunoassay (Inmunocap 250, Thermofisher Scientific, Waltham, MA, USA) with a normal range under IU/mL.

4.4. Isolation of Peripheral Blood Mononuclear Cells

Peripheral blood mononuclear cells (PBMCs) were obtained from heparinized venous blood and were separated by Ficoll-Hypaque (Lymphoprep™, Axis-Shield, Oslo, Norway) gradient centrifugation [47]. They were then resuspended in RPMI-1640 with 10% heat-inactivated fetal calf serum (Gibco, Life Technologies Limited, Renfrew, UK), 25mM HEPES and 1% penicillin-streptomycin (Biowhittaker, Lonza, Barcelona, Spain). Cell enumeration was performed as previously described [48]. The PBMCs of each patients or control were adjusted to 1 10^6 cells/mL prior to antibody staining.

The cell number counts of lymphocytes subsets were calculated by the percentage of each subpopulation in the PBMCs determined by flow cytometry multiplied by the total number of lymphocytes per microliter obtained by a complete blood count from a conventional hemogram measured by Beckman Coulter, Inc (Brea, CA, USA).

4.5. In Vitro Culture

The spontaneous and stimulated T-lymphocyte subset expression of IFNγ, IL-17A and IL-4 was assessed by in vitro intracytoplasmic staining in the presence of 2mM monensin. The PBMCs were stimulated with 50 ng/mL phorbol-12-myristate-13-acetate (PMA, Sigma-Aldrich, MerkMillipore, Boston, MA, USA) plus 1μg/mL ionomycin (Calbiochem, MerkMillipore, Boston, MA, USA) for 6 h. Spontaneous cytokine expression was determined in parallel cultures in the absence of exogenous stimuli.

4.6. Surface and Intracellular Lymphocyte Staining

T-lymphocytes were studied in PBMCs by nine-color flow cytometry. PBMCs were incubated with the next surface-labeled monoclonal-antibodies, CD3-PercP, CCR7-PECY7 (Becton-Dickinson, BD, CA, USA), CD8-Alexa405, CD45RA-APC (Caltag, Carlsbad, CA, USA) and CD27-APCAlexa780 (eBioscience, San Diego, CA, USA).

For intracytoplasmic staining, cells were fixed and permeabilized (Fix and Perm, Caltag, Carlsbad, CA, USA), and cytokines were stained with IL-4-PE, IFNγ-Alexa700 and IL-17A-FITC (Becton-Dickinson, BD, CA, USA). All samples were stained with a dead cell-discriminator simultaneously with antibody addition (Fixable aqua dead cell stain kit for 405 nm excitation; Molecular Probes, Eugene, OR, USA).

Samples were acquired in a FacsAria-II flow cytometer and were analyzed using FacsDiva 5.0 and Flow-Jo 7.0 software (Becton-Dickinson, BD, San Jose, CA, USA).

4.7. Cytokines Serum Levels

Samples were obtained in sterile clotting tubes from peripheral blood by ante-cubital venipuncture. These samples were centrifuged at 863× *g* for 20 min at 4 °C, aliquoted, identified and labeled, and frozen at −80 °C. Then, they were thawed and evaluated using the high sensitivity human MILLIPLEX® kit to simultaneously measure IFNγ, IL-4 and IL-17A (Millipore) following the manufacturer's instructions and revealing the results by Luminex (MAGPIX® system). The tested cytokines had the following sensitivity limits (0.48 pg/mL for IFNγ, 1.12 pg/mL for IL-4 and 0.33 pg/mL for IL-17A). The results were analyzed using Analyst 5.1 software MILLIPLEX® (MerkMillipore, Boston, MA, USA).

4.8. STATs Flow Cytometry

The spontaneous and stimulated CD4$^+$T-lymphocyte subset expression of STAT-1, STAT-3 and STAT-6 was assessed by in vitro phosphoprotein intracytoplasmic staining. To evaluate STAT-1, STAT-3 and STAT-6 phosphorylation, PBMCs were stimulated for 15′ with 40.000 U/mL of IFNα for STAT-1, 0.1μg/mL of IL-6 for STAT-3 and 0.1 μg/mL of IL-4 for STAT-6. Additionally, the total STAT-1, STAT-3 and STAT-6 protein was analyzed in CD4$^+$T-lymphocyte subsets.

Surface and intracellular lymphocyte staining. For intracytoplasmic STAT staining, PBMCs were fixed, permed (BDPhosphoflow, Becton-Dickinson, BD, San Jose, CA, USA) and stained with the subsequent surface-labeled monoclonal-antibodies CD4-FITC, CD27-PE, CD3-Percp (Becton-Dickinson, BD, San Jose, CA, USA) CD45RA-Alexa405 (eBioscience, San Diego, CA, USA) and with the STAT1-FITC, STAT3-Pacificblue or STAT6-PE (Becton-Dickinson, BD, San Jose, CA, USA) intracellular-labeled monoclonal-antibodies against phosphorylated or total STAT protein.

The quality control of the flow cytometer was performed daily according to the manufacturer's instructions (Becton-Dickinson, BD, San Jose, CA, USA). The staining protocol and quality and analysis controls were performed by 'fluorescence minus one control' as described by Roederer et al. [49], and the flow cytometry results were presented following the guidelines of the International Society of Advancement of Cytometry (ISAC) [50].

4.9. Statistical Analysis

Analyses were performed using SPSS-22 software (SPSS-IBM, Armonk, NY, USA). Since most variables did not fulfill the normality hypothesis, the Mann–Whitney U-test for nonparametric data was used to analyze differences between groups, and analysis of variance followed by Wilcoxon tests were used for within group analyses. The significance level was set at $p < 0.05$.

5. Conclusions

The results revealed a heterogeneous function of CD4+ T-lymphocytes subsets in the early clinical stages of RA with potential pathogenic relevance:

The numbers of circulating Th1, Th2 or Th17 CD4$^+$T-lymphocytes subsets in the early clinical stages of RA show two different profiles of cytokine producing CD4$^+$ T-lymphocyte subsets associated to a response or not associated to the MTX treatment of the RA patients.

The pattern of IL-17$^+$, IFNγ^+ and IL-4$^+$ CD4$^+$ T production detected in new-onset DMARD-naïve RA patients could be modified by MTX treatment.

Results may offer a way of identifying which patients will respond, or not, to MTX treatment.

Author Contributions: M.Á.-M. and J.M.S. were responsible for the study conception and design, J.M.S. and A.M.G. for the data acquisition, and M.Á.-M., J.M.S., D.D., C.B., A.M., A.P., L.R., A.I.S. and F.A. for the data analysis and interpretation. J.M.S., M.Á.-M., C.B. and I.S. drafted the manuscript. All authors read and approved the final manuscript.

Funding: This work was partially supported by grants from the Fondo de Investigación de la Seguridad Social, Instituto de Salud Carlos III (PI18/01726), Spain and the Programa de Actividades de I+D de la Comunidad de Madrid en Biomedicina (MITIC-CM, S2017/BMD-3804), Madrid, Spain.

Acknowledgments: The authors would like to thank all the medical doctors, nurses and technical staff of the Immune System Diseases-Rheumatology Service of the Hospital Universitario Principe de Asturias and the Department of Medicine of the University of Alcalá for their careful and generous collaboration while doing this work.

Conflicts of Interest: The authors declare no conflict of interest.

Abbreviations

IFNg	Interferon gamma
IL-4	Interleukin-4
IL-17	Interleukin-17a
RA	Rheumatoid arthritis
DMARDs	Disease-Modifying antirheumatic drugs
PBMC	Peripheral blood mononuclear cells
FITC	Fluorescein-Isothiocyanate
PE	Phycoerythrin
Apc-Alexa780	Allophycocyanin-alexa-780
Pe-Cy7	Phycoerythrin-Cyanine Seven
mAb	Monoclonal antibodies
MTX	Methrotexate
Th	T helper
T_N	T naïve
T_{CM}	T central memory
T_{EM}	T effector memory
T_E	T effector
PMA	Phorbol-12-Myristate-13-Acetate

References

1. Scott, D.L.; Wolfe, F.; Huizinga, T.W.J. Rheumatoid arthritis. *Lancet* **2010**, *376*, 1094–1108. [CrossRef]
2. Weyand, C.M.; Goronzy, J. Pathogenesis of rheumatoid arthritis. *Med. Clin. N. Am.* **1997**, *81*, 29–55. [CrossRef]
3. Cope, A.P. T cells in rheumatoid arthritis. *Arthritis Res. Ther.* **2008**, *10*, S1. [CrossRef]
4. Okada, R.; Kondo, T.; Matsuki, F.; Takata, H.; Takiguchi, M. Phenotypic classification of human CD4+ T cell subsets and their differentiation. *Int. Immunol.* **2008**, *20*, 1189–1199. [CrossRef]
5. Sallusto, F.; Lenig, D.; Forster, R.; Lipp, M.; Lanzavecchia, A. Two subsets of memory T lymphocytes with distinct homing potentials and effector functions. *Nature* **1999**, *401*, 708–712. [CrossRef]
6. Sallusto, F.; Monticelli, S. The many faces of CD4 T cells: Roles in immunity and disease. *Semin. Immunol.* **2013**, *25*, 249–251. [CrossRef]
7. Schmitt, N.; Ueno, H. Regulation of human helper T cell subset differentiation by cytokines. *Curr. Opin. Immunol.* **2015**, *34*, 130–136. [CrossRef] [PubMed]
8. Toh, M.-L.; Miossec, P. The role of T cells in rheumatoid arthritis: New subsets and new targets. *Curr. Opin. Rheumatol.* **2007**, *19*, 284–288. [CrossRef]
9. Lönnberg, T.; Chen, Z.; Lahesmaa, R. From a gene-centric to whole-proteome view of differentiation of T helper cell subsets. *Brief. Funct. Genomics.* **2013**, *12*, 471–482. [CrossRef]
10. Vahedi, G.; Takahashi, H.; Nakayamada, S.; Sun, H.-W.; Sartorelli, V.; Kanno, Y.; O'Shea, J.J. STATs shape the active enhancer landscape of T cell populations. *Cell* **2012**, *151*, 981–993. [CrossRef]
11. Maecker, H.T.; McCoy, J.P.; Nussenblatt, R. Standardizing immunophenotyping for the Human Immunology Project. *Nat. Rev. Immunol.* **2012**, *12*, 191–200. [CrossRef] [PubMed]
12. Kaech, S.M.; Wherry, E.J.; Ahmed, R. Effector and memory T-cell differentiation: Implications for vaccine development. *Nat. Rev. Immunol.* **2002**, *2*, 251–262. [CrossRef] [PubMed]
13. Sallusto, F.; Geginat, J.; Lanzavecchia, A. Central Memory and Effector Memory T Cell Subsets: Function, Generation, and Maintenance. *Annu. Rev. Immunol.* **2004**, *22*, 745–763. [CrossRef] [PubMed]
14. Taylor, J.J.; Jenkins, M.K. CD4+ memory T cell survival. *Curr. Opin. Immunol.* **2011**, *23*, 319–323. [CrossRef] [PubMed]
15. Sallusto, F.; Lanzavecchia, A. Heterogeneity of CD4+ memory T cells: Functional modules for tailored immunity. *Eur. J. Immunol.* **2009**, *39*, 2076–2082. [CrossRef]
16. Monserrat, J.; Bohórquez, C.; Lahoz, A.M.G.; Movasat, A.; Pérez, A.; Ruíz, L.; Diaz, D.; Chara, L.; Sánchez, A.I.; Albarrán, F.; et al. The Abnormal CD4+T Lymphocyte Subset Distribution and Vbeta Repertoire in New-onset Rheumatoid Arthritis Can Be Modulated by Methotrexate Treament. *Cells* **2019**, *8*, 871. [CrossRef]

17. Wehrens, E.J.; Prakken, B.J.; Wijk, F.V. T cells out of control—Impaired immune regulation in the inflamed joint. *Nat. Rev. Rheumatol.* **2012**, *9*, 34–42. [CrossRef]
18. Alex, P.; Szodoray, P.; Knowlton, N.; Dozmorov, I.M.; Turner, M.; Frank, M.B.; Arthur, R.E.; Willis, L.; Flinn, D.; Hynd, R.F.; et al. Multiplex serum cytokine monitoring as a prognostic tool in rheumatoid arthritis. *Clin. Exp. Rheumatol.* **2007**, *25*, 584–592.
19. Arroyo-Villa, I.; Bautista-Caro, M.-B.; Balsa, A.; Aguado-Acín, P.; Nuño, L.; Bonilla-Hernán, M.-G.; Puig-Kröger, A.; Martín-Mola, E.; Miranda-Carus, M.-E. Frequency of Th17 CD4+ T Cells in Early Rheumatoid Arthritis: A Marker of Anti-CCP Seropositivity. *PLoS ONE* **2012**, *7*, e42189. [CrossRef]
20. Deane, K.D.; O'Donnell, C.I.; Hueber, W.; Majka, D.S.; Lazar, A.A.; Derber, L.A.; Gilliland, M.W.R.; Edison, J.; Norris, J.M.; Robinson, W.H.; et al. The number of elevated cytokines and chemokines in preclinical seropositive rheumatoid arthritis predicts time to diagnosis in an age-dependent manner. *Arthritis Rheum.* **2010**, *62*, 3161–3172. [CrossRef]
21. Kokkonen, H.; Söderström, I.; Rocklöv, J.; Hallmans, G.; Lejon, K.; Rantapää-Dahlqvist, S.; Söderström, I.; Rocklöv, J. Up-regulation of cytokines and chemokines predates the onset of rheumatoid arthritis. *Arthritis Rheum.* **2010**, *62*, 383–391. [CrossRef] [PubMed]
22. Kosmaczewska, A.; Swierkot, J.; Ciszak, L.; Szteblich, A.; Chrobak, A.; Karabon, L.; Partyka, A.; Szechinski, J.; Wiland, P.; Frydecka, I. Patients with the most advanced rheumatoid arthritis remain with Th1 systemic defects after TNF inhibitors treatment despite clinical improvement. *Rheumatol. Int.* **2013**, *34*, 243–253. [CrossRef] [PubMed]
23. Wu, C.; Goodall, J.C.; Busch, R.; Gaston, H. Relationship of CD146 expression to secretion of interleukin (IL)-17, IL-22 and interferon-γ by CD4(+) T cells in patients with inflammatory arthritis. *Clin. Exp. Immunol.* **2015**, *179*, 378–391. [CrossRef]
24. Adamson, A.S.; Collins, K.; Laurence, A.; O'Shea, J. The Current STATus of lymphocyte signaling: New roles for old players. *Curr. Opin. Immunol.* **2009**, *21*, 161–166. [CrossRef]
25. Kuuliala, K.; Kuuliala, A.; Koivuniemi, R.; Oksanen, S.; Hämäläinen, M.; Moilanen, E.; Kautiainen, H.; Leirisalo-Repo, M.; Repo, H. Constitutive STAT3 Phosphorylation in Circulating CD4+ T Lymphocytes Associates with Disease Activity and Treatment Response in Recent-Onset Rheumatoid Arthritis. *PLoS ONE* **2015**, *10*, e0137385. [CrossRef] [PubMed]
26. Kuuliala, K.; Kuuliala, A.; Koivuniemi, R.; Kautiainen, H.; Repo, H.; Leirisalo-Repo, M. STAT6 and STAT1 Pathway Activation in Circulating Lymphocytes and Monocytes as Predictor of Treatment Response in Rheumatoid Arthritis. *PLoS ONE* **2016**, *11*, e0167975. [CrossRef]
27. Ramiro, S.; Landewé, R.; Breedveld, F.C.; Buch, M.; Burmester, G.; Dougados, M.; Emery, P.; Gaujoux-Viala, C.; Gossec, L.; Nam, J.; et al. EULAR recommendations for the management of rheumatoid arthritis with synthetic and biological disease-modifying antirheumatic drugs: 2013 update. *Ann. Rheum. Dis.* **2013**, *73*, 492–509. [CrossRef]
28. Firestein, G.S. Immunologic Mechanisms in the Pathogenesis of Rheumatoid Arthritis. *J. Clin. Rheumatol.* **2005**, *11*, S39–S44. [CrossRef]
29. Fekete, A.; Soos, L.; Szekanecz, Z.; Szabo, Z.; Szodoray, P.; Barath, S.; Lakos, G. Disturbances in B- and T-cell homeostasis in rheumatoid arthritis: Suggested relationships with antigen-driven immune responses. *J. Autoimmun.* **2007**, *29*, 154–163. [CrossRef]
30. Kohem, C.L.; Brezinschek, R.I.; Wisbey, H.; Tortorella, C.; Lipsky, P.E.; Oppenheimer-Marks, N. Enrichment of differentiated CD45RBdim. *Arthritis Rheum.* **1996**, *39*, 844–854. [CrossRef]
31. Neidhart, M.; Pataki, F.; Schönbächler, J.; Brühlmann, P. Flow cytometric characterisation of the "false naive" (CD45RA+, CD45R0-, CD29 bright+) peripheral blood T-lymphocytes in health and in rheumatoid arthritis. *Rheumatol. Int.* **1996**, *16*, 77–87. [CrossRef] [PubMed]
32. Neidhart, M.; Fehr, K.; Pataki, F.; Michel, B.A. The levels of memory (CD45RA?, RO+) CD4+ and CD8+ peripheral blood T-lymphocytes correlate with IgM rheumatoid factors in rheumatoid arthritis. *Rheumatol. Int.* **1996**, *15*, 201–209. [CrossRef] [PubMed]
33. Ponchel, F.; Morgan, A.W.; Bingham, S.J.; Quinn, M.; Buch, M.; Verburg, R.J.; Henwood, J.; Douglas, S.H.; Masurel, A.; Conaghan, P.G.; et al. Dysregulated lymphocyte proliferation and differentiation in patients with rheumatoid arthritis. *Blood* **2002**, *100*, 4550–4556. [CrossRef] [PubMed]

34. Kotake, S.; Nanke, Y.; Yago, T.; Kawamoto, M.; Kobashigawa, T.; Yamanaka, H. Ratio of Circulating IFNγ + "Th17 Cells" in Memory Th Cells Is Inversely Correlated with the Titer of Anti-CCP Antibodies in Early-Onset Rheumatoid Arthritis Patients Based on Flow Cytometry Methods of the Human Immunology Project. *BioMed Res. Int.* **2016**, *2016*, 9694289. [CrossRef] [PubMed]
35. Raza, K.; Falciani, F.; Curnow, S.J.; Ross, E.J.; Lee, C.-Y.; Akbar, A.N.; Lord, J.; Gordon, C.; Buckley, C.D.; Salmon, M. Early rheumatoid arthritis is characterized by a distinct and transient synovial fluid cytokine profile of T cell and stromal cell origin. *Arthritis Res. Ther.* **2005**, *7*, R784–R795. [CrossRef]
36. Chara, L.; Sánchez-Atrio, A.; Pérez, A.; Cuende, E.; Albarrán, F.; Turrión, A.; Chevarria, J.; Barco, A.A.D.; Sánchez, M.A.; Monserrat, J.; et al. The number of circulating monocytes as biomarkers of the clinical response to methotrexate in untreated patients with rheumatoid arthritis. *J. Transl. Med.* **2015**, *13*, 2. [CrossRef]
37. Rossol, M.; Kraus, S.; Pierer, M.; Baerwald, C.; Wagner, U. The CD14brightCD16+ monocyte subset is expanded in rheumatoid arthritis and promotes expansion of the Th17 cell population. *Arthritis Rheum.* **2012**, *64*, 671–677. [CrossRef]
38. Cosmi, L.; De Palma, R.; Santarlasci, V.; Maggi, L.; Capone, M.; Frosali, F.; Rodolico, G.; Querci, V.; Abbate, G.; Angeli, R.; et al. Human interleukin 17–producing cells originate from a CD161+CD4+ T cell precursor. *J. Exp. Med.* **2008**, *205*, 1903–1916. [CrossRef]
39. Kotake, S.; Yago, T.; Kobashigawa, T.; Nanke, Y. The Plasticity of Th17 Cells in the Pathogenesis of Rheumatoid Arthritis. *J. Clin. Med.* **2017**, *6*, 67. [CrossRef]
40. Wessels, J.A.M.; Guchelaar, H.-J.; Huizinga, T.W.J. Recent insights in the pharmacological actions of methotrexate in the treatment of rheumatoid arthritis. *Rheumatol. Oxf.* **2007**, *47*, 249–255. [CrossRef]
41. Möller, B.; Kukoc-Zivojnov, N.; Okamgba, S.; Kessler, U.; Puccetti, E.; Ottmann, O.G.; Kaltwasser, J.P.; Hoelzer, D.; Ruthardt, M. Folinic acid antagonizes methotrexate-induced differentiation of monocyte progenitors. *Rheumatol. Int.* **2002**, *22*, 60–67. [CrossRef] [PubMed]
42. Phillips, D.C.; Woollard, K.J.; Griffiths, H.R. The anti-inflammatory actions of methotrexate are critically dependent upon the production of reactive oxygen species. *Br. J. Pharmacol.* **2003**, *138*, 501–511. [CrossRef] [PubMed]
43. Strauss, G.; Osen, W.; Debatin, K.-M. Induction of apoptosis and modulation of activation and effector function in T cells by immunosuppressive drugs. *Clin. Exp. Immunol.* **2002**, *128*, 255–266. [CrossRef] [PubMed]
44. Aletaha, D.; Neogi, T.; Silman, A.J.; Funovits, J.; Felson, D.T.; Bingham, C.O.; Birnbaum, N.S.; Burmester, G.R.; Bykerk, V.P.; Cohen, M.D.; et al. 2010 Rheumatoid arthritis classification criteria: An American College of Rheumatology/European League against Rheumatism collaborative initiative. *Arthritis Rheum.* **2010**, *62*, 2569–2581. [CrossRef]
45. González, V.M.; Stewart, A.; Ritter, P.L.; Lorig, K. Translation and validation of arthritis outcome measures into Spanish. *Arthritis Rheum.* **1995**, *38*, 1429–1446. [CrossRef]
46. Gestel, A.M.V.; Prevoo, M.L.L.; Hof, M.A.V.; Rijswijk, M.H.V.; De Putte, L.B.A.V.D.; Riel, P.L.C.M.V. Development and validation of the european league against rheumatism response criteria for rheumatoid arthritis: Comparison with the preliminary american college of rheumatology and the world health organization/international league against rheumatism criteria. *Arthritis Rheum.* **1996**, *39*, 34–40. [CrossRef]
47. Böyum, A. Isolation of mononuclear cells and granulocytes from human blood. Isolation of monuclear cells by one centrifugation, and of granulocytes by combining centrifugation and sedimentation at 1 g. *Scand. J. Clin. Lab. Invest. Suppl.* **1968**, *97*, 77–89.
48. Monserrat, J.; De Pablo, R.; Reyes, E.; Diaz, D.; Barcenilla, H.; Zapata, M.R.; De La Hera, A.; Prieto, A.; Alvarez-Mon, M. Clinical relevance of the severe abnormalities of the T cell compartment in septic shock patients. *Crit. Care* **2009**, *13*, R26. [CrossRef]
49. Roederer, M. Compensation in Flow Cytometry. *Curr. Protoc. Cytom.* **2002**, *22*, 1–14. [CrossRef]
50. Roederer, M.; Darzynkiewicz, Z.; Parks, D.R. Guidelines for the Presentation of Flow Cytometric Data. *Methods Cell Biol.* **2004**, *75*, 241–256. [CrossRef]

International Journal of *Molecular Sciences*

MDPI

Article

Antibiotic Treatment Prior to Injury Improves Post-Traumatic Osteoarthritis Outcomes in Mice

Melanie E. Mendez [1], Deepa K. Murugesh [1], Aimy Sebastian [1], Nicholas R. Hum [1,2], Summer A. McCloy [1], Edward A. Kuhn [1], Blaine A. Christiansen [3] and Gabriela G. Loots [1,2,*]

[1] Lawrence Livermore National Laboratories, Physical and Life Sciences Directorate, Livermore, CA 94550, USA; mendez20@llnl.gov (M.E.M.); murugesh2@llnl.gov (D.K.M.); sebastian4@llnl.gov (A.S.); hum3@llnl.gov (N.R.H.); mccloy2@llnl.gov (S.A.M.); kuhn7@llnl.gov (E.A.K.)

[2] UC Merced, School of Natural Sciences, Merced, CA 95343, USA

[3] UC Davis Medical Center, Department of Orthopedic Surgery, Sacramento, CA 95817, USA; bchristiansen@ucdavis.edu

* Correspondence: loots1@llnl.gov; Tel.: +1-925-423-0923

Received: 24 July 2020; Accepted: 29 August 2020; Published: 3 September 2020

Abstract: Osteoarthritis (OA) is a painful and debilitating disease characterized by the chronic and progressive degradation of articular cartilage. Post-traumatic OA (PTOA) is a secondary form of OA that develops in ~50% of cases of severe articular injury. Inflammation and re-occurring injury have been implicated as contributing to the progression of PTOA after the initial injury. However, there is very little known about external factors prior to injury that could affect the risk of PTOA development. To examine how the gut microbiome affects PTOA development we used a chronic antibiotic treatment regimen starting at weaning for six weeks prior to ACL rupture, in mice. A six-weeks post-injury histological examination showed more robust cartilage staining on the antibiotic (AB)-treated mice than the untreated controls (VEH), suggesting slower disease progression in AB cohorts. Injured joints also showed an increase in the presence of anti-inflammatory M2 macrophages in the AB group. Molecularly, the phenotype correlated with a significantly lower expression of inflammatory genes *Tlr5, Ccl8, Cxcl13*, and *Fozo6* in the injured joints of AB-treated animals. Our results indicate that a reduced state of inflammation at the time of injury and a lower expression of Wnt signaling modulatory protein, *Rspo1*, caused by AB treatment can slow down or improve PTOA outcomes.

Keywords: osteoarthritis; PTOA; gene expression; RNA-seq; cartilage degeneration; tibial compression; gut microbiome; antibiotics; LPS

1. Introduction

The individual microbial cells that constitute the human gut microbiome outnumber our cells by a factor of 10 [1]. In utero, most fetuses are free of microorganisms [2]; the first exposure babies have to microbes is during birth as they move through the birth canal, hence babies born in natural birth are inoculated with microorganisms by their mothers. The gut microbiome initiates with breast feeding and builds complexity as the baby's diet evolves from milk to other types of foods [3]. It reaches dynamic stability by the age of 3, and while a person's gut biome is relatively stable, there are many genetic and environmental factors that influence its composition and dynamic change in each person [4]. The microorganisms living in our gut that do not cause harm, and may even have a beneficial contribution to human health, are called commensals. The gut microbiome composition can be disrupted by dietary changes, antibiotic treatment or pathogenic infections, and in reciprocal interactions changes to the composition and abundance of commensals could affect the entire system by producing unwarranted gastrointestinal and immune diseases [5–7].

Published literature suggests that the gut microbiome has an indirect effect on bone through changes to the immune system and inflammatory cytokines [8,9]. Commensals aid in immune-regulation by releasing microbial associated molecular patterns (MAMPs) such as lipopolysaccharides (LPSs) that bind and activate toll-like receptors (*Tlr*); LPSs have been shown to bind to *Tlr4* [9–14]. This activation causes an inflammatory cascade that releases inflammatory cytokines and interferons which act as transcription factors to induce naïve immune cells to mature [15–17]. Studies have suggested that gut biome dysbiosis can promote aggressive bone destruction mediated by osteoclasts due to an increase in tumor necrosis factor alpha (TNF-α) [18–20]. Furthermore, we have previously shown that elevated levels of LPSs negatively impact bone by promoting bone loss and accelerate post-traumatic osteoarthritis (PTOA) development. We also showed that LPS administration prior to injury elevates *Tlr5/7/8* transcription in the joint [10,21]. TNF-α promotes osteoclastogenesis by increasing RANK-L expression in bone marrow cells and therefore elevating the number of osteoclast precursor cells [20,22–24].

In the context of PTOA, it has been shown that when the gut microbiome of obese mice is modified by supplementing oligofructose, OA phenotypes diminish, which correlates with a reduction in the levels of inflammation in the colon and cytokine levels circulating in the serum and present in the knee [25]. Cyclic compressive loading in mice on a high-fat diet have promoted more severe PTOA phenotypes than mice on a normal diet, while *Tlr5*$^{-/-}$ mice treated with ampicillin and neomycin have shown improvement in the cartilage phenotype post injury [26]. Germ-free mice have also been shown to have a better OA outcome after destabilization of the medial meniscus, and modifications to the gut microbiome have improved PTOA phenotype in obese mice [25,27,28]. Tibial compression induced injury in 20-week-old germ-free mice has shown an increase in bone volume [29]. Therefore, a precedent exists in support of the gut microbiome composition as a potential risk factor for the development of PTOA, but additional studies are required to elucidate potential mechanisms that contribute to the unwarranted PTOA phenotypes.

Most PTOA-related studies to date have examined factors likely to exacerbate or accelerate the development of osteoarthritis post injury, if administered at the time of injury or shortly thereafter [30]. Since bone and cartilage sometimes exhibit an inverse relationship to insult, such that what is anabolic for bone is catabolic for cartilage and vice versa [31], we speculated that gut biome modifications would slow down or improve PTOA outcomes. Therefore, this study aimed to examine how partial elimination of the gut microbiome through antibiotic treatment prior to injury would influence PTOA outcomes. Studying the effects of medication administered before an injury is of high biomedical importance because, clinically, most concerns are centered on side-effects due to co-administration. Currently, however, standards of medical care do not consider gut biome status, nor is gut dysbiosis a recoded clinical parameter. Research that can show the prognostic and diagnostic value of gut biome status could potentially lead to new standards of care. In addition, antibiotics are widely prescribed to teens and young adults who may be active in sports and therefor more susceptible to joint injuries. According to the CDC, in 2016, 64.9 million oral antibiotic prescriptions were issued to people under the age of 20, the equivalent of 790 per 1000 people; therefore, gut dysbiosis may be more common than expected in young athletes suffering an articular injury [32]. As the population of the USA ages there will be an increase in PTOA cases; studying how antibiotics modify PTOA phenotypes will be helpful to finding preventative treatments in the future for both young and old patients.

2. Results

2.1. Antibiotic Treatment Prior to Injury Delays Cartilage Resorption in Injured Joints

Using an established, noninvasive, tibial compression PTOA mouse model [33–37], we examined whether a six-week course of antibiotics (ampicillin (1.0 g/L)/neomycin (0.5 g/L)) [26] would impact OA outcomes, post injury. C57Bl/6J mice were examined histologically at six weeks post injury. Examination of the uninjured, contralateral femoral heads revealed a more intense Safranin-O staining throughout the articular cartilage of the antibiotic (AB)-treated group compared to untreated controls (VEH), but both AB and VEH joints displayed normal morphology (Figure 1A,C). A slightly less mineralized area, characterized by large pockets of bone marrow, was observed in the femoral condyle of AB-treated, injured joints, relative to the VEH injured group (Figure 1B,D). Consistent with the AB uninjured control, the femoral condyle of the injured AB group (Figure 1d; arrow, asterisk) appeared to also have an increase in Safranin-O staining intensity as well as a thicker articular cartilage layer than the injured VEH, suggesting higher levels of proteoglycans and reduced chondrocyte apoptosis in the injured joints of AB-treated animals (Figure 1b; arrow, asterisk). The meniscus (Figure 1bb,dd; arrow, asterisk) of injured AB joints showed a thicker hyperplastic morphology with enhanced cellular infiltration. The meniscus in the injured VEH group also showed cellular infiltration but at a significantly lower level than the AB injured group. Examination of the sagittal views of the joints by a modified Osteoarthritis Research Society International (OARSI) grading scale determined that AB-treated injured joints had a significantly lower cartilage score than VEH-treated injured joints with a p-value of 0.038 (Figure 1E). These results imply that modifying the gut microbiome through the administration of an ampicillin/neomycin antibiotic cocktail prior to injury was sufficient to improve the cartilage phenotype subsequent to trauma, and reduce PTOA outcomes.

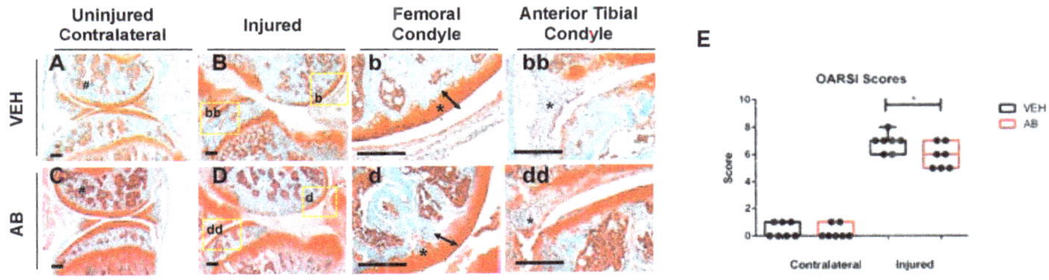

Figure 1. Characterization of post traumatic osteoarthritis (PTOA)-associated structural changes of antibiotic-treated animals in the knee. (**A**) Histological evaluation of vehicle (VEH) contralateral, (**B–bb**) VEH injured, (**C**) Antibiotic treated (AB) contralateral, and (**D–dd**) AB injured joints conducted at six weeks post injury using Safranin-O and Fast Green staining (scale bars indicate 200 mm). High magnification images corresponding to yellow boxes (**B**,**D**) are provided b, bb, d, dd. (**E**) PTOA severity was quantified using a modified OARSI scoring system (* p-value < 0.05).

2.2. Antibiotic Treatment Has a Negative Effect on Bone, Post Injury

The bone phenotypes of AB- and VEH-treated mice were characterized by micro-computed tomography (μCT) to quantify subchondral trabecular bone mass and osteophyte volume at six weeks post injury. Consistent with prior published results, VEH injured joints had significantly less subchondral bone volume (BV/TV) by ~17.28% and ~11.31% when compared to contralateral and uninjured controls, respectively (Figure 2A). Antibiotic-treated injured joints lost 13.67% when compared to contralateral AB treated and 17.42% when compared to uninjured AB-treated controls. The subchondral bone volume (BV/TV) fraction of AB group had ~0.2%, ~7.1%, and ~10.9% lower BV/TV than the VEH group when comparing the uninjured, injured, and contralateral groups; the contralateral group was the only one that was statistically significant, suggesting that AB treatment does not elevate BV/TV in the uninjured leg (Figure 2A). Trabecular number (Tb.N) of the AB group had ~0.2% and ~0.4% higher Tb.N on the uninjured and injured groups, respectively, compared to the VEH; the contralateral had ~1.1% lower Tb.N on the VEH. Tb.N was not statistically significant (Figure 2B). Trabecular thickness (Tb.Th) showed the VEH group had ~2.9%, ~7.6%, and ~10.6 higher Tb.Th than uninjured, injured, and contralateral AB cohorts; injured and contralateral were significant (Figure 2C). Trabecular spacing (Tb.Sp) AB showed ~1%, ~0.4%, and ~2.2% larger Tb.Sp than the VEH uninjured, injured, and contralateral groups, respectively; none were statistically significant (Figure 2D). The VEH group had ~39.7% significantly higher osteophyte volume (Op.V) compared to the AB cohort (Figure 2E). Visual representations of Op.V showed a larger amount of osteophytes in VEH joints, consistent with the quantification data (Figure 2F).

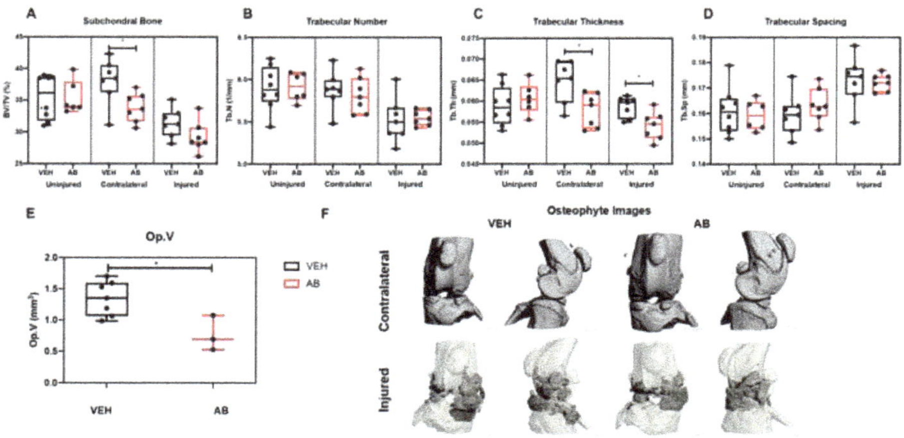

Figure 2. Bone phenotype of antibiotic-treated injured mice. (**A**) Subchondral trabecular bone volume fraction (BV/TV) of the distal femoral epiphysis. (**B**) Trabecular number was measured using the average number of trabeculae per unit length. (**C**) Trabecular thickness was measured using the mean thickness of trabeculae assessed using direct 3D methods. (**D**) Trabecular spacing was measured using the mean distance between trabeculae, assessed using direct 3D methods [38]. (**E**) Osteophyte volume at six weeks post injury. (**F**) Osteophyte imaging using μCT. (* $p < 0.05$).

2.3. LPS Treatment Compared to AB Treatment

Lipopolysaccharides (LPSs) administered five days prior to the joint injury did not elicit any significant changes in the bone phenotype when compared to the AB-treated uninjured bones. However, as previously reported [10], LPS administration alone was sufficient to modulate the cartilage phenotype on both the contralateral and injured joints towards a more severe phenotype (Figure 3E,F). LPS injured joints showed an enhanced thinning of the femoral cartilage that was distinguishable from the cartilage of the VEH and AB injured groups (Figure 3b,d,f). The damage to the cartilage in the LPS injured joints corresponded with a significantly higher OARSI score than the VEH and AB injured joints (Figure 3I). There was an increase in cellular infiltration on the AB- and LPS-treated joints compared to the VEH (Figure 3bb,dd,ff). Combination of the AB treatment and LPS challenge (AB+LPS) significantly improved the LPS-mediated phenotype, reverting the contralaterals back to the OARSI scores recorded for the VEH injured and uninjured groups (Figure 3A,B,G,H). These results indicate that the effects of LPSs are blunted by the AB treatment, where statistical analysis does not distinguish between VEH and AB+LPS in either the uninjured or injured groups (Figure 3I).

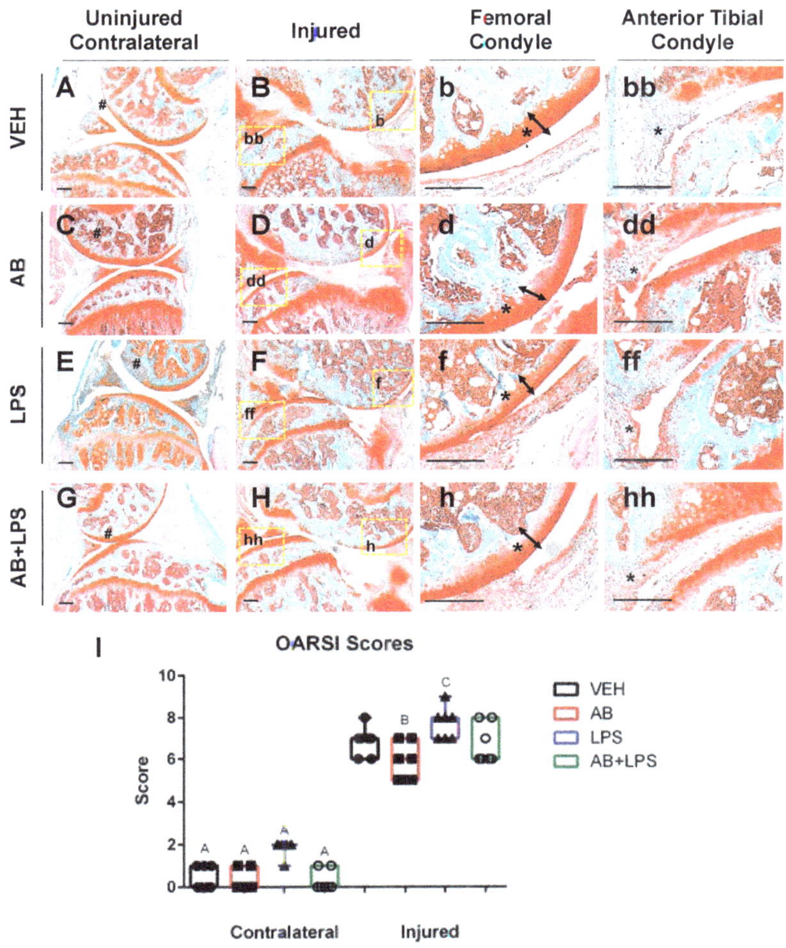

Figure 3. Characterization of PTOA-associated structural changes in the injured VEH, AB, LPS, and AB+LPS groups. (**A**–**hh**) Histological evaluation of uninjured and injured joints at six weeks post injury using Safranin-O and Fast Green staining. Black scale bars indicate 200 μm. Numeral sign indicates the femoral condyle (**A**,**C**,**E**,**G**). High magnification images corresponding to yellow boxes (**B**,**D**,**F**,**H**) are provided (**b**, **bb**, **d**, **dd**, **f**, **ff**, **h**, **hh**). Arrows and asterisks indicate the thickness of the cartilage in the femoral condyle (**b**, **d**, **f**, **h**). Asterisks indicate cellularity in the synovium (**bb**, **dd**, **ff**, **hh**). (**I**) OARSI scores (* p-value < 0.05).

Macrophages Associated with Healing Are Increased in Antibiotic-Treated Joints

Tissue resident macrophages are essential in providing innate immune defenses and regulating tissue and organ homeostasis [39]. Macrophages and other inflammatory cells are recruited to injury sites where they also play key roles in tissue remodeling and repair [40,41]. In the joint there is a population of inactive macrophages residing in the synovium [42]. These cells are activated under certain conditions such as injury or inflammation. Macrophages can be found using the marker F4/80, which is a marker for cells of mononuclear phagocyte lineage in mice [43]. Macrophages can be both pro-inflammatory (M1) and anti-inflammatory (M2), and the co-action of these subtypes can repair damaged tissue through specific cytokine secretion. Identification of both macrophage populations was done using F4/80 and iNOS as an M1 marker while using CD206 as a M2 marker. In the joint, however, a change in the M1/M2 ratio may be critical in PTOA progression and development. Histological examination of the injured joints indicated a hyperplastic synovium that appeared to have significant cellular infiltration on LPS- and AB-treated injured joints (Figure 3dd,ff; asterisk), and this morphology was similar to that of LPS-treated injured joints previously described [10]. To determine whether AB treatment prior to ACL rupture altered the composition of M1 and M2 cells in the injured joint, we used M1/M2 specific antibody markers to distinguish these subtypes by immunohistochemistry (Figure 4). On the meniscus, we observed a slightly higher staining of anti iNOS antibody indicative of some M1 macrophage infiltration in the AB injured joints compared to the VEH injured joints (Figure 4A,B). The M1 macrophage infiltration presence in AB injured joints was less than that of LPS injured joints (Figure 4B,C). In contrast, we observed a higher level of anti CD206 antibody staining in AB injured joints when compared to VEH and LPS injured, indicative of higher levels of M2 macrophages present in the injured joints of AB-treated animals (Figure 4D–F). These results suggest that while there is an increase in macrophages for both LPS and AB treatments, the LPS-treated joints have an increase in pro-inflammatory macrophages while AB-treated joints have an increase in anti-inflammatory macrophages that may be helping mitigate the PTOA phenotype.

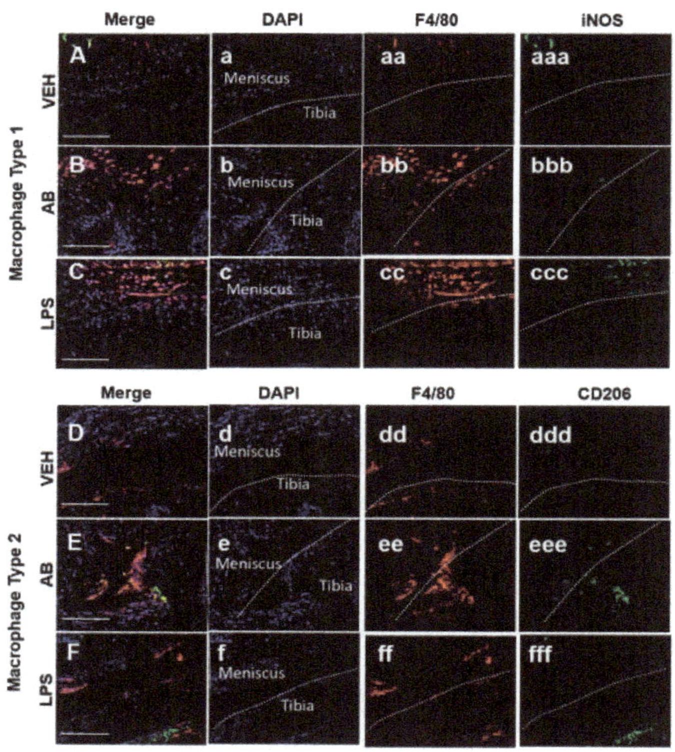

Figure 4. Macrophage infiltration analysis of the VEH-, AB-, and LPS-treated injured joints. (**A–C**) Fluorescent immunohistochemistry (IHC) of macrophage type 1 markers F4/80 and iNOS. (**D–F**) Fluorescent IHC of macrophage type 2 markers F4/80 and CD205. Dashed line in white represents the surface of the anterior tibial condyle for all images. (**a–f**) DAPI; (**aa–ff**) F4/80; (**aaa–ccc**) iNOS; (**ddd–fff**) CD206. White scale bar represents 100 μm.

2.4. Gene Expression Changes Associated with Chronic Antibiotic Treatment

To determine antibiotic treatment-related molecular changes in knee joints we compared the transcriptome of 10-week-old mice that had been treated with AB in their drinking water to VEH controls. We found 620 significantly upregulated genes in uninjured AB compared to the uninjured VEH group; the majority of genes accounting for these transcriptional changes were associated with immune responses. Some of the groups we found were of genes associated with collagen (*C1qb* [44], and *Fcna* [45]), regulators of adaptive immunity (*Btla* [46], *Lax1* [47], *Tnfrsf13c* [48], *Lat* [49], and *Cd40* [50]), and genes associated with the major histocompatibility complex type II (*Tnfrsf14* [51], *Cd86* [52], and *Cd8b1* [53]). We found 737 significantly downregulated genes in the AB uninjured group compared to the VEH uninjured group. These genes included regulators of skeletal development (*Alpl* [37], *Col6a1* [54], *Col6a2* [55], *Sox9* [37], *Sox11* [56], and *Wnt9a* [57]), Hippo signaling (*Tead1*, *Tead4* [58], and *Yap1* [59]), muscle contraction (*Myh8*, *Myh2*, and *Myom2*), and inflammatory response (*Tlr5* [60], *Ccl8* [61], *Cxcl13* [37], *C5ar1* [62], *Cxcr1* [63], and *Foxo6* [64]). Inflammatory gene comparison between AB injured and uninjured groups compared to the corresponding VEH groups are shown in Figure 5A and Table 1.

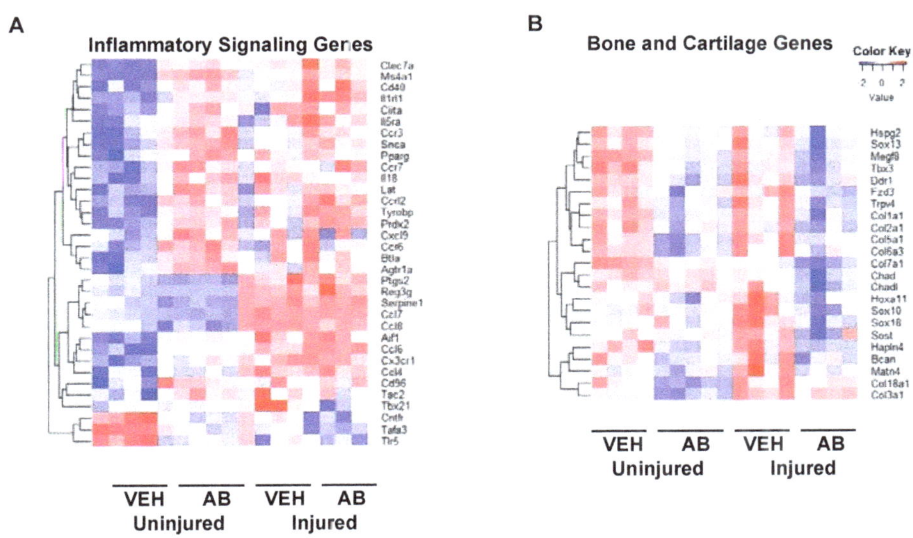

Figure 5. Gene expression changes associated with antibiotic treatment. (**A**) Genes associated with inflammatory process modified by AB treatment and AB with injury compared to VEH uninjured and injured. (**B**) Genes associated with bone and cartilage formation modified by AB treatment along with injury compared to VEH uninjured and injured.

Table 1. Inflammatory gene overlap between the AB and VEH groups, showing the expression levels. Fold change (log2 scale) values are shown in the table (FDR < 0.05 for all genes). Changes that were not significant are denoted as ns.

Gene	Uninjured	Injured
Agtr1a	0.898	ns
Aif1	0.740	ns
Btla	0.880	ns
Ccl4	1.437	ns
Ccl6	0.679	ns
Ccl7	−1.600	ns
Ccl8	−0.790	ns
Ccr3	0.998	ns
Ccr6	1.522	ns
Ccr7	0.931	ns
Ccrl2	0.691	ns
Cd40	0.829	ns
Cd96	1.028	ns
Ciita	1.033	ns
Clec7a	0.863	ns
Cntfr	−1.117	−0.870
Cx3cr1	0.856	ns
Cxcl9	0.653	ns
Il18	0.846	ns
Il1rl1	0.685	0.696
Il5ra	0.762	0.719
Lat	0.768	ns
Lat	0.768	ns
Ms4a1	1.293	ns
Pparg	0.665	ns
Prdx2	0.905	0.607
Ptgs2	−0.934	ns
Reg3g	−1.769	ns
Serpine1	−0.974	ns
Snca	1.135	ns
Tac2	0.789	ns
Tafa3	−1.234	−0.905
Tbx21	ns	−0.913
Tlr5	−0.987	ns
Tyrobp	0.645	ns

We also found 185 genes significantly upregulated when comparing the AB injured to the VEH injured group. Among these we found negative regulators of cytokine production (*Arg1* and *Sars*) and small molecule catabolic processes (*Bad* and *Galk1*). We found 284 genes significantly downregulated when comparing the AB injured group to the VEH injured group. Among these we found regulators of the Wnt signaling pathway (*Sost* [35,65], *Fzd3*), Notch signaling pathway (Notch4), collagen-associated genes (*Chad*, *Col16a1*, and *Lep*), and transcription factors known to be involved in cellular differentiation processes (*Sox18*, *Foxd2*, and *Sox10*). Genes associated with bone and cartilage formation are shown in Figure 5B and Table 2.

Table 2. Bone and cartilage gene overlap between the AB and VEH groups, showing expression levels. Fold change (log2 scale) values are shown in the table (FDR < 0.05 for all genes). Changes that were not significant are denoted as ns.

Gene	Uninjured	Injured
Bcan	−0.921	−1.072
Chad	ns	−0.910
Chadl	ns	−0.617
Col18a1	−0.923	ns
Col1a1	−0.740	−0.782
Col2a1	−0.608	−0.752
Col3a1	−0.666	ns
Col5a1	−0.800	−0.660
Col6a3	−1.055	−0.598
Col7a1	−0.689	ns
Ddr1	ns	−0.603
Fzd3	ns	−0.624
Hapln4	−0.903	−0.988
Hoxa11	ns	−0.696
Hspg2	−0.805	−0.660
Matn4	ns	−0.596
Megf8	−0.693	−0.615
Sost	ns	−0.655
Sox10	ns	−1.405
Sox13	ns	−0.705
Sox18	ns	−0.826
Tbx3	−0.846	−0.750
Trpv4	ns	−0.627

There were 78 genes upregulated in both AB groups when compared to their corresponding VEH control groups, including *C1qb* [44] and *Cd3d* [66]. There were 151 genes downregulated in both AB groups compared to the VEH group. These included skeletal muscle contraction (*Myh1*, *Myh3* [67], *Myh14* [68], and *Myom3* [69]), and extracellular matrix proteins found in bone and cartilage (*Col1a1*, *Col2a1*, *Col5a1*, *Col6a3* [37], and *Col7a1* [70]). *Tbx5* and *Klhl40* were upregulated in the AB injured group and downregulated in the AB uninjured group when compared to their corresponding VEH groups. *Cd209a* and *Rspo1* were downregulated in the AB injured group and upregulated in the AB uninjured group when compared to their corresponding VEH groups. Comparing the AB uninjured and AB injured groups showed that bone formation genes like *Cthrc1* were upregulated in the AB injured group. *Mmp3* [37], *Lox*, *Loxl3*, *Mmp10*, and *Mmp19*, were downregulated in the AB uninjured group when compared to the AB injured group.

Comparison of Gene Expression Changes Between Chronic Antibiotic Treatment and LPS Treatment

In order to compare treatment-related molecular changes in the joint we compared the expression of AB and LPS to VEH of the same injury. We found 32 genes that were upregulated in both the AB and LPS groups compared to the uninjured VEH group. Among these we found genes related to the inflammatory and immune system (*Cx3cr1*, *Cd3d*, *Ccl4*, and *Ccl6*). We found *Rspo1* [71] to be upregulated in both the AB and LPS groups compared to the VEH groups, and downregulated in the AB injured group when compared to the injured VEH group. There were three genes (*Fgfbp1*, *Tnnc1*, and *Rab20*) found to be upregulated in the injured AB and LPS groups compared to the injured VEH. We found 18 genes downregulated in the AB and LPS uninjured groups when compared to the corresponding VEH groups. Genes related to the immune system were among these (*Bcl3*, *Prtn3*, *Tnfsf9*, and *Ifitm1*). We found seven genes to be upregulated in the uninjured LPS group while downregulated in the uninjured AB group when compared to the corresponding VEH groups. These genes are *Tlr5*, *C5ar1*, *Aqp4*, *Ryr3*, *Mdga1*, *Foxo6*, and *Kcng4*. We found two genes (*Cd209a* and *Lep*) downregulated in both injured the AB and LPS groups compared to the injured vehicle. We found marker *Cd209a*, which is present in macrophages and dendritic cells, to be upregulated in the uninjured AB and LPS groups and downregulated in the injured AB and LPS groups when compared to the corresponding VEH groups. Gene expression between the AB and LPS groups compared to the VEH groups is found in Table 3.

Table 3. Overlap of upregulated genes between the AB and LPS groups compared to the VEH showing the expression levels. Fold change (log2 scale) values are shown in the table (FDR < 0.05 for all genes). Changes that were not significant are denoted as ns.

Gene	VEH Uninjured		VEH Injured	
	AB Uninjured	LPS Uninjured	AB Injured	LPS Injured
4921531C22Rik	0.680	0.945	ns	ns
Aldh3b2	1.289	0.963	ns	ns
Aldh3b3	0.783	1.204	ns	ns
Alox15	0.652	0.674	ns	ns
Arhgef3	0.592	0.602	ns	ns
Arl11	0.652	1.176	ns	ns
Ccl4	1.437	2.782	ns	ns
Ccl6	0.679	1.222	ns	ns
Cd209a	1.336	0.901	−0.592	−0.669
Cd3d	1.285	1.012	0.858	ns
Cd84	0.673	0.776	ns	ns
Cd8b1	1.480	ns	ns	ns
Clec7a	0.863	1.204	ns	ns
Csta2	1.172	1.269	ns	ns
Cstdc4	1.338	1.411	ns	ns
Cx3cr1	0.856	1.127	ns	ns
Cyp2ab1	1.010	1.803	ns	ns

Table 3. *Cont.*

Gene	VEH Uninjured		VEH Injured	
	AB Uninjured	LPS Uninjured	AB Injured	LPS Injured
Fgfbp1	ns	ns	1.518	1.753
Gzma	1.587	1.392	0.610	ns
Jaml	0.638	1.826	ns	ns
Klrc2	0.784	1.324	ns	ns
Lep	−0.701	−0.682	ns	ns
N4bp2l1	0.685	0.780	ns	ns
Nat8l	0.729	1.402	ns	ns
Neurl3	0.782	0.984	ns	ns
P2rx2	1.304	1.411	ns	ns
Ptpro	0.780	1.169	ns	ns
Rab20	ns	ns	0.702	0.608
Rspo1	0.768	1.592	−0.751	ns
Sirpb1a	0.803	1.056	ns	ns
Sirpb1b	0.667	1.096	ns	ns
Sirpb1c	0.780	1.109	ns	ns
Skint3	0.922	1.670	ns	ns
Tmem71	0.745	1.000	ns	ns
Tnnc1	ns	ns	0.881	0.780
Tyrobp	0.645	0.695	ns	ns
Vnn3	0.941	1.210	ns	ns

3. Discussion

The role of chronic antibiotic treatment prior to injury on the development of PTOA has not been previously investigated. Previous studies associating gut biome changes with skeletal phenotypes have focused primarily on bone, and have shown that the gut microbiome can influence osteoclastogenesis and affect bone volume [23]. Previous studies have also described the changes in the gut microbiome and bone using the same antibiotic cocktail [25,72]; however, our study is the first to examine how depletion of the gut biome with an ampicillin/neomycin antibiotics cocktail affects the development of osteoarthritis following a traumatic joint injury. Although morphologically our data indicate increased cellular infiltration in the synovium of injured joints of antibiotic-treated cohorts, reminiscent of synovitis induced by LPS administration [10], AB treatment did not have a significant effect on the BV/TV of the injured joint, resulting in no significant changes in BV/TV between the injured VEH and injured AB groups. The only significant bone phenotype was observed when contralateral were compared, where VEH-treated mice had an increase in BV/TV relative to uninjured control. AB-treated mice had a slight, but significant decrease in BV/TV. However, AB treatment improved the cartilage phenotype as reflected by a significantly lower OARSI score in these mice. There are several possible explanations for this outcome. The cellularity was examined using Ly6G and Ly6C markers, which highlighted an increase in the presence of monocytes, neutrophils, and granulocytes. In order to increase specificity, we stained with M1 and M2 markers, which showed an increase in the frequency of pro-inflammatory macrophages in the LPS-treated joints, while more anti-inflammatory macrophages were present in the AB-treated group. This correlation supports the conclusion that different macrophage subtypes could have influenced the exacerbation of PTOA in the LPS-treated cohorts, while deaccelerating PTOA progression in AB-treated cohorts.

It is also possible that chronic antibiotic treatment in juvenile mice (starting at four weeks of age) is anabolic to the articular cartilage, and during the six weeks of AB treatment prior to the injury the cartilage of these animals produced significantly more extracellular matrix. Furthermore, the cartilage of AB-treated animals may also display slightly different biomechanical properties than VEH controls. This theory is in part supported by the observation that uninjured joints of AB-treated animals stained more intensely with Safranin-O than the VEH uninjured joints (Figure 1A,C). If the cartilage of AB-treated animals acquired different mechanical properties, including increased stiffness or increased elastic modulus, cartilage degradation in these mice may have proceeded at a slower pace than the VEH, accounting for the milder phenotype in these injured joints. Additionally, we see a downregulation of gene *Rspo1* in injured AB joints when compared to injured VEH. This could be the reasoning for the decrease in OA progression, as *Rspo1* has previously been shown to have a role during OA progression [71]. Future studies examining the biomechanical properties of cartilage at different ages and in different treatment groups will have to be conducted to confirm whether significant differences in these properties exist.

Alternatively, the observed PTOA outcomes may be driven primarily by molecular changes. We observed 113 genes, including inflammatory genes *Bmper*, *Ccl2*, *Ccl7*, *Ccl8*, *Cxcl5*, *IL6*, *IL11*, *IL33*, and *Cxcl10*, that overlapped between the injured VEH, LPS, and AB groups and the uninjured groups of their respective treatments with significantly elevated expression in the injured joints; however, the blunted effect was present only in the AB injured group, suggesting that these molecules have a less potent effect in when mice are treated with AB prior to injury. Gene expression data indicate that the inflammatory genes *Ptgs2*, *Reg3g*, and *Serpine1* were downregulated in uninjured AB-treated mice, while *Tbx21* was found to be downregulated in injured AB joints. Two inflammatory genes found to be downregulated in both the injured and uninjured AB groups as compared to the corresponding VEH were *Tafa3* and *Cntfr*, which are both associated with the immune and nervous system. These genes have not been studied in the context of PTOA, and their influence on injury outcome would be interesting to study. When examining molecular changes in the immune system in prior reports, we have shown that elevated and persistent immune activation accelerates osteoarthritis phenotypes post injury [10]. Furthermore, we have shown that systemic LPS administration five days prior to injury negatively impacts PTOA, resulting in a more severe phonotype [10]. We have also shown that LPS-treated mice display highly elevated levels of toll-like receptors 5, 7, and 8 (*Tlr5*, *Tlr7*, *Tlr8*), and we hypothesized that the enhanced PTOA phenotype in LPS-treated mice may be due in part to increased signaling through these receptors. One complementary transcriptional result derived from the RNA-seq data examined herein is the discovery that *Tlr5* is significantly downregulated in AB-treated uninjured joints. Kim et al. showed that *Tlr5* in rheumatoid arthritis promotes monocyte presence and osteoclast formation due to the cross regulation of the *Tlr5* and TNF-α pathways [73]. If *Tlr5* similarly modulates the expression of inflammatory genes that are directly involved in cartilage degradation post injury, the observed transcriptional suppression of *Tlr5* in uninjured joints may promote a molecular resistance to inflammatory cytokines. Future studies will have to evaluate whether *Tlr5* receptor antagonists can prevent or slow down the development of OA post ACL rupture.

The current literature presents conflicting evidence on the effects of antibiotic treatment and the gut microbiome on bone, showing that modifications may have no significant changes in BV/TV after injury when compared to untreated control mice, but have a lowering effect when compared to uninjured treated mice [26]. In germ-free mice, AB treatment can increase the BV/TV after injury compared to injured controls, but these mice also have a lower BV/TV when compared to uninjured germ-free mice [29]. Our results showed no changes in BV/TV on injured AB-treated mice when compared to the injured VEH, but did show a decrease in in BV/TV when compared to the AB contralateral. These results are similar to the decrease in BV/TV observed after tibial compression (TC) injury in strains that are resistant to PTOA, like *MRL/MpJ* [36,74]. Our AB group showed an improvement in cartilage, and though these mice are not OA-resistant to the extent of *MRL/MpJ* mice, we observed similarities in the expression of T-cell markers like *Cd3d* and *Cd8b1* [36]. Although inflammation is resolved quicker in *MRL/MpJ* mice, bone resorption still occurs, similar to the C57Bl6 strain, due to the presence of pro-inflammatory cytokines and matrix metalloproteinases (MMPs) that promote osteoclastogenesis and extracellular matrix degradation [75–77]. The similarity of T-cell markers could potentially enhance healing and accelerate inflammation resolution in AB-treated mice, which could diminish the PTOA phenotype.

Our study uniquely examines the impact of long-term antibiotic treatment on OA outcomes subsequent to joint trauma. Prior to this study, we did not know if there were any PTOA changes caused by the administration of antibiotics. While we found that this particular AB regime had a beneficial effect on the health of injured and uninjured joints, it still remains to be elucidated whether short term AB treatment can be prophylactic; most importantly, questions remain about whether AB treatment post injury would have the same beneficial effect. This study highlights the importance of how the body works as a system and how systemic and local factors present prior to injury can significantly impact how our body heals and responds to trauma. This study highlights the importance of the gut biome in modulating PTOA, specifically by affecting toll-like receptors transcriptional levels that may in turn influence PTOA outcome after injury.

4. Materials and Methods

4.1. Tibial Compression Overload

C57Bl/6J mice were purchased from the Jackson Laboratory (Bar Harbor, ME, USA; Stock No: 000664) at four weeks of age and randomized into experimental groups ($n >= 4$). The antibiotic (AB) -treated group received treatment (ampicillin [78,79] (1.0g/L; Sigma; A9518-25G; St. Louis, MO, USA); neomycin [80–82] (0.5 g/L; Sigma; N1876-25G; St. Louis, MO, USA) in drinking water starting at weaning (four weeks of age) for six weeks; the untreated group (VEH) was provided with regular drinking water. Five days prior to injury at 10 weeks of age, cohorts of mice were separated into three groups (VEH, AB, and lipopolysaccharide (LPS)). The LPS group received an intraperitoneal (IP) injection of LPS (1 mg/kg; Sigma; L6529-1MG; St. Louis, MO, USA), while the VEH and AB groups received an IP injection of saline of an equivalent volume. On the day of injury, all groups were subjected to non-invasive ACL rupture using a single dynamic tibial compressive overload using an electromagnetic material testing system (ElectroForce 3200, TA Instruments, New Castle, DE, USA) as previously described [35,74,83]. Cohorts were placed under anesthesia using isoflourane prior to injury [84]. ACL injury was performed by placing the mouse in the system and applying a compressive load at 1 mm/s until ACL rupture (typically 12N-14N); the uninjured group was placed in the system and received a non-injury compressive force (2N-3N). After injury, mice cohorts were given saline (0.05 mL) and buprenorphine (0.05 mg/kg) and returned to normal cage activity as previously described [34–36,74]. All animal experiments were approved by the Lawrence Livermore National Laboratory and University of California, Davis Institutional Animal Care and Use Committee (approved on 14/07/2016), and conformed to the Guide for the care and use of laboratory animals under protocol 250.

4.2. Micro-Computed Tomography (μCT)

Injured joints, contralateral joints from injured mice, and bilateral joints from uninjured mice were collected six weeks post injury for all groups. Samples were dissected and fixed for 72 h at 4 °C using 10% neutral buffer formalin; samples were stored in 70% ethanol at 4 °C until scanned. Whole knees were scanned using a SCANO μCT 35 (Bassersdorf, Switzerland) according to the rodent bone structure analysis guidelines (X-ray tube potential = 55 kVp, intensity = 114 mA, 10 μm isotropic nominal voxel size, integration time = 900 ms) [34]. Trabecular bone in the distal femoral epiphysis was analyzed by manually drawing contours on 2D transverse slides to designate the region of trabecular bone enclosed by the growth plate and subchondral cortical bone plate. We quantified trabecular bone volume fraction (BV/TV), trabecular thickness (Tb.Th), trabecular number (Tb.N), and trabecular separation (Tb.Sp) [38]. Mineralized osteophyte volume in injured and contralateral joints was also quantified by drawing contours around all heterotopic mineralized tissue attached to the distal femur and proximal tibia as well as the whole fabellae, menisci, and patella. Total mineralized osteophyte volume was then determined as the volumetric difference in mineralized tissue between injured and uninjured joints. Statistical analysis was performed using two-way ANOVA and a Student's t-test with a two-tailed distribution, with two-sample equal variance (homoscedastic test). For all tests, $p < 0.05$ was considered statistically significant.

4.3. Histological Assessment of Articular Cartilage and Joint Degeneration

VEH-, AB-, and LPS-treated injured, contralateral, and uninjured joints were dissected six weeks post injury, then fixed, dehydrated, paraffin-embedded, and sectioned as previously described [74]. The cartilage was visualized in sagittal 6-μm paraffin serial using Safranin-O (0.1%, Sigma; S8884; St. Louis, MO, USA) and Fast Green (0.05%, Sigma; F7252; St. Louis, MO, USA) as previously described [35]. OA severity was evaluated using a modified Osteoarthritis Research Society International (OARSI) scoring scale as previously described [85]. Cartilage scoring began ~0.4 mm out from the start of synovium to the articular cartilage. Blinded slides were evaluated by seven scientists (six with and one without expertise in OA) utilizing modified (sagittal) OARSI scoring parameters due to the severe phenotype caused by TC loading-destabilization that promotes mechanical-induced tibial degeneration on injured joints [74,85]. Modified scores: (0) for intact cartilage staining with strong red staining on the femoral condyle and tibia; (1) minor fibrillation without cartilage loss; (2) clefts below the superficial zone; (3) cartilage thinning on the femoral condyle and tibia; (4) lack of staining on the femoral condyle and tibia; (5) staining present on 90% of the entire femoral condyle with tibial degeneration; (6) staining present on over 80% of the femoral condyle with tibial degeneration; (7) staining present on 75% of the femoral condyle with tibial degeneration; (8) staining present on over 50% of the femora condyle with tibial degeneration; (9) staining present in 25% of the femoral condyle with tibial degeneration; (10) staining present in less than 10% of the femoral condyle with tibial degeneration.

4.4. Immunofluorescent Staining

Six-micrometer sections from injured samples from both treatment groups of *C57Bl/6J* were used. Unitrieve was used as an antigen retrieval method for 30 min at 65 °C [86]. Primary antibodies: Anti-F4/80 (Abcam, ab16911(1:50)), Anti-CD206 (Abcam, ab64693(1:500)), and Anti-iNOS (Abcam, ab15323(1:100)) were used and incubated overnight at room temperature in a dark humid chamber. Negative control slides were incubated with secondary antibody only. Stained slides were mounted with Prolong Gold with DAPI (Molecular Probes, Eugene, OR, USA). Slides were imaged using a Leica DM5000 microscope. ImagePro Plus V7.0 Software and a QIClick CCD camera (QImaging, Surrey, BC, Canada) were used for imaging and photo editing.

4.5. RNA Sequencing and Data Analysis

C57Bl/6J injured and uninjured joints from VEH-, AB-, and LPS-treated male and female mice were collected 24 h after injury ($n >= 4$). Joints were dissected and cut at the edges of the joint region with small traces of soft tissue to preserve the articular integrity. RNA was isolated and sequenced as previously described [36]. RNA-seq data quality was checked using FastQC software (version 0.11.5). Sequence reads were aligned to the mouse reference genome (mm10) using STAR (version 2.6). After read mapping, 'featureCounts' from Rsubread package (version 1.30.5) was used to perform read summarization to generate gene-wise read counts. Differentially expressed genes (DEGs) were identified using edgeR (version 3.22.3). Genes with a false discovery rate (FDR) corrected p-value less than 0.05 and fold change greater than 1.5 were considered as DEGs. Heatmaps were generated using heatmap.2 function in R package 'gplots'.

5. Conclusions

Chronic antibiotic administration known to deplete some gram negative bacteria, primarily Bacteroidetes, while expanding the Proteobacteria phylum provided protective benefit from the development of post-traumatic osteoarthritis after joint injury.

Author Contributions: Study design: M.E.M. and G.G.L.; Data acquisition: M.E.M., D.K.M., N.R.H., S.A.M., E.A.K., and B.A.C. Data analysis and interpretation: M.E.M., A.S., B.A.C., and G.G.L., M.E.M. and G.G.L. wrote the manuscript. All authors have read and agreed to the published version of the manuscript.

Funding: M.E.M: D.K.M, A.S, N.R.H and G.G.L were supported by Lawrence Livermore National Laboratory LDRD grants 20-LW-002 and 16-ERD-007. G.G.L was also supported in part by DOD grant PR180268.

Acknowledgments: This work was performed under the auspices of the U.S. Department of Energy by Lawrence Livermore National Laboratory under Contract DE-AC52-07NA27344. LLNL-JRNL-812395.

Conflicts of Interest: The authors declare no conflict of interest.

Abbreviations

AB	Antibiotic group
ACL	Anterior cruciate ligament
BV.TV	Subchondral bone volume
ECM	Extracellular matrix
LPS	Lipopolysaccharide group
MMP	Metalloproteinase
OA	Osteoarthritis
PTOA	Post-traumatic osteoarthritis
RNA-seq	RNA sequencing
Tb.N	Trabecular number
Tb.Sp	Trabecular spacing
Tb.Th	Trabecular thickness
TC	Tibial compression
μCT	Microcomputed tomography
VEH	Vehicle group

References

1. Bull, M.J.; Plummer, N.T. Part 1: The Human Gut Microbiome in Health and Disease. *Integr. Med. (Encinitas)* **2014**, *13*, 17–22. [PubMed]
2. Sender, R.; Fuchs, S.; Milo, R. Revised Estimates for the Number of Human and Bacteria Cells in the Body. *PLoS Biol.* **2016**, *14*, e1002533. [CrossRef] [PubMed]
3. Van den Elsen, L.W.J.; Garssen, J.; Burcelin, R.; Verhasselt, V. Shaping the Gut Microbiota by Breastfeeding: The Gateway to Allergy Prevention? *Front. Pediatr.* **2019**, *7*, 47. [CrossRef]
4. Tanaka, M.; Nakayama, J. Development of the gut microbiota in infancy and its impact on health in later life *Allergol. Int.* **2017**, *66*, 515–522. [CrossRef] [PubMed]
5. Clemente, J.C.; Ursell, L.K.; Parfrey, L.W.; Knight, R. The impact of the gut microbiota on human health: An integrative view. *Cell* **2012**, *148*, 1258–1270. [CrossRef] [PubMed]
6. Liang, D.; Leung, R.K.-K.; Guan, W.; Au, W.W. Involvement of gut microbiome in human health and disease: Brief overview, knowledge gaps and research opportunities. *Gut Pathog.* **2018**, *10*, 3. [CrossRef]
7. Mohajeri, M.H.; Brummer, R.J.M.; Rastall, R.A.; Weersma, R.K.; Harmsen, H.J.M.; Faas, M.; Eggersdorfer, M. The role of the microbiome for human health: From basic science to clinical applications. *Eur. J. Nutr.* **2018**, *57*, 1–14. [CrossRef]
8. McAleer, J.P.; Vella, A.T. Understanding how lipopolysaccharide impacts CD4 T-cell immunity. *Crit. Rev. Immunol.* **2008**, *28*, 281–299.
9. Bahar, B.; O'Doherty, J.V.; Vigors, S.; Sweeney, T. Activation of inflammatory immune gene cascades by lipopolysaccharide (LPS) in the porcine colonic tissue ex-vivo model. *Clin. Exp. Immunol.* **2016**, *186*, 266–276. [CrossRef]

10. Mendez, M.E.; Sebastian, A.; Murugesh, D.K.; Hum, N.R.; McCool, J.L.; Hsia, A.W.; Christiansen, B.A.; Loots, G.G. LPS-induced Inflammation Prior to Injury Exacerbates the Development of Post-Traumatic Osteoarthritis in Mice. *J. Bone Miner. Res.* **2020**. [CrossRef]
11. Soares, J.-B.; Pimentel-Nunes, P.; Roncon-Albuquerque, R.; Leite-Moreira, A. The role of lipopolysaccharide/toll-like receptor 4 signaling in chronic liver diseases. *Hepatol. Int.* **2010**, *4*, 659–672. [CrossRef] [PubMed]
12. Calil, I.L.; Zarpelon, A.C.; Guerrero, A.T.G.; Alves-Filho, J.C.; Ferreira, S.H.; Cunha, F.Q.; Cunha, T.M.; Verri, W.A. Lipopolysaccharide induces inflammatory hyperalgesia triggering a TLR4/MyD88-dependent cytokine cascade in the mice paw. *PLoS ONE* **2014**, *9*, e90013. [CrossRef] [PubMed]
13. Mogensen, T.H. Pathogen recognition and inflammatory signaling in innate immune defenses. *Clin. Microbiol. Rev.* **2009**, *22*, 240–273. [CrossRef] [PubMed]
14. Maslanik, T.; Tannura, K.; Mahaffey, L.; Loughridge, A.B.; Beninson, L.; Benninson, L.; Ursell, L.; Greenwood, B.N.; Knight, R.; Fleshner, M. Commensal bacteria and MAMPs are necessary for stress-induced increases in IL-1β and IL-18 but not IL-6, IL-10 or MCP-1. *PLoS ONE* **2012**, *7*, e50636. [CrossRef] [PubMed]
15. Chen, Y.; Haines, C.J.; Gutcher, I.; Hochweller, K.; Blumenschein, W.M.; McClanahan, T.; Hämmerling, G.; Li, M.O.; Cua, D.J.; McGeachy, M.J. Foxp3(+) regulatory T cells promote T helper 17 cell development in vivo through regulation of interleukin-2. *Immunity* **2011**, *34*, 409–421. [CrossRef] [PubMed]
16. Chu, H.; Mazmanian, S.K. Innate immune recognition of the microbiota promotes host-microbial symbiosis. *Nat. Immunol.* **2013**, *14*, 668–675. [CrossRef] [PubMed]
17. Kim, C.H. Host and microbial factors in regulation of T cells in the intestine. *Front. Immunol.* **2013**, *4*, 141. [CrossRef]
18. Kitaura, H.; Kimura, K.; Ishida, M.; Kohara, H.; Yoshimatsu, M.; Takano-Yamamoto, T. Immunological Reaction in TNF-α-Mediated Osteoclast Formation and Bone Resorption In Vitro and In Vivo. *Clin. Dev. Immunol.* **2013**, *2013*, 181849. [CrossRef]
19. McCabe, L.R.; Irwin, R.; Schaefer, L.; Britton, R.A. Probiotic use decreases intestinal inflammation and increases bone density in healthy male but not female mice. *J. Cell. Physiol.* **2013**, *228*, 1793–1798. [CrossRef]
20. Collins, F.L.; Schepper, J.D.; Rios-Arce, N.D.; Steury, M.D.; Kang, H.J.; Mallin, H.; Schoenherr, D.; Camfield, G.; Chishti, S.; McCabe, L.R.; et al. Immunology of Gut-Bone Signaling. *Adv. Exp. Med. Biol.* **2017**, *1033*, 59–94. [CrossRef]
21. Teramachi, J.; Inagaki, Y.; Shinohara, H.; Okamura, H.; Yang, D.; Ochiai, K.; Baba, R.; Morimoto, H.; Nagata, T.; Haneji, T. PKR regulates LPS-induced osteoclast formation and bone destruction in vitro and in vivo. *Oral. Dis.* **2017**, *23*, 181–188. [CrossRef] [PubMed]
22. Iqbal, J.; Yuen, T.; Sun, L.; Zaidi, M. From the gut to the strut: Where inflammation reigns, bone abstains. *J. Clin. Investig.* **2016**, *126*, 2045–2048. [CrossRef] [PubMed]
23. Charles, J.F.; Ermann, J.; Aliprantis, A.O. The intestinal microbiome and skeletal fitness: Connecting bugs and bones. *Clin. Immunol.* **2015**, *159*, 163–169. [CrossRef] [PubMed]
24. Schepper, J.D.; Collins, F.L.; Rios-Arce, N.D.; Raehtz, S.; Schaefer, L.; Gardinier, J.D.; Britton, R.A.; Parameswaran, N.; McCabe, L.R. Probiotic Lactobacillus reuteri Prevents Postantibiotic Bone Loss by Reducing Intestinal Dysbiosis and Preventing Barrier Disruption. *J. Bone Miner. Res.* **2019**, *34*, 681–698. [CrossRef] [PubMed]
25. Schott, E.M.; Farnsworth, C.W.; Grier, A.; Lillis, J.A.; Soniwala, S.; Dadourian, G.H.; Bell, R.D.; Doolittle, M.L.; Villani, D.A.; Awad, H.; et al. Targeting the gut microbiome to treat the osteoarthritis of obesity. *JCI Insight* **2018**, *3*. [CrossRef]
26. Guss, J.D.; Ziemian, S.N.; Luna, M.; Sandoval, T.N.; Holyoak, D.T.; Guisado, G.G.; Roubert, S.; Callahan, R.L.; Brito, I.L.; van der Meulen, M.C.H.; et al. The effects of metabolic syndrome, obesity, and the gut microbiome on load-induced osteoarthritis. *Osteoarthr. Cartil.* **2019**, *27*, 129–139. [CrossRef]
27. Ulici, V.; Kelley, K.L.; Azcarate-Peril, M.A.; Cleveland, R.J.; Sartor, R.B.; Schwartz, T.A.; Loeser, R.F. Osteoarthritis induced by destabilization of the medial meniscus is reduced in germ-free mice. *Osteoarthr. Cartil.* **2018**, *26*, 1098–1109. [CrossRef]
28. Szychlinska, M.A.; Di Rosa, M.; Castorina, A.; Mobasheri, A.; Musumeci, G. A correlation between intestinal microbiota dysbiosis and osteoarthritis. *Heliyon* **2019**, *5*, e01134. [CrossRef]
29. Hahn, A.K.; Wallace, C.W.; Welhaven, H.D.; Brooks, E.; McAlpine, M.; Christiansen, B.A.; Walk, S.T.; June, R.K. The microbiome mediates subchondral bone loss and metabolomic changes after acute joint trauma. *bioRxiv* **2020**, 2020.05.08.084822. [CrossRef]

30. Carbone, A.; Rodeo, S. Review of current understanding of post-traumatic osteoarthritis resulting from sports injuries. *J. Orthop. Res.* **2017**, *35*, 397–405. [CrossRef]
31. Hardcastle, S.A.; Dieppe, P.; Gregson, C.L.; Davey Smith, G.; Tobias, J.H. Osteoarthritis and bone mineral density: Are strong bones bad for joints? *Bonekey Rep.* **2015**, *4*, 624. [CrossRef] [PubMed]
32. *Outpatient Antibiotic Prescriptions — United States, 2017*; Center for Disease Control and Prevention: Atlanta, GA, USA, 2017.
33. Christiansen, B.A.; Anderson, M.J.; Lee, C.A.; Williams, J.C.; Yik, J.H.N.; Haudenschild, D.R. Musculoskeletal changes following non-invasive knee injury using a novel mouse model of post-traumatic osteoarthritis. *Osteoarthr. Cartil.* **2012**, *20*, 773–782. [CrossRef] [PubMed]
34. Lockwood, K.A.; Chu, B.T.; Anderson, M.J.; Haudenschild, D.R.; Christiansen, B.A. Comparison of loading rate-dependent injury modes in a murine model of post-traumatic osteoarthritis. *J. Orthop. Res.* **2014**, *32*, 79–88. [CrossRef] [PubMed]
35. Chang, J.C.; Christiansen, B.A.; Murugesh, D.K.; Sebastian, A.; Hum, N.R.; Collette, N.M.; Hatsell, S.; Economides, A.N.; Blanchette, C.D.; Loots, G.G. SOST/Sclerostin Improves Posttraumatic Osteoarthritis and Inhibits MMP2/3 Expression After Injury: SOST OVEREXPRESSION IMPROVES PTOA OUTCOMES. *J. Bone Miner. Res.* **2018**, *33*, 1105–1113. [CrossRef]
36. Sebastian, A.; Chang, J.C.; Mendez, M.E.; Murugesh, D.K.; Hatsell, S.; Economides, A.N.; Christiansen, B.A.; Loots, G.G. Comparative Transcriptomics Identifies Novel Genes and Pathways Involved in Post-Traumatic Osteoarthritis Development and Progression. *Int. J. Mol. Sci.* **2018**, *19*, 2657. [CrossRef] [PubMed]
37. Sebastian, A.; Murugesh, D.K.; Mendez, M.E.; Hum, N.R.; Rios-Arce, N.D.; McCool, J.L.; Christiansen, B.A.; Loots, G.G. Global Gene Expression Analysis Identifies Age-Related Differences in Knee Joint Transcriptome during the Development of Post-Traumatic Osteoarthritis in Mice. *Int. J. Mol. Sci.* **2020**, *21*, 364. [CrossRef]
38. Bouxsein, M.L.; Boyd, S.K.; Christiansen, B.A.; Guldberg, R.E.; Jepsen, K.J.; Müller, R. Guidelines for assessment of bone microstructure in rodents using micro-computed tomography. *J. Bone Miner. Res.* **2010**, *25*, 1468–1486. [CrossRef]
39. Klar, A.S.; Michalak-Mićka, K.; Biedermann, T.; Simmen-Meuli, C.; Reichmann, E.; Meuli, M. Characterization of M1 and M2 polarization of macrophages in vascularized human dermo-epidermal skin substitutes in vivo. *Pediatr. Surg. Int.* **2018**, *34*, 129–135. [CrossRef]
40. Fairweather, D.; Cihakova, D. Alternatively activated macrophages in infection and autoimmunity. *J. Autoimmun.* **2009**, *33*, 222–230. [CrossRef]
41. Wynn, T.A.; Barron, L.; Thompson, R.W.; Madala, S.K.; Wilson, M.S.; Cheever, A.W.; Ramalingam, T. Quantitative Assessment of Macrophage Functions in Repair and Fibrosis. In *Current Protocols in Immunology*; Coligan, J.E., Bierer, B.E., Margulies, D.H., Shevach, E.M., Strober, W., Eds.; John Wiley & Sons, Inc.: Hoboken, NJ, USA, 2011; ISBN 978-0-471-14273-7.
42. Culemann, S.; Grüneboom, A.; Nicolás-Ávila, J.Á.; Weidner, D.; Lämmle, K.F.; Rothe, T.; Quintana, J.A.; Kirchner, P.; Krljanac, B.; Eberhardt, M.; et al. Locally renewing resident synovial macrophages provide a protective barrier for the joint. *Nature* **2019**, *572*, 670–675. [CrossRef]
43. Dos Anjos Cassado, A. F4/80 as a Major Macrophage Marker: The Case of the Peritoneum and Spleen. *Results Prob. Cell Differ.* **2017**, *62*, 161–179. [CrossRef]
44. Lubbers, R.; van Schaarenburg, R.A.; Kwekkeboom, J.C.; Levarht, E.W.N.; Bakker, A.M.; Mahdad, R.; Monteagudo, S.; Cherifi, C.; Lories, R.J.; Toes, R.E.M.; et al. Complement component C1q is produced by isolated articular chondrocytes. *Osteoarthr. Cartil.* **2020**, *28*, 675–684. [CrossRef] [PubMed]
45. Jarlhelt, I.; Genster, N.; Kirketerp-Møller, N.; Skjoedt, M.-O.; Garred, P. The ficolin response to LPS challenge in mice. *Mol. Immunol.* **2019**, *108*, 121–127. [CrossRef] [PubMed]
46. Lin, S.-C.; Kuo, C.-C.; Chan, C.-H. Association of a BTLA gene polymorphism with the risk of rheumatoid arthritis. *J. Biomed. Sci.* **2006**, *13*, 853–860. [CrossRef] [PubMed]
47. Wang, X.; Ning, Y.; Guo, X. Integrative meta-analysis of differentially expressed genes in osteoarthritis using microarray technology. *Mol. Med. Rep.* **2015**, *12*, 3439–3445. [CrossRef]
48. Smulski, C.R.; Eibel, H. BAFF and BAFF-Receptor in B Cell Selection and Survival. *Front. Immunol.* **2018** *9*, 2285. [CrossRef]
49. Bacchelli, C.; Moretti, F.A.; Carmo, M.; Adams, S.; Stanescu, H.C.; Pearce, K.; Madkaikar, M.; Gilmour, K.C.; Nicholas, A.K.; Woods, C.G.; et al. Mutations in linker for activation of T cells (LAT) lead to a novel form of severe combined immunodeficiency. *J. Allergy Clin. Immunol.* **2017**, *139*, 634–642.e5. [CrossRef]

50. Gotoh, H.; Kawaguchi, Y.; Harigai, M.; Hara, M.; Saito, S.; Yamaguchi, T.; Shimada, K.; Kawamoto, M.; Tomatsu, T.; Kamatani, N. Increased CD40 expression on articular chondrocytes from patients with rheumatoid arthritis: Contribution to production of cytokines and matrix metalloproteinases. *J. Rheumatol.* **2004**, *31*, 1506–1512. [PubMed]
51. Perdigones, N.; Vigo, A.G.; Lamas, J.R.; Martínez, A.; Balsa, A.; Pascual-Salcedo, D.; de la Concha, E.G.; Fernández-Gutiérrez, B.; Urcelay, E. Evidence of epistasis between TNFRSF14 and TNFRSF6B polymorphisms in patients with rheumatoid arthritis. *Arthritis Rheum.* **2010**, *62*, 705–710. [CrossRef]
52. Liu, M.F.; Kohsaka, H.; Sakurai, H.; Azuma, M.; Okumura, K.; Saito, I.; Miyasaka, N. The presence of costimulatory molecules CD86 and CD28 in rheumatoid arthritis synovium. *Arthritis Rheum.* **1996**, *39*, 110–114. [CrossRef]
53. Gwon, S.-Y.; Rhee, K.-J.; Sung, H.J. Gene and Protein Expression Profiles in a Mouse Model of Collagen-Induced Arthritis. *Int. J. Med. Sci.* **2018**, *15*, 77–85. [CrossRef] [PubMed]
54. Alexopoulos, L.G.; Youn, I.; Bonaldo, P.; Guilak, F. Developmental and osteoarthritic changes in Col6a1-knockout mice: Biomechanics of type VI collagen in the cartilage pericellular matrix. *Arthritis Rheum.* **2009**, *60*, 771–779. [CrossRef] [PubMed]
55. Lv, M.; Zhou, Y.; Polson, S.W.; Wan, L.Q.; Wang, M.; Han, L.; Wang, L.; Lu, X.L. Identification of Chondrocyte Genes and Signaling Pathways in Response to Acute Joint Inflammation. *Sci. Rep.* **2019**, *9*, 93. [CrossRef] [PubMed]
56. Xu, S.; Yu, J.; Wang, Z.; Ni, C.; Xia, L.; Tang, T. SOX11 promotes osteoarthritis through induction of TNF-α. *Pathol. Res. Pract.* **2019**, *215*, 152442. [CrossRef] [PubMed]
57. Teufel, S.; Köckemann, P.; König, U.; Hartmann, C. Loss of Wnt9a and Wnt4 causes degenerative joint alterations. *Osteoarthr. Cartil.* **2018**, *26*, S94–S95. [CrossRef]
58. Fu, L.; Hu, Y.; Song, M.; Liu, Z.; Zhang, W.; Yu, F.-X.; Wu, J.; Wang, S.; Izpisua Belmonte, J.C.; Chan, P.; et al. Up-regulation of FOXD1 by YAP alleviates senescence and osteoarthritis. *PLoS Biol.* **2019**, *17*, e3000201. [CrossRef]
59. Zhang, Q.; Fang, X.; Zhao, W.; Liang, Q. The transcriptional coactivator YAP1 is overexpressed in osteoarthritis and promotes its progression by interacting with Beclin-1. *Gene* **2019**, *689*, 210–219. [CrossRef]
60. Chamberlain, N.D.; Vila, O.M.; Volin, M.V.; Volkov, S.; Pope, R.M.; Swedler, W.; Mandelin, A.M.; Shahrara, S. TLR5, a novel and unidentified inflammatory mediator in rheumatoid arthritis that correlates with disease activity score and joint TNF-α levels. *J. Immunol.* **2012**, *189*, 475–483. [CrossRef]
61. Zhang, X.; Chen, L.; Dang, W.-Q.; Cao, M.-F.; Xiao, J.-F.; Lv, S.-Q.; Jiang, W.-J.; Yao, X.-H.; Lu, H.-M.; Miao, J.-Y.; et al. CCL8 secreted by tumor-associated macrophages promotes invasion and stemness of glioblastoma cells via ERK1/2 signaling. *Lab. Investig.* **2020**, *100*, 619–629. [CrossRef]
62. Mödinger, Y.; Rapp, A.; Pazmandi, J.; Vikman, A.; Holzmann, K.; Haffner-Luntzer, M.; Huber-Lang, M.; Ignatius, A. C5aR1 interacts with TLR2 in osteoblasts and stimulates the osteoclast-inducing chemokine CXCL10. *J. Cell. Mol. Med.* **2018**, *22*, 6002–6014. [CrossRef]
63. Ha, H.; Debnath, B.; Neamati, N. Role of the CXCL8-CXCR1/2 Axis in Cancer and Inflammatory Diseases. *Theranostics* **2017**, *7*, 1543–1588. [CrossRef] [PubMed]
64. Wang, R.; Zhang, S.; Previn, R.; Chen, D.; Jin, Y.; Zhou, G. Role of Forkhead Box O Transcription Factors in Oxidative Stress-Induced Chondrocyte Dysfunction: Possible Therapeutic Target for Osteoarthritis? *Int. J. Mol. Sci.* **2018**, *19*, 3794. [CrossRef] [PubMed]
65. Yee, C.S.; Manilay, J.O.; Chang, J.C.; Hum, N.R.; Murugesh, D.K.; Bajwa, J.; Mendez, M.E.; Economides, A.E.; Horan, D.J.; Robling, A.G.; et al. Conditional Deletion of Sost in MSC-Derived Lineages Identifies Specific Cell-Type Contributions to Bone Mass and B-Cell Development. *J. Bone Miner. Res.* **2018**, *33*, 1748–1759. [CrossRef] [PubMed]
66. Zhang, R.; Yang, X.; Wang, J.; Han, L.; Yang, A.; Zhang, J.; Zhang, D.; Li, B.; Li, Z.; Xiong, Y. Identification of potential biomarkers for differential diagnosis between rheumatoid arthritis and osteoarthritis via integrative genome-wide gene expression profiling analysis. *Mol. Med. Rep.* **2018**. [CrossRef] [PubMed]
67. Weiss, A.; Leinwand, L.A. The mammalian myosin heavy chain gene family. *Annu. Rev. Cell Dev. Biol.* **1996**, *12*, 417–439. [CrossRef]
68. Rossi, A.C.; Mammucari, C.; Argentini, C.; Reggiani, C.; Schiaffino, S. Two novel/ancient myosins in mammalian skeletal muscles: MYH14/7b and MYH15 are expressed in extraocular muscles and muscle spindles. *J. Physiol. (Lond.)* **2010**, *588*, 353–364. [CrossRef]

69. Arvanitidis, A.; Henriksen, K.; Karsdal, M.A.; Nedergaard, A. Neo-epitope Peptides as Biomarkers of Disease Progression for Muscular Dystrophies and Other Myopathies. *J. Neuromuscul. Dis.* **2016**, *3*, 333–346. [CrossRef]
70. Chou, C.-H.; Lee, C.-H.; Lu, L.-S.; Song, I.-W.; Chuang, H.-P.; Kuo, S.-Y.; Wu, J.-Y.; Chen, Y.-T.; Kraus, V.B.; Wu, C.-C.; et al. Direct assessment of articular cartilage and underlying subchondral bone reveals a progressive gene expression change in human osteoarthritic knees. *Osteoarthr. Cartil.* **2013**, *21*, 450–461. [CrossRef]
71. Lee, Y.H.; Sharma, A.R.; Jagga, S.; Lee, S.S.; Nam, J.S. Differential Expression Patterns of Rspondin Family and Leucine-Rich Repeat-Containing G-Protein Coupled Receptors in Chondrocytes and Osteoblasts. *Cell J.* **2021**, *22*, 437–449. [CrossRef]
72. Rios-Arce, N.D.; Schepper, J.D.; Dagenais, A.; Schaefer, L.; Daly-Seiler, C.S.; Gardinier, J.D.; Britton, R.A.; McCabe, L.R.; Parameswaran, N. Post-antibiotic gut dysbiosis-induced trabecular bone loss is dependent on lymphocytes. *Bone* **2020**, *134*, 115269. [CrossRef]
73. Kim, S.-J.; Chen, Z.; Chamberlain, N.D.; Essani, A.B.; Volin, M.V.; Amin, M.A.; Volkov, S.; Gravallese, E.M.; Arami, S.; Swedler, W.; et al. Ligation of TLR5 promotes myeloid cell infiltration and differentiation into mature osteoclasts in rheumatoid arthritis and experimental arthritis. *J. Immunol.* **2014**, *193*, 3902–3913. [CrossRef] [PubMed]
74. Chang, J.C.; Sebastian, A.; Murugesh, D.K.; Hatsell, S.; Economides, A.N.; Christiansen, B.A.; Loots, G.G. Global molecular changes in a tibial compression induced ACL rupture model of post-traumatic osteoarthritis: GLOBAL MOLECULAR CHANGES AFTER ACL INJURY. *J. Orthop. Res.* **2017**, *35*, 474–485. [CrossRef]
75. Paiva, K.B.S.; Granjeiro, J.M. Bone tissue remodeling and development: Focus on matrix metalloproteinase functions. *Arch. Biochem. Biophys.* **2014**, *561*, 74–87. [CrossRef] [PubMed]
76. Nakatani, T.; Chen, T.; Partridge, N.C. MMP-13 is one of the critical mediators of the effect of HDAC4 deletion on the skeleton. *Bone* **2016**, *90*, 142–151. [CrossRef] [PubMed]
77. Klein, T.; Bischoff, R. Physiology and pathophysiology of matrix metalloproteases. *Amino Acids* **2011**, *41*, 271–290. [CrossRef]
78. Kaushik, D.; Mohan, M.; Borade, D.M.; Swami, O.C. Ampicillin: Rise fall and resurgence. *J. Clin. Diagn. Res.* **2014**, *8*, ME01–ME03. [CrossRef]
79. Chudobova, D.; Dostalova, S.; Blazkova, I.; Michalek, P.; Ruttkay-Nedecky, B.; Sklenar, M.; Nejdl, L.; Kudr, J.; Gumulec, J.; Tmejova, K.; et al. Effect of ampicillin, streptomycin, penicillin and tetracycline on metal resistant and non-resistant Staphylococcus aureus. *Int. J. Environ. Res. Public Health* **2014**, *11*, 3233–3255. [CrossRef]
80. Waksman, S.A.; Lechevalier, H.A.; Harris, D.A. Neomycin-production and antibiotic properties. *J. Clin. Investig.* **1949**, *28*, 934–939. [CrossRef]
81. Masur, H.; Whelton, P.K.; Whelton, A. Neomycin toxicity revisited. *Arch. Surg.* **1976**, *111*, 822–825. [CrossRef]
82. Macdonald, R.H.; Beck, M. Neomycin: A review with particular reference to dermatological usage. *Clin. Exp. Dermatol.* **1983**, *8*, 249–258. [CrossRef]
83. Christiansen, B.A.; Guilak, F.; Lockwood, K.A.; Olson, S.A.; Pitsillides, A.A.; Sandell, L.J.; Silva, M.J.; van der Meulen, M.C.H.; Haudenschild, D.R. Non-invasive mouse models of post-traumatic osteoarthritis. *Osteoarthr. Cartil.* **2015**, *23*, 1627–1638. [CrossRef] [PubMed]
84. Prys-Roberts, C. Isoflurane. *Br. J. Anaesth* **1981**, *53*, 1243–1245. [CrossRef] [PubMed]
85. Glasson, S.S.; Chambers, M.G.; Van Den Berg, W.B.; Little, C.B. The OARSI histopathology initiative-recommendations for histological assessments of osteoarthritis in the mouse. *Osteoarthr. Cartil.* **2010**, *18* (Suppl. 3), S17–S23. [CrossRef]
86. Yee, C.S.; Xie, L.; Hatsell, S.; Hum, N.; Murugesh, D.; Economides, A.N.; Loots, G.G.; Collette, N.M. Sclerostin antibody treatment improves fracture outcomes in a Type I diabetic mouse model. *Bone* **2016**, *82*, 122–134. [CrossRef] [PubMed]

International Journal of
Molecular Sciences

MDPI

Article

Ameliorated Autoimmune Arthritis and Impaired B Cell Receptor-Mediated Ca^{2+} Influx in Nkx2-3 Knock-out Mice

Esam Khanfar [1], Katalin Olasz [1], Fanni Gábris [1,2], Erzsébet Gajdócsi [1], Bálint Botz [3,4], Tamás Kiss [4,5], Réka Kugyelka [1], Tímea Berki [1], Péter Balogh [1,2] and Ferenc Boldizsár [1,*]

1 Department of Immunology and Biotechnology, Medical School, University of Pécs, 7624 Pécs, Hungary; esam.khanfar@pte.hu (E.K.); olasz.katalin@pte.hu (K.O.); gabris.fanni@pte.hu (F.G.); gajdocsi.erzsebet@pte.hu (E.G.); reka.kugyelka@gmail.com (R.K.); berki.timea@pte.hu (T.B.); balogh.peter@pte.hu (P.B.)

2 Lymphoid Organogenesis Research Group, János Szentágothai Research Centre, University of Pécs, 7624 Pécs, Hungary

3 Department of Medical Imaging, Medical School, University of Pécs, 7624 Pécs, Hungary; balint.botz@gmail.com

4 Molecular Pharmacology Research Group, János Szentágothai Research Centre and Centre for Neuroscience, University of Pécs, 7624 Pécs, Hungary; kiss891012@gmail.com

5 Department of Pharmacology and Pharmacotherapy, Medical School, University of Pécs, 7624 Pécs, Hungary

* Correspondence: boldizsar.ferenc@pte.hu; Tel.: +36-72-536-288

Received: 23 July 2020; Accepted: 25 August 2020; Published: 26 August 2020

Abstract: B cells play a crucial role in the pathogenesis of rheumatoid arthritis. In Nkx2-3-deficient mice (Nkx2-$3^{-/-}$) the spleen's histological structure is fundamentally changed; therefore, B cell homeostasis is seriously disturbed. Based on this, we were curious, whether autoimmune arthritis could be induced in Nkx2-$3^{-/-}$ mice and how B cell activation and function were affected. We induced arthritis with immunization of recombinant human proteoglycan aggrecan G1 domain in Nkx2-$3^{-/-}$ and control BALB/c mice. We followed the clinical picture, characterized the radiological changes, the immune response, and intracellular Ca^{2+} signaling of B cells. Incidence of the autoimmune arthritis was lower, and the disease severity was milder in Nkx2-$3^{-/-}$ mice than in control BALB/c mice. The radiological changes were in line with the clinical picture. In Nkx2-$3^{-/-}$ mice, we measured decreased antigen-induced proliferation and cytokine production in spleen cell cultures; in the sera, we found less anti-CCP-IgG2a, IL-17 and IFNγ, but more IL-1β, IL-4 and IL-6. B cells isolated from the lymph nodes of Nkx2-$3^{-/-}$ mice showed decreased intracellular Ca^{2+} signaling compared to those isolated from BALB/c mice. Our findings show that the transcription factor Nkx2-3 might regulate the development of autoimmune arthritis most likely through modifying B cell activation.

Keywords: autoimmune arthritis; Nkx2-3; B cell activation

1. Introduction

Rheumatoid arthritis (RA) is the most frequent systemic autoimmune disease in the Western-European and North-American countries [1]. The disease primarily affects the small joints, where a chronic, progressive inflammation leads to cartilage and bone destruction, associated with severe pain and disability [1]. Despite intensive research, no definitive cause(s) of the disease are known and therefore, unfortunately, no curative treatment is available to date [2]. So, finding the potential pathogenic factors and mechanisms in the background of RA is of utmost importance because they might provide a basis for future therapies. In this regard, mouse models of RA are extremely useful because several aspects of the disease can be studied more efficiently than in humans [3]. Especially those models are beneficial, which share many features of RA, like proteoglycan-aggrecan-induced arthritis (PGIA) [4] and its refined version, recombinant human G1 domain-induced arthritis (GIA) [5]. (P)GIA is similar to RA in many respect: (i) clinical picture [4,5], (ii) histological changes [4,5], (iii) radiological changes [4,6], (iv) autoreactive T cell activation [7], (v) Th1 and Th17 differentiation [8], (vi) production of autoantibodies (both against the mouse cartilage aggrecan and citrullinated antigens) [5] and (vii) proinflammatory cytokines was described [5].

RA is a chronic, progressive disease, usually lasting for decades [2,9,10]. According to our present view on RA pathogenesis, the patients are diagnosed only in the final inflammatory/destructive phase of the disease, when the typical symptoms (pain, swollen joints) appear [10]. However, the loss of tolerance and the development of symptomless autoimmunity precedes this usually by several years [10]. The dysregulation of the immune system might be the result of the interplay between genetic (*MHC* and *non-MHC* genes), epigenetic and environmental factors (infections, diet, smoking) [9,10]. The development of autoreactive T cells and starting of autoantibody production might be the key elements of this preclinical/latent phase of RA [10] and likewise, during the initiation period of its model PGIA [8]. These processes most likely take place not only locally, in the joints, but, importantly, in the lymphatic tissues like the lymph nodes and the spleen [2,8].

The spleen is well known for its function in the degradation of red blood cells and the immune response against blood-borne antigens, especially those of encapsulated bacteria [11,12]. Moreover, the spleen is critical for B cell development and, uniquely, all major peripheral B cell populations (B1a-, B1b-, B2-, marginal zone (MZ) B cells) can be found here. Not much is known about the exact role of the spleen in RA, however, based on mouse models of GIA and collagen-induced arthritis (CIA), we might suspect a potential involvement: increased size and more activated cells can be detected in spleens from both GIA (own unpublished observation) or CIA mice [13].

Nirenberg-Kim (NK) 2 homeobox 3 (Nkx2-3) is a homeodomain transcription factor, which is essential for the normal development of the spleen, Peyer's patches and small intestine [14–17]. Along with its role in the development of intestinal lymphoid tissues. Nkx2-3 is crucial for the expression and regulation of the mucosal addressin cell adhesion molecule-1 (MADCAM-1) on the spleen sinus lining cells and on high endothelial venules of the mesenteric lymph nodes and Peyer's patches [17–20]. Nkx2-3 has an important role in spleen organization and function, since it controls the correct micro-environment for B cell maturation and T-cell-dependent (TD) immune reaction [14,21]. Its absence results in disorganized germinal center (GC) formation leading to abnormal secondary B cell differentiation and decreased antibody response with minimal affinity maturation [21,22]. Nkx2-3-deficient mice (Nkx2-3$^{-/-}$) are either asplenic or have a significantly reduced spleen size with a lack of the marginal zone [21]. In response to the TD antigen, the number of circulating lymphocytes of the Nkx2-3$^{-/-}$ mice was found to be increased compared to both Nkx2-3$^{+/-}$ and Nkx2-3$^{+/+}$ [21] indicating their altered distribution between peripheral lymphoid tissues. Moreover, Nkx2-3$^{-/-}$ mice showed an elevation in the number of the B cells in mesenteric lymph nodes which may be due to the abnormal development of the small intestine and the Peyer's patches of these mice, and also a significant increase in the number of the IgM$^+$ B cells in the bone marrow (BM) [21].

In humans, overexpression of Nkx2-3 was found to be associated with both Crohn's disease and ulcerative colitis through its effect on the regulation of PTPN2 expression, VEGF and MADCAM-1 signaling, and the production of endothelin-1 [16,18,23,24]. Additionally, Robles and colleagues reported that chromosomal translocation of *Nkx2-3* gene alongside with immunoglobulin heavy chain gene (*IGH*), resulted in irregular B cell receptor signaling leading to the MZ B cell lymphomagenesis, through the activation of the NF-KB and PI3K-AKT pathways [25].

Our aim in this study was to investigate the effect of Nkx2-3 deficiency in GIA, a mouse model of autoimmune arthritis, and study the effect of Nkx2-3 absence on B cell signaling and activation. Here, we report for the first time that GIA can be induced in Nkx2-3$^{-/-}$ mice, although with lower incidence, decreased severity and less joint destruction. We measured decreased T cell proliferation and cytokine production in spleen cultures. We found less anti-CCP-IgG2a, IL-17 and IFNγ, but more IL-1β, IL-4 and IL-6 in the sera. Finally, B cells of Nkx2-3$^{-/-}$ mice showed decreased intracellular Ca^{2+} signaling compared to those isolated from BALB/c mice. Collectively, these data indicate that Nkx2-3 mice are relatively resistant to GIA-induction which correlates with their impaired in vitro B cell responsiveness.

2. Results

2.1. Decreased Severity and Incidence of rhG1-Induced Arthritis in Nkx2-3 Knock-Out Mice

The spleen plays a critical role in the correct development and recirculation of B cell populations. The connection between the peritoneal B cell pool and the splenic B cells is also well established [26]. Recombinant human G1-induced arthritis is provoked by repeated intraperitoneal injections of the aggrecan G1 domain in the dimethyl-dioctadecyl-ammonium (DDA) adjuvant. By intraperitoneal immunization the first antigen encounter occurs in the peritoneal cavity, but soon the antigen is transported to other lymphoid tissues like the local lymph nodes through lymph vessels and the spleen through blood vessels. In GIA, both the local peritoneal activation of immune cells and the activation of the splenic cells are thought to be critical for the development of autoimmune arthritis [8].

Since Nkx2-3 knock-out mice were present with severe splenic developmental defects, we were curious to test whether rhG1-induced arthritis could be observed in them. To this end, we immunized Nkx2-3$^{-/-}$ and wild-type control BALB/c mice side-by-side. Nkx2-3$^{-/-}$ mice developed arthritis; however, to a lesser extent than the control BALB/c mice indicated by both the lower clinical severity scores (9.2 ± 1.0 in Nkx2-3$^{-/-}$ versus 13.0 ± 0.9 in BALB/c controls at Day 61) (Figure 1A) and the lower incidence (~70% in Nkx2-3$^{-/-}$ versus >90% in BALB/c controls after the third immunization) (Figure 1B). The clinical scores were supported by the limb thickness measurements, too. We measured the wrist (Figure 1(Ca)), leg (Figure 1(Cb)) and ankle (Figure 1(Cc)) thickness two weeks after the third immunization. We found that in arthritic Nkx2-3$^{-/-}$ mice, the limbs were significantly less swollen (Figure 1(Ca–Cc)) indicating a lower degree of inflammatory edema. Interestingly, in Nkx2-3$^{-/-}$ mice, the disease progression was also different from that seen in BALB/c mice: in GIA, typically, the arthritis develops progressively and once established it will not regress, however, in the case of Nkx2-3$^{-/-}$ mice we have seen the undulation of paw inflammation in some cases.

2.2. Micro-CT Imaging Confirmed Decreased Cartilage and Bone Destruction in Arthritic Nkx2-3 Knock-Out Mice

Next, we wanted to visualize the radiological changes induced by GIA in Nkx2-3$^{-/-}$ and control BALB/c mice. RA causes not only cartilage destruction but the adjacent bone is always affected as a result of the inflammation-induced osteoclast activity. Typical changes associated with RA are bone loss, osteophyte formation and, in the latter stages of the disease, ankylosis. So, we performed a micro-CT analysis of arthritic Nkx2-3$^{-/-}$ and control BALB/c mice. As shown by the pseudocolor enhanced micro-CT images wild-type mice demonstrated marked osteophyte formation and bone surface irregularity predominantly in the tarsal and metatarsal region (Figure 2A,C,E) In comparison, Nkx2-3$^{-/-}$ animals showed less severe detrimental bone structural damage secondary to the autoimmune arthritis manifested by a more limited surface porosity and periarticular inflammatory osteoporosis (Figure 2A,C,E).

We also analyzed the micro-CT scans for some quantitative markers of the bone microarchitecture, e.g., number (Po.N), volume (Po.V) and surface of bone pores (Po.S), and the bone surface/Total Volume (BS/TV) values. In arthritic Nkx2-3 KO mice, the slightly decreased Po.N together with the increased Po.V and Po.S values could be due to decreased reactive bone formation, whereas the slightly decreased BS/TV value might indicate less osteophyte formation, all of which correlate with the milder arthritis (Figure A1).

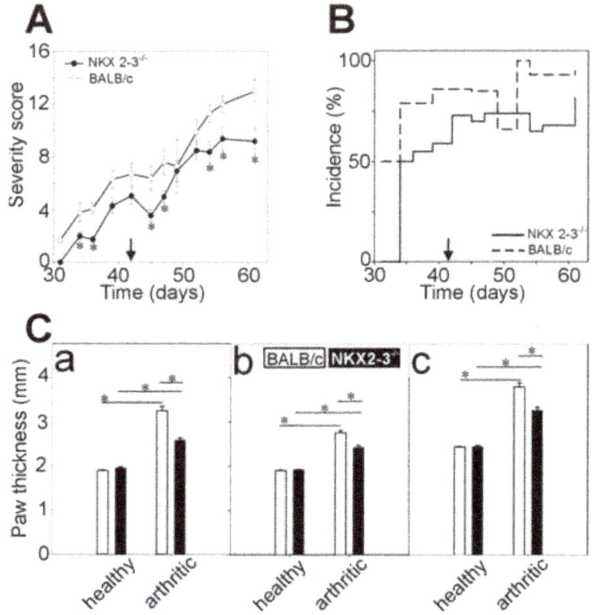

Figure 1. The comparison of the clinical parameters of recombinant human G1 (rhG1)-induced arthritis (GIA) in Nkx2-3$^{-/-}$ and control BALB/c mice. Female Nkx2-3$^{-/-}$ (n = 40) and control BALB/c (n = 27) mice were immunized with rhG1 and dimethyl-dioctadecyl-ammonium (DDA) adjuvant intraperitoneally three times every third week. The severity score (**A**) and incidence (**B**) of the induced arthritis is shown on the diagrams. Black arrows show the time of the third immunization (Day 42). Severity of the disease was determined every second day with the help of a scoring system ranging from 1 to 4, based on the swelling, redness and ankylosis of the joints of the paws. Clinical scores are visualized as mean ± standard error of mean (SEM). The thickness of the limbs (**C**) were measured with a digital caliper two weeks after the third immunization. The diagrams show the thickness values of the wrist (**C/a**), legs (**C/b**) and ankles (**C/c**) as mean ± SEM. Statistically significant differences ($* p < 0.05$) are indicated.

2.3. Comparison of the G1-Specific Immune Response between Nkx2-3$^{-/-}$ and BALB/c Mice

Given the lower severity and incidence of autoimmune arthritis in the Nkx2-3$^{-/-}$ mice, next, we wanted to characterize the immune response against the G1 antigen and correlate it to the clinical picture. At the end of the experiments, mice were sacrificed and their spleens and sera were harvested for in vitro assays similarly to previous studies [5,27]. In the in vitro studies, we divided the Nkx2-3$^{-/-}$ mice into arthritic and nonarthritic subgroups to see the possible differences in the immunological parameters.

First, we characterized the antigen-induced proliferation of spleen cells. We found significantly decreased proliferation in both arthritic and nonarthritic Nkx2-3$^{-/-}$ mice compared to the arthritic BALB/c mice (Figure 3A). Since Th1, Th2 and Th17 cytokines play a pivotal role in the regulation of GIA [8,28], next, we measured the cytokine production of the rhG1-stimulated spleen cell cultures (Figure 3B). We found that Nkx2-3$^{-/-}$ spleen cells produced significantly less IL-4, IL-6 and IFNγ and markedly, but not significantly, less IL-17 than the corresponding BALB/c spleen cells (Figure 3B). There was no difference in the TNFα production of splenocytes isolated from Nkx2-3$^{-/-}$ or control BALB/c mice (Figure 3B). Of note, nonarthritic Nkx2-3$^{-/-}$ spleen cells produced no detectable amount of the tested cytokines even in the presence of rhG1.

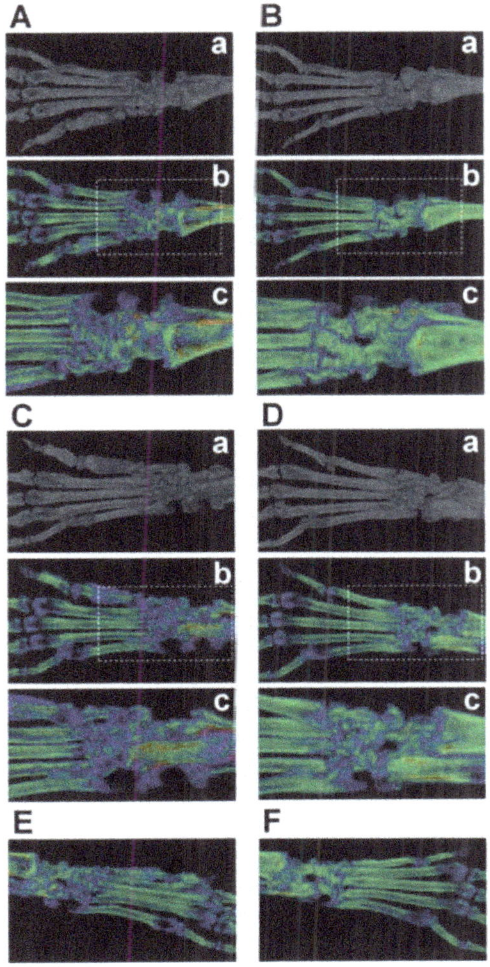

Figure 2. The comparison of the bone microarchitectural changes caused by GIA in Nkx2-3$^{-/-}$ and control BALB/c mice. Arthritic Nkx2-3$^{-/-}$ (n = 2) and control BALB/c (n = 2) mice were anesthetized and micro-CT scans were made from the right hind limbs. Representative images show the dorsal (**A**) and (**B**) or plantar (**C**,**D**) or side views (**E**,**F**) of the arthritic legs from BALB/c (**A**,**C**,**E**) and Nkx2-3$^{-/-}$ (**B**,**D**,**F**) mice, respectively. Pseudocolored images (**A**/**b**,**c**, **B**/**b**,**c**, **C**/**b**,**c**, **D**/**b**,**c**, **E**,**F**) show the bone densities (violet and blue colors indicate low density-; yellow, red and green colors indicate high-density areas, respectively). The white dashed line-surrounded rectangular areas indicated in **A**/**b**, **B**/**b**, **C**/**b** and **D**/**b** are shown with higher magnification in **A**/**c**, **B**/**c**, **C**/**c** and **D**/**d**.

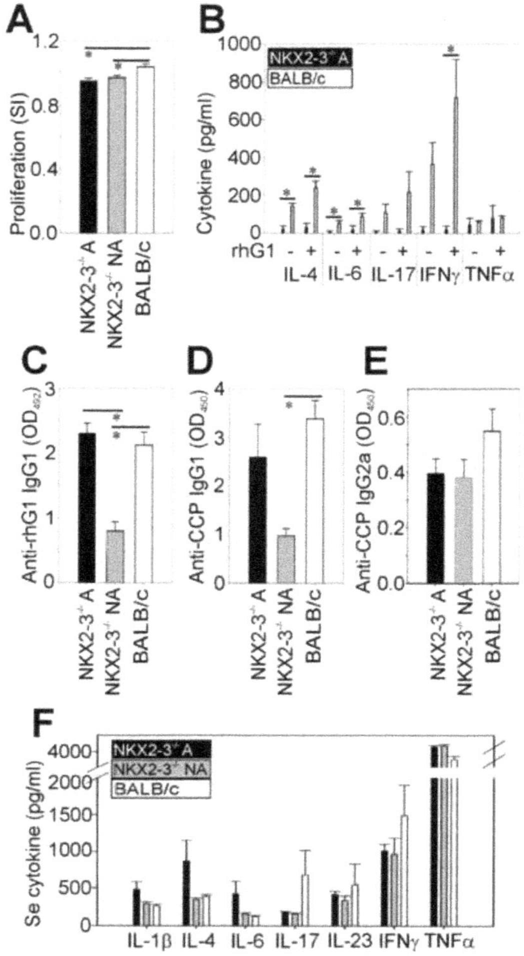

Figure 3. The comparison of the rhG1-induced immune response in Nkx2-3$^{-/-}$ (n = 9) and control BALB/c (n = 9) mice. Nkx2-3$^{-/-}$ mice were divided into arthritic (n = 5) and nonarthritic (n = 4) subgroups during the analysis. In all diagrams (**A–F**), bars show the mean ± SEM values calculated from n = 5 arthritic Nkx2-3$^{-/-}$ mice (black), n = 4 nonarthritic Nkx2-3$^{-/-}$ mice (gray) and n = 9 arthritic control BALB/c mice (white). Statistically significant differences ($*\ p < 0.05$) are indicated. (**A**) Proliferation of spleen cells was tested after incubation in the presence or absence of rhG1 for 5d in vitro. Bars represent the stimulation index (SI) calculated as a ratio of stimulated/nonstimulated values of the same mice. (**B**) In vitro cytokine production of spleen cells was tested after incubation in the presence or absence of rhG1 for 5 d. Cell culture supernatants were harvested and the specific cytokine concentrations were measured by sandwich ELISA. Note, spleen cells from the nonarthritic Nkx2-3$^{-/-}$ group did not produce any measurable amount of cytokines. (**C**) The serum anti-rhG1-specific IgG1 antibodies were measured using indirect ELISA. Sera were diluted at 1:8000. Bars show the optical density values measured at 492 nm. (**D,E**) The serum anti-CCP-specific IgG1 and IgG2a antibodies were measured using indirect ELISA. Sera were not diluted. Bars show the optical density values measured at 450 nm. (**F**) Serum cytokine levels were measured with sandwich ELISA.

Antibody production is an important laboratory parameter of GIA correlating with the severity of the disease [5]. So, after the characterization of the cellular immune response, we went on to measure the joint inflammation-related serum antibody levels of Nkx2-3$^{-/-}$ and BALB/c mice. We found significantly decreased anti-rhG1 (Figure 3C) and anti-CCP (Figure 3D) IgG1 levels in the nonarthritic Nkx2-3$^{-/-}$ mice sera compared to the arthritic BALB/c controls. The arthritic Nkx2-3$^{-/-}$ mice had similar levels of anti-rhG1 (Figure 3C) and anti-CCP (Figure 3D) IgG1 to the arthritic BALB/c mice. Furthermore, the anti-CCP-IgG2a levels were lower (but not significantly) in both arthritic and nonarthritic Nkx2-3$^{-/-}$ mice than in arthritic BALB/c controls (Figure 3E). In line with our expectations, we found that the sera of nonarthritic Nkx2-3$^{-/-}$ mice contained lower levels of anti-rhG1 and anti-CCP IgG1 when compared to the arthritic Nkx2-3$^{-/-}$ sera (Figure 3C,D). In contrast, there was no significant difference between the anti-CCP IgG2a levels of the sera from arthritic or nonarthritic Nkx2-3$^{-/-}$ mice (Figure 3E).

Finally, we compared the serum pro- and anti-inflammatory cytokine concentrations of Nkx2-3$^{-/-}$ and BALB/c mice. We found markedly, but not significantly, elevated serum levels of IL-1β, IL-4, IL-6 and TNFα and markedly decreased IL-17 and IFNγ in arthritic Nkx2-3$^{-/-}$ mice when compared to the arthritic BALB/c controls (Figure 3F). In the case of IL-1β, IL-4 and IL-6, the serum concentrations were markedly, but not significantly, higher in the arthritic than in the nonarthritic Nkx2-3$^{-/-}$ sera (Figure 3F).

2.4. Comparison of the Ca^{2+}-Signaling in B and T Cells of Nkx2-3$^{-/-}$ and BALB/c Mice

Since we found significant differences in the rhG1-induced immune responses of the Nkx2-3$^{-/-}$ and BALB/c mice, we were curious about what could be in the background of such variations. In the case of GIA, similarly to RA, close cooperation between T and B cells is necessary for the development of autoimmunity [7]. Since the Nkx2-3 mutation affects mostly the B lymphocyte development and recirculation, we hypothesized that the activation of B cells might be impaired, which, in turn, led to ameliorated arthritis. To characterize the activation of the B cells, we isolated the inguinal and mesenteric lymph nodes from Nkx2-3$^{-/-}$ or BALB/c control mice and loaded the lymphocytes with the Ca^{2+}-specific indicator Fluo-3. Then, we activated the B cells with cross-linking of the BcR with anti-IgM or IgG antibodies and followed the intracellular Ca^{2+} signals (Figure 4).

We found significantly lower anti-IgM or anti-IgG-induced Ca^{2+}-signal in the B cells isolated from the inguinal lymph nodes of Nkx2-3$^{-/-}$ mice than those from BALB/c (Figure 4A,C). Similarly, B cells isolated from the mesenteric lymph nodes, showed decreased Ca^{2+}-signal both after anti-IgM or anti-IgG-activation (Figure 4B,D) when compared to BALB/c controls, however, these differences did not reach statistical significance. Finally, although we were not expecting any changes in the T cell activation in Nkx2-3$^{-/-}$ mice, we tested the Ca^{2+}-signal of T cells after anti-CD3 cross-linking. As we expected, the Ca^{2+}-signals of T cells isolated from both the inguinal and mesenteric lymph nodes were similar in Nkx2-3$^{-/-}$ and BALB/c mice indicating that, indeed, the Nkx2-3 mutation caused an activation perturbance specifically in B cells.

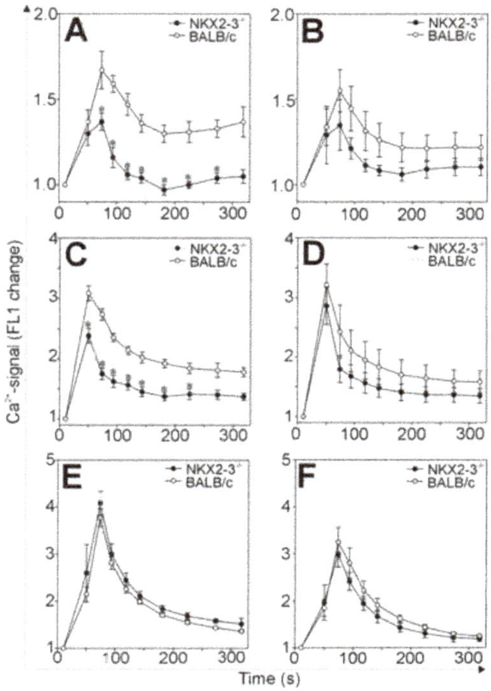

Figure 4. The comparison of the Ca^{2+}-signals of B and T cells in Nkx2-3$^{-/-}$ and control BALB/c mice. Cells were isolated from the inguinal (**A**,**C**,**E**) or mesenteric (**B**,**D**,**F**) lymph nodes of Nkx2-3$^{-/-}$ and BALB/c mice and loaded with the Ca^{2+}-specific indicator Fluo-3. Activation of B cells was induced by anti-IgM (**A**,**B**) or anti-IgG (**C**,**D**), activation of T cells was induced by anti-CD3 cross-linking (**E**,**F**). The changes in the intracellular Ca^{2+} levels of B or T cells were measured with a flow cytometer in the FL1 channel for five and a half minutes. Graphs show the time-dependent changes in the FL1 fluorescence (ratiometric with the intracellular Ca^{2+} level) as mean ± SEM values calculated from the data of n = 3 Nkx2-3$^{-/-}$ and n = 3 BALB/c mice. * $p < 0.05$.

3. Discussion

In the present study, we set out to study how Nkx2-3-deficiency impacted the development of autoimmune arthritis. To answer this question, we used a mouse RA model, GIA, whereby we immunized Nkx2-3$^{-/-}$ and BALB/c control mice side-by-side with the rhG1 antigen. While the spleen plays important roles in the T-dependent immune responses [11,29], and in GIA it also serves as an activation niche for autoreactive lymphocytes [8,30], in Nkx2-3$^{-/-}$ mice, with severely damaged spleen, GIA could still be induced. This result shows that in GIA the spleen's role is not exclusive in the activation of autoreactive lymphocytes, and confirms that the lymph nodes and perhaps other lymphatic or extralymphatic tissues [8] may play an equally important role in the disease induction. On the other hand, we observed lower incidence and decreased arthritis severity in the Nkx2-3$^{-/-}$ mice compared to the wild-type controls, thus, the splenic defects had a significant impact on the rhG1-induced immune reaction. During the induction of (P)GIA, we immunized the mice with PG extracts/rhG1 and DDA intraperitoneally which led to the local activation of T lymphocytes both in the peritoneal cavity and the mesenteric lymph nodes followed by the systemic immune response in which the spleen is involved [8]. The local activation of Th1 and Th17 cells in the peritoneal cavity is of special importance because it was a specific feature of BALB/c mice which are the only susceptible mouse strain for (P)GIA [8]. The present results in Nkx2-3$^{-/-}$ mice might also support this: the local peritoneal activation could remain unchanged, however, the systemic response, developing in the spleen is missing, which could be responsible for the weaker arthritis.

As it was previously described there is a significant B cell trafficking between the peritoneal cavity and the spleen [26]. Although there was a preferential homing of the peritoneal B1 and B2 cells towards other serosa surfaces like the pleura, however, some B1 and B2 cells migrated from the peritoneal cavity into the spleen [26]. Since in Nkx2-3$^{-/-}$ mice, the spleen microarchitecture is seriously defective, with abnormal adhesion molecule expression and vessel formation [29] most likely, the above-mentioned B cell trafficking is defective [29], in addition to the absence of MZ B cells involved in antigen delivery for GC initiation [21]. B lymphocytes not only play a role as precursors for antibody-producing plasma cells in autoimmune arthritis but have an equally important role as antigen-presenting cells [31]. Based on the above-mentioned works [26,29], we propose that the local, peritoneal antigen presentation by B cells could remain unchanged, however, due to the potential lack of splenic homing (and the severely reduced GC formation in the spleen upon T-dependent antigen challenge [21]), the systemic activation could be impaired. The subsequently weaker immune response is mirrored in the decreased splenic proliferation and cytokine production. This was particularly pronounced in the case of lymphocyte-derived cytokines (IL-4, IL-6, IL-17 and IFNγ), but, in the case of TNFα, we measured approximately equal amounts in Nkx2-3$^{-/-}$ and control BALB/c spleen cell cultures, showing that the macrophages were not affected.

In humans, the potential pathogenic role of the Nkx2-3 transcription factor was found in inflammatory bowel diseases (Crohn's and ulcerative colitis) so far [23,24] and also suggested in spondylarthritis more recently [32]. In mice, the absence of Nkx2-3 proved to be protective in DSS-induced colitis through an IL-22-independent mechanism [18]. To our knowledge, this was the first experiment where the Nkx2-3$^{-/-}$ mutation was investigated in the context of autoimmune arthritis. Based on the data presented in this study, Nkx2-3 is not only involved in intestinal inflammatory diseases, but also affects autoimmune arthritis.

An important finding of the present study was that not all Nkx2-3$^{-/-}$ mice developed arthritis upon rhG1 immunization: in all experiments, 20–40% of Nkx2-3$^{-/-}$ mice remained healthy contrary to BALB/c mice (>90% incidence, as seen here and in previous studies [5,27]). To decipher what could be the reason why certain immunized mice did not develop arthritis, we analyzed their immune response parameters separately. We measured considerably lower anti-rhG1 and anti-CCP IgG1 antibody levels in the sera of nonarthritic than in the sera of arthritic Nkx2-3$^{-/-}$ mice, respectively. This alone could explain the differences in the arthritis, since it has been shown in several earlier studies that the serum antibody levels against the proteoglycan aggrecan (and its immunodominant region: G1 domain) and CCP show the strongest correlation with the severity of GIA [33,34]. Furthermore, in nonarthritic Nkx2-3$^{-/-}$ mice, the serum concentrations of IL-1β, IL-4 and IL-6 were lower than in arthritic Nkx2-3$^{-/-}$ mice. We hypothesize that in those Nkx2-3$^{-/-}$ mice, which did not develop arthritis, the B cell activation and/or antigen presentation was inadequate to induce sufficient antibody production and autoreactive T cell activation. However, further and more detailed investigation would be needed to adequately answer this question.

Even in those Nkx2-3$^{-/-}$ mice which did develop GIA, there were significantly milder symptoms (lower clinical scores, lesser edema, radiologically decreased cartilage and bone destruction). This was in line with those serum parameters which were clearly different from the control BALB/c mice. Specifically, although the anti-rhG1 and anti-CCP-IgG1 antibody levels were similar in the arthritic Nkx2-3$^{-/-}$ mice and the controls, the anti-CCP-IgG2a antibodies were produced in lesser amounts. Additionally, the concentrations of signature cytokines of GIA [5], and likewise, RA [2], IFNγ and IL-17 were markedly lower, whereas the concentrations of IL-1β, IL-4 and IL-6 were markedly higher in Nkx2-3$^{-/-}$ than in BALB/c mice. Overall, these markers suggest a stronger Th2 activation (primarily indicated by IL-4 and anti-CCP IgG2a) in Nkx2-3$^{-/-}$ mice instead of the characteristic Th1/Th17 dominated immune response seen in GIA of BALB/c mice [5,8,28]. Since Th2 cytokines have primarily anti-inflammatory effects [11] and have been shown to ameliorate PGIA [35], we suggest that this slight shift towards Th2 measured in Nkx2-3$^{-/-}$ mice might explain the milder arthritis.

As described here, and earlier [5], similarly to RA, in GIA mice significant anti-CCP antibody production can be detected. The process of citrullination and the role of autoantibodies against these modified antigens is of special interest in RA. ACPA production is promoted by environmental factors like smoking and genetic predispositions such as *HLA-DRB1* [36]. Several studies reported that ACPA positive patients are prone to have more joint erosions [36,37]. ACPA form immune complexes with the citrullinated peptides leading to the activation of macrophages and proinflammatory cytokine production, as well as osteoclastogenesis [36,37]. ACPA is highly specific to RA and can be early detected, even before the onset of RA. Therefore, it is used as a specific diagnostic marker for RA [38]. Recently, it was also found that the pathogenic ACPA are hyperglycosylated which might be regulated by Th17 cells [37]. Since in GIA Th17 activation was observed it is tempting to speculate that altered glycosylation might also occur which could contribute to the pathologic immune reaction against the cartilage antigen components.

Finally, to find a cellular mechanism in the background of the above-detailed immune response differences, we turned our attention to the activation of B cells. B cell activation starts with the engagement of the BcR by the antigen and followed by a well-characterized line of biochemical events including the phosphorylation of cytoplasmic signaling proteins and the transient elevation of the cytoplasmic Ca^{2+}-level [11]. We studied the latter and found that in mesenteric and inguinal lymph node B cells of Nkx2-3$^{-/-}$ mice, in vitro stimulation with both anti-mouse IgM and anti-mouse IgG caused a weaker Ca^{2+}-signal compared to BALB/c controls. At the same time, the Ca^{2+}-signal in Nkx2-3$^{-/-}$ T cells remained unchanged, showing that this was a B-cell-specific alteration. This decreased B cell activation capacity of Nkx2-3$^{-/-}$ mice was also seen on phospho-blots from some preliminary experiments (data not shown), however, further analysis is needed to clarify which protein(s) could be involved in the signaling changes. These data are in harmony with those described earlier: increased expression of Nkx2-3 in B cells led to Syk and Lyn phosphorylation, elevated basal Ca^{2+}-level and anti-IgM-induced Ca^{2+}-signal [25], the exact opposite to what we found here, in the absence of Nkx2-3. The decreased antigen-driven B cell activation could lead to weaker B cell proliferation and differentiation which, in turn, could explain the less pronounced immune response and the consequently milder autoimmune arthritis.

In conclusion, the complex immune response changes in Nkx2-3$^{-/-}$ mice due to the defective spleen structure and function could explain the reduced severity and lower incidence of autoimmune arthritis. At the cellular level, we found weaker B cell activation which might, at least in part, be responsible for the altered immune response. These data add to our knowledge about the significance of the spleen in the development of autoimmunity, and hopefully serve as a starting point for future studies.

4. Materials and Methods

4.1. Mice

We used 4–5 months old [39] female Nkx2-3-deficient (Nkx2-3$^{-/-}$) [29] and BALB/c mice. Animals were kept and bred in the transgenic mouse facility of the Department of Immunology and Biotechnology under conventional conditions at 24 ± 2 °C with a controlled 12/12 h light/dark cycle. Mice used in experiments were housed in groups of five and they received acidified water and food ad libitum.

All animal experiments were performed in accordance with the regulations set out by the Animal Welfare Committee of the University of Pécs (BA02/2000-48/2017 (06/27/2017)).

4.2. Induction and Assessment of Recombinant Human G1-Induced Arthritis

To induce arthritis, Nkx2-3$^{-/-}$ and BALB/c mice were immunized side-by-side as described previously [5]. Briefly, mice received intraperitoneal injections of 40 μg rhG1 antigen mixed with dimethyl-dioctadecyl-ammonium (DDA) adjuvant dissolved in PBS, on Days 0, 21 and 42. The clinical signs of arthritis were monitored regularly after the second immunization: all mice were examined every second day and the symptoms were quantified using a clinical scoring system ranging from 0 to 4 based on the swelling, redness and ankylosis of the joints of the paws (maximum possible score 16) as described before [4,5]. The diameters of the inflamed front and hind paws and ankles were measured using digital calipers with an accuracy of 0.01 mm two weeks after the third immunization. Three weeks after the last immunization, mice were sacrificed, then blood sera, spleens and lymph nodes were collected for further in vitro studies.

4.3. Micro-CT

The right hind paws of mice were scanned under anesthesia with i.p. ketamine (120 mg/kg; Calypsol, Gedeon Richter, Budapest, Hungary) and xylazine (6 mg/kg; Sedaxylan, Eurovet Animal Health, Bladel, The Netherlands) using a SkyScan 1176 in vivo micro-CT system (Bruker, Kontich, Belgium). A 0.5 mm Al filter was used, the voxel size was 17.5 µm, tube voltage was 50 kV, tube current was set to 500 µA. 3D reconstructions of the scans were made with the CT Analyzer software, and representative pseudocolor images were generated to highlight bone erosions and osteophyte formation.

4.4. In Vitro Spleen Cell Culture

Spleens were isolated and homogenized mechanically, then the spleen cells were cultured in DMEM supplemented with 10% fetal calf serum on 48-well plates (1.8×10^6 cells in 600 µL medium/well), in the presence or absence of 1.5 µg rhG1 antigen for 5 d. Supernatants were collected and stored in −20 °C and later used for ELISA measurements.

4.5. Antigen-Specific Proliferation Assay

Another part of the spleen cells were cultured in DMEM supplemented with 10% fetal calf serum, in the presence or absence of 1.5 µg rhG1 antigen in triplicates on 96-well plates (3×10^5 cells in 200 µL medium/well) for 5 d. Promega CellTiter96® Nonradioactive Cell Proliferation Assay (Promega, Madison, WI, USA) was used to measure the proliferation rate according to the manufacturer's instructions.

4.6. ELISA Measurements

The specific cytokine concentrations (IL-1β, IL-4, IL-6, IL-17, IL-23, IFN-γ and TNF-α) were measured in the blood sera and the supernatants of in vitro-cultured spleen cells using sandwich ELISA (R&D Systems, Minneapolis, MN, USA), according to the manufacturer's instructions.

The serum-concentration of rhG1 antigen-specific antibodies was measured using indirect ELISA as described earlier [27]. Briefly, 96-well ELISA plates were coated overnight at room temperature with the rhG1 antigen (0.1 µg/well in 100 µL carbonate coating buffer). After overnight incubation, plates were incubated for 1 h with 1.5% nonfat dry milk (NFDM) in PBS blocking buffer, followed by washing 5 times with 0.5% Tween in PBS. Next, diluted sera were added to the plate and incubated for 2 h at room temperature, then washed 5 times with 0.5% Tween in PBS. After that, anti-IgG1-peroxidase (BD Bioscience, San Jose, CA, USA) secondary antibody was added to the plate and incubated for 2 h at room temperature. The results were detected using orthophenylenediamine chromophore and H_2O_2 substrate.

The anti-CCP IgG1 and IgG2a antibody levels of sera were determined using the commercially available Immunoscan CCP Plus ELISA kit (SVAR, Malmö, Sweden) with slight modification. For the development of the reactions, we used anti-mouse-IgG1-peroxidase or anti-mouse-IgG2a-peroxidase (both from BD Bioscience, San Jose, CA, USA) secondary antibody instead of the kit's secondary reagent.

4.7. Ca^{2+} Signaling Measurements

The intracellular Ca^{2+} levels were measured using a flow cytometer with the Fluo-3 indicator as described before [40,41]. Briefly, single-cell suspensions were prepared from the lymph nodes of the arthritic mice and suspended in RPMI supplemented with 5% FBS and 2M $CaCl_2$ (1×10^6 cells/mL). Cells were loaded with Fluo-3-AM (Invitrogen, Carlsbad, CA, USA) for 30 min at 37 °C in humidified air with 5% CO_2. Using a flow cytometer, we gated on the lymphocytes based on FSC/SSC parameter distribution. The Fluo-3 fluorescence which is proportional to the intracellular Ca^{2+} level [40] was detected in the FL1 channel. The baseline Fluo-3 fluorescence was measured for 1 min, then cells were stimulated with anti-mouse-IgM, IgG, or anti-mouse CD3 followed by secondary anti-hamster antibodies, measurements for five and a half minutes. Data were analyzed by the Cell Quest software (BD Biosciences, San Jose, CA, USA). The FL1 mean fluorescence intensity values were calculated along the time axis of the plots, and these were divided by the baseline fluorescence value, thereby the Ca^{2+} signal was expressed as FL1 change [41]. Please note that all Ca^{2+} measurements were performed using unsorted lymph node cells and the B or T cell activation was only distinguished based on the specific nature of the activation: anti-mouse-IgM or IgG activates only B cells through the BcR, whereas anti-CD3 cross-linking activates T cells selectively.

4.8. Statistical Analysis

All values are presented as mean ± standard error of mean (SEM). Student's t-test was used to compare the experimental groups. p-values < 0.05 were considered statistically significant.

Author Contributions: Conceptualization, F.B, P.B., T.B.; methodology, E.K., K.O., R.K., F.G., F.B., B.B., T.K., E.G.; software, B.B., T.K.; validation, F.B., K.O. and T.B.; formal analysis, E.K., F.B.; investigation, E.K., K.O., K.R., E.G.; resources, F.B., P.B., T.B.; data curation, F.B.; writing—original draft preparation, E.K., F.B.; writing—review and editing, F.B.; visualization, B.B., T.K.; supervision, F.B.; project administration, F.B.; funding acquisition, F.B., T.B. All authors have read and agreed to the published version of the manuscript.

Funding: This research was funded by by the European Union, cofinanced by the European Social Fund: Projects "Comprehensive Development for Implementing Smart Specialization Strategies at the University of Pécs" (EFOP-3.6.1.-16-2016-00004) and "PEPSYS—Complexity of peptide-signalization and its role in systemic diseases" (GINOP 2.3.2-15-2016-00050). This work was supported by grants EFOP-3.6.1-16-2016-00004 "Stay Alive", and GINOP-2.3.2.-15-2016-00048. B.B. was supported by the János Bolyai Research Scholarship of The Hungarian Academy of Sciences (BO/00501/19/5) and the ÚNKP-19-4-P-PTE-458 New National Excellence Program of the Ministry for Innovation and Technology.

Acknowledgments: The micro-CT studies were performed in the Small Animal In Vivo Imaging Core Facility of the Szentagothai Research Centre, University of Pecs. The authors express their gratitude to Tibor T. Glant, now retired, formerly at Rush University Medical Center, Chicago, IL, USA for providing us with the rhG1 antigen-producing CHO cell line and also for the several year-long fruitful scientific collaboration.

Conflicts of Interest: The authors declare no conflict of interest.

Abbreviations

a-CCP	Anticyclic citrullinated peptide antibody
APCs	Antigen-presenting cells
Ca^{2+}	Calcium
CD	cluster of differentiation
DDA	Dimethyl-Dioctadecyl-ammonium adjuvant
DMEM	Dulbecco's modified Eagle's medium
ELISA	Enzyme-linked immunosorbent assay
FCS	Fetal calf serum
FSC	Forward scatter
GC	Germinal center
GIA	Recombinant human G1-induced arthritis
i.p	Intraperitoneal
IFN-γ	Interferon γ
IGH	Immunoglobulin heavy chain gene

IL	Interleukin
MADCAM-1	Mucosal vascular addressin cell adhesion molecule 1
MZ	Marginal zone
NFDM	Nonfat dry milk
NF-kB	Nuclear factor kappa-light-chain-enhancer of activated B cells
Nkx2-3	Nirenberg-Kim (NK) 2 homeobox 3
Nkx2-3$^{-/-}$	Nkx2-3-deficient mouse (homozygous)
PBS	Phosphate buffer solution
PI3K	Phosphoinositide 3-kinases
PKB	Protein Kinase B
PTPN2	Tyrosine-protein phosphatase nonreceptor type 2
RA	Rheumatoid arthritis
rhG1	Recombinant human G1
RPMI	Roswell Park Memorial Institute Medium
SSC	Side scatter
TF	Transcription factor
Th	T helper cell
TNF-α	Tumor necrosis factor α
VEGF	Vascular endothelial growth factor

Appendix A

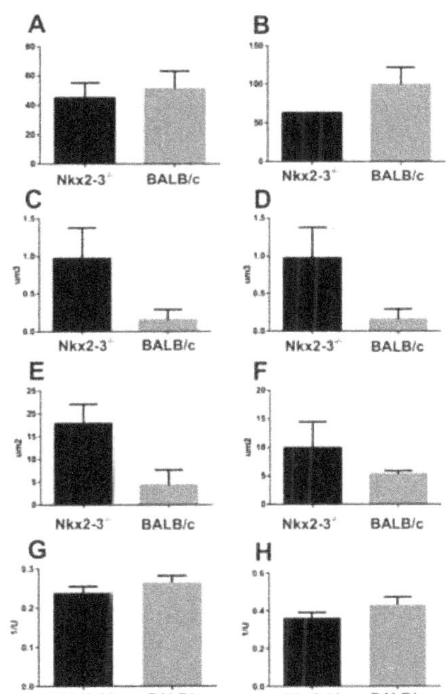

Figure A1. Comparison of the quantitative markers of bone microarchitecture in arthritic Nkx2-3$^{-/-}$ and BALB/c mice based on the micro-CT scans (representative images are shown in Figure 2). We compared the bone pore number (Po.N) (**A**,**B**), volume (Po.V) (**C**,**D**) and surface (Po.S) (**E**,**F**), and the Bone Surface/Total Volume (BS/TV) values (**G**,**H**) of the metatarsal (**A**,**C**,**E**,**G**) and tarsal (**B**,**D**,**F**,**H**) regions from arthritic Nkx2-3$^{-/-}$ (black bars) and BALB/c (gray bars) mice, respectively. Bars show the mean ± SEM values calculated from the data of 2 Nkx2-3$^{-/-}$ and 2 BALB/c mice.

References

1. Scott, D.L.; Wolfe, F.; Huizinga, T.W.J. Rheumatoid arthritis. *Lancet* **2010**, *376*, 1094–1108. [CrossRef]
2. Lin, Y.-J.; Anzaghe, M.; Schülke, S. Update on the Pathomechanism, Diagnosis, and Treatment Options for Rheumatoid Arthritis. *Cells* **2020**, *9*, 880. [CrossRef] [PubMed]
3. Kugyelka, R.; Kohl, Z.; Olasz, K.; Mikecz, K.; Rauch, T.A.; Glant, T.T.; Boldizsar, F. Enigma of IL-17 and Th17 cells in rheumatoid arthritis and in autoimmune animal models of arthritis. *Mediat. Inflamm.* **2016**, *2016*, 6145810. [CrossRef]
4. Glant, T.T.; Mikecz, K.; Arzoumanian, A.; Poole, A.R. Proteoglycan-induced arthritis in BALB/c mice. Clinical features and histopathology. *Arthritis Rheum.* **1987**, *30*, 201–212. [CrossRef] [PubMed]
5. Glant, T.T.; Radacs, M.; Nagyeri, G.; Olasz, K.; Laszlo, A.; Boldizsar, F.; Hegyi, A.; Finnegan, A.; Mikecz, K. Proteoglycan-induced arthritis and recombinant human proteoglycan aggrecan G1 domain-induced arthritis in BALB/c mice resembling two subtypes of rheumatoid arthritis. *Arthritis Rheum.* **2011**, *63*, 1312–1321. [CrossRef] [PubMed]
6. Horváth, Á.; Borbély, É.; Bölcskei, K.; Szentes, N.; Kiss, T.; Belák, M.; Rauch, T.; Glant, T.; Zákány, R.; Juhász, T.; et al. Regulatory role of capsaicin-sensitive peptidergic sensory nerves in the proteoglycan-induced autoimmune arthritis model of the mouse. *J. Neuroinflamm.* **2018**, *15*, 335. [CrossRef] [PubMed]
7. Hanyecz, A.; Olasz, K.; Tarjanyi, O.; Nemeth, P.; Mikecz, K.; Glant, T.T.; Boldizsar, F. Proteoglycan aggrecan conducting T cell activation and apoptosis in a murine model of rheumatoid arthritis. *Biomed. Res. Int.* **2014**, *2014*, 942148. [CrossRef]
8. Boldizsar, F.; Tarjanyi, O.; Nemeth, P.; Mikecz, K.; Glant, T.T. Th1/Th17 polarization and acquisition of an arthritogenic phenotype in arthritis-susceptible BALB/c, but not in MHC-matched, arthritis-resistant DBA/2 mice. *Int. Immunol.* **2009**, *21*, 511–522. [CrossRef]
9. McInnes, I.B.; Schett, G. Pathogenetic insights from the treatment of rheumatoid arthritis. *Lancet* **2017**, *389*, 2328–2337. [CrossRef]
10. Smolen, J.S.; Aletaha, D.; Barton, A.; Burmester, G.R.; Emery, P.; Firestein, G.S.; Kavanaugh, A.; McInnes, I.B.; Solomon, D.H.; Strand, V.; et al. Rheumatoid arthritis. *Nat. Rev. Dis. Prim.* **2018**, *4*, 18001. [CrossRef]
11. Abbas, A.; Lichtman, A.; Pillai, S. *Cellular and Molecular Immunology*; Elsevier: Amsterdam, The Netherlands, 2017; Available online: https://www.elsevier.com/books/cellular-and-molecular-immunology/abbas/978-0-323-47978-3 (accessed on 15 June 2020).
12. Crane, G.M.; Liu, Y.-C.; Chadburn, A. Spleen: Development, anatomy and reactive lymphoid proliferations. *Semin. Diagn. Pathol.* **2020**. [CrossRef] [PubMed]
13. Tsuji, F.; Yoshimi, M.; Katsuta, O.; Takai, M.; Ishihara, K.; Aono, H. Point mutation of tyrosine 759 of the IL-6 family cytokine receptor, gp130, augments collagen-induced arthritis in DBA/1J mice. *BMC Musculoskelet. Disord.* **2009**, *10*, 23. [CrossRef] [PubMed]
14. Yu, W.; Hegarty, J.P.; Berg, A.; Chen, X.; West, G.; Kelly, A.A.; Wang, Y.; Poritz, L.S.; Koltun, W.A.; Lin, Z. NKX2-3 transcriptional regulation of endothelin-1 and VEGF signaling in human intestinal microvascular endothelial cells. *PLoS ONE* **2011**, *6*, e20454. [CrossRef] [PubMed]
15. Nagel, S.; Drexler, H.G. Deregulated NKL Homeobox Genes in B-Cell Lymphoma. *Cancers* **2019**, *11*, 1874. [CrossRef]
16. Kerkhofs, C.; Williams, A.P.; Brunner, H.G.; Faust, S.N.; Rae, W.; Wurm, P.; Fockens, P.; Laass, M.; Kokke, F. Mutations in RPSA and NKX2—3 link development of the spleen and intestinal vasculature. *Hum. Mutat.* **2020**, *41*, 196–202. [CrossRef]
17. Vojkovics, D.; Kellermayer, Z.; Kajtár, B.; Roncador, G.; Vincze, Á.; Balogh, P. Nkx2-3-A Slippery Slope From Development Through Inflammation Toward Hematopoietic Malignancies. *Biomark. Insights* **2018**, *13*. [CrossRef]
18. Kellermayer, Z.; Vojkovics, D.; Dakah, T.A.; Bodó, K.; Botz, B.; Helyes, Z.; Berta, G.; Kajtár, B.; Schippers, A.; Wagner, N.; et al. IL-22-Independent Protection from Colitis in the Absence of Nkx2.3 Transcription Factor in Mice. *J. Immunol.* **2019**, *202*, 1833–1844. [CrossRef]
19. Kuhbandner, K.; Hammer, A.; Haase, S.; Terbrack, E.; Hoffmann, A.; Schippers, A.; Wagner, N.; Hussain, R.Z.; Miller-Little, W.A.; Koh, A.Y.; et al. MAdCAM-1-Mediated Intestinal Lymphocyte Homing Is Critical for the Development of Active Experimental Autoimmune Encephalomyelitis. *Front. Immunol.* **2019**, *10*, 903. [CrossRef]

20. Myint, P.K.; Park, E.J.; Gaowa, A.; Kawamoto, E.; Shimaoka, M. Targeted remodeling of breast cancer and immune cell homing niches by exosomal integrins. *Diagn. Pathol.* **2020**, *15*, 38. [CrossRef]
21. Tarlinton, D.; Light, A.; Metcalf, D.; Harvey, R.P.; Robb, L. Architectural defects in the spleens of Nkx2-3-deficient mice are intrinsic and associated with defects in both B cell maturation and T cell-dependent immune responses. *J. Immunol.* **2003**, *170*, 4002–4010. [CrossRef]
22. Pabst, O. NKX2.3 is required for MAdCAM-1 expression and homing of lymphocytes in spleen and mucosa-associated lymphoid tissue. *EMBO J.* **2000**, *19*, 2015–2023. [CrossRef] [PubMed]
23. Parkes, M.; Barrett, J.C.; Prescott, N.J.; Tremelling, M.; Anderson, C.A.; Fisher, S.A.; Roberts, R.G.; Nimmo, E.R.; Cummings, F.R.; Soars, D.; et al. Sequence variants in the autophagy gene IRGM and multiple other replicating loci contribute to Crohn's disease susceptibility. *Nat. Genet.* **2007**, *39*, 830–832. [CrossRef] [PubMed]
24. Fisher, S.A.; Tremelling, M.; Anderson, C.A.; Gwilliam, R.; Bumpstead, S.; Prescott, N.J.; Nimmo, E.R.; Massey, D.; Berzuini, C.; Johnson, C.; et al. Genetic determinants of ulcerative colitis include the ECM1 locus and five loci implicated in Crohn's disease. *Nat. Genet.* **2008**, *40*, 710–712. [CrossRef] [PubMed]
25. Robles, E.F.; Mena-Varas, M.; Barrio, L.; Merino-Cortes, S.V.; Balogh, P.; Du, M.-Q.; Akasaka, T.; Parker, A.; Roa, S.; Panizo, C.; et al. Homeobox NKX2-3 promotes marginal-zone lymphomagenesis by activating B-cell receptor signalling and shaping lymphocyte dynamics. *Nat. Commun.* **2016**, *7*, 11889. [CrossRef] [PubMed]
26. Lábadi, A.; Balogh, P. Differential preferences in serosal homing and distribution of peritoneal B-cell subsets revealed by in situ CFSE labeling. *Int. Immunol.* **2009**, *21*, 1047–1056. [CrossRef] [PubMed]
27. Kugyelka, R.; Prenek, L.; Olasz, K.; Kohl, Z.; Botz, B.; Glant, T.T.; Berki, T.; Boldizsár, F. ZAP-70 Regulates Autoimmune Arthritis via Alterations in T Cell Activation and Apoptosis. *Cells* **2019**, *8*, 504. [CrossRef]
28. Holló, K.; Glant, T.T.; Garzó, M.; Finnegan, A.; Mikecz, K.; Buzás, E. Complex pattern of Th1 and Th2 activation with a preferential increase of autoreactive Th1 cells in BALB/c mice with proteoglycan (aggrecan)-induced arthritis. *Clin. Exp. Immunol.* **2000**, *120*, 167–173.
29. Czömpöly, T.; Lábadi, A.; Kellermayer, Z.; Olasz, K.; Arnold, H.-H.; Balogh, P. Transcription factor Nkx2-3 controls the vascular identity and lymphocyte homing in the spleen. *J. Immunol.* **2011**, *186*, 6981–6989. [CrossRef]
30. Buzás, E.I.; Végvári, A.; Murad, Y.M.; Finnegan, A.; Mikecz, K.; Glant, T.T. T-cell recognition of differentially tolerated epitopes of cartilage proteoglycan aggrecan in arthritis. *Cell. Immunol.* **2005**, *235*, 98–108. [CrossRef]
31. O'Neill, S.K.; Shlomchik, M.J.; Glant, T.T.; Cao, Y.; Doodes, P.D.; Finnegan, A. Antigen-specific B cells are required as APCs and autoantibody-producing cells for induction of severe autoimmune arthritis. *J. Immunol.* **2005**, *174*, 3781–3788. [CrossRef]
32. Gracey, E.; Vereecke, L.; McGovern, D.; Fröhling, M.; Schett, G.; Danese, S.; De Vos, M.; Van den Bosch, F.; Elewaut, D. Revisiting the gut–joint axis: Links between gut inflammation and spondyloarthritis. *Nat. Rev. Rheumatol.* **2020**, *16*, 415–433. [CrossRef] [PubMed]
33. Mikecz, K.; Glant, T.T.; Poole, A.R. Immunity to cartilage proteoglycans in BALB/c mice with progressive polyarthritis and ankylosing spondylitis induced by injection of human cartilage proteoglycan. *Arthritis Rheum.* **1987**, *30*, 306–318. [CrossRef] [PubMed]
34. Olasz, K.; Boldizsar, F.; Kis-Toth, K.; Tarjanyi, O.; Hegyi, A.; van Eden, W.; Rauch, T.A.; Mikecz, K.; Glant, T.T. T cell receptor (TCR) signal strength controls arthritis severity in proteoglycan-specific TCR transgenic mice. *Clin. Exp. Immunol.* **2012**, *167*, 346–355. [CrossRef] [PubMed]
35. Cao, Y.; Brombacher, F.; Tunyogi-Csapo, M.; Glant, T.T.; Finnegan, A. Interleukin-4 regulates proteoglycan-induced arthritis by specifically suppressing the innate immune response. *Arthritis Rheum.* **2007**, *56*, 861–870. [CrossRef]
36. Grosse, J.; Allado, E.; Roux, C.; Pierreisnard, A.; Couderc, M.; Clerc-Urmes, I.; Remen, T.; Albuisson, É.; De Carvalho-Bittencourt, M.; Chary-Valckenaere, I.; et al. ACPA-positive versus ACPA-negative rheumatoid arthritis: Two distinct erosive disease entities on radiography and ultrasonography. *Rheumatol. Int.* **2020**, *40*, 615–624. [CrossRef]
37. Coutant, F. Pathogenic effects of anti-citrullinated protein antibodies in rheumatoid arthritis—Role for glycosylation. *Jt. Bone Spine* **2019**, *86*, 562–567. [CrossRef]
38. Sakaguchi, W.; To, M.; Yamamoto, Y.; Inaba, K.; Yakeishi, M.; Saruta, J.; Fuchida, S.; Hamada, N.; Tsukinoki, K. Detection of anti-citrullinated protein antibody (ACPA) in saliva for rheumatoid arthritis using DBA mice infected with Porphyromonas gingivalis. *Arch. Oral Biol.* **2019**, *108*, 104510. [CrossRef]

39. Tarjanyi, O.; Boldizsar, F.; Nemeth, P.; Mikecz, K.; Glant, T.T. Age-related changes in arthritis susceptibility and severity in a murine model of rheumatoid arthritis. *Immun. Ageing* **2009**, *6*, 8. [CrossRef]
40. Minta, A.; Kao, J.P.; Tsien, R.Y. Fluorescent indicators for cytosolic calcium based on rhodamine and fluorescein chromophores. *J. Biol. Chem.* **1989**, *264*, 8171–8178.
41. Boldizsár, F.; Berki, T.; Miseta, A.; Németh, P. Effect of hyperglycemia on the basal cytosolic free calcium level, calcium signal and tyrosine-phosphorylation in human T-cells. *Immunol. Lett.* **2002**, *82*, 159–164. [CrossRef]

International Journal of
Molecular Sciences

MDPI

Article

Identification of Novel Targets of Knee Osteoarthritis Shared by Cartilage and Synovial Tissue

Chenshuang Li [1] and Zhong Zheng [2,*]

1 Department of Orthodontics, School of Dental Medicine, University of Pennsylvania, Philadelphia, PA 19104, USA; lichens@upenn.edu

2 Section of Orthodontics, Dental and Craniofacial Research Institute and Division of Growth and Development, School of Dentistry, University of California, Los Angeles, CA 90095, USA

* Correspondence: zzheng@dentistry.ucla.edu; Tel.: +1-(310)-206-5646

Received: 5 August 2020; Accepted: 19 August 2020; Published: 22 August 2020

Abstract: Arthritis is the leading cause of disability among adults, while osteoarthritis (OA) is the most common form of arthritis that results in cartilage loss. However, accumulating evidence suggests that the protective hyaline cartilage should not be the sole focus of OA treatment. Particularly, synovium also plays essential roles in OA's initiation and progression and warrants serious consideration when battling against OA. Thus, biomarkers with similar OA-responsive expressions in cartilage and synovium should be the potential targets for OA treatment. On the other hand, molecules with a distinguished response during OA in cartilage and synovium should be ruled out as OA therapeutic(s) to avoid controversial effects in different tissues. Here, to pave the path for developing a new generation of OA therapeutics, two published transcriptome datasets of knee articular cartilage and synovium were analyzed in-depth. Genes with statistically significantly different expression in OA and healthy cartilage were compared with those in the synovium. Thirty-five genes with similar OA-responsive expression in both tissues were identified while recognizing three genes with opposite OA-responsive alteration trends in cartilage and synovium. These genes were clustered based on the currently available knowledge, and the potential impacts of these clusters in OA were explored.

Keywords: osteoarthritis; cartilage; synovium; whole transcriptome sequencing; biomarker

1. Introduction

Arthritis appears in over 100 identified diseases that can damage any joint in the body, causing inflammation that results in pain, stiffness, swelling, and decreased motion [1,2]. As the leading cause of disability among adults [3], arthritis has been diagnosed in approximately 54.4 million people in the U.S. alone [2,3]. Since arthritis affects people of all ages, sex, and races, its prevalence is expected to increase sharply shortly and turns to be a tremendous economic burden on patients and society [3–5]. Especially, osteoarthritis (OA) is the most common form of arthritis and affects around 18% of women and 10% of men over 60 [4,6]. Alarmingly, recent studies suggest that younger adults are also suffering from OA [7] associated with trauma and occupation-related joint stress [8]. Unfortunately, there are currently no approved disease-modifying osteoarthritis drugs (DMOADs) that can prevent, stop, or even restrain the progression of OA [4,9,10]. Thus, the Osteoarthritis Research Society International (OARSI) recognizes OA as an incurable condition [4]. When considering productivity loss due to OA, estimates are between 0.25% and 0.50% of the gross domestic product (GDP) [11]. Therefore, the biomedical burden of OA is enormous, growing, and inadequately addressed.

Since OA is primarily characterized by disordered articular cartilage homeostasis with subsequent inflammation and degradation, the major effects of developing an ideal OA-combating agent were focused on protecting and reestablishing the hyaline cartilage [12]. However, due to the development of the imaging and diagnosis techniques, synovitis has also been recognized as common in OA in the past decade and offers another potential target for treatment [13]. In response to this finding, glucocorticoids and non-steroidal anti-inflammatory drugs (NSAIDs) are the most prescribed OA medications [14]. For instance, glucocorticoids, such as prednisone and cortisone, are broadly used for current arthritis treatment due to their anti-inflammatory potency [15–17] and achieving short-term improvement in symptoms of OA [18,19]. However, the effect may vary substantially in different patient groups [18,20]. More importantly, multiple adverse side-effects in the musculoskeletal, cardiovascular, and gastrointestinal systems [20–22] challenge the application of glucocorticoids as a safe treatment option. Meanwhile, NSAIDs do not adequately control OA progression [23], while their long-term usage is associated with potentially harmful adverse effects [24]. Even more disappointing, the efficacy of disease-modifying antirheumatic drugs (DMARDs) that postpone rheumatoid arthritis (RA) progression by slowing or suppressing inflammation has not been replicated in OA clinical trials via systemic or local administration [25–27], which may be attributed to their failure on directly managing cartilage destruction—the primary cause of OA [4,28].

Although hyaline cartilage and synovium can cross-talk via synovial fluid [14] and share some inflammatory signaling pathways [29], it is worth noting that they are two distinct types of tissues and may respond differently to the same stimulation, such as OA. Strategically, the agents benefiting one tissue with the expense of another should be avoided for OA treatment. On the other hand, the biomarker(s) has/have similar OA-responsive expressions in cartilage and synovium should be a more suitable marker for OA progression than those only altered in one of these two types of tissues. Moreover, the bioactive molecule that defends and rebuilds both hyaline cartilage and synovium is favorable for OA control and treatment with no doubt. Therefore, publicly available transcriptome datasets of knee articular cartilage and synovial tissue were integrated and analyzed in the current study to gain insight into developing the new generation of DMOADs that promote both cartilage and synovium.

2. Results

2.1. Initial Evaluation of the Synovial and Cartilage RNA-seq Data Sets

By using the keywords "osteoarthritis" in the https://www.ncbi.nlm.nih.gov/gds with the selection of "*Homo sapiens*" under the column of "Top Organisms" and "Expression profiling by high throughput sequencing" under the column of "study type", 499 items were identified which containing 4 datasets, 72 series, and 423 samples. After reviewing all the items, one dataset (GSE114007) containing transcriptome data of human knee cartilage from 18 healthy (5 females, 13 males) and 20 OA (11 females, 9 males) samples, and one dataset (GSE89408) containing transcriptome data of human synovium from 28 healthy (14 females, 14 males) and 22 OA (13 females, 9 males) samples that cover the U.S. population were included in the current study. After removing the samples with an overall alignment rate ≤75%, there were 11 human healthy cartilage samples (4 females, 9 males), 14 human OA cartilage samples (8 females, 6 males), 22 human healthy synovium samples (10 females, 12 males) and 20 human OA synovium (12 females, 8 males) samples underwent further analysis (Table S1).

By distinguishing the gene expression pattern between cartilage and synovium, multidimensional scaling (MDS) and principal component analysis (PCA) on the transcriptome profiling validated the quality of the included samples with minimum tissue contamination as expected (Figure 1).

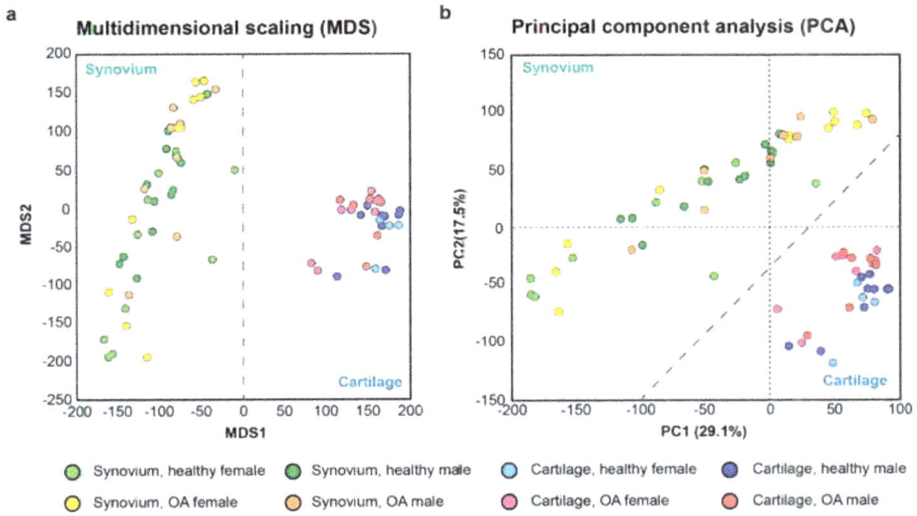

Figure 1. Multidimensional scaling (MDS) (**a**) and principal component analysis (PCA) (**b**) distinguish transcriptome of synovium and cartilage samples included in the current study.

2.2. *Identification of the Common OA-Responsive Genes in Both Cartilage and Synovium*

Heatmaps of the differential expression genes (DEGs) in cartilage and synovium samples were generated, respectively, visualizing the gene expression changes between healthy and OA samples (Figure 2). In both cartilage and synovium, healthy samples could be easily distinguished from OA samples. Interestingly, cartilage displays more gene alteration in response to OA than synovium: 761 DEGs (414 increased, 347 decreased) were identified when comparing OA cartilage samples to their healthy counterparts and 372 OA-responsive DEGs (188 increased, 184 decreased) in synovium samples (Figures 2 and 3). Then, by comparing the OA-responsive DEGs in cartilage and synovium, we recognized 24 upregulated and 11 downregulated genes shared by these two tissues (Figure 3). In addition, there were 3 genes that exhibited different expression trends in cartilage and synovium in OA (Figure 3).

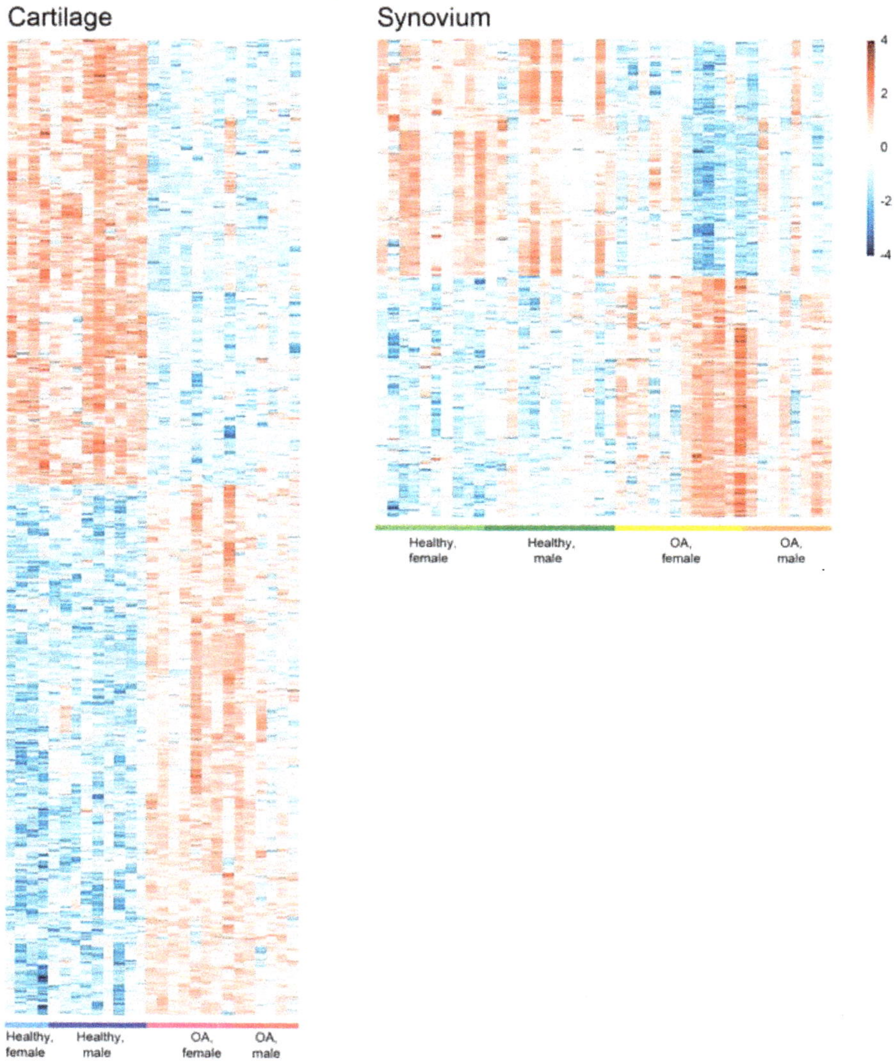

Figure 2. Heatmaps visualize the osteoarthritis (OA)-responsive differential expressed genes (DEGs) in cartilage and synovium, respectively.

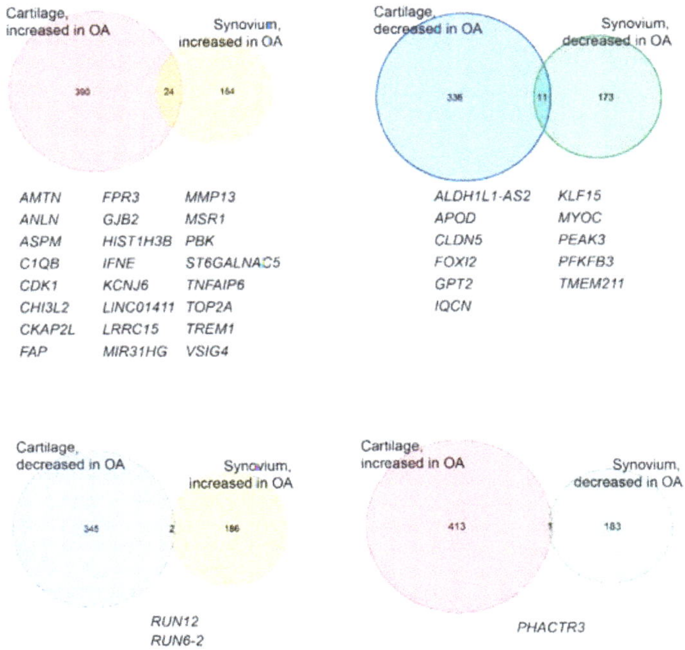

Figure 3. Venn diagrams visualize the osteoarthritis (OA)-responsive differential expressed genes (DEGs) with the same or different expression trends in cartilage and synovium. *AMTN—Amelotin; ANLN—Anillin; ASPM—Abnormal spindle-like microcephaly-associated protein; C1QB—complement C1q subcomponent subunit B; CDK1—cyclin-dependent kinase 1; CHI3L2—Chitinase-3-like protein 2; CKAP2L—cytoskeleton-associated protein 2 like; FAP—fibroblast activation protein alpha; FPR3—N-formyl peptide receptor 3; GJB2—Gap junction beta-2 protein; H1ST1H3B—histone cluster 1 H3 family member b; IFNE—Interferon epsilon; KCNJ6—G protein-activated inward rectifier potassium channel 2/Potassium voltage-gated channel subfamily J member 6; LINC01411—long intergenic non-protein coding RNA 1411; LRRC15—Leucine-rich repeat-containing protein 15; MIR31HG—MIR31 host gene; MMP13—Matrix metallopeptidase-13; MSR1—Macrophage scavenger receptor types I and II; PBK—Lymphokine-activated killer T-cell-originated protein kinase; ST6GALNAC5—Alpha-N-acetylgalactosaminide alpha-2,6-sialyltransferase 5; TNFAIP6—Tumor necrosis factor-inducible gene 6 protein; TOP2A—DNA topoisomerase 2-alpha; TREM1—Triggering receptor expressed on myeloid cell 1; VSIG4—V-set and immunoglobulin domain containing 4; ALDH1L1-AS2—ALDH1L1 antisense RNA 2; APOD—Apolipoprotein; CLDN5—Claudin-5; FOXI2—forkhead box I2; GPT2—Glutamate pyruvate transaminase 2/Alanine aminotransferase 2; IQCN—IQ motif containing N; KLF15—Krueppel-like factor 15; MYOC—Myocilin; PEAK3—PEAK family member 3; PFKFB3—6-phosphofructo-2-kinase/fructose-2,6-biphosphatase 3; TMEM211—transmembrane protein 211; RUN12-RNA U12 small nuclear; RUN6-2—RNA U6 small nuclear 2; PHACTR3—Phosphatase and actin regulator 3.*

2.3. Pathway Enrichment and Protein-Protein Interaction Cluster

Firstly, pathway enrichment against the Reactome knowledgebase [30] was employed to get insight into the potential underlying regulation pathways. Nineteen of the total 35 DEGs were successfully enriched in 276 pathways among 21 clusters (Figure 4a and Table S2). Among them, 4 pathways, including "G0 and early G1" and "mitotic G1 phase and G1/S transition" pathways of the "cell cycle" cluster, "alanine metabolism" of the "metabolism" cluster, and "RUNX1 regulates expression of components of tight junctions" pathway of the "gene expression (Transcription)" cluster, display a false discovery rate (FDR) value less than 0.05 (Figure 4b), highlighting themselves as the potential vital OA-responsive pathways in both cartilage and synovium. Noticeably, 16 other DEGs, including *Leucine-rich repeat-containing protein 15* (*LRRC15*), *Myocilin* (*MYOC*), *cytoskeleton-associated protein 2 like* (*CKAP2L*), *forkhead box I2* (*FOXI2*), *ALDH1L1 antisense RNA 2* (*ALDH1L1-AS2*), *IQ motif containing N* (*IQCN*), *transmembrane protein 211* (*TMEM211*), *anillin actin-binding protein* (*ANLN*), *abnormal spindle microtubule assembly* (*ASPM*), *PEAK family member 3* (*PEAK3*), *Interferon epsilon* (*IFNE*), *Chitinase-3-like protein 2* (*CHI3L2*), *Lymphokine-activated killer T-cell-originated protein kinase* (*PBK*), *V-set and immunoglobulin domain containing 4* (*VSIG4*), *long intergenic non-protein coding RNA 1411* (*LINC01411*), and *MIR31 host gene* (*MIR31HG*), were not picked by the pathway database, which indicates that our current understanding of OA pathogenesis is dreadfully inadequate.

a

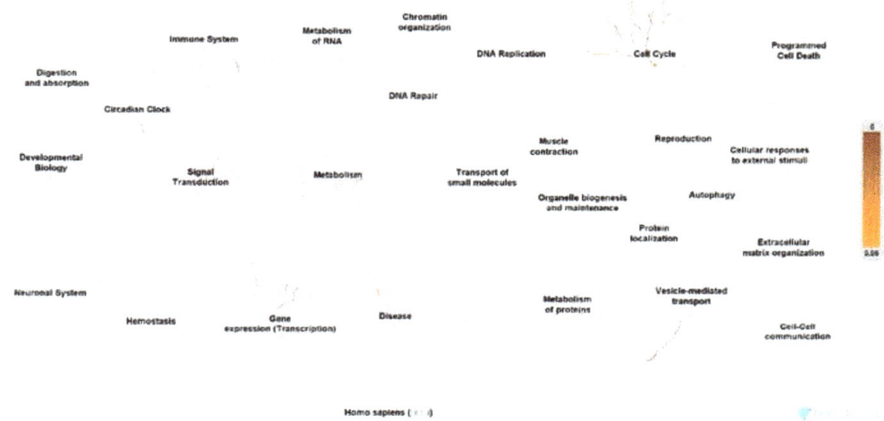

b

Pathway identifier	Pathway name	#Entities found	#Entities total	Entities ratio	Entities pValue	Entities FDR	#Reactions found	#Reactions total	Reactions ratio	Submitted entities found
R-HSA-1538133	G0 and Early G1	4	38	0.00259	7.99E-06	0.00229	4	27	0.002083	TOP2A;CDK1
R-HSA-8964540	Alanine metabolism	2	6	4.09E-04	1.86E-04	0.02341	4	4	3.09E-04	GPT2
R-HSA-453279	Mitotic G1 phase and G1/S transition	5	173	0.01179	2.56E-04	0.02341	14	99	0.007638	TOP2A;CDK1
R-HSA-8935964	RUNX1 regulates expression of components of tight junctions	2	8	5.45E-04	3.30E-04	0.02341	2	6	4.63E-04	CLDN5

Figure 4. Pathway enrichment of the 35 common osteoarthritis (OA)-responsive differential expressed genes (DEGs) in cartilage and synovium has been conducted against the Reactome database. (**a**) The diagram of the distribution of the identified pathways. (**b**) The list of the identified pathways with a false discovery rate (FDR) less than 0.05. *TOP2A—DNA topoisomerase 2-alpha; CDK1—cyclin-dependent kinase 1; GPT2—Glutamate pyruvate transaminase 2/Alanine aminotransferase 2; CLDN5—Claudin-5.*

Since only 19 of 35 (54.3%) common OA-responsive DEGs in cartilage and synovium were picked by Reactome knowledgebase, manually align these 35 DEGs was achieved for further functional clustering. As inflammation is the primary and tissue shared event during OA, we first checked the DEGs that could relate to immune regulation. Based on the functional information collected in the Uniprot database [31] (Table S3), 10 DEGs, including *Apolipoprotein* (*APOD*), *complement C1q subcomponent subunit B* (*C1QB*), *N-formyl peptide receptor 3* (*FPR3*), *histone cluster 1 H3 family member b* (*HIST1H3B*), *IFNE*, *Macrophage scavenger receptor type I and II* (*MSR1*), *PBK*, *Tumor necrosis factor-inducible gene 6 protein* (*TNFAIP6*), *Triggering receptor expressed on myeloid cell 1* (*TREM1*), and *VSIG4*, were categorized to the inflammation-modulating group (Table 1). Protein-protein interactions among APOD, C1QB, FPR3, VSIG4, and MSR1 have also been assembled by the STRING networks [32]. These interactions, albeit weak (such as "textmining" and "co-expression"), were gathered in the biological processes related to "regulation of immune system process", "response to stress", "regulation of inflammatory response", and "response to the stimulus" (Figure 5).

Table 1. Ten common DEGs related to "inflammation modulating".

Symbol	Gene Name	Healthy vs. OA				Expression	Function in Uniprot
		Synovium		Cartilage			
		logFC	*p* Value	logFC	*p* Value		
APOD	*Apolipoprotein D*	−2.30916619	0.025415	−3.64045	0.000375	Extracellular region or secreted	Aging, angiogenesis, brain development, glucose metabolic process, lipid metabolic process, negative regulation of cytokine production involved in inflammatory response, negative regulation of focal adhesion assembly, negative regulation of lipoprotein lipid oxidation, negative regulation of monocyte chemotactic protein-1 production, negative regulation of platelet-derived growth factor receptor signaling pathway, negative regulation of protein import into nucleus, negative regulation of smooth muscle cell-matrix adhesion, negative regulation of smooth muscle cell proliferation, negative regulation of T cell migration, peripheral nervous system axon regeneration, response to axon injury, response to drug, response to reactive oxygen species, tissue regeneration
C1QB	*Complement C1q subcomponent subunit B*	1.71705429	0.036863	2.74003	0.042712	Extracellular region or secreted	Complement activation, classical pathway; innate immune response, inner ear development, regulation of complement activation, synapse pruning
FPR3	*N-formyl peptide receptor 3*	2.00718964	0.004814	2.587989	0.045465	Plasma membrane	Chemotaxis, complement receptor mediated signaling pathway, G protein-coupled receptor signaling pathway, inflammatory response, phospholipase C-activating G protein-coupled receptor signaling pathway, positive regulation of cytosolic calcium ion concentration, signal transduction
HIST1H3B	*Histone cluster 1 H3 family member b*	1.89596286	0.033674	2.685807	0.025722	Nucleus	Blood coagulation, cellular protein metabolic process, chromatin organization, chromatin silencing at rDNA, DNA replication-dependent nucleosome assembly, interleukin-7 mediated signaling pathway, negative regulation of gene expression, epigenetic, nucleosome assembly, regulation of gene silencing by miRNA, regulation of megakaryocyte differentiation, telomere organization

Table 1. *Cont.*

Symbol	Gene Name	Healthy vs. OA				Expression	Function in Uniprot
		Synovium		Cartilage			
		logFC	*p* Value	logFC	*p* Value		
IFNE	*Interferon epsilon*	2.74670721	0.001932	3.545149	0.000413	Extracellular region or secreted	Adaptive immune response, B cell differentiation, B cell proliferation, cytokine-mediated signaling pathway, defense response to bacterium, defense response to virus, humoral immune response, natural killer cell activation involved in immune response, positive regulation of peptidyl-serine phosphorylation of STAT protein, response to exogenous dsRNA, T cell activation involved in immune response
MSR1	*Macrophage scavenger receptor types I and II*	2.00838663	0.011941	3.360986	0.015031	-	Amyloid-beta clearance, cholesterol transport, negative regulation of gene expression, phagocytosis, engulfment, plasma lipoprotein particle clearance, positive regulation of cholesterol storage, positive regulation of macrophage derived foam cell differentiation, receptor-mediated endocytosis
PBK	*Lymphokine-activated killer T-cell-originated protein kinase*	1.94190515	0.035765	2.802857	0.011073	Nucleus	Cellular response to UV, mitotic cell cycle, negative regulation of inflammatory response, negative regulation of proteasomal ubiquitin-dependent protein catabolic process, negative regulation of stress-activated MAPK cascade
TNFAIP6	*Tumor necrosis factor-inducible gene 6 protein*	2.42594431	0.004714	4.335193	0.000138	Extracellular region or secreted	Hyaluronic acid binding; cell adhesion, cell-cell signaling, inflammatory response, negative regulation of inflammatory response, neutrophil degranulation, ovulation, positive regulation of cell migration, signal transduction
TREM1	*Triggering receptor expressed on myeloid cells 1*	1.77423941	0.042306	4.671057	3.93×10^{-5}	Extracellular region or secreted, Plasma membrane	Acute inflammatory response, humoral immune response, innate immune response, intracellular signal transduction, leukocyte migration, regulation of immune response
VSIG4	*V-set and immunoglobulin domain-containing protein 4*	1.90947583	0.019372	3.174618	0.024179	-	Negative regulation of complement activation, alternative pathway; negative regulation of interleukin-2 production, negative regulation of macrophage activation, negative regulation of T cell proliferation

OA—osteoarthritis; logFC—log fold change; rDNA—Recombinant DNA; miRNA—microRNA; STAT—signal transducer and activator of transcription; dsRNA—Double-stranded RNA; UV—Ultraviolet; MAPK—mitogen-activated protein kinase.

a

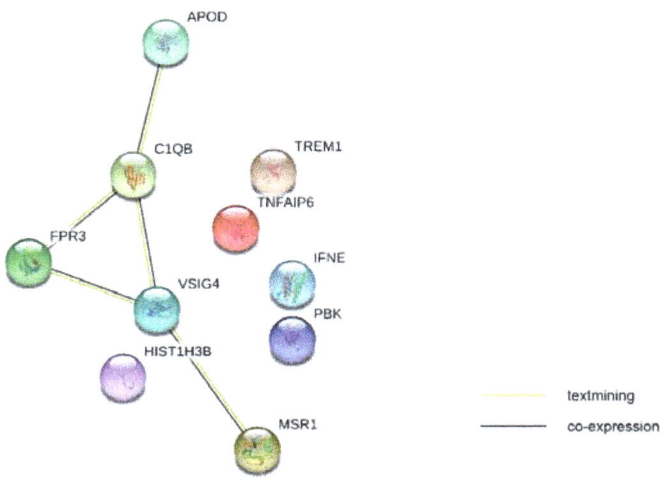

b

#term ID	term description	observed gene count	background gene count	false discovery rate	matching proteins in the network (labels)
GO:0006952	defense response	6	1234	0.0029	C1QB,FPR3,IFNE,TNFAIP6,TREM1,VSIG4
GO:0006959	humoral immune response	4	252	0.0029	C1QB,IFNE,TREM1,VSIG4
GO:0002682	regulation of immune system process	6	139[illegible]	0.003	APOD,C1QB,FPR3,HIST1H3B,TREM1,VSIG4
GO:0006950	response to stress	8	3267	0.003	APOD,C1QB,FPR3,HIST1H3B,IFNE,TNFAIP6, TREM1,VSIG4
GO:0050727	regulation of inflammatory response	4	338	0.003	APOD,C1QB,PBK,TNFAIP6
GO:0050728	negative regulation of inflammatory response	3	117	0.003	APOD,PBK,TNFAIP6
GO:0048583	regulation of response to stimulus	8	3822	0.0054	APOD,C1QB,FPR3,IFNE,PBK,TNFAIP6,TREM1, VSIG4
GO:0006956	complement activation	2	49	0.0146	C1QB,VSIG4
GO:0045087	innate immune response	4	676	0.0146	C1QB,IFNE,TREM1,VSIG4
GO:0002376	immune system process	6	2370	0.0157	C1QB,FPR3,IFNE,TNFAIP6,TREM1,VSIG4
GO:0006955	immune response	5	1560	0.0198	C1QB,IFNE,TNFAIP6,TREM1,VSIG4
GO:0050776	regulation of immune response	4	873	0.021	C1QB,FPR3,TREM1,VSIG4
GO:0072376	protein activation cascade	2	74	0.021	C1QB,VSIG4
GO:0002252	immune effector process	4	927	0.0241	C1QB,IFNE,TNFAIP6,VSIG4
GO:0002253	activation of immune response	3	393	0.0241	C1QB,FPR3,VSIG4
GO:0050896	response to stimulus	9	7824	0.0429	APOD,C1QB,FPR3,HIST1H3B,IFNE,PBK, TNFAIP6,TREM1,VSIG4

Figure 5. STRING database displayed the protein-protein interaction network among the 10 common differential expressed genes (DEGs) in cartilage and synovium that related to inflammation modulating. (**a**) the diagram generated from the STRING data based to demonstrate the potential interactions. (**b**) The list contains identified pathways with a false discovery rate (FDR) less than 0.05. *APOD—Apolipoprotein; C1QB—complement C1q subcomponent subunit B; FPR3—N-formyl peptide receptor 3; HIST1H3B—histone cluster 1 H3 family member b; IFNE—Interferon epsilon; MSR1—Macrophage scavenger receptor type I and II; PBK—Lymphokine-activated killer T-cell-originated protein kinase; TNFAIP6—Tumor necrosis factor-inducible gene 6 protein; TREM1—Triggering receptor expressed on myeloid cell 1; VSIG4—V-set and immunoglobulin domain containing 4.*

Additionally, 7 genes, including *MYOC*, *Amelotin* (*AMTN*), *CHI3L2*, *Prolyl endopeptidase FAP* (*Fibroblast activation protein alpha*; *FAP*), *LRRC15*, *MMP13*, and *TNFAIP6*, were grouped based on their functions related to "extracellular matrix (ECM) binding, formation, degradation" listed in the Uniprot database (Table 2). Although the STRING network could assemble no direct protein-protein interaction with statistical significance, several biological processes were detected, such as "fibronectin binding", "collagen binding", and "metalloendopeptidase activity" (Figure 6).

Table 2. Seven common DEGs related to "extracellular matrix (ECM) binding, formation, degradation."

Symbol	Gene Name	Healthy vs. OA				Expression	Function in Uniprot
		Synovium		Cartilage			
		logFC	*p* Value	logFC	*p* Value		
MYOC	*Myocilin*	−3.2029017	0.00068	−4.11544	0.002817	Extracellular region or secreted, Golgi apparatus, mitochondrion, rough endoplasmic reticulum	Bone development, clustering of voltage-gated sodium channels, ERBB2-ERBB3 signaling pathway, myelination in peripheral nervous system, negative regulation of cell-matrix adhesion, negative regulation of Rho protein signal transduction, negative regulation of stress fiber assembly, neuron projection development, non-canonical Wnt signaling pathway via JNK cascade, osteoblast differentiation, positive regulation of cell migration, positive regulation of focal adhesion assembly, positive regulation of mitochondrial depolarization, positive regulation of phosphatidylinositol 3-kinase signaling, positive regulation of protein kinase B signaling, positive regulation of stress fiber assembly, positive regulation of substrate adhesion-dependent cell spreading, regulation of MAPK cascade, skeletal muscle hypertrophy
AMTN	*Amelotin*	3.91241415	0.002914	5.414278	0.000259	Extracellular region or secreted	Biomineral tissue development, cell adhesion, cellular protein metabolic process, odontogenesis of dentin-containing tooth, positive regulation of biomineral tissue development, positive regulation of enamel mineralization, post-translational protein modification
CHI3L2	*Chitinase-3-like protein 2*	2.17945593	0.023414	3.223409	0.000902	Extracellular region or secreted	Carbohydrate metabolic process, chitin catabolic process
FAP	*Prolyl endopeptidase FAP/Fibroblast activation protein alpha*	1.68745632	0.044592	2.264122	0.013885	Extracellular region or secreted, plasma membrane	Angiogenesis, cell adhesion, endothelial cell migration, melanocyte apoptotic process, melanocyte proliferation, mitotic cell cycle arrest, negative regulation of cell proliferation involved in contact inhibition, negative regulation of extracellular matrix disassembly, negative regulation of extracellular matrix organization, positive regulation of cell cycle arrest, positive regulation of execution phase of apoptosis, proteolysis, proteolysis involved in cellular protein catabolic process, regulation of collagen catabolic process, regulation of fibrinolysis
LRRC15	*Leucine-rich repeat-containing protein 15*	2.10204668	0.016016	5.236099	2.11×10^{-5}	Extracellular region or secreted	Collagen binding, fibronectin binding, laminin binding; negative regulation of protein localization to plasma membrane, positive regulation of cell migration, receptor-mediated virion attachment to host cell
MMP13	*Matrix metallopeptidase-13/ Collagenase 3*	3.48223529	7.54×10^{-5}	3.194238	0.001586	Extracellular region or secreted	Bone mineralization, bone morphogenesis, cellular protein metabolic process, collagen catabolic process, endochondral ossification, extracellular matrix disassembly, extracellular matrix organization, growth plate cartilage development, proteolysis, response to amyloid-beta
TNFAIP6	*Tumor necrosis factor-inducible gene 6 protein*	2.42594431	0.004714	4.335193	0.000138	Extracellular region or secreted	Hyaluronic acid binding; cell adhesion, cell-cell signaling, inflammatory response, negative regulation of inflammatory response, neutrophil degranulation, ovulation, positive regulation of cell migration, signal transduction

OA—osteoarthritis; logFC—log fold change; ERBB—epidermal growth factor; Wnt—Wingless-related integration site; JNK-c—Jun N-terminal kinases; MAPK—mitogen-activated protein kinase.

a

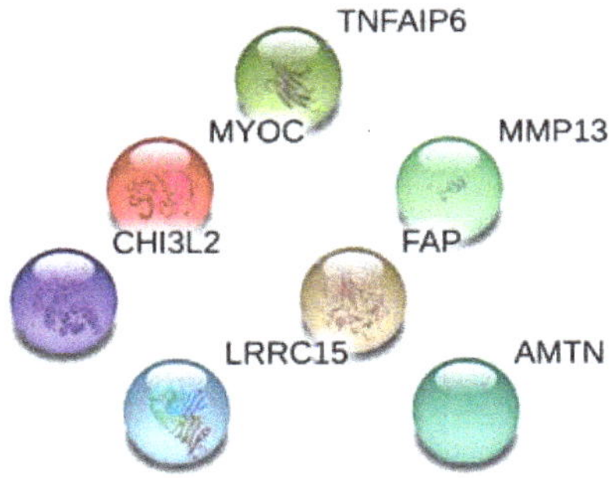

b

#term ID	term description	observed gene	background gene count	false discovery rate	matching proteins in the network (labels)
GO:0001968	fibronectin binding	2	26	0.0025	LRRC15,MYOC
GO:0005518	collagen binding	2	61	0.0065	LRRC15,MMP13
GO:0004222	metalloendopeptidase activity	2	110	0.0136	FAP,MMP13
GO:0004252	serine-type endopeptidase activity	2	180	0.0267	FAP,MMP13
GO:0044877	protein-containing complex binding	3	968	0.0279	FAP,LRRC15,MMP13

Figure 6. The clustering results from the STRING database by inputting 7 extracellular matrix related genes. (**a**) the diagram generated from the STRING data based to demonstrate the potential interactions. (**b**)The list contains identified pathways with a false discovery rate less than 0.05. *MYOC: Myocilin, AMTN: Amelotin, CHI3L2: Chitinase-3-like protein 2, FAP: Fibroblast activation protein alpha, LRRC15: Leucine-rich repeat-containing protein 15, MMP13: Matrix metallopeptidase-13, TNFAIP6: Tumor necrosis factor-inducible gene 6 protein.*

On the other hand, functions of the 3 DEGs whose OA-induced responses are different in synovium and cartilage were also examined. However, only *Phosphatase and actin regulator 3* (*PTACTR3*) could be found in the Uniprot database. As a protein expressed in the cell nucleus, PTACTR3 functions in "actin binding", "protein phosphatase 1 binding" and "protein phosphatase inhibitor activity" (Table S4). No known OA-related function of the other two noncoding DEGs, *RNA, U12 small nuclear* (*RNU12*), and *RNA, U6 small nuclear 2* (*RNU6-2*) again highlights the lack of sufficient knowledge related to OA.

3. Discussion

It is no wonder that *matrix metallopeptidase 13* (*MMP13*), a broadly investigated critical OA-related gene [33,34], is one of the 35 DEGs that respond to OA the same trend in both cartilage and synovium, demonstrating the reliability of the current study. In addition to MMP13, some of these OA-responsive DEGs shared by cartilage and synovium have also been studied in the arena against arthritis, although their function may only be investigated solely in cartilage or synovium. For example, CHI3L2 (also known as YKL-39) has been identified as a biochemical marker for the OA progression in human cartilage since 2002 [35,36]. Functionally, CHI3HL2 has been shown to enhance the proliferation and type II collagen expression in ATDC5 mouse chondrogenic cells [37]. With the successful generation of polyclonal and monoclonal antibodies against CHI3L2, strong activation of the CHI3L2 was detected not only in human T lymphocyte cell lines and monocytes but in the synovial fluid of an OA patient [38]. More importantly, autoimmunity against CHI3L2 was also detected in OA patients [39]. However, its function on synovium tissue is still unknown.

On the other hand, as a transmembrane serine protease that is known to be associated with cell migration and cell invasiveness [40], FAP has been associated with arthritic synovium and cartilage. FAP-deficiency in hTNFtg mice led to less cartilage degradation [40], while highly expressed FAP has been detected in the rheumatoid synovium [41]. A radiolabeled anti–FAP antibody has even been used as a noninvasive strategy to monitor the course of collagen-induced arthritis in mice [41]. For the therapeutic drug development, targeted photodynamic therapy (tPDT) using the anti-FAP antibody 28H1 coupled to the photosensitizer IRDye700DX moderately delayed the collagen-induced arthritis development in mice [42]. Meanwhile, TREM-1 has also been identified as a biomarker of synovitis in RA [43] and predicting the therapeutic response to methotrexate in RA [44]. Inhibiting the expression of TREM-1 could suppress the chondrocyte injury induce by IL-1β in vitro [45], and ameliorate collagen-induced arthritis and protect bone and cartilage damage in vivo [46]. Although these published functional tests were predominantly archived in the RA scenario, especially with the RA synovial fibroblasts, our current study identified expression of FAP and TREM-1 significantly upregulated in both synovium and cartilage of OA patients, strongly suggesting that lowering FAP and TREM-1 might be beneficial for both RA and OA patients.

Besides, MSR1 is a multifunctional receptor expressed primarily on cells of the myeloid lineage [47]. It positively regulates the activation of macrophages and thus promoting the inflammation [48]. The genetic deficiency of *Msr1* decreased the incidence and severity of autoimmune arthritis in the K/BxN T cell receptor (TCR) transgenic mouse model [47]. It is well known that the immune system plays a critical role in OA pathogenesis, and previous studies have acknowledged that the application of immunomodulatory drugs is a potential avenue for OA treatments [49–51]. With the identification of MSR1 in the current study, we may further prove the immune processes' participation within the OA joint and synovium [9].

TNFAIP6 (also known as TSG-6) is an upregulated OA-responsive DEG shared by cartilage and synovium. It is a multifunctional protein with anti-inflammatory and tissue-protective biopotencies [52]. It has been shown that intra-articular delivery of TNFAIP6 could reduce cartilage damage in a rat model of OA [53]. However, in the current study, the expression of TNFAIP6 is increased in both cartilage and synovium tissue during OA. These controversial findings could be explained by the article from Chou et al. published in 2018 [54]: TNFAIP6 was highly expressed in damaged articular and meniscal cartilage and cytokine-treated chondrocytes; functionally, TNFAIP6 impairs hyaluronan-aggrecan assembly, but TNFAIP6 mediated hyaluronan-heavy chain formation reduced this adverse effect. Thus, whether TNFAIP6 could be utilized for OA treatment or if it could worsen OA prognosis still needs further investigations.

Meanwhile, our finding is in line with the previous publication that 6-phosphofructo-2-kinase/fructose2,6-bisphosphatase 3 (PFKFB3) expression was down-regulated in human OA cartilage tissues [55]. PFKFB3 is a glycolytic regulator modulating glycolytic metabolism, alleviating endoplasmic reticulum stress, reducing caspase 3 activation, and promoting aggrecan and type II collagen expressions in human OA cartilage [55]. Interestingly, PFKFB3 expression was increased in RA patients' synovial tissue but not in those of OA patients [56]. Moreover, inhibition of PFKFB3 suppresses the synovial inflammation and joint destruction in RA [56]. The distinct expression patterns and entirely opposite functions of PFKFB3 in OA and RA may set PFKFB3 as a biomarker for clinical differential diagnosis and may explain why some DMARDs are failing to improve OA.

Notably, we also identified multiple molecules that had not been correlated to OA. Nevertheless, their functions in chondrogenesis or inflammation make them as the novel targets for OA investigations in the future. For instance, APOD has been identified to be a downstream gene regulated by SRY-box transcription factor 9 (SOX9), an essential transcription factor for chondrocyte phenotype maintaining [57], in human chondrocytic cell line (SW1353) and primary human articular chondrocytes (hARCs) [58]. Particularly, *SOX9* downregulation in OA cartilage is followed by reduced expression of *APOD* [58]. Our finding is consistent with this publication that the expression of *APOD* lowered in OA cartilage tissue, and we also found that *APOD* is decreased in OA synovium. Interestingly, *SOX9* is not one of the 35 common OA-responsive DEGs shared by cartilage and synovium, suggesting that SOX9 may not play a critical role in OA's synovium. Thus, APOD may participate in other SOX9-independent signaling pathways in the synovium tissue during OA progression. A recent study identified APOD as one of the novel molecular markers of human Th17 cells [59]. Although Th17 cells were initially investigated in RA due to their potency against autoimmune diseases [59], accumulating evidence suggests they are also increased in the OA [60]. Additionally, the high APOD protein level in the round ligament fat depot of severely obese women is associated with an improved inflammatory profile [61]. Thus, APOD may manage OA through chondrogenesis in articular cartilage and immune regulation in the synovium. Further functional investigations are necessary to verify this hypothesis.

Another example is C1QB, one of the C1Q genes which transcript component C1B predispose to RA [62]. The newly published paper demonstrated that primary hARCs express *C1QA*, *C1QB*, *C1QC*, and secret C1Q to the extracellular medium, while this expression is regulated by proinflammatory cytokines stimulations [63]. C1Q could bond to the chondrocytes in vitro, altering the expression of collagens [63]. C1Q can also bond to the cartilage matrix components, such as fibromodulin (FMOD), and activate the complement system to eliminate pathogens and damaged cells for tissue recovery and reconstruction [64]. Since the STRING database identified the biological process of "regulating the immune system process" the role of complement activation in both synovium and articular cartilage during OA might be worth more attention.

CDK1 is another commonly increased DEG in OA cartilage and synovium. As a member of the cyclin-dependent kinase family that plays a pivotal role in controlling the cell cycle [65], CDK1 is not only a hub node of the protein-protein interaction network of the 1,25-dihydroxy-vitamin D3 treated primary OA chondrocytes [66]; its expression is also related to the pathogenesis of RA [67]. It is interesting to find that CDK1 is one of the top 10 hub genes identified from the database of "osteoarthritic degenerative meniscal lesions" [65]. Thus, our current study supports the hypothesis that CDK1 plays an essential role in all three of cartilage, synovium, and meniscus. However, the "cell cycle" cluster has a broad range of effects on a diversity of biological events, and thus CDK1 may not be a unique biomarker for OA diagnosis or treatment.

FPR3 has two isoforms FPR1 and FPR2. The FPRs belong to the classical chemotactic G-protein-coupled receptor family that has recently been recognized to play critical roles in inflammation regulation in response to pathogen- or damage-associated chemotactic molecular patterns [68]. The FPRs agonists have been broadly investigated as a potential treatment strategy for various inflammation-related diseases [68]. Recently, the investigation of FPR agonists has extended to RA [69]. Thus, the anti-inflammation effect of FPR agonists might be utilized in OA targeting both the synovium and cartilage based on the finding in our research.

Our current finding is consistent with the previous studies demonstrating that the expression of KLF15 is significantly lower in chondrocytes from OA patients than from healthy subjects [70]. KLF15 is a transcriptional factor that could promote the chondrogenic differentiation of human mesenchymal stem cells by binding to the promoter of SOX9 and activating its expression [71]. Moreover, KLF15 could reduce the TNF-α-induced expression of MMP-3, a well-known cartilage-degrading enzyme [70]. On the other hand, KFL15 activation could negatively regulate inflammations in several cell types [72–75]. Thus, elevating KLF15 levels in OA may also achieve the dual effects of pro-chondrogenesis and anti-inflammation.

Last but not least, several identified genes have even not been correlated to joints so far. With the rapid development and advancement in the research fields, their OA correlations would be gradually established sooner or later. For example, amelotin (AMTN) is a novel secreted protein firstly identified in 2005 and was thought to be specific for ameloblasts [76]. Later on, most research about this protein was focused on its expression in gingival epithelial cells regulated by proinflammatory cytokines [77,78]. Since the current study distinguished *AMTN* as one of the upregulated genes in both synovium and cartilage in response to OA, its functional involvement in OA, particularly in inflammatory reactions, may be worth assessed. Additionally, KCNJ6 (also known as GIRK2) is a potassium channel regulator that holds potential as a pain-reducing target in OA patients [79,80].

It is well known that sex is an essential factor that significantly alters the gene expression in OA pathogenesis. In humans, the prevalence of OA is knowingly higher in women than men [4,6], while women typically present with worse symptoms, including more significant complaints of pain and disability [81,82]. Meanwhile, although OA is not an inevitable consequence of growing old, older age is the most significant risk factor for OA due to the accumulation of a diversity of OA inducers, such as joint injury, obesity, genetics, and anatomical factors that affect joint mechanics [83]. It is also possible that age-related cell senescence plays a critical role in promoting OA initiation and progression. Unfortunately, currently available transcriptome datasets are not collected to reflect the influence of ages, limiting our ability to draw the "blueprint" of age-related OA gene expression. Clearly, it is an urgent task to conquer in future investigations. On the other hand, as the current study aims to identify the potential unisex markers in OA synovium and cartilage and to get the insight into novel OA therapies effective in both male and female OA patients with all ages, we believe that the identified targets mentioned above are valid for the new generation of DMOAD developing.

4. Materials and Methods

SRA files of healthy and OA human knee cartilage (GEO accession number: GSE114007) and health and OA synovium (GEO accession number: GSE89408) RNA-seq data were downloaded from https://www.ncbi.nlm.nih.gov/sra. Data analyses were performed on the Galaxy platform (UseGalaxy.org, [84]). The FASTQC RNA-seq reads were aligned to the human genome (GRCh38) using HISAT2 aligner (Galaxy v. 2.1.0+galaxy 5) with default parameters [85]. Samples with an overall alignment rate >75% were used for further analysis. Raw counts of sequencing read for the feature of genes were extracted by featureCounts (Galaxy v. 1.6.4+galaxy1) [86]. Then, the limma package (Galaxy v. 3.38.3+galaxy3) was used to identify DEGs with its voom method [87,88]. Expressed genes were selected as their counts per million (CPM) value not less than 1 in at least two samples across the entire experiment, while lowly expressed genes were removed for the flowing analyses. Quasi-likelihood F-tests (ANOVA-like analysis) were achieved to identify DEGs [89]. Genes with fold change (FC) more than 2 and false discovery rate (FDR) less than 0.01 were assigned as DEGs. Heatmap, multidimensional scaling (MDS), principal component analysis (PCA), and the Venn diagram were conducted in R (v. 3.6.3) [90] with packages pheatmap (v. 1.0.12), vegan (v. 2.5-6), ggplot2 (v. 3.3.0), and VennDiagram (v. 1.6.20). Pathway enrichment of identified DEGs was firstly performed against the Reactome knowledgebase [30]. In addition, the summary of the known biofunctions for these genes was searched in the Uniprot database [31] for manually functional annotation. The STRING network [32] was also utilized for the protein-protein association and interaction assembling.

5. Conclusions

In summary, our current study identified several novel genes as the potential biomarkers or treatment targets for OA, which will benefit both synovium and cartilage. In combination with the excellent works published by worldwide researchers, we hope our work could pave the path for developing the new generation of DMOADs.

Supplementary Materials: Supplementary materials can be found at http://www.mdpi.com/1422-0067/21/17/6033/s1. Table S1. The information of the samples included in the current study; Table S2. The list of the identified pathways from the Reactome database; Table S3. The biological processes described in the Uniprot database for the genes with the same expression trends in response to OA; Table S4. The biological processes described in the Uniprot database for the genes with different expression trends in response to OA.

Author Contributions: Conceptualization, C.L.; methodology, C.L. and Z.Z.; validation, C.L. and Z.Z.; formal analysis, Z.Z.; writing—original draft preparation, C.L.; writing—review and editing, Z.Z. All authors have read and agreed to the published version of the manuscript.

Funding: This research received no external funding.

Conflicts of Interest: The authors declare no conflict of interest.

References

1. National Health Service, UK, Arthritis. Available online: https://www.nhs.uk/conditions/arthritis/ (accessed on 19 August 2020).
2. Centres for Disease Control and Prevention, USA, Arthritis Types. Available online: https://www.cdc.gov/arthritis/basics/types.html (accessed on 19 August 2020).
3. Arthritis Foundation. Understanding Arthritis. Available online: https://www.arthritis.org/about-arthritis/understanding-arthritis/ (accessed on 19 August 2020).
4. Osteoarthritis Research Society International. Osteoarthritis: A serious Disease. 2016, pp. 1–103. Available online: https://www.oarsi.org/sites/default/files/docs/2016/oarsi_white_paper_oa_serious_disease_121416_1.pdf (accessed on 19 August 2020).
5. Hootman, J.M.; Helmick, C.G.; Barbour, K.E.; Theis, K.A.; Boring, M.A. Updated Projected Prevalence of Self-Reported Doctor-Diagnosed Arthritis and Arthritis-Attributable Activity Limitation Among US Adults, 2015–2040. *Arthritis Rheumatol.* **2016**, *68*, 1582–1587. [CrossRef] [PubMed]
6. Hunter, D.J.; Bierma-Zeinstra, S. Osteoarthritis. *Lancet* **2019**, *393*, 1745–1759. [CrossRef]
7. Kopec, J.A.; Rahman, M.M.; Berthelot, J.M.; Le Petit, C.; Aghajanian, J.; Sayre, E.C.; Cibere, J.; Anis, A.H.; Badley, E.M. Descriptive epidemiology of osteoarthritis in British Columbia, Canada. *J. Rheumatol.* **2007**, *34*, 386–393. [PubMed]
8. Lohmander, L.S.; Englund, P.M.; Dahl, L.L.; Roos, E.M. The long-term consequence of anterior cruciate ligament and meniscus injuries: Osteoarthritis. *Am. J. Sports Med.* **2007**, *35*, 1756–1769. [CrossRef] [PubMed]
9. Sokolove, J.; Lepus, C.M. Role of inflammation in the pathogenesis of osteoarthritis: Latest findings and interpretations. *Ther. Adv. Musculoskelet. Dis.* **2013**, *5*, 77–94. [CrossRef]
10. Karsdal, M.A.; Michaelis, M.; Ladel, C.; Siebuhr, A.S.; Bihlet, A.R.; Andersen, J.R.; Guehring, H.; Christiansen, C.; Bay-Jensen, A.C.; Kraus, V.B. Disease-modifying treatments for osteoarthritis (DMOADs) of the knee and hip: Lessons learned from failures and opportunities for the future. *Osteoarthr. Cartil.* **2016**, *24*, 2013–2021. [CrossRef]
11. Puig-Junoy, J.; Ruiz, A. Socio-economic costs of osteoarthritis: A systematic review of cost-of-illness studies. *Semin. Arthritis Rheu.* **2015**, *44*, 531–541. [CrossRef]
12. Medvedeva, E.V.; Grebenik, E.A.; Gornostaeva, S.N.; Telpuhov, V.I.; Lychagin, A.V.; Timashev, P.S.; Chagin, A.S. Repair of Damaged Articular Cartilage: Current Approaches and Future Directions. *Int. J. Mol. Sci.* **2018**, *19*, 2366. [CrossRef]
13. Wenham, C.Y.; Conaghan, P.G. The role of synovitis in osteoarthritis. *Ther. Adv. Musculoskelet. Dis.* **2010**, *2*, 349–359. [CrossRef]
14. Mathiessen, A.; Conaghan, P.G. Synovitis in osteoarthritis: Current understanding with therapeutic implications. *Arthritis Res. Ther.* **2017**, *19*, 18. [CrossRef]
15. Caplan, L.; Wolfe, F.; Russell, A.S.; Michaud, K. Corticosteroid use in rheumatoid arthritis: Prevalence, predictors, correlates, and outcomes. *J. Rheumatol.* **2007**, *34*, 696–705. [PubMed]
16. Hammer, M.; Schwarz, T.; Ganser, G. Intra-articular injection of cortisone. *Z. Rheumatol.* **2015**, *74*, 774–779. [CrossRef] [PubMed]
17. Chandrappa, M.; Biswas, S. Glucocorticoids in Management of Adult Rheumatoid Arthritis-Current Prescribing Practices and Perceptions of Physicians in India: GLUMAR Survey. *Rheumatology* **2017**, *7*, 1000220. [CrossRef]
18. Saltychev, M.; Mattie, R.; McCormick, Z.; Laimi, K. The Magnitude and Duration of the Effect of Intra-articular Corticosteroid Injections on Pain Severity in Knee Osteoarthritis: A Systematic Review and Meta-Analysis. *Am. J. Phys. Med. Rehabil.* **2020**, *99*, 617–625. [CrossRef]
19. Arroll, B.; Goodyear-Smith, F. Corticosteroid injections for osteoarthritis of the knee: Meta-analysis. *BMJ* **2004**, *328*, 869. [CrossRef]
20. Savvidou, O.; Milonaki, M.; Goumenos, S.; Flevas, D.; Papagelopoulos, P.; Moutsatsou, P. Glucocorticoid signaling and osteoarthritis. *Mol. Cell Endocrinol.* **2019**, *480*, 153–166. [CrossRef]

21. Cooper, C.; Bardin, T.; Brandi, M.L.; Cacoub, P.; Caminis, J.; Civitelli, R.; Cutolo, M.; Dere, W.; Devogelaer, J.P.; Diez-Perez, A.; et al. Balancing benefits and risks of glucocorticoids in rheumatic diseases and other inflammatory joint disorders: New insights from emerging data. An expert consensus paper from the European Society for Clinical and Economic Aspects of Osteoporosis and Osteoarthritis (ESCEO). *Aging Clin. Exp. Res.* **2016**, *28*, 1–16. [CrossRef]
22. Compston, J. Glucocorticoid-induced osteoporosis: An update. *Endocrine* **2018**, *61*, 7–16. [CrossRef]
23. Scott, D.L. Arthritis in the Elderly. In *Brocklehurst's Textbook of Geriatric Medicine and Gerontology*, 7th ed.; Fillit, H.M., Rockwood, K., Woodhouse, K., Eds.; Saunders, Elsevier: Philadelphia, PA, USA, 2010; pp. 566–576.
24. Brosseau, L.; Taki, J.; Desjardins, B.; Thevenot, O.; Fransen, M.; Wells, G.A.; Mizusaki Imoto, A.; Toupin-April, K.; Westby, M.; Alvarez Gallardo, I.C.; et al. The Ottawa panel clinical practice guidelines for the management of knee osteoarthritis. Part two: Strengthening exercise programs. *Clin. Rehabil.* **2017**, *31*, 596–611. [CrossRef]
25. Verbruggen, G.; Wittoek, R.; Cruyssen, B.V.; Elewaut, D. Tumour necrosis factor blockade for the treatment of erosive osteoarthritis of the interphalangeal finger joints: A double blind, randomised trial on structure modification. *Ann. Rheum. Dis.* **2012**, *71*, 891–898. [CrossRef]
26. Chevalier, X.; Ravaud, P.; Maheu, E.; Baron, G.; Rialland, A.; Vergnaud, P.; Roux, C.; Maugars, Y.; Mulleman, D.; Lukas, C.; et al. Adalimumab in patients with hand osteoarthritis refractory to analgesics and NSAIDs: A randomised, multicentre, double- blind, placebo-controlled trial. *Ann. Rheum. Dis.* **2015**, *74*, 1697–1705. [CrossRef] [PubMed]
27. Chevalier, X.; Goupille, P.; Beaulieu, A.D.; Burch, F.X.; Bensen, W.G.; Conrozier, T.; Loeuille, D.; Kivitz, A.J.; Silver, D.; Appleton, B.E. Intraarticular Injection of Anakinra in Osteoarthritis of the Knee: A Multicenter, Randomized, Double-Blind, Placebo-Controlled Study. *Arthrit. Rheum.-Arthr.* **2009**, *61*, 344–352. [CrossRef] [PubMed]
28. Appleton, C.T. Osteoarthritis year in review 2017: Biology. *Osteoarthr. Cartil.* **2018**, *26*, 296–303. [CrossRef] [PubMed]
29. Wojdasiewicz, P.; Poniatowski, L.A.; Szukiewicz, D. The role of inflammatory and anti-inflammatory cytokines in the pathogenesis of osteoarthritis. *Mediat. Inflamm.* **2014**, *2014*, 561459. [CrossRef] [PubMed]
30. Jassal, B.; Matthews, L.; Viteri, G.; Gong, C.; Lorente, P.; Fabregat, A.; Sidiropoulos, K.; Cook, J.; Gillespie, M.; Haw, R.; et al. The reactome pathway knowledgebase. *Nucleic Acids Res.* **2020**, *48*, 498–503. [CrossRef]
31. UniProt, C. UniProt: A worldwide hub of protein knowledge. *Nucleic Acids Res.* **2019**, *47*, 506–515. [CrossRef]
32. Szklarczyk, D.; Gable, A.L.; Lyon, D.; Junge, A.; Wyder, S.; Huerta-Cepas, J.; Simonovic, M.; Doncheva, N.T.; Morris, J.H.; Bork, P.; et al. STRING v11: Protein-protein association networks with increased coverage, supporting functional discovery in genome-wide experimental datasets. *Nucleic Acids Res.* **2019**, *47*, D607–D613. [CrossRef]
33. Li, H.; Wang, D.; Yuan, Y.; Min, J. New insights on the MMP-13 regulatory network in the pathogenesis of early osteoarthritis. *Arthritis Res. Ther.* **2017**, *19*, 248. [CrossRef]
34. Wang, M.; Sampson, E.R.; Jin, H.; Li, J.; Ke, Q.H.; Im, H.J.; Chen, D. MMP13 is a critical target gene during the progression of osteoarthritis. *Arthritis Res. Ther.* **2013**, *15*, 5. [CrossRef]
35. Steck, E.; Breit, S.; Breusch, S.J.; Axt, M.; Richter, W. Enhanced expression of the human chitinase 3-like 2 gene (YKL-39) but not chitinase 3-like 1 gene (YKL-40) in osteoarthritic cartilage. *Biochem. Biophys. Res. Commun.* **2002**, *299*, 109–115. [CrossRef]
36. Knorr, T.; Obermayr, F.; Bartnik, E.; Zien, A.; Aigner, T. YKL-39 (chitinase 3-like protein 2), but not YKL-40 (chitinase 3-like protein 1), is up regulated in osteoarthritic chondrocytes. *Ann. Rheum Dis* **2003**, *62*, 995–998. [CrossRef] [PubMed]
37. Miyatake, K.; Tsuji, K.; Yamaga, M.; Yamada, J.; Matsukura, Y.; Abula, K.; Sekiya, I.; Muneta, T. Human YKL39 (chitinase 3-like protein 2), an osteoarthritis-associated gene, enhances proliferation and type II collagen expression in ATDC5 cells. *Biochem. Biophys. Res. Commun.* **2013**, *431*, 52–57. [CrossRef] [PubMed]
38. Ranok, A.; Khunkaewla, P.; Suginta, W. Human cartilage chitinase 3-like protein 2: Cloning, expression, and production of polyclonal and monoclonal antibodies for osteoarthritis detection and identification of potential binding partners. *Monoclon. Antibodies Immunodiagn. Immunother.* **2013**, *32*, 317–325. [CrossRef]

39. Tsuruha, J.; Masuko-Hongo, K.; Kato, T.; Sakata, M.; Nakamura, H.; Sekine, T.; Takigawa, M.; Nishioka, K. Autoimmunity against YKL-39, a human cartilage derived protein, in patients with osteoarthritis. *J. Rheumatol.* **2002**, *29*, 1459–1466. [PubMed]
40. Waldele, S.; Koers-Wunrau, C.; Beckmann, D.; Korb-Pap, A.; Wehmeyer, C.; Pap, T.; Dankbar, B. Deficiency of fibroblast activation protein alpha ameliorates cartilage destruction in inflammatory destructive arthritis. *Arthritis Res. Ther.* **2015**, *17*, 12. [CrossRef]
41. Van der Geest, T.; Laverman, P.; Gerrits, D.; Walgreen, B.; Helsen, M.M.; Klein, C.; Nayak, T.K.; Storm, G.; Metselaar, J.M.; Koenders, M.I.; et al. Liposomal Treatment of Experimental Arthritis Can Be Monitored Noninvasively with a Radiolabeled Anti-Fibroblast Activation Protein Antibody. *J. Nucl. Med.* **2017**, *58*, 151–155. [CrossRef]
42. Dorst, D.N.; Rijpkema, M.; Boss, M.; Walgreen, B.; Helsen, M.M.A.; Bos, D.L.; Brom, M.; Klein, C.; Laverman, P.; van der Kraan, P.M.; et al. Targeted photodynamic therapy selectively kills activated fibroblasts in experimental arthritis. *Rheumatology* **2020**. [CrossRef]
43. Gorlier, C.; Gottenberg, J.E.; Laurans, L.; Simon, T.; Ait-Oufella, H.; Sellam, J. Serum level of soluble triggering receptor expressed on myeloid cells-1 (sTREM-1) is a biomarker of synovitis in rheumatoid arthritis. *Int. J. Rheum. Dis.* **2019**, *22*, 1616–1618. [CrossRef]
44. Gamez-Nava, J.I.; Bonilla-Lara, D.; Ponce-Guarneros, J.M.; Zuniga-Mora, J.A.; Perez-Guerrero, E.E.; Murillo-Vazquez, J.D.; Becerra-Alvarado, I.N.; Rodriguez-Jimenez, N.A.; Saldana-Cruz, A.M.; Vazquez-Villegas, M.L.; et al. Utility of soluble triggering receptor expressed on myeloid cells-1 (sTREM-1) as biomarker to predict therapeutic response to methotrexate in rheumatoid arthritis. *Innate Immun.* **2017**, *23*, 606–614. [CrossRef]
45. Tang, J.; Dong, Q. Knockdown of TREM-1 suppresses IL-1beta-induced chondrocyte injury via inhibiting the NF-kappaB pathway. *Biochem. Biophys. Res. Commun.* **2017**, *482*, 1240–1245. [CrossRef]
46. Shen, Z.T.; Sigalov, A.B. Rationally designed ligand-independent peptide inhibitors of TREM-1 ameliorate collagen-induced arthritis. *J. Cell. Mol. Med.* **2017**, *21*, 2524–2534. [CrossRef]
47. Haasken, S.; Auger, J.L.; Taylor, J.J.; Hobday, P.M.; Goudy, B.D.; Titcombe, P.J.; Mueller, D.L.; Binstadt, B.A. Macrophage scavenger receptor 1 (Msr1, SR-A) influences B cell autoimmunity by regulating soluble autoantigen concentration. *J. Immunol.* **2013**, *191*, 1055–1062. [CrossRef] [PubMed]
48. Guo, M.; Hartlova, A.; Gierlinski, M.; Prescott, A.; Castellvi, J.; Losa, J.H.; Petersen, S.K.; Wenzel, U.A.; Dill, B.D.; Emmerich, C.H.; et al. Triggering MSR1 promotes JNK-mediated inflammation in IL-4-activated macrophages. *EMBO J.* **2019**, *38*. [CrossRef] [PubMed]
49. Kalaitzoglou, E.; Griffin, T.M.; Humphrey, M.B. Innate Immune Responses and Osteoarthritis. *Curr. Rheumatol. Rep.* **2017**, *19*, 45. [CrossRef] [PubMed]
50. Millerand, M.; Berenbaum, F.; Jacques, C. Danger signals and inflammaging in osteoarthritis. *Clin. Exp. Rheumatol* **2019**, *37*, 48–56.
51. Lopes, E.B.P.; Filiberti, A.; Husain, S.A.; Humphrey, M.B. Immune Contributions to Osteoarthritis. *Curr. Osteoporos. Rep.* **2017**, *15*, 593–600. [CrossRef]
52. Day, A.J.; Milner, C.M. TSG-6: A multifunctional protein with anti-inflammatory and tissue-protective properties. *Matrix Biol.* **2019**, *78–79*, 60–83. [CrossRef]
53. Tellier, L.E.; Trevino, E.A.; Brimeyer, A.L.; Reece, D.S.; Willett, N.J.; Guldberg, R.E.; Temenoff, J.S. Intra-articular TSG-6 delivery from heparin-based microparticles reduces cartilage damage in a rat model of osteoarthritis. *Biomater. Sci.* **2018**, *6*, 1159–1167. [CrossRef]
54. Chou, C.H.; Attarian, D.E.; Wisniewski, H.G.; Band, P.A.; Kraus, V.B. TSG-6—A double-edged sword for osteoarthritis (OA). *Osteoarthr. Cartil.* **2018**, *26*, 245–254. [CrossRef]
55. Qu, J.; Lu, D.; Guo, H.; Miao, W.; Wu, G.; Zhou, M. PFKFB3 modulates glycolytic metabolism and alleviates endoplasmic reticulum stress in human osteoarthritis cartilage. *Clin. Exp. Pharmacol. Physiol.* **2016**, *43*, 312–318. [CrossRef]
56. Zou, Y.; Zeng, S.; Huang, M.; Qiu, Q.; Xiao, Y.; Shi, M.; Zhan, Z.; Liang, L.; Yang, X.; Xu, H. Inhibition of 6-phosphofructo-2-kinase suppresses fibroblast-like synoviocytes-mediated synovial inflammation and joint destruction in rheumatoid arthritis. *Br. J. Pharmacol.* **2017**, *174*, 893–908. [CrossRef] [PubMed]
57. Lefebvre, V.; Dvir-Ginzberg, M. SOX9 and the many facets of its regulation in the chondrocyte lineage. *Connect. Tissue Res.* **2017**, *58*, 2–14. [CrossRef] [PubMed]

58. Tew, S.R.; Clegg, P.D.; Brew, C.J.; Redmond, C.M.; Hardingham, T.E. SOX9 transduction of a human chondrocytic cell line identifies novel genes regulated in primary human chondrocytes and in osteoarthritis. *Arthritis Res. Ther.* **2007**, *9*, 107. [CrossRef] [PubMed]
59. Salkowska, A.; Karas, K.; Karwaciak, I.; Walczak-Drzewiecka, A.; Krawczyk, M.; Sobalska-Kwapis, M.; Dastych, J.; Ratajewski, M. Identification of Novel Molecular Markers of Human Th17 Cells. *Cells* **2020**, 9. [CrossRef]
60. Zhu, W.; Zhang, X.; Jiang, Y.; Liu, X.; Huang, L.; Wei, Q.; Huang, Y.; Wu, W.; Gu, J. Alterations in peripheral T cell and B cell subsets in patients with osteoarthritis. *Clin. Rheumatol.* **2020**, *39*, 523–532. [CrossRef]
61. Desmarais, F.; Bergeron, K.F.; Lacaille, M.; Lemieux, I.; Bergeron, J.; Biron, S.; Rassart, E.; Joanisse, D.R.; Mauriege, P.; Mounier, C. High ApoD protein level in the round ligament fat depot of severely obese women is associated with an improved inflammatory profile. *Endocrine* **2018**, *61*, 248–257. [CrossRef]
62. Trouw, L.A.; Daha, N.; Kurreeman, F.A.; Bohringer, S.; Goulielmos, G.N.; Westra, H.J.; Zhernakova, A.; Franke, L.; Stahl, E.A.; Levarht, E.W.; et al. Genetic variants in the region of the C1q genes are associated with rheumatoid arthritis. *Clin. Exp. Immunol.* **2013**, *173*, 76–83. [CrossRef]
63. Lubbers, R.; van Schaarenburg, R.A.; Kwekkeboom, J.C.; Levarht, E.W.N.; Bakker, A.M.; Mahdad, R.; Monteagudo, S.; Cherifi, C.; Lories, R.J.; Toes, R.E.M.; et al. Complement component C1q is produced by isolated articular chondrocytes. *Osteoarthr. Cartil.* **2020**, *28*, 675–684. [CrossRef]
64. Li, C.; Ha, P.; Jiang, W.; Haveles, C.S.; Zheng, Z.; Zou, M. Fibromodulin—A New Target of Osteoarthritis Management? *Front. Pharmacol.* **2019**, *10*, 1475. [CrossRef]
65. Huan, X.; Jinhe, Y.; Rongzong, Z. Identification of Pivotal Genes and Pathways in Osteoarthritic Degenerative Meniscal Lesions via Bioinformatics Analysis of the GSE52042 Dataset. *Med. Sci. Monit.* **2019**, *25*, 8891–8904. [CrossRef]
66. Zhang, G.; Gu, M.; Xu, Y.; Wu, Z. A comprehensive analysis on the effects of 1,25(OH)2D3 on primary chondrocytes cultured from patients with osteoarthritis. *Gene* **2020**, *730*, 144322. [CrossRef] [PubMed]
67. Fattah, S.A.; Abdel Fattah, M.A.; Mesbah, N.M.; Saleh, S.M.; Abo-Elmatty, D.M.; Mehanna, E.T. The expression of zinc finger 804a (ZNF804a) and cyclin-dependent kinase 1 (CDK1) genes is related to the pathogenesis of rheumatoid arthritis. *Arch. Physiol. Biochem.* **2020**, 1–6. [CrossRef]
68. Chen, K.; Bao, Z.; Gong, W.; Tang, P.; Yoshimura, T.; Wang, J.M. Regulation of inflammation by members of the formyl-peptide receptor family. *J. Autoimmun.* **2017**, *85*, 64–77. [CrossRef] [PubMed]
69. Crocetti, L.; Vergelli, C.; Guerrini, G.; Cantini, N.; Kirpotina, L.N.; Schepetkin, I.A.; Quinn, M.T.; Parisio, C.; Di Cesare Mannelli, L.; Ghelardini, C.; et al. Novel formyl peptide receptor (FPR) agonists with pyridinone and pyrimidindione scaffolds that are potentially useful for the treatment of rheumatoid arthritis. *Bioorg. Chem.* **2020**, *100*, 103880. [CrossRef] [PubMed]
70. Li, Y.; Zhao, M.; Xiao, W. KLF15 Regulates the Expression of MMP-3 in Human Chondrocytes. *J. Interferon Cytokine Res.* **2018**, *38*, 356–362. [CrossRef]
71. Song, Z.; Lian, X.; Wang, Y.; Xiang, Y.; Li, G. KLF15 regulates in vitro chondrogenic differentiation of human mesenchymal stem cells by targeting SOX9. *Biochem. Biophys. Res. Commun.* **2017**, *493*, 1082–1088. [CrossRef]
72. Lu, Y.; Zhang, L.; Liao, X.; Sangwung, P.; Prosdocimo, D.A.; Zhou, G.; Votruba, A.R.; Brian, L.; Han, Y.J.; Gao, H.; et al. Kruppel-like factor 15 is critical for vascular inflammation. *J. Clin. Investig.* **2013**, *123*, 4232–4241. [CrossRef]
73. Jung, D.Y.; Chalasani, U.; Pan, N.; Friedline, R.H.; Prosdocimo, D.A.; Nam, M.; Azuma, Y.; Maganti, R.; Yu, K.; Velagapudi, A.; et al. KLF15 is a molecular link between endoplasmic reticulum stress and insulin resistance. *PLoS ONE* **2013**, *8*, e77851. [CrossRef]
74. Mallipattu, S.K.; Guo, Y.; Revelo, M.P.; Roa-Pena, L.; Miller, T.; Ling, J.; Shankland, S.J.; Bialkowska, A.B.; Ly, V.; Estrada, C.; et al. Kruppel-Like Factor 15 Mediates Glucocorticoid-Induced Restoration of Podocyte Differentiation Markers. *J. Am. Soc. Nephrol.* **2017**, *28*, 166–184. [CrossRef]
75. Lu, Y.Y.; Li, X.D.; Zhou, H.D.; Shao, S.; He, S.; Hong, M.N.; Liu, J.C.; Xu, Y.L.; Wu, Y.J.; Zhu, D.L.; et al. Transactivation domain of Kruppel-like factor 15 negatively regulates angiotensin II-induced adventitial inflammation and fibrosis. *FASEB J.* **2019**, *33*, 6254–6268. [CrossRef]
76. Iwasaki, K.; Bajenova, E.; Somogyi-Ganss, E.; Miller, M.; Nguyen, V.; Nourkeyhani, H.; Gao, Y.; Wendel, M.; Ganss, B. Amelotin—A Novel Secreted, Ameloblast-specific Protein. *J. Dent. Res.* **2005**, *84*, 1127–1132. [CrossRef] [PubMed]

77. Nakayama, Y.; Tsuruya, Y.; Noda, K.; Yamazaki-Takai, M.; Iwai, Y.; Ganss, B.; Ogata, Y. Negative feedback by SNAI2 regulates TGFbeta1-induced amelotin gene transcription in epithelial-mesenchymal transition. *J. Cell. Physiol.* **2019**, *234*, 11474–11489. [CrossRef] [PubMed]
78. Yamazaki, M.; Mezawa, M.; Noda, K.; Iwai, Y.; Matsui, S.; Takai, H.; Nakayama, Y.; Ogata, Y. Transcriptional regulation of human amelotin gene by interleukin-1beta. *FEBS Open Bio* **2018**, *8*, 974–985. [CrossRef] [PubMed]
79. Nockemann, D.; Rouault, M.; Labuz, D.; Hublitz, P.; McKnelly, K.; Reis, F.C.; Stein, C.; Heppenstall, P.A. The K(+) channel GIRK2 is both necessary and sufficient for peripheral opioid-mediated analgesia. *EMBO Mol. Med.* **2013**, *5*, 1263–1277. [CrossRef]
80. Tsantoulas, C. Emerging potassium channel targets for the treatment of pain. *Curr. Opin. Support. Palliat. Care* **2015**, *9*, 147–154. [CrossRef]
81. McAlindon, T.E.; Cooper, C.; Kirwan, J.R.; Dieppe, P.A. Knee pain and disability in the community. *Br. J. Rheumatol.* **1992**, *31*, 189–192. [CrossRef]
82. Cho, H.J.; Chang, C.B.; Yoo, J.H.; Kim, S.J.; Kim, T.K. Gender Differences in the Correlation between Symptom and Radiographic Severity in Patients with Knee Osteoarthritis. *Clin. Orthop. Relat. Res.* **2010**, *468*, 1749–1758. [CrossRef]
83. Shane Anderson, A.; Loeser, R.F. Why is osteoarthritis an age-related disease? *Best Pract. Res. Clin. Rheumatol* **2010**, *24*, 15–26. [CrossRef]
84. Afgan, E.; Baker, D.; Batut, B.; van den Beek, M.; Bouvier, D.; Cech, M.; Chilton, J.; Clements, D.; Coraor, N.; Gruning, B.A.; et al. The Galaxy platform for accessible, reproducible and collaborative biomedical analyses: 2018 update. *Nucleic Acids Res.* **2018**, *46*, 537–544. [CrossRef]
85. Kim, D.; Langmead, B.; Salzberg, S.L. HISAT: A fast spliced aligner with low memory requirements. *Nat. Methods* **2015**, *12*, 357–360. [CrossRef]
86. Liao, Y.; Smyth, G.K.; Shi, W. featureCounts: An efficient general purpose program for assigning sequence reads to genomic features. *Bioinformatics* **2014**, *30*, 923–930. [CrossRef] [PubMed]
87. Smyth, G.K. limma: Linear Models for Microarray Data. In *Bioinformatics and Computational Biology Solutions Using R and Bioconductor. Statistics for Biology and Health*; Gentleman, R., Carey, V.J., Huber, W., Irizarry, R.A., Dudoit, S., Eds.; Springer: New York, NY, USA, 2005; Available online: https://doi.org/10.1007/0-387-29362-0_23 (accessed on 19 August 2020).
88. Law, C.W.; Chen, Y.; Shi, W.; Smyth, G.K. voom: Precision weights unlock linear model analysis tools for RNA-seq read counts. *Genome Biol.* **2014**, *15*, 29. [CrossRef] [PubMed]
89. Lun, A.T.; Chen, Y.; Smyth, G.K. It's DE-licious: A Recipe for Differential Expression Analyses of RNA-seq Experiments Using Quasi-Likelihood Methods in edgeR. *Methods Mol. Biol.* **2016**, *1418*, 391–416. [CrossRef] [PubMed]
90. *A Language and Environment for Statistical Computing*; Version 3.6.3; The R Foundation: Vienna, Austria, 2020; Available online: http://www.R-project.org/ (accessed on 19 August 2020).

International Journal of *Molecular Sciences*

MDPI

Article

Infrapatellar Fat Pad Gene Expression and Protein Production in Patients with and without Osteoarthritis

Elisa Belluzzi [1,†], Veronica Macchi [2,3,†], Chiara Giulia Fontanella [4,5], Emanuele Luigi Carniel [5,6], Eleonora Olivotto [7], Giuseppe Filardo [8], Gloria Sarasin [2], Andrea Porzionato [2,3], Marnie Granzotto [9], Assunta Pozzuoli [1], Antonio Berizzi [10], Manuela Scioni [11], Raffaele De Caro [2,3], Pietro Ruggieri [10], Roberto Vettor [9], Roberta Ramonda [12], Marco Rossato [9,*] and Marta Favero [12,13]

1 Musculoskeletal Pathology and Oncology Laboratory, Orthopedic and Traumatologic Clinic, Department of Surgery, Oncology and Gastroenterology (DISCOG), University of Padova, 35128 Padova, Italy; elisa.belluzzi@gmail.com (E.B.); assunta.pozzuoli@unipd.it (A.P.)

2 Institute of Human Anatomy, Department of Neurosciences, University of Padova, 35121 Padova, Italy; veronica.macchi@unipd.it (V.M.); gloria.sarasin@unipd.it (G.S.); andrea.porzionato@unipd.it (A.P.); raffaele.decaro@unipd.it (R.D.C.)

3 L.i.f.e. L.a.b. Program, Consorzio per la Ricerca Sanitaria (CORIS), Veneto Region, 35128 Padova, Italy

4 Department of Civil, Environmental and Architectural Engineering, University of Padova, 35131 Padova, Italy; chiaragiulia.fontanella@unipd.it

5 Centre for Mechanics of Biological Materials, University of Padova, 35131 Padova, Italy; emanueleluigi.carniel@unipd.it

6 Department of Industrial Engineering, University of Padova, 35131 Padova, Italy

7 RAMSES Laboratory, RIT Department, IRCCS Istituto Ortopedico Rizzoli, 40136 Bologna, Italy; eleonora.olivotto@ior.it

8 Applied and Translational Research (ATR) Center, IRCCS Istituto Ortopedico Rizzoli, 40136 Bologna, Italy; g.filardo@biomec.ior.it

9 Clinica Medica 3, Department of Medicine—DIMED, University of Padova, School of Medicine, 35128 Padova, Italy; marnie.granzotto@unipd.it (M.G.); roberto.vettor@unipd.it (R.V.)

10 Orthopaedic and Traumatologic Clinic, Department of Surgery, Oncology and Gastroenterology (DiSCOG), University of Padova, 35128 Padova, Italy; antonio berizzi@unipd.it (A.B.); pietro.ruggieri@unipd.it (P.R.)

11 Department of Statistical Sciences, University of Padova, 35121 Padova, Italy; scioni@stat.unipd.it

12 Rheumatology Unit, Department of Medicine-DIMED, University—Hospital of Padova, Via Giustiniani, 2, 35128 Padova, Italy; roberta.ramonda@unipd.it (R.R.); faveromarta@gmail.com (M.F.)

13 Internal Medicine I, Cà Foncello Hospital, 31100 Treviso, Italy

* Correspondence: marco.rossato@unipd.it; Tel.: +39-049-8218747

† These authors contributed equally to this work.

Received: 24 July 2020; Accepted: 19 August 2020; Published: 21 August 2020

Abstract: Osteoarthritis (OA) is one of the most common joint disorders. Evidence suggests that the infrapatellar fat pad (IFP) is directly involved in OA pathology. However, a comparison between OA versus non-OA IFP is still missing. Thus, the aim of this study was to compare IFP molecular, adipocytes and extracellular matrix characteristics of patients affected by OA, and patients undergoing anterior cruciate ligament (ACL) reconstruction. We hypothesized that not only inflammation but also changes in adipocytes and extracellular matrix (ECM) composition might be involved in OA pathogenesis. Fifty-three patients were enrolled. IFP biopsies were obtained, evaluating: (a) lymphocytic infiltration and vascularization; (b) adipocytes area and number; (c) adipo-cytokines and extracellular matrix gene expression levels, (d) IL-6 and VEGF protein production; (e) collagen fibers distribution. OA IFP was more inflamed and vascularized compared to ACL IFP. OA IFP adipocytes were larger and numerically lower (1.3-fold) than ACL IFP adipocytes. An increase of gene expression of typical white adipose tissue genes was observed in OA compared to ACL

IFP. Collagen-types distribution was different in the OA IFP group compared to controls, possibly explaining the change of the biomechanical characteristics found in OA IFP. Statistical linear models revealed that the adipocyte area correlated with BMI in the OA group. In conclusion, inflammation and fibrotic changes of OA IFP could represent novel therapeutic targets to counteract OA.

Keywords: adipocyte; infrapatellar fat pad; osteoarthritis; anterior cruciate ligament; inflammation

---

1. Introduction

Osteoarthritis (OA) is one of the most frequent forms of arthritis and an important cause of pain and disability in elderly people [1]. The most affected joint is the knee, with a worldwide estimated radiographic prevalence of 3.8% [2].

Nowadays, OA is considered a whole joint disease involving cartilage, meniscus, synovial membrane, and infrapatellar fat pad (IFP) [3–6]. It is well-known that OA is characterized by synovial inflammation, determined by synoviocytes, which secrete pro-inflammatory cytokines that induce chondrocytes to produce degradative enzymes of the extracellular matrix (ECM) and inhibit both tissue repair and regeneration [7]. Actually, there is no cure for this pathology and the OA management relies on symptomatic interventions. Total joint replacement represents the only treatment available for end-stage OA. However, physical activity and nutrition supplements are considered as nonpharmacological and preventive treatment for OA and sarcopenia [7–9].

Recently, attention has focused on the role of the IFP in OA pathophysiology [3,10,11]. It has been shown that IFP produces pro-inflammatory mediators inducing synovial inflammation and seems to act as an anatomo-functional unit with synovial membrane contributing to OA onset and progression [3,10–14].

Moreover, during the last years, research has focused on the study of IFP-derived stem cells for regenerative medicine [15]. Recently, we showed that OA-IFP stem cells seem to be primed by the pathological environment and to exert incomplete protective activity from OA inflammation [16].

A decrease of IFP volume and an increase of hypointense signal at the magnetic resonance imaging (hallmarks of fibrosis) were described in OA patients compared to controls [17]. It has been reported that IFP signal intensity alterations were associated with the incidence of radiographic OA [18] and that IFP hypointense signals were associated with increased knee cartilage defects and bone marrow lesions [19]. Moreover, IFP undergoes biomechanical changes in OA, showing a nonorganized distribution of the stresses within the interlobular septa affecting the mechanical (and possibly functional) response of the adipose lobules [20]. Usually, gene expression of OA IFP is compared with that of subcutaneous adipose tissue of the same subject, although these depots are very different. In this regard, the comparison of different IFP conditions could allow us to better understand and quantify the specific disease-related changes of the IFP.

The aim of the present study was to compare the histological, morphometric, and molecular characteristics of IFP of patients undergoing total knee replacement (TKR) for end-stage OA with those of patients undergoing anterior cruciate ligament reconstruction (ACLR) after traumatic rupture. We hypothesized that not only inflammation but also changes in adipocytes and extracellular matrix (ECM) composition might be involved in OA pathogenesis.

2. Results

2.1. Demographic and Clinical Characteristics of Patients

Twenty-eight patients undergoing ACLR for traumatic rupture and twenty-five patients undergoing TKR for end-stage OA were enrolled. Patients' characteristics are summarized in Table S2, Supplementary Materials. The time between the injury and the surgery of patients with

ACLR was at least 6 months (median 8 months; interquartile range (IQR), 14.5–6). Males were 75% in the ACL group and 28% in the OA group ($p = 0.001$). Moreover, ACL subjects were statistically younger (median age 31; IQR, 42–22) compared to OA patients (median age 68; IQR, 75–62) ($p < 0.0001$). The BMI of the ACL group (median BMI 23.04; IQR, 25.26–20.57) was statistically lower than that of OA patients (median 29.52; IQR, 32.25–25.95) ($p < 0.0001$).

2.2. Histopathological Grading

The IFP histopathological grading was evaluated in 23 ACL IFP and 25 OA IFP (Table 1). It was not possible to perform the histological analysis in 3 ACL samples due to the small volume of the biopsies. Lymphocytic infiltration was substantially absent in all ACL IFP (grade 0) except for one, which was graded as 1. On the contrary, lymphocytic infiltration was present in the majority of OA IFP: 28% of the OA IFP was graded as 1 and 52% as 2. Lymphocytic infiltration was found to be statistically different between the two groups ($p < 0.0001$). Vascularity was increased in OA IFP (median 30.6; 42.9–30.6) compared to ACL IFP (median 8.9; 17.5–7.2) ($p < 0.0001$).

Table 1. Infrapatellar fat pad histopathological scoring system.

IFP Histopathological Grading	ACL ($n = 23$)	End-Stage OA ($n = 25$)	p-Value
Lymphocytic Infiltration, number (%)	1 (3.6)	20 (80)	
Grade 0, number (%)	22 (95.7)	5 (20)	<0.0001
Grade 1, number (%)	1 (3.6)	7 (28)	
Grade 2, number (%)	0 (0)	13 (52)	
Vascularity, median (IQR)	8.9 (17.5–7.2)	30.6 (42.9–30.6)	<0.0001

ACL = anterior cruciate ligament; OA = osteoarthritis. Data are expressed as number (%) or median (IQR).

2.3. Adipocyte Morphology Evaluation

Adipocytes dimension in ACL and OA IFP was quantified, showing an increase of the cell area in adipocytes of OA IFP compared to ACL IFP ($p < 0.0001$) (Figure 1a,b and Table 2). The number of adipocytes was evaluated, revealing a decrease in OA compared to ACL IFP ($p = 0.0013$) consistent with the increase of the adipocyte area in OA (Figure 1c).

Table 2. Infrapatellar fat pad adipocytes characteristics.

IFP Adipocytes	ACL ($n = 24$)	End-Stage OA ($n = 25$)	p-Value
Area (μm^2), median (IQR)	1798.03 (2362.46–1113.82)	3128.72 (3632.46–2583.45)	<0.0001
Major axis (μm), median (IQR)	53.60 (62.68–42.47)	72.16 (78.98–66.45)	<0.0001
Minor axis (μm), median (IQR)	39.79 (49.43–32.63)	52.73 (58.90–48.70)	<0.0001
eccentricity, median (IQR)	0.66 (0.70–0.63)	0.67 (0.70–0.64)	0.211

ACL = anterior cruciate ligament; OA = osteoarthritis. Data are expressed as median (IQR).

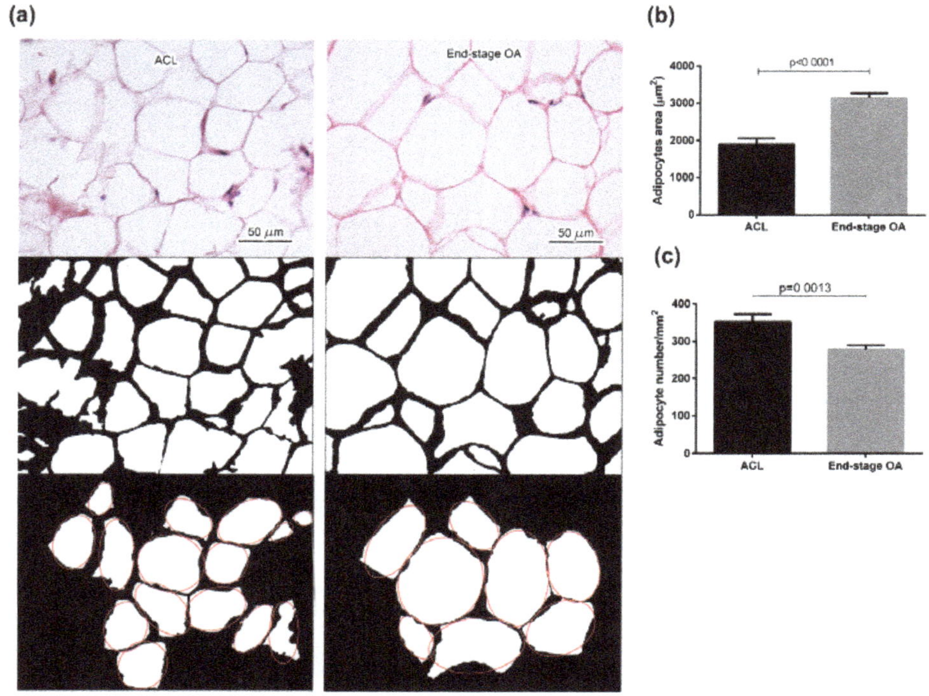

Figure 1. Adipocytes morphology evaluation. (**a**) ACL (on the left) and end-stage OA (on the right) adipocytes were reported from HE stained sections and then converted into the corresponding binary images. For each image, adipocytes areas (white regions) were identified and approximated to ellipses (red line). The comparison between adipocytes area (**b**) and number (**c**) for ACL and end-stage OA (Median and IQR) showed the increment of adipocytes size and the decrease of adipocytes number in OA IFP. ACL = anterior cruciate ligament; OA = osteoarthritis.

2.4. Gene Expression Analysis and Immunohistochemistry

2.4.1. Inflammation and Vascularization

In order to compare cytokines and chemokines gene expression of ACL IFP to OA IFP, qRT-PCR was performed in eight samples for each group (Figures S1 and S2 Supplementary Materials).

The median age and BMI were statistically different between the two subgroups as well as in the whole population ($p < 0.0001$ and $p = 0.010$, respectively).

A statistical difference was observed between the two subgroups in *IL-6* and *VEGF* gene expression levels ($p = 0.0039$ and $p = 0.0183$, respectively) (Figure 2a–d), while no differences were observed in *MCP-1/CCL-2* and *TNF-α* expression (Figure S1, Supplementary Materials). A decrease in *TGF-β* gene expression levels was determined in OA IFP compared to ACL IFP ($p = 0.0368$) (Figure S1, Supplementary Materials). On the basis of these results, IL-6 and VEGF proteins were evaluated by IHC or HE in a group of patients confirming the difference detected by gene expression between ACL ($n = 21$) and OA IFP ($n = 14$) (Figure 2b,c,e,f) (Table S3, Supplementary Materials).

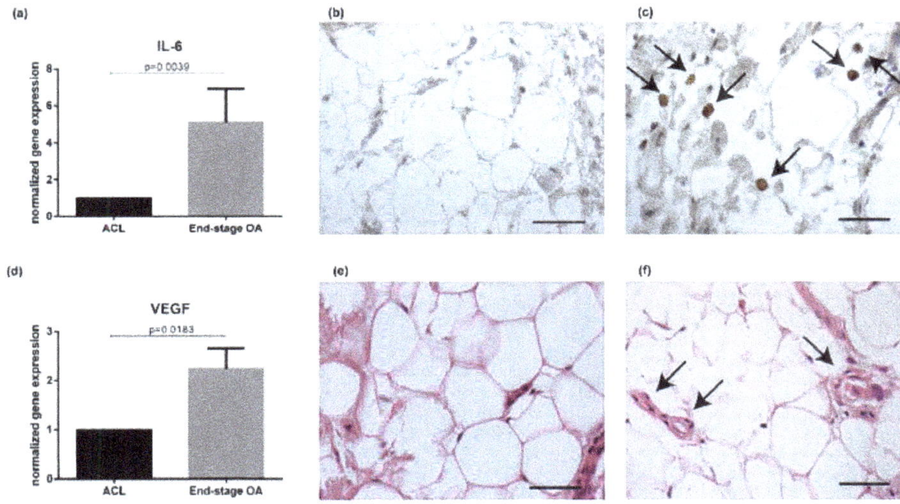

Figure 2. Evaluation of inflammation and vascularization in IFP of ACL and end-stage OA patients. *IL-6* gene expression revealed an increase of *IL-6* expression in end-stage OA IFP (n = 8) compared to ACL IFP (n = 8) (**a**). Immunohistochemistry of IL-6 end-stage OF IFP showed a marked positivity (highlighted by the arrows) (**c**) compared to ACL IFP (**b**). *VEGF* gene expression levels were increased in end-stage OA (n = 8) compared to ACL IFP (n = 8) (**d**). Hematoxylin–eosin image showed an increased in end-stage OA IFP (highlighted by the arrows) (**f**) compared to ACL IFP (**e**). Scale bar b = 50 μm; c = 23.8 μm; e,f = 37.5 μm. IL = interleukin; ACL = anterior cruciate ligament; IFP = infrapatellar fat pad; OA = osteoarthritis; VEGF = vascular endothelial grow factor.

2.4.2. Adipokines

Gene expression analysis of different adipokines was performed comparing ACL and OA IFP samples (Figure 3). There was an increase of white adipose tissue typical genes (*adiponectin*, *leptin*, and *FAB4*) in end-stage OA compared to ACL IFP (p = 0.0167, p = 0.0122, and p = 0.0056, respectively), while no differences were observed regarding *PPAR-γ* (p = 0.1590). The expression of *GPMNB* was evaluated, showing a decrease in end-stage OA compared to ACL IFP (p = 0.0007). On the contrary, an increase of *ITH5* gene expression was shown in end-stage OA compared to ACL IFP (p = 0.0277). No differences were evident in *SERPIN2* gene expression between the two groups (Figure S1, Supplementary Materials).

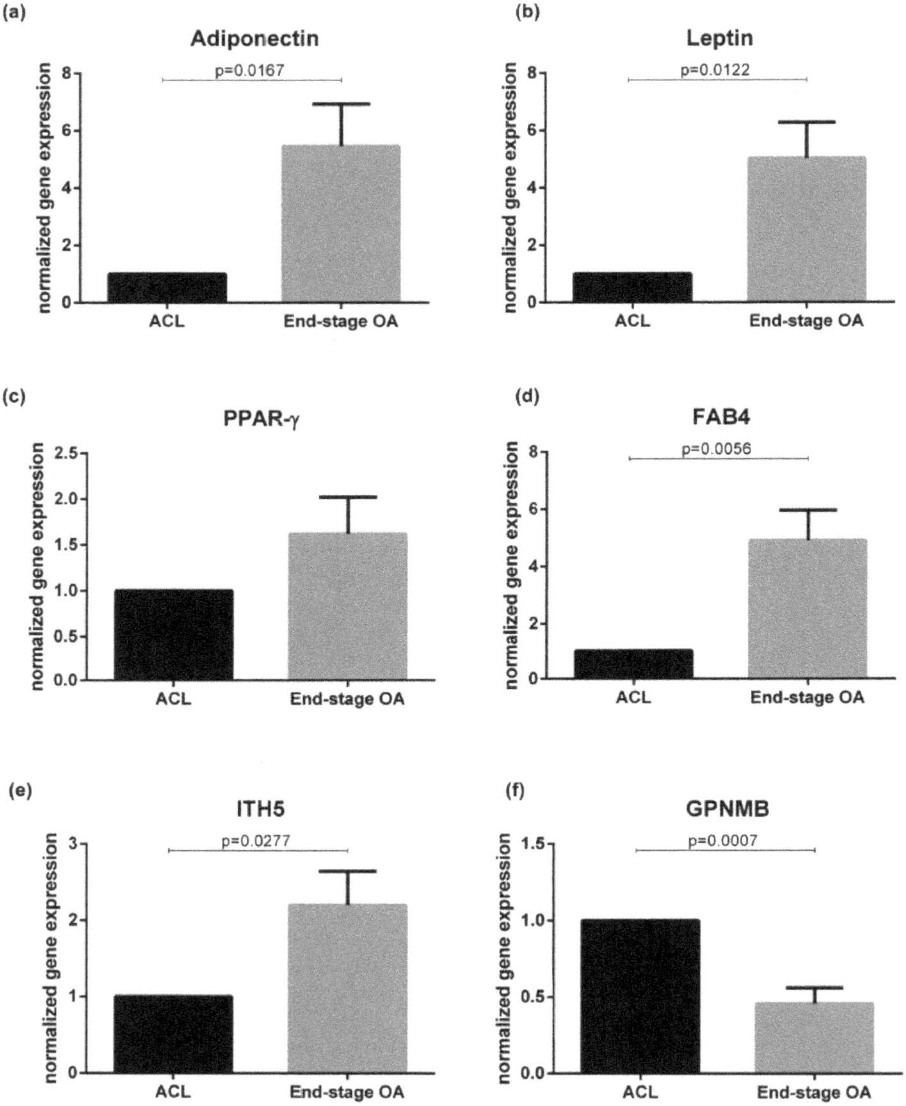

Figure 3. Adipokines evaluation in IFP ACL (n = 8) and end-stage OA patients (n = 8). (**a**) *Adiponectin* gene expression levels were increased in end-stage OA compared to ACL IFP. (**b**) *Leptin* gene expression levels were increased in end-stage OA compared to ACL IFP. (**c**) *PPAR-γ* gene expression levels were increased in end-stage OA compared to ACL IFP. (**d**) *FAB4* gene expression levels were increased in end-stage OA compared to ACL IFP. (**e**) *ITH5* gene expression was higher in end-stage OA IFP. (**f**) *GPNMB* gene expression was higher in ACL IFP. IFP = infrapatellar fat pad; ACL = anterior cruciate ligament; OA = osteoarthritis; PPAR-γ = peroxisome proliferative activated receptor gamma; FABP4 = fatty acid-binding protein 4; ITH5 = inter-α-trypsin inhibitor heavy chain 5; GPNMB = transmembrane glycoprotein NMB.

2.4.3. Extracellular Matrix Remodeling

The analysis of the expression of genes involved in ECM remodeling revealed a decrease of *COLI* expression in end-stage OA compared to ACL IFP ($p = 0.0156$) (Figure 4a), while no differences were detected in both *COLIII* (Figure 4c) and *COLVI* (Figure S2, Supplementary Materials) gene expression ($p = 0.1289$ and $p = 0.598$, respectively). COLI and COLIII were evaluated also by Sirius red (Figure 4) showing a decrease of both collagen proteins in OA ($n = 14$) compared to ACL IFP ($n = 18$) ($p = 0.001$, $p < 0.0001$, respectively).

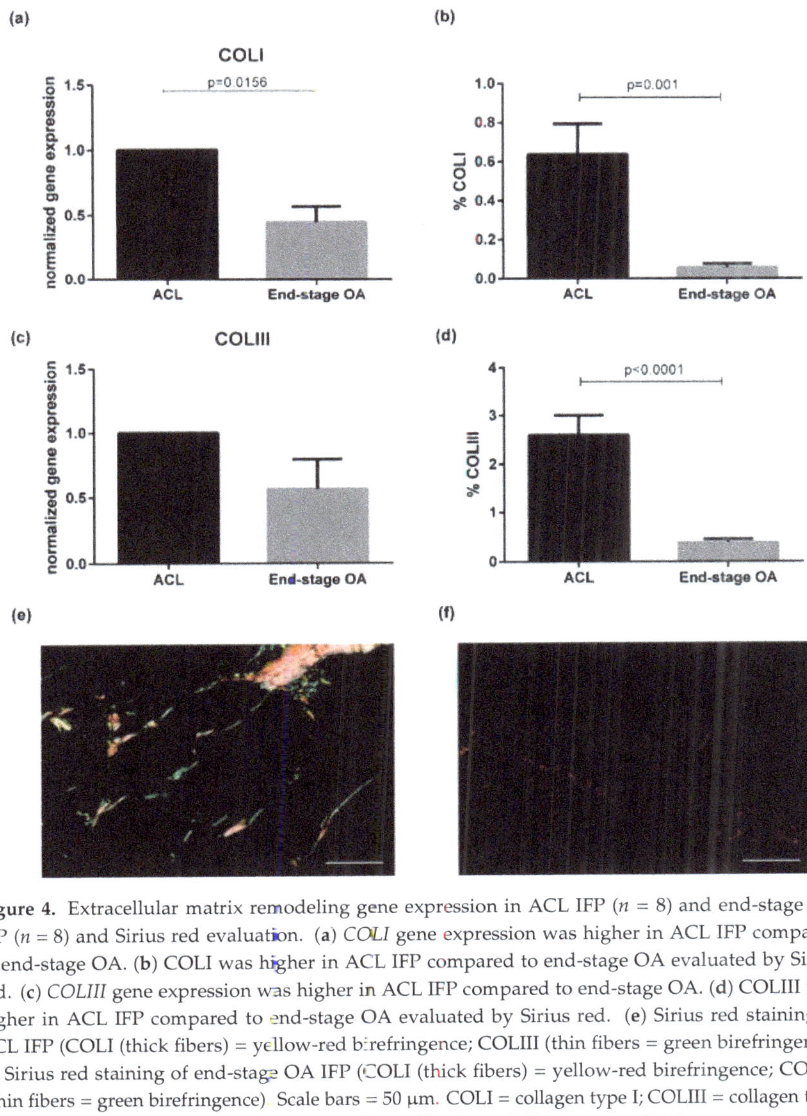

Figure 4. Extracellular matrix remodeling gene expression in ACL IFP ($n = 8$) and end-stage OA IFP ($n = 8$) and Sirius red evaluation. (**a**) *COLI* gene expression was higher in ACL IFP compared to end-stage OA. (**b**) COLI was higher in ACL IFP compared to end-stage OA evaluated by Sirius red. (**c**) *COLIII* gene expression was higher in ACL IFP compared to end-stage OA. (**d**) COLIII was higher in ACL IFP compared to end-stage OA evaluated by Sirius red. (**e**) Sirius red staining of ACL IFP (COLI (thick fibers) = yellow-red birefringence; COLIII (thin fibers = green birefringence). (**f**) Sirius red staining of end-stage OA IFP (COLI (thick fibers) = yellow-red birefringence; COLIII (Thin fibers = green birefringence). Scale bars = 50 µm. COLI = collagen type I; COLIII = collagen type 3; ACL = anterior cruciate ligament; IFP = infrapatellar fat pad; OA = osteoarthritis.

2.5. Correlations Between Histological Data and Morphometric Analysis

The age of overall cohort correlated positively with the adipocyte area ($r = 0.591$, $p < 0.0001$), and negatively with the adipocyte number ($r = -0.412$, $p = 0.003$) (Figure S3a,b, Supplementary Materials). However, considering the two groups separately, both correlations were not maintained. The adipocytes area was positively correlated with BMI of overall cohort ($r = 0.621$, $p < 0.0001$) (Figure S3c, Supplementary Materials) while, separating the two groups, this correlation was present only in end-stage OA IFP ($r = 0.413$, $p = 0.040$) (Figure S3e,f, Supplementary Materials). The number of adipocytes of the overall cohort was negatively correlated with BMI ($r = -0.427$, $p = 0.003$) (Figure S3d, Supplementary Materials) and this correlation was maintained only in the OA group ($r = -0.514$, $p = 0.009$) (Figure S3g,h, Supplementary Materials).

2.6. Influence of BMI and Age

Since well-known risk factors for OA, such as BMI and age, were not equally distributed between the two patient groups, we applied linear models to control their influence (Tables S4–S6, Supplementary Materials). Vascularity did not fit a normal distribution, and so it was log-transformed before being modeled. Lymphocytic infiltration, IL-6 immunohistochemical grading, vascularity, and adipocyte numbers were all independent from BMI and age. Furthermore, BMI and age did not have any significant effect on the response variables, whether analyzing OA and ACL rupture separately or combined. Only the adipocyte area was almost associated with BMI in the OA group ($p = 0.057$) and significantly associated when the two patient groups were considered together ($p = 0.033$).

3. Discussion

This is the first study investigating the histological, morphometric, and molecular characteristics of end-stage OA IFP compared to ACL IFP. In particular, we have explored not only IFP inflammation but also adipocytes and ECM changes in these two groups. The studies published so far mostly focalized on IFP inflammation and utilized the subcutaneous adipose tissue of the knee region as "healthy" control, which might not be an optimal "healthy" control because of the differences in physiological functions and biomechanical characteristics of these fat depots [21]. Furthermore, OA IFP characterization is of great importance to unravel its role in OA pathology as occurred for other tissues such as synovial membrane and cartilage [22,23].

The important novelty of this study is the evidence that, beyond inflammation, also adipocytes and ECM characteristics of OA patients are different compared to IFP derived from ACL patients. In particular, these data suggest that OA pathology induces molecular changes in IFP, affecting the cells and ECM composition in addition to the increase of inflammation.

Regarding the adipocyte characteristics, we observed that the adipocyte area was 1.7-fold higher in end-stage OA compared to ACL IFP, while the adipocyte number was lower in end-stage OA compared to ACL IFP. Interestingly, the adipocyte area of IFP was positively correlated with BMI, while adipocyte number was negatively correlated with BMI, but only the adipocyte area was confirmed to be associated with the BMI at linear regression model in the overall population and in the end-stage OA group. The absence of the correlation in the ACL IFP group between BMI and adipocyte area could be explained, considering that all these subjects were lean.

Previous studies evaluated the adipocyte area in OA IFP subgrouping the patients according to BMI, observing that the area was smaller in lean OA patients (BMI < 25 kg/m^2) compared to severely obese OA patients (BMI ≥ 35 kg/m^2) [24]. In contrast, de Jon et al. did not observe any difference in adipocyte size of OA IFP related to patient BMI, reporting that adipocyte volume and size of OA IFP were smaller compared to subcutaneous adipose tissue used as control [25]. The influence of BMI on the adipocyte area was not confirmed in other studies, both in animals and humans. Barboza et al. showed an increase of IFP volume in mice with high-fat diet-induced obesity compared to controls. In contrast, no difference was reported in the adipocyte area, suggesting that obesity does not influence this IFP feature [26]. In addition, other authors demonstrated that BMI did not exhibit any effect on adipocyte area in humans [27].

In general, the adipocyte area has been studied from all adipose tissue anatomical locations and in both sexes. The adipocyte area increases in size along with adiposity level, reaching a plateau in massively obese subjects [28]. Here, we showed that age was positively associated with the adipocyte area and negatively with the adipocyte number of IFP, although these findings were not confirmed by the linear regression model. No specific studies have been published so far evaluating the effects of age on IFP adipocyte characteristics. However, no significant association was observed between age and adipocyte size distribution parameters in omental and subcutaneous adipose tissue [29].

We observed an increase of lymphocytic infiltration as well as of vascularity in end-stage OA IFP compared to ACL IFP, confirming our previous data obtained comparing end-stage OA IFP with that of cadavers considered as healthy controls [30]. Increased lymphocytic infiltration and vascularity were independent of age and BMI in both groups in the linear models, suggesting that these inflammatory features play an important role in OA pathology. Moreover, in agreement with the histological IFP scores, we observed an increase of *IL-6* and *VEGF* mRNA expression levels in OA compared to ACL IFP. The increase of IL-6 expression was also confirmed by IHC in agreement with our previous results [30]. Surprisingly, we did not observe increased MCP-1 expression levels in OA IFP compared to ACL IFP, at variance with what we observed in a previous study using IHC [30]. The expression of all classical adipose tissue markers was increased in OA IFP compared to ACL IFP, in agreement with previously published data showing an increase of adipogenesis genes in end-stage OA IFP compared to early OA IFP [31].

The expression of other genes putatively involved in adipose tissue ECM organization and cell differentiation, such as *SERPIN2, GPNMB,* and *ITH5* considered as novel adipokines, was investigated only in OA IFP patients without any comparison with controls [32]. Differences in *GPNMB* and *ITH5* expression were observed between the OA and ACL IFP, with no differences for *SERPIN2*. Several studies highlighted the presence of fibrosis in OA IFP compared to non-OA tissues and subcutaneous adipose tissue [13,30]. GPNMB is a transmembrane protein involved in adipose tissue-derived inflammation in a mouse model of obesity [33]. We showed an increase of *GPNMB* in OA compared with ACL IFP with the increase of the inflammatory pattern in OA IFP. ITIs proteins are directly involved in the stabilization of ECM forming complexes binding hyaluronic acid molecules [34]. ITIH5 is highly expressed in white adipose tissue, and the expression seems to be increased in obese subjects [35]. Here, we observed an increase in its expression in OA IFP, in agreement with the increase of fibrosis. However, we cannot exclude that the differences observed in GPNMB and ITIH5 expression could be influenced by BMI, an important risk factor for OA.

The expression of other genes involved in the ECM composition was also investigated. ECM of adipose tissue is composed of several types of collagen and is particularly rich in COLVI that is positively correlated with BMI [36]. We evaluated *COLI, III,* and *COLVI,* showing that *COLI* and *COLIII* levels were decreased in OA compared to ACL IFP, while no differences were detected in *COLVI* expression. The differences in COLI and COLIII were also confirmed at the protein level, supporting the hypothesis of a change in ECM composition in OA, leading to the fibrotic phenotype of OA IFP [24,30]. This could also explain the reason why OA IFP has a biomechanical behavior different from that of healthy IFP [20].

Our study pointed out for the first time that OA pathology has a direct impact on IFP ECM and, in particular, on the expression of collagens and adipokines involved in the fibrotic process. These findings might open the possibility that fibrosis could be the target of a novel therapeutic strategy to counteract the OA progression and related pain in OA patients. This is also supported by a recently published paper by Onuma et al. that established a novel inflammation-induced knee pain model in rats and showed that the inflammation-induced fibrotic changes in the IFP were associated with the prolongation of joint pain [37]. The main limitation of our work is the age and BMI differences between the two groups of subjects, due to their specific categorization, given the fact that ACL rupture usually occurs in young, lean athletes, while OA occurs mainly in aging females. However, we showed that our analysis was not influenced by these confounders by general linear models except for the adipocyte area in the OA group and the overall cohort. In particular, inflammatory features such as lymphocytic infiltration, vascularization, and IL-6 protein expression as evaluated by IHC were increased in OA IFP compared to controls independently from BMI, suggesting an important role of IFP inflammation in OA pathogenesis. Unfortunately, it was not possible to apply the linear models to the gene expression analysis due to the small sample size. In addition, we cannot exclude that the acute trauma occurring during ACL rupture influenced our analysis [38]. However, in our study, we have enrolled patients who underwent ACLR at least 6 months after the injury in order to avoid the inflammatory phase occurring after the trauma. Bigoni et al. analyzed cytokines levels in synovial fluid of patients with ACL tears divided in the study population into 4 groups according to the time elapsed from the injury. Those authors demonstrated that there was an increased level of pro-inflammatory cytokines in the acute phase of inflammation, followed by a decrease with a minimum of three months after injury [39]. Current studies on patients with ACLR are mainly focused on the evaluation of inflammatory markers in the synovial fluid. Heilmeier et al. correlated the synovial fluid inflammatory markers with the IFP/synovial membrane abnormalities detected by MRI [40]. They found that the degree of IFP abnormality correlated positively with the synovial fluid levels of the inflammatory cytokine markers and with chondro-destructive markers as MMP-1 and −3. Since these Authors did not analyze IFP and synovial membrane inflammatory cytokines expression, it is not possible to discern the contribution of each joint tissue in the secretion of these inflammatory markers [40].

4. Materials and Methods

4.1. Study Population

Patients undergoing ACLR were enrolled at the IRCSS Rizzoli Orthopedic Institute (Bologna, Italy), while patients undergoing TKR for end-stage OA were enrolled at the Orthopaedic Clinic (University-Hospital of Padova, Padova, Italy). The Local Ethical Committees approved the study protocol and all patients signed written informed consent (approval code: 4510/AO/18, approval date: 18 July 2019). Patients or the public were not involved in the design, or conduct, or report, or disseminate plans of our research. Patients with previous knee surgery or other significant pathologies were excluded from the study. For each patient, demographic and clinical data were recorded.

Small biopsies of IFP were obtained during knee arthroscopy for ACLR or TKR surgery.

4.2. Histology and Immunohistochemistry

From the paraffin-embedded samples, 10 μm thick sections were obtained and stained with hematoxylin–eosin (HE) and Sirius red. For each case the IFP's score was applied considering the presence of lymphocytic infiltration and vascularization as published [21]. The adipose lobules dimension and the thickness of the interlobular septa were not evaluated due to the small volume of the IFP biopsies obtained from the ACL patients and gene expression analysis was not performed in all patients of this group.

All sections were analyzed under a DM4500-B light microscope (Leica Microsystems, Wetzlar, Germany) and recorded in full color (24 bit) with a digital camera (DFC 480, Leica Microsystems).

Collagen subtypes were studied on sections stained with Sirius red and quantified as previously described [41].

For immunohistochemical (IHC) analysis, an anti-IL-6 antibody (polyclonal mouse antibody, Thermo Fisher) was used at 1:200 without antigen retrieval. Tissue sections were incubated using the DAKO Autostainer System (EnVision™ FLEX, High pH). The presence of positive cells was evaluated and graded as follows: grade 0 = absence of positive cells, grade 1 = weak positive cells, grade 1 = rare strong positive cells, grade 2 = clustered strong positive cells, grade 3 = diffuse strong positive cells.

4.3. Morphometric Analysis

After digitizing the images acquired at 10× magnification from HE stained sections, images were converted to binary images (black-white) for the elaboration with a Programming Language Software (Matlab R2018b, The MathWorks, Inc., Natick, MA, USA). A specific procedure was adopted to identify the boundary of the adipocytes, considering the connected regions of similar intensity in the grayscale images [20,30,41]. The white regions represent the adipocytes and the black region, the boundary.

In each image, adipocytes were approximated to ellipses, and areas and major/minor axes were calculated. A count of the number of adipocytes for each image was calculated.

4.4. Gene Expression Analysis

Total RNA was extracted from IFP away from the synovial membrane using QIAMP mini kit (Qiagen, Hilden, Germany) following the manufacturer's protocol. First-strand cDNAs were synthesized from equal amounts of total RNA using random primers and M-MLV reverse transcriptase (Promega, Madison, WI, USA). Quantitative real-time PCR (qRT-PCR) for adipokines (leptin, adiponectin, peroxisome proliferative activated receptor gamma2 [PPARγ], fatty acid binding protein 4 [FABP4]), cytokines (IL-6, TNF-α, monocyte chemotactic protein 1 [MCP-1]), vascular endothelial growth factor (VEGF), chemokines (C-X-C motif chemokine ligand 8 [CXCL8]), genes involved in extracellular matrix remodeling (collagen type I [COLI], collagen type III [COLIII], and collagen type VI [COLVI], transmembrane glycoprotein NMB [GPNMB], inter-α-trypsin inhibitor heavy chain 5 [ITH5], serine proteinase inhibitor 2 [SERPIN2]), and transforming growth factor (TGF-β) was performed using Sybr-Green fluorophore and specific primers (Table S1, Supplementary Materials). Reaction efficiency was established for each set of primers and for an endogenous unregulated reference gene (18 s), after quantification of six different dilutions of the cDNA pool and calculated from the slope according to the equation $E = 10^{-1}/\text{slope}$ [42]. qRT-PCR was performed in triplicate for each gene and carried out in duplicate for each sample by DNA Engine Opticon 2 (MJ Research, Waltham, MA, USA). Melting curves confirmed the specificity of the amplification signal target of our gene. Data were calculated using the comparative (ΔΔCt) method as the ratio of each gene to the expression of the housekeeping gene and are represented as fold-change versus controls.

4.5. Statistical Analysis

The Shapiro–Wilk's test was used to determine whether data were distributed normally. Chi-square (χ^2) test or Fisher's exact test were performed to compare categorical and dichotomous data. Mann–Whitney test or unpaired *t*-test were used to compare continuous variables. Spearman's or Pearson's correlations were performed to analyze associations between continuous variables. One-way ANOVA or Kruskal–Wallis, with Tukey's post-hoc test, were used to analyze categorical data. Continuous variables were reported as median ± interquartile range (IQR), while categorical variables were reported as frequency and percentage. Generalized linear regression models were applied to investigate the association of the ACL and OA IFP variables with BMI and age. A $p < 0.05$ was considered as statistically significant. All analyses were performed with SPSS version 23.0 or R [43].

5. Conclusions

In conclusion, we confirmed that OA IFP is more inflamed and vascularized compared to ACL IFP, both at the histological and molecular levels. Moreover, we found that OA IFP adipocytes are larger and numerically lower than ACL IFP adipocytes. ECM collagen types distribution in the OA IFP group is different compared to controls, possibly explaining the biomechanical characteristics changes of OA IFP tissue. This study supports the hypothesis that IFP is involved in OA pathology. The clinical relevance of this work is that inflammation and fibrosis of IFP could represent possible therapeutic targets to counteract OA pathology. In this regard, future studies targeting inflammation and/or fibrosis of OA IFP are needed.

Supplementary Materials: Supplementary materials can be found at http://www.mdpi.com/1422-0067/21/17/6016/s1.

Author Contributions: Conceptualization, E.B., V.M., M.R., and M.F.; formal analysis, E.B. and M.S.; investigation, E.B., C.G.F., E.L.C., M.G., G.S., and A.P. (Assunta Pozzuoli); resources, E.B., A.P. (Assunta Pozzuoli), E.O., G.F., A.B., and P.R.; data curation, E.B., V.M., and M.F.; writing—original draft preparation, E.B. and M.F.; writing—review and editing, E.B., V.M., C.G.F., M.S., M.R., E.O., G.F., and M.F.; supervision, V.M., M.R., R.R., R.V., P.R., and M.F.; funding acquisition, M.R., V.M., A.P. (Andrea Porzionato), and R.D.C. All authors have read and agreed to the published version of the manuscript.

Funding: This research was funded by the L.i.f.e.L.a.b. Program of the 'Consorzio per la Ricerca Sanitaria' (CORIS) of the Veneto Region, Italy, grant number DGR1017, 17 July 2018.

Acknowledgments: Part of these data were first presented as a poster at the 2019 Congress of the Italian Society of Anatomy and Histology (SIAI) (Naples, 22–24 September). The authors are grateful to Diego Guidolin for the collagen analysis.

Conflicts of Interest: The authors declare no conflict of interest. The funders had no role in the design of the study, in the collection, analyses, or interpretation of data; in the writing of the manuscript, or in the decision to publish the results.

Abbreviations

ACLR	anterior cruciate ligament reconstruction
COLI	collagen Type I
COLIII	collagen Type Iii
COLVI	collagen Type Vi
CXCL8	C-X-C motif chemokine ligand 8
FABP4	fatty acid-binding protein 4
GPNMB	transmembrane glycoprotein NMB
HE	hematoxylin–eosin
IFP	infrapatellar fat pad
IL-6	interleukin-6
ITH5	inter-A-trypsin inhibitor heavy chain 5
MCP-1	monocyte chemotactic protein 1
OA	osteoarthritis
PPARγ	peroxisome proliferative activated receptor gamma
QRT-PCR	quantitative real-time PCR
SERPIN2	serine proteinase inhibitor 2
TGF-B	transforming growth factor B
TNF-A	tumor necrosis factor-A
TKR	total knee replacement
VEGF	vascular endothelial growth factor

References

1. Global Burden of Disease Study 2013 Collaborators. Global, regional, and national incidence, prevalence, and years lived with disability for 301 acute and chronic diseases and injuries in 188 countries, 1990–2013: A systematic analysis for the Global Burden of Disease Study 2013. *Lancet Lond. Engl.* **2015**, *386*, 743–800. [CrossRef]
2. Cross, M.; Smith, E.; Hoy, D.; Nolte, S.; Ackerman, I.; Fransen, M.; Bridgett, L.; Williams, S.; Guillemin, F.; Hill, C.L.; et al. The global burden of hip and knee osteoarthritis: Estimates from the global burden of disease 2010 study. *Ann. Rheum. Dis.* **2014**, *73*, 1323–1330. [CrossRef] [PubMed]
3. Belluzzi, E.; El Hadi, H.; Granzotto, M.; Rossato, M.; Ramonda, R.; Macchi, V.; De Caro, R.; Vettor, R.; Favero, M. Systemic and local adipose tissue in knee osteoarthritis. *J. Cell Physiol.* **2017**, *232*, 1971–1978. [CrossRef] [PubMed]

4. Loeser, R.F.; Goldring, S.R.; Scanzello, C.R.; Goldring, M.B. Osteoarthritis: A disease of the joint as an organ. *Arthritis Rheum.* **2012**, *64*, 1697–1707. [CrossRef]
5. Favero, M.; Belluzzi, E.; Trisolino, G.; Goldring, M.B.; Goldring, S.R.; Cigolotti, A.; Pozzuoli, A.; Ruggieri, P.; Ramonda, R.; Grigolo, B.; et al. Inflammatory molecules produced by meniscus and synovium in early and end-stage osteoarthritis: A coculture study. *J. Cell Physiol.* **2019**, *234*, 11176–11187. [CrossRef]
6. Favero, M.; Ramonda, R.; Goldring, M.B.; Goldring, S.R.; Punzi, L. Early knee osteoarthritis. *RMD Open* **2015**, *1*, e000062. [CrossRef]
7. Castrogiovanni, P.; Di Rosa, M.; Ravalli, S.; Castorina, A.; Guglielmino, C.; Imbesi, R.; Vecchio, M.; Drago, F.; Szychlinska, M.A.; Musumeci, G. Moderate physical activity as a prevention method for knee osteoarthritis and the role of synoviocytes as biological key. *Int. J. Mol. Sci.* **2019**, *20*, 511. [CrossRef] [PubMed]
8. Castrogiovanni, P.; Trovato, F.M.; Loreto, C.; Nsir, H.; Szychlinska, M.A.; Musumeci, G. Nutraceutical supplements in the management and prevention of osteoarthritis. *Int. J. Mol. Sci.* **2016**, *17*, 2042. [CrossRef]
9. Szychlinska, M.A.; Castrogiovanni, P.; Trovato, F.M.; Nsir, H.; Zarrouk, M.; Lo Furno, D.; Di Rosa, M.; Imbesi, R.; Musumeci, G. Physical activity and mediterranean diet based on olive tree phenolic compounds from two different geographical areas have protective effects on early osteoarthritis, muscle atrophy and hepatic steatosis. *Eur. J. Nutr.* **2019**, *58*, 565–581. [CrossRef]
10. Belluzzi, E.; Stocco, E.; Pozzuoli, A.; Granzotto, M.; Porzionato, A.; Vettor, R.; De Caro, R.; Ruggieri, P.; Ramonda, R.; Rossato, M.; et al. Contribution of infrapatellar fat pad and synovial membrane to knee osteoarthritis pain. *BioMed Res. Int.* **2019**, *2019*, 18. [CrossRef]
11. Belluzzi, E.; Olivotto, E.; Toso, G.; Cigolotti, A.; Pozzuoli, A.; Biz, C.; Trisolino, G.; Ruggieri, P.; Grigolo, B.; Ramonda, R.; et al. Conditioned media from human osteoarthritic synovium induces inflammation in a synoviocyte cell line. *Connect. Tissue Res.* **2019**, *60*, 136–145. [CrossRef] [PubMed]
12. Eymard, F.; Pigenet, A.; Citadelle, D.; Flouzat-Lachaniette, C.H.; Poignard, A.; Benelli, C.; Berenbaum, F.; Chevalier, X.; Houard, X. Induction of an inflammatory and prodegradative phenotype in autologous fibroblast-like synoviocytes by the infrapatellar fat pad from patients with knee osteoarthritis. *Arthritis Rheumatol.* **2014**, *66*, 2165–2174. [CrossRef] [PubMed]
13. Eymard, F.; Pigenet, A.; Citadelle, D.; Tordjman, J.; Foucher, L.; Rose, C.; Flouzat Lachaniette, C.H.; Rouault, C.; Clement, K.; Berenbaum, F.; et al. Knee and hip intra-articular adipose tissues (IAATs) compared with autologous subcutaneous adipose tissue: A specific phenotype for a central player in osteoarthritis. *Ann. Rheum. Dis.* **2017**, *76*, 1142–1148. [CrossRef]
14. Macchi, V.; Stocco, E.; Stecco, C.; Belluzzi, E.; Favero, M.; Porzionato, A.; De Caro, R. The infrapatellar fat pad and the synovial membrane: An anatomo-functional unit. *J. Anat.* **2018**, *233*, 146–154. [CrossRef]
15. Zhong, Y.C.; Wang, S.C.; Han, Y.H.; Wen, Y. Recent advance in source, property, differentiation, and applications of infrapatellar fat pad adipose-derived stem cells. *Stem Cells Int.* **2020**, *2020*, 2560174. [CrossRef]
16. Stocco, E.; Barbon, S.; Piccione, M.; Belluzzi, E.; Petrelli, L.; Pozzuoli, A.; Ramonda, R.; Rossato, M.; Favero, M.; Ruggieri, P.; et al. Infrapatellar fat pad stem cells responsiveness to microenvironment in osteoarthritis: From morphology to function. *Front. Cell Dev. Biol.* **2019**, *7*, 323. [CrossRef] [PubMed]
17. Fontanella, C.G.; Belluzzi, E.; Rossato, M.; Olivotto, E.; Trisolino, G.; Ruggieri, P.; Rubini, A.; Porzionato, A.; Natali, A.; De Caro, R.; et al. Quantitative MRI analysis of infrapatellar and suprapatellar fat pads in normal controls, moderate and end-stage osteoarthritis. *Ann. Anat. Anat. Anz. Off. Organ Anat. Ges.* **2019**, *221*, 108–114. [CrossRef]
18. Wang, K.; Ding, C.; Hannon, M.J.; Chen, Z.; Kwoh, C.K.; Hunter, D.J. Quantitative signal intensity alteration in infrapatellar fat pad predicts incident radiographic osteoarthritis: The osteoarthritis initiative. *Arthritis Care Res.* **2019**, *71*, 30–38. [CrossRef]
19. Han, W.; Aitken, D.; Zhu, Z.; Halliday, A.; Wang, X.; Antony, B.; Cicuttini, F.; Jones, G.; Ding, C. Hypointense signals in the infrapatellar fat pad assessed by magnetic resonance imaging are associated with knee symptoms and structure in older adults: A cohort study. *Arthritis Res. Ther.* **2016**, *18*, 234. [CrossRef]
20. Fontanella, C.G.; Macchi, V.; Carniel, E.L.; Frigo, A.; Porzionato, A.; Picardi, E.E.E.; Favero, M.; Ruggieri, P.; de Caro, R.; Natali, A.N. Biomechanical behavior of Hoffa's fat pad in healthy and osteoarthritic conditions: Histological and mechanical investigations. *Australas. Phys. Eng. Sci. Med.* **2018**, *41*, 657–667. [CrossRef]
21. Fontanella, C.G.; Carniel, E.L.; Frigo, A.; Macchi, V.; Porzionato, A.; Sarasin, G.; Rossato, M.; De Caro, R.; Natali, A.N. Investigation of biomechanical response of Hoffa's fat pad and comparative characterization. *J. Mech. Behav. Biomed. Mater.* **2017**, *67*, 1–9. [CrossRef]

22. Pauli, C.; Whiteside, R.; Heras, F.L.; Nesic, D.; Koziol, J.; Grogan, S.P.; Matyas, J.; Pritzker, K.P.; D'Lima, D.D.; Lotz, M.K. Comparison of cartilage histopathology assessment systems on human knee joints at all stages of osteoarthritis development. *Osteoarthr. Cartil.* **2012**, *20*, 476–485. [CrossRef]
23. Benito, M.J.; Veale, D.J.; FitzGerald, O.; van den Berg, W.B.; Bresnihan, B. Synovial tissue inflammation in early and late osteoarthritis. *Ann. Rheum. Dis.* **2005**, *64*, 1263–1267. [CrossRef]
24. Harasymowicz, N.S.; Clement, N.D.; Azfer, A.; Burnett, R.; Salter, D.M.; Simpson, A. Regional differences between perisynovial and infrapatellar adipose tissue depots and their response to class II and class III obesity in patients with osteoarthritis. *Arthritis Rheumatol* **2017**, *69*, 1396–1406. [CrossRef]
25. de Jong, A.J.; Klein-Wieringa, I.R.; Andersen, S.N.; Kwekkeboom, J.C.; Herb-van Toorn, L.; de Lange-Brokaar, B.J.E.; van Delft, D.; Garcia, J.; Wei, W.; van der Heide, H.J.L.; et al. Lack of high BMI-related features in adipocytes and inflammatory cells in the infrapatellar fat pad (IFP). *Arthritis Res. Ther.* **2017**, *19*, 186. [CrossRef]
26. Barboza, E.; Hudson, J.; Chang, W.P.; Kovats, S.; Towner, R.A.; Silasi-Mansat, R.; Lupu, F.; Kent, C.; Griffin, T.M. Profibrotic infrapatellar fat pad remodeling without M1 macrophage polarization precedes knee osteoarthritis in mice with diet-induced obesity. *Arthritis Rheumatol* **2017**, *69*, 1221–1232. [CrossRef]
27. Garcia, J.; Wei, W.; Runhaar, J.; Wright, K.; Mennan, C.; Roberts, S.; Van Osch, G.; Bastiaansen-Jenniskens, Y. Obesity does not affect the size of infrapatellar fat pad adipocytes: Implications for the pathogenesis of knee osteoarthritis. *Osteoarthr. Cartil.* **2016**, *24*, S334–S335. [CrossRef]
28. Mansour, M.F.; Chan, C.-W.J.; Laforest, S.; Veilleux, A.; Tchernof, A. Sex differences in body fat distribution. In *Adipose Tissue Biology*; Symonds, M.E., Ed.; Springer International Publishing: Cham, Switzerland, 2017; pp. 257–300.
29. Michaud, A.; Laforest, S.; Pelletier, M.; Nadeau, M.; Simard, S.; Daris, M.; Lebœuf, M.; Vidal, H.; Géloën, A.; Tchernof, A. Abdominal adipocyte populations in women with visceral obesity. *Endocrinology* **2016**, *174*, 227–239. [CrossRef]
30. Favero, M.; El-Hadi, H.; Belluzzi, E.; Granzotto, M.; Porzionato, A.; Sarasin, G.; Rambaldo, A.; Iacobellis, C.; Cigolotti, A.; Fontanella, C.G.; et al. Infrapatellar fat pad features in osteoarthritis: A histopathological and molecular study. *Rheumatol. Oxf.* **2017**, *56*, 1784–1793. [CrossRef]
31. Gandhi, R.; Takahashi, M.; Virtanen, C.; Syed, K.; Davey, J.R.; Mahomed, N.N. Microarray analysis of the infrapatellar fat pad in knee osteoarthritis: Relationship with joint inflammation. *J. Rheumatol.* **2011**, *38*, 1966–1972. [CrossRef]
32. Conde, J.; Scotece, M.; Abella, V.; Gomez, R.; Lopez, V.; Villar, R.; Hermida, M.; Pino, J.; Gomez-Reino, J.J.; Gualillo, O. Identification of novel adipokines in the joint. Differential expression in healthy and osteoarthritis tissues. *PLoS ONE* **2015**, *10*, e0123601. [CrossRef]
33. Gabriel, T.L.; Tol, M.J.; Ottenhof, R.; van Roomen, C.; Aten, J.; Claessen, N.; Hooibrink, B.; de Weijer, B.; Serlie, M.J.; Argmann, C.; et al. Lysosomal stress in obese adipose tissue macrophages contributes to MITF-dependent Gpnmb induction. *Diabetes* **2014**, *63*, 3310–3323. [CrossRef]
34. Rugg, M.S.; Willis, A.C.; Mukhopadhyay, D.; Hascall, V.C.; Fries, E.; Fulop, C.; Milner, C.M.; Day, A.J. Characterization of complexes formed between TSG-6 and inter-alpha-inhibitor that act as intermediates in the covalent transfer of heavy chains onto hyaluronan. *J. Biol. Chem.* **2005**, *280*, 25674–25686. [CrossRef]
35. Anveden, A.; Sjoholm, K.; Jacobson, P.; Palsdottir, V.; Walley, A.J.; Froguel, P.; Al-Daghri, N.; McTernan, P.G.; Mejhert, N.; Arner, P.; et al. ITIH-5 expression in human adipose tissue is increased in obesity. *Obes. Silver Spring Md.* **2012**, *20*, 708–714. [CrossRef]
36. Pasarica, M.; Gowronska-Kozak, B.; Burk, D.; Remedios, I.; Hymel, D.; Gimble, J.; Ravussin, E.; Bray, G.A.; Smith, S.R. Adipose tissue collagen VI in obesity. *J. Clin. Endocrinol. Metab.* **2009**, *94*, 5155–5162. [CrossRef]
37. Onuma, H.; Tsuji, K.; Hoshino, T.; Inomata, K.; Udo, M.; Nakagawa, Y.; Katagiri, H.; Miyatake, K.; Watanabe, T.; Sekiya, I.; et al. Fibrotic changes in the infrapatellar fat pad induce new vessel formation and sensory nerve fiber endings that associate prolonged pain. *J. Orthop. Res.* **2020**, *38*, 1296–1306. [CrossRef]
38. Punzi, L.; Galozzi, P.; Luisetto, R.; Favero, M.; Ramonda, R.; Oliviero, F.; Scanu, A. Post-traumatic arthritis: Overview on pathogenic mechanisms and role of inflammation. *RMD Open* **2016**, *2*, e000279. [CrossRef]
39. Bigoni, M.; Sacerdote, P.; Turati, M.; Franchi, S.; Gandolla, M.; Gaddi, D.; Moretti, S.; Munegato, D.; Augusti, C.A.; Bresciani, E.; et al. Acute and late changes in intraarticular cytokine levels following anterior cruciate ligament injury. *J. Orthop. Res. Off. Publ. Orthop. Res. Soc.* **2013**, *31*, 315–321. [CrossRef]

40. Heilmeier, U.; Mamoto, K.; Amano, K.; Eck, B.; Tanaka, M.; Bullen, J.A.; Schwaiger, B.J.; Huebner, J.L.; Stabler, T.V.; Kraus, V.B.; et al. Infrapatellar fat pad abnormalities are associated with a higher inflammatory synovial fluid cytokine profile in young adults following ACL tear. *Osteoarthr. Cartil.* **2020**, *28*, 82–91. [CrossRef]
41. Macchi, V.; Porzionato, A.; Sarasin, G.; Petrelli, L.; Guidolin, D.; Rossato, M.; Fontanella, C.G.; Natali, A.; De Caro, R. The infrapatellar adipose body: A histotopographic study. *Cells Tissues Organs* **2016**, *201*, 220–231. [CrossRef]
42. Pfaffl, M.W.; Tichopad, A.; Prgomet, C.; Neuvians, T.P. Determination of stable housekeeping genes, differentially regulated target genes and sample integrity: BestKeeper—Excel-based tool using pair-wise correlations. *Biotechnol. Lett.* **2004**, *26*, 509–515. [CrossRef]
43. R Core Team. *R: A Language and Environment for Statistical Computing*; R Foundation for Statistical Computing: Vienna, Austria, 2014.

International Journal of *Molecular Sciences*

MDPI

Article

Inflammatory Cytokine-Producing Cells and Inflammation Markers in the Synovium of Osteoarthritis Patients Evidenced in Human Herpesvirus 7 Infection

Valerija Groma [1,*], Mihails Tarasovs [1,2], Sandra Skuja [1], Sofija Semenistaja [1], Zaiga Nora-Krukle [3], Simons Svirskis [3] and Modra Murovska [3]

1 Joint Laboratory of Electron Microscopy, Institute of Anatomy and Anthropology, Riga Stradins University, Kronvalda blvd 9, LV-1010 Riga, Latvia; mihails.tarasovs@rsu.lv (M.T.); Sandra.skuja@rsu.lv (S.S.); sofijasem@inbox.lv (S.S.)

2 Department of Internal Diseases, Riga Stradins University, Hipokrata str. 2, LV-1038 Riga, Latvia

3 Institute of Microbiology and Virology, Riga Stradins University, Ratsupites str. 5, LV-1067 Riga, Latvia; Zaiga.nora@rsu.lv (Z.N.-K.); ssvirskis@latnet.lv (S.S.); modra.murovska@rsu.lv (M.M.)

* Correspondence: valerija.groma@rsu.lv; Tel.: +371-673-20421

Received: 1 July 2020; Accepted: 19 August 2020; Published: 20 August 2020

Abstract: A direct association between joint inflammation and the progression of osteoarthritis (OA) has been proposed, and synovitis is considered a powerful driver of the disease. Among infections implicated in the development of joint disease, human herpesvirus 7 (HHV-7) infection remains poorly characterized. Therefore, we assessed synovitis in OA patients; determined the occurrence and distribution of the HHV-7 antigen within the synovial membrane of OA-affected subjects; and correlated plasma levels of the pro-inflammatory cytokines tumor necrosis factor (TNF), interleukin-6 (IL-6), and TNF expressed locally within lesioned synovial tissues with HHV-7 observations, suggesting differences in persistent latent and active infection. Synovial HHV-7, CD4, CD68, and TNF antigens were detected immunohistochemically. The plasma levels of TNF and IL-6 were measured by an enzyme-linked immunosorbent assay. Our findings confirm the presence of persistent HHV-7 infection in 81.5% and reactivation in 20.5% of patients. In 35.2% of patients, virus-specific DNA was extracted from synovial membrane tissue samples. We evidenced the absence of histopathologically detectable synovitis and low-grade changes in the majority of OA patients enrolled in the study, in both HHV-7 PCR+ and HHV-7 PCR- groups. The number of synovial CD4-positive cells in the HHV-7 polymerase chain reaction (PCR)+ group was significantly higher than that in the HHV-7 PCR- group. CD4- and CD68-positive cells were differently distributed in both HHV-7 PCR+ and HHV-7 PCR- groups, as well as in latent and active HHV-7 infection. The number of TNF+ and HHV-7+ lymphocytes, as well as HHV-7+ vascular endothelial cells, was strongly correlated. Vascular endothelial cells, especially in the case of infection reactivation, appeared vulnerable. The balance between virus latency and reactivation is a long-term relationship between the host and infectious agent, and the immune system appears to be involved in displaying overreaction when a shift in the established equilibrium develops.

Keywords: osteoarthritis; synovium; cytokines; HHV-7; PCR; ELISA; immunohistochemistry

1. Introduction

Joint diseases are recognized as common, widespread disabling pathologies all over the globe [1]. Among chronic rheumatic diseases having a substantial impact on population health, osteoarthritis (OA) is the one destined to increase and become the most prevalent [2]. It is estimated that among persons with OA, about 80% have some degree of movement limitation and 25% are unable to perform daily activities [3]. Previous studies have accentuated the role of OA as the major cause of hip and knee replacement surgeries [4]. Osteoarthritis has long been viewed as a degenerative disease of cartilage, but accumulating evidence indicates that inflammation has a crucial role in its pathogenesis [5,6]. A direct association between joint inflammation and the progression of OA has been proposed [7,8], and synovitis has been considered a powerful driver of the OA process [9].

The synovial membrane comprises a tissue enclosing the synovial cavity around the opposing surfaces of articular cartilage. It contains a superficial layer, called the intima, composed of two types of synoviocytes—macrophages or type A cells and fibroblast-like or type B cells—and underneath is layer of subintima which houses blood vessels and nerves. Synoviocytes manufacture, secrete, absorb, and adjust the contents of the joint cavity by producing and remodeling the extracellular matrix molecules (ECMs), both collagenous and ground substance/adhesion molecules, thus controlling local homeostasis [10,11]. Intimal cells are essential producers of cytokines, including the pro-inflammatory factors tumor necrosis factor (TNF), interleukin-1β (IL-1β), and interleukin-6 (IL-6) [12–14]. Cytokines diffusing through the synovial fluid into the articular cartilage may further activate chondrocytes and synoviocytes, thus sustaining inflammation [15].

Arthritogenic viruses implicated in the development of joint pathologies [16], including those manifesting with synovial damage, have been explored [16–19]. A viral etiology is evident for approximately 1% of all cases of acute arthritis [20]. Human herpesviruses are ubiquitous pathogens establishing a persistent infection in the host for life, but their contribution to articular damage and the etiopathogenesis of OA remains obscure [21–24].

The results of several studies have confirmed the presence of human herpesvirus 6 (HHV-6) and 7 (HHV-7) DNA and viral antigens by polymerase chain reaction (PCR) techniques, in situ hybridization, immunohistochemistry, and electron microscopy in blood plasma, peripheral blood mononuclear cells, the brain, and skin [25–30]. Furthermore, our earlier study reported on the presence of human HHV-6 and HHV-7 infection markers in synovial fluid and synovial tissues of rheumatoid arthritis (RA)-affected patients [31]. HHV-6A, HHV-6B, and HHV-7 are genetically related to human cytomegalovirus (HCMV) constituting the β-herpesvirus subfamily [22,32]. There is evidence suggesting that Epstein–Barr virus (EBV) and HCMV infection contribute to the pathogenesis of RA [18]. Furthermore, the presence of DNA from varicella zoster (VZV), herpes simplex virus (HSV), EBV, and HHV-6 has been confirmed in the synovial fluid and peripheral blood mononuclear cells of patients with RA, OA, and axial spondyloarthritis. In RA and spondyloarthritis, the authors found that the PCR results were concordant with the inflammatory activity of the disease [33,34]. The frequency and extent of synovial inflammation in OA linked to the assessment of inflammatory cytokine-producing cells evidenced in the presence of HHV-7 infection has not yet been elucidated, including the latency and reactivation conditions.

2. Results

2.1. Nested Polymerase Chain Reaction

Qualitative nested PCR (nPCR) testing was performed on 54 patients. The presence of persistent HHV-7 infection (the presence of the HHV-7 genomic sequence in DNA extracted from whole peripheral blood (WPB)) was detected in 44/54 (81.5%) OA patients. Out of 44 OA patients, the HHV-7 sequence in WPB DNA samples was detected in 27 females and 17 males. In 19/54 (35.2%) patients, virus-specific DNA was also present in DNA extracted from synovial membrane tissue samples (Figure 1a). All samples from patients with HHV-7 genomic sequences in whole blood DNA were analyzed for viral infection reactivation (viral genomic sequences in cell-free blood plasma DNA). HHV-7 reactivation was found in 9/44 (20.5%) patients. Interestingly, in seven out of nine patients with an active viral infection, the HHV-7 specific genomic sequence was also found in both WPB and synovial membrane DNA (Figure 1b).

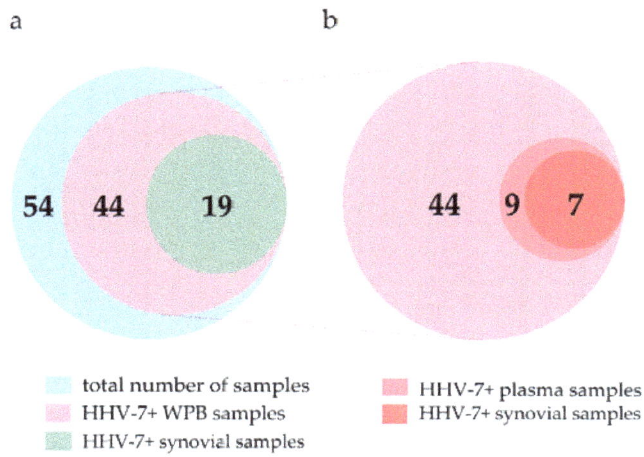

Figure 1. Distribution of patients enrolled in the study according to nested PCR data. (**a**) Venn diagram circles are scaled according to the number of samples and depict the total number, the number of human herpesvirus 7 (HHV-7)-positive whole peripheral blood (WPB), and the synovial membrane tissue samples. (**b**) Extract from the HHV-7 PCR+ group depicts the number of positive samples detected in the case of persistent and active viral infection (blood plasma and synovial membrane samples).

2.2. Plasma Levels of TNF and IL-6

The plasma levels of both pro-inflammatory cytokines greatly varied from 0 to 58 pg/mL and from 0 to 100 pg/mL for TNF and IL-6, respectively. No significant difference in the plasma levels for TNF or IL-6 was determined when the HHV-7 PCR+ and HHV-7 PCR− groups were compared. Plots representing the distributions of IL-6 and TNF cytokine plasma levels found in OA patients of both study groups, consisting of HHV-7 PCR+ and HHV-7 PCR−, can be seen in Figure 2.

2.3. Assessment of Synovitis Applying the Krenn Scoring System

Forty-eight OA patients out of a cohort of 54 presented with materials sufficient for further analyses and were stratified into two groups: Nineteen HHV-7 PCR+ subjects (39.6%) and 29 HHV-7 PCR− subjects (60.4%). Seventeen HHV-7 PCR− and 25 HHV-7 PCR− subjects presented with tissues suitable for assessing synovitis. HHV-7 PCR+ OA subjects presented with a median synovitis score of 3 (IQR 2–4), whereas HHV-7 PCR− OA subjects had a median synovitis score of 2 (IQR 1–4). The trend towards higher Krenn scores in the HHV-7 PCR+ group when compared to the HHV-7 PCR− group was confirmed (Figure 3a). There was no significant difference found in synovitis scores estimated for the HHV-7 PCR+ and HHV-7 PCR− groups (p = 0.483). Six (35%), 10 (59%), and 1 (6%) and 12 (48%), 10 (40%), and 3 (12%) OA patients presented without histopathologically detectable synovitis, low-grade synovitis, and high-grade synovitis in the HHV-7 PCR+ and HHV-7 PCR− study groups, respectively (Figure 3b).

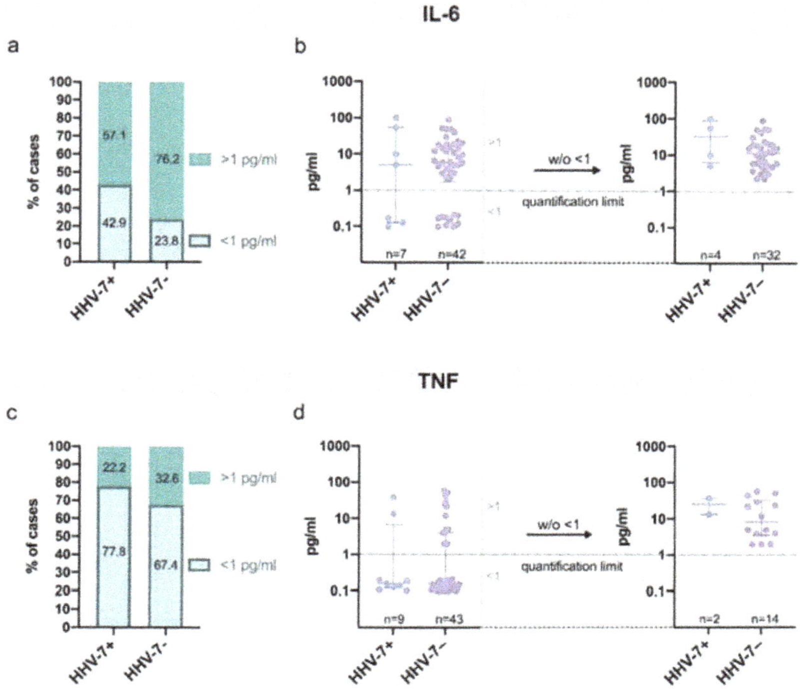

Figure 2. Assessment of plasma levels of pro-inflammatory cytokines—tumor necrosis factor (TNF) and interleukin-6 (IL-6)—in osteoarthritis (OA) patients in both study groups, HHV-7 PCR+ and HHV-7 PCR−. Plots depict the distributions of IL-6 (**a**) and TNF (**c**) plasma levels demonstrated in OA patients in both study groups—HHV-7 PCR+ and HHV-7 PCR−. (**b**,**d**) Dot plots represent the quantified data for IL-6 (**b**) and TNF (**d**) plasma levels. (**b**) Each dot represents a single data point; blue dots represent IL-6 plasma levels assessed in the HHV-7 PCR+ group, and violet dots represent IL-6 plasma levels assessed in the HHV-7 PCR− group. (**d**) Each dot represents a single data point; blue dots represent TNF plasma levels assessed in the HHV-7 PCR+ group, and violet dots represent TNF plasma levels assessed in the HHV-7 PCR− group. The quantification limit (QL) for the assay of cytokine assessment was set as 1 pg/mL. Cytokine levels below QL (<1) were uniformly set as random values around QL/10. The right part of graph (**b**) and graph (**d**) represent data excluding values below the detection (quantification) level (w/o < 1), i.e., data without values of less than 1 (w/o < 1). W/o—without (write-off).

2.4. Histopathology and Immunohistochemical Detection of Antigens within the Synovial Membrane

To better explore the extent of synovitis and the contribution of cells to the development of inflammation, we performed a microscopical analysis of the synovial membrane tissue samples. In the first set of histopathological examinations, we assessed the synovial morphology in HHV-7 PCR+ and HHV-7 PCR− groups when inflammation was not confirmed microscopically. Histopathologically, the lining cells formed one layer, the synovial stroma revealed normal cellularity, and no inflammatory infiltrates were present. In contrast, the synovial lesions consistent with low-grade synovitis demonstrated an increase in thickness of the lining layer and stromal cellularity, and the presence of a few, mostly perivascular lymphocytes or/and plasma cells (Figure 3c). Comparatively, high-grade synovitis was distinguished by the presence of a greatly thickened lining; the appearance of ulceration and multinucleated giant cells; greatly increased stromal cellularity; and, finally, the presence of numerous lymphocytes and plasma cells, often forming follicle-like aggregates (Figure 3d).

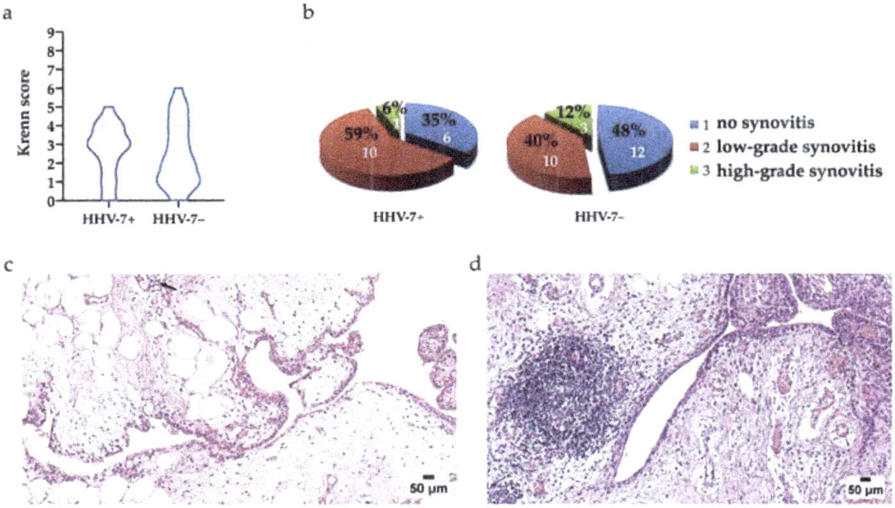

Figure 3. The presence of synovitis assessed by Krenn scores (**a**), statistically (**b**), and morphologically (**c**). (**a**) Violin plots depict the differences in median values demonstrated in the histopathological assessment of Krenn scores from the study groups. Synovitis revealed in the tissue samples of HHV-7 PCR+ OA patients presented with a median value of 3 (IQR 2–4), whereas HHV-7 PCR− OA patients presented with a median value of 2 (IQR 1–4). There was no significant difference found in the synovitis scores estimated for the HHV-7 PCR+ and HHV-7 PCR− groups ($p = 0.483$). Simultaneously, Krenn scores tended to be higher in the HHV-7 PCR+ group when compared to the HHV-7 PCR− group. (**b**) Frequencies of the absence of synovitis and the presence of low- and high-grade synovitis detected during histopathological assessment of the synovial membrane tissue samples from the study groups. The estimation confirms that OA patients commonly present without histopathologically detectable synovitis or demonstrate low-grade synovial inflammation. (**c**) A representative image depicting low-grade synovitis in OA. The synovial lining layer is slightly thickened, and the stromal density is slightly increased; few perivascular lymphocytes are evident (arrow). Hematoxylin and eosin staining. (**d**) A low-power image demonstrating high-grade synovitis in OA. The synovial lining layer is moderately thickened, and some lymphocytes are evident; stroma reveals moderate activation, whereas perivascular inflammatory cells and lymphatic follicle characterize the inflammatory component. Hematoxylin and eosin staining. Scale bars: 50 μm.

To further explore synovitis, we specified the cellular contributors by the use of immunohistochemistry. The small number of synovial CD4-positive lymphocytes found in the samples of both study groups, consisting of HHV-7 PCR+ and HHV-7 PCR−, was in line with low-grade synovitis (Figure 4a). Even in the absence of severe synovial inflammation, a statistically significant difference between the number of CD4-positive cells in HHV-7 PCR+ and HHV-7 PCR- groups was confirmed (Figure 4b).

To better assess the local expression of the pro-inflammatory marker TNF, we compared the numbers of TNF-positive cells in HHV-7 PCR+ and HHV-7 PCR− OA, and found no statistically significant differences between the groups. Similarly, no correlation was established when plasma cytokine levels were compared to the data depicting immunohistochemistry findings. Furthermore, we used the Wilcoxon matched-pairs signed rank test to compute the matched pairs, TNF-positive cell number, and HHV-7-positive cell number, submitting synovial samples of the HHV-7 PCR+ group to the test (Figure 4c). Simultaneously, in the HHV-7 PCR+ group, changes in the TNF-positive and HHV-7-positive cell count had a significant, positive correlation ($r = 0.593$, $p = 0.0453$) when assessed by Spearman's rank correlation (Figure 4d).

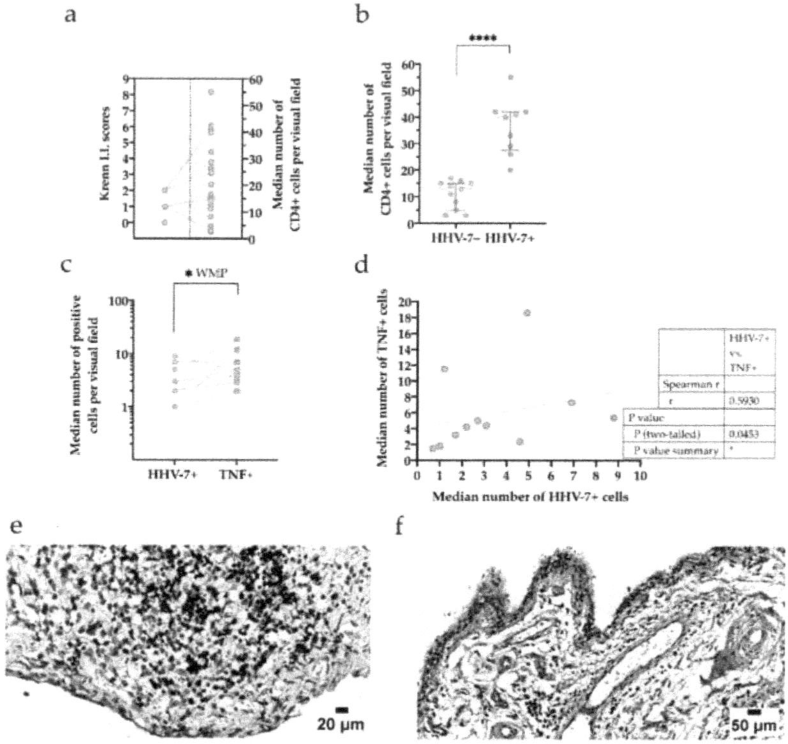

Figure 4. Assessment of synovial CD4-positive lymphocytes and TNF-positive cells in both study groups—HHV-7 PCR+ and HHV-7 PCR−—and HHV-7-positive cells in the HHV-7 PCR+ group. (**a**) The absence of synovitis graded as 0–1, and the presence of a small number of synovial CD4-positive lymphocytes found in the samples of both study groups—HHV-7 PCR+ and HHV-7 PCR−—consistent with low-grade synovitis (grade "2"). Grade "2" synovitis presented with a higher number of CD4-positive lymphocytes when compared to the lower grades. I.I. Krenn—inflammatory infiltration as a substantial part of the Krenn score (inflammatory infiltration, cellular hyperplasia of the lining layer, and cellular density of the sublining layer summed up to provide the Krenn score). Each dot represents a single data point. (**b**) The median number of CD4-positive cells per visual field in the synovial samples obtained from the HHV-7 PCR+ group is significantly higher than that in the HHV-7 PCR− group. Asterisks represent the significance level (**** $p < 0.0001$). (**c**) Median numbers assessed for immunohistochemically confirmed that positive cells are plotted for TNF and HHV-7 antigens. WMP—Wilcoxon matched-pairs signed rank test. The asterisk represents the significance level (* $p < 0.05$). Each dot represents a single data point; blue dots represent HHV-7+ cells, and violet squares represent TNF+ cells. (**d**) Correlation of the median number of HHV-7+ and TNF+ cells expressed per visual field and detected in the samples of the HHV-7 PCR+ group; $r = 0.593$, $p = 0.0453$. An increase in the number of HHV-7+ cells reveals the elevation in the number of TNF+ cells. (**e**) CD4 immunohistochemistry. A representative image demonstrating T-lymphocytes decorated by the anti-CD4 antibody and recognized by the presence of brown reaction products in a follicle-like lymphocytic inflammatory infiltrate found in the synovial sample of HHV-7 PCR+ subjects. Scale bar 20 µm. (**f**) Through the use of TNF immunohistochemistry, the synovial lining presents TNF-positive cells interspersed by TNF-negative cells, whereas the sublining demonstrates mostly perivascular positivity observed in a sample of HHV-7 PCR+ patients. Scale bar: 50 µm.

When submitting the synovial samples obtained from both study groups for microscopical analysis, the lymphocytes and plasma cells colonizing the sublining layer demonstrated either diffusely scattered patterns of distribution, or compact and mostly perivascular patterns. Often, the presence of small follicle-like lymphocytic inflammatory infiltrates was confirmed (Figure 4e). Simultaneously, when assessed immunohistochemically, TNF-positive cells were distributed across the synovial lining and sublining and often demonstrated perivascular localization (Figure 4f).

To better recognize and estimate residential cells, synovial macrophages, and their role in the production of pro-inflammatory cytokines, we labeled cells with the anti-CD68 antibody. Furthermore, we compared the presence and number of CD68-positive and CD4-positive cells. The distribution of inflammatory cells bearing CD68 and CD4 labeling varied in both HHV-7 PCR+ and HHV-7 PCR− groups; however, the difference was not statistically significant (Figure 5a). Opposingly, the distribution of synovial CD68-positive cells and CD4-positive cells differed to a greater extent when latent and active HHV-7 infection was referred (Figure 5c). Simultaneously, no correlation was established when CD68 immunohistochemistry data were compared to the results depicting plasma pro-inflammatory cytokine levels (TNF and IL-6). Under the microscope, CD68-positive cells presented in both synovial subdivisions, the lining and sublining layers were diffusely distributed in both HHV-7 PCR− (Figure 5b) and HHV-7 PCR+ (Figure 5d) groups, and more local patterns of distribution were acquired when contributing to follicle-like inflammatory infiltrates.

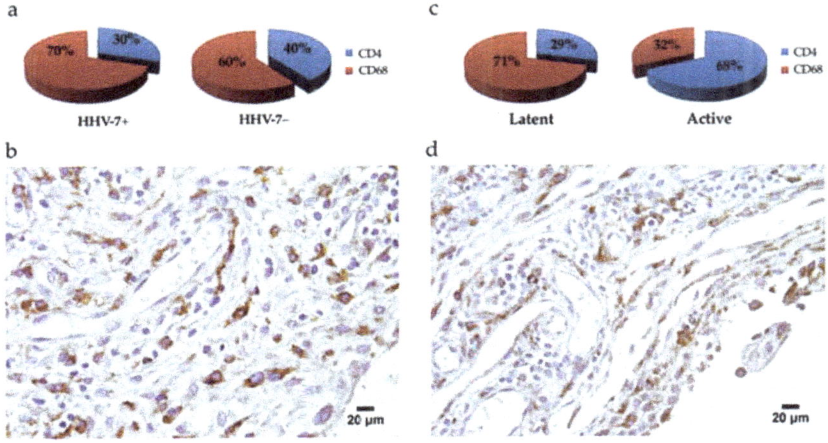

Figure 5. Comparison of the distribution of synovial CD68- and CD4-positive inflammatory cells by the use of statistics (**a**,**c**), and the microscopical assessment of CD68-positive cells (**b**,**d**). (**a**) The distribution of CD68- and CD4-positive cells in both HHV-7 PCR+ and HHV-7 PCR− groups: CD68-positive cells constituted almost two-thirds (70%) of inflammatory cells found in HHV-7 PCR− samples, whereas, for CD68- and CD4-positive cells, 60 and 40%, respectively, were more equally distributed in HHV-7 PCR+. (**c**) CD68-positive cells represented a major part (71%) of inflammatory cells in latent HHV-7 infection, whereas these were opposingly distributed in active HHV-7 infection, with 68% and 32% of CD4- and CD68-positive cells, respectively. (**b**,**d**) CD68 immunohistochemistry; a representative image ((**b**), HHV-7 PCR− sample; (**d**), HHV-7 PCR+ sample) demonstrating CD68-positive cells decorated by the anti-CD68 antibody and developed brown reaction products in the synoviocytes of lining layer and the macrophages of sublining layer. The immunohistochemical decoration reflects the presence of lysosome-specific proteins involved in sorting in the trans-Golgi region, targeting to lysosomes, and fusion with the plasma membrane.

Fourteen of 19 HHV-7 PCR+ OA patients presented with synovium applicable for further immunohistochemical studies and tissue detection of the antigen. Furthermore, HHV-7-positive lymphocytes and macrophages were distinguished by their cytological appearance. To better explore the relationship between synovial cells bearing the HHV-7 antigen and TNF-producing cells, we computed the matched pairs' TNF-positive cell number and HHV-7-positive cell number, similar to Figure 4c,d but stratified into cellular types (Figure 6a,c). We determined a statistically significant, positive correlation (r = 0.6629, p = 0.0367) between HHV-7-positive lymphocytes and TNF-positive cells (Figure 6b), whereas a negative correlation (r = −0.6797, p = 0.0351) was found between HHV-7-positive endotheliocytes and TNF-positive cells (Figure 6d).

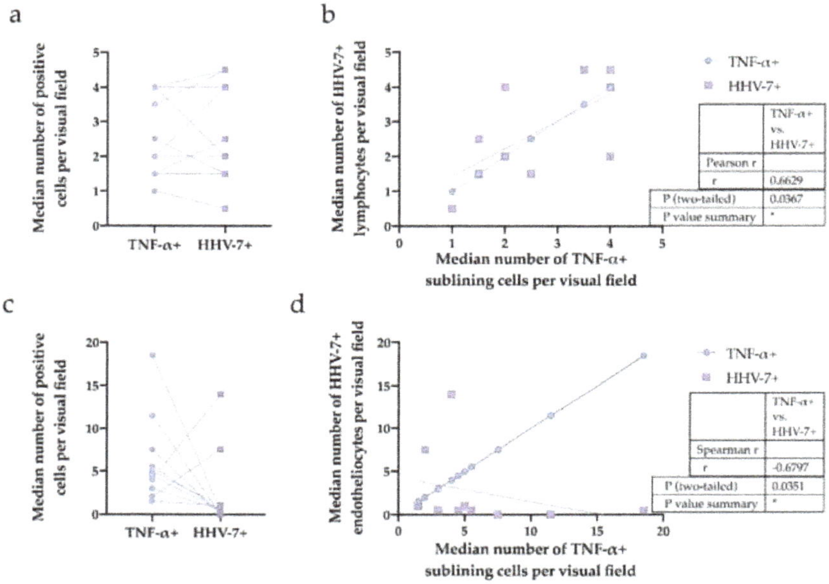

Figure 6. Assessment of synovial HHV-7-positive cells—lymphocytes (panel (**a**) and (**b**)) and vascular endothelial cells (panel (**c**) and (**d**)), and TNF-positive cells in the HHV-7 PCR+ group. (**a**) Median numbers assessed for immunohistochemically confirmed positive cells are plotted for the TNF and HHV-7 antigen. Each dot represents a single data point; blue dots represent TNF+ cells, and violet squares represent HHV-7+ lymphocytes. (**b**) Correlation between the median number of TNF+ cells and HHV-7+ lymphocytes expressed per visual field and detected in the samples of the HHV-7 PCR+ group; r = 0.6629, p = 0.0367. Each dot represents a single data point; blue dots represent TNF+ cells, and violet squares represent HHV-7+ lymphocytes. Correlations determined by Pearson's rank correlation test. (**c**) Median numbers assessed for immunohistochemically confirmed positive cells are plotted for the TNF and HHV-7 antigen. Each dot represents a single data point; blue dots represent TNF+ cells, and violet squares represent HHV-7+ endotheliocytes. (**d**) Correlation between the median number of TNF+ cells and HHV-7+ endotheliocytes expressed per visual field and detected in the samples of the HHV-7 PCR+ group; r = −0.6797, p = 0.0351. Each dot represents a single data point; blue dots represent TNF+ cells, and violet squares represent HHV-7+ endotheliocytes. Correlations were determined by the Spearman's rank correlation test.

Finally, HHV-7 immunohistochemistry data were compared for patients presenting with latent and active infection. When assessed quantitatively, HHV-7-positive lymphocytes, endotheliocytes, and macrophages constituted 58, 27, and 15% and 32, 67, and 1% of the cases of latent and active HHV-7 infection, respectively (Figure 7a,b). The immunohistochemical estimation of synovial HHV-7-positive cells applied for the HHV-7 PCR+ group demonstrated that cells labeled with the anti-HHV-7 antibody were localized in the sublining layer, both peri- and intravascularly (Figure 7c,d), and in the lining layer

(Figure 7e,f). Moreover, some endothelial cells constituting the internal lining of blood vessels found in the synovial membrane stroma were positively stained with the anti-HHV-7 antibody. Furthermore, evidence of the presence of HHV-7 expression in synovial tissue correlated with nPCR data.

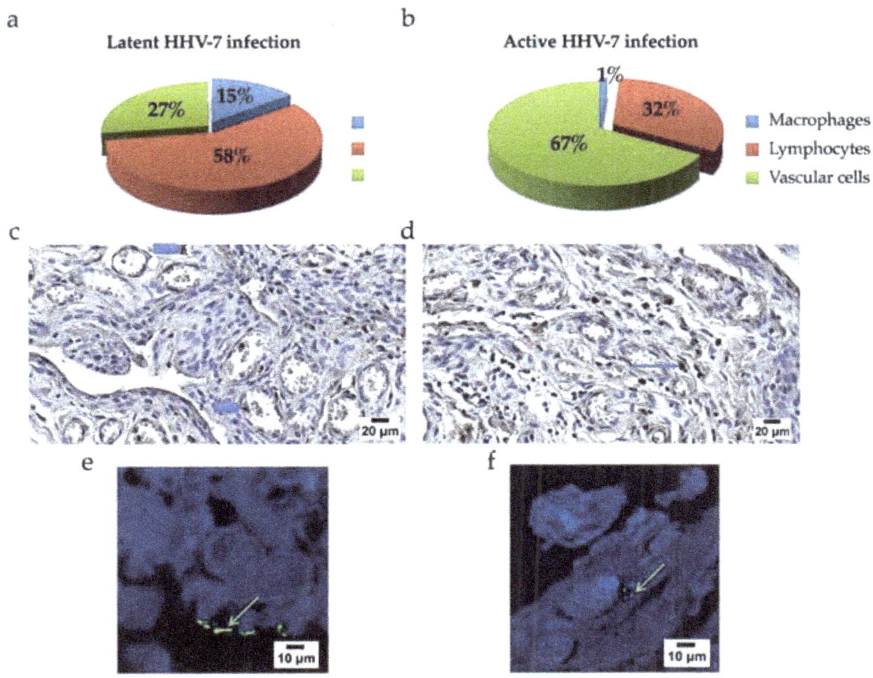

Figure 7. The assessment of the HHV-7 antigen in the synovial membrane. (**a**,**b**) Frequencies of HHV-7-positive lymphocytes, vascular endotheliocytes, and macrophages based on immunohistochemistry data and compared for patients presenting with latent (**a**) and active infection (**b**). When assessed quantitatively, HHV-7-positive lymphocytes constituted a significant cellular fraction affected by the virus in latent HHV-7 infection and reached 58%. In contrast, vascular endotheliocytes forming the innermost layer of vascular beds appeared the most vulnerable in active HHV-7 infection, demonstrating a 67% involvement. There was a significant difference found between the distribution of HHV-7-positive endotheliocytes estimated for latent and active HHV-7 infections ($p = 0.028$). (**c**) Immunohistochemical detection of the HHV-7 antigen in the case of latent HHV-7 infection. Intravascular HHV-7-positive cells recognized by brown coloration (blue arrowheads) localized in the lumen of congested blood vessels. Cellular nuclei counterstained with Mayer's hematoxylin (blue). Scale bar: 20 μm. (**d**) Numerous perivascular (blue arrow) and vascular endothelial HHV-7-positive cells localized in the sublining layer. Cellular nuclei counterstained with Mayer's hematoxylin (blue). Scale bar: 20 μm. Detection of the tegument protein pp85 of HHV-7 by immunofluorescence (HHV-7-immunopositive products, green), confocal microscopy; 1% toluidine blue was added to the fluorophore, and it resulted in near infra-red fluorescence in the cellular cytoplasmic compartment. Green arrows indicate the presence of viral protein at the top of synovial macrophages (**e**) and within the cell cytoplasm (**f**). Scale bar: 10 μm.

3. Discussion

Chronic, low-grade, local inflammation underlining the OA process has been considered as an essential feature of the disease [6,8,9,35]. Furthermore, the action of an inflamed synovium as a trigger of the OA process has been suggested and points at cells recruited in intra-articular changes [36].

Therefore, the assessment of synovial lesions has been encouraged by both research and clinical practice [37–39].

Previous studies have explored the molecular mechanisms of the cell entry of betaherpesviruses; some authors have designated CD46 as an entry receptor in the case of HHV-6 infection and demonstrated the presence of it on a major target cell—activated T lymphocytes [40]. Alternatively, other authors have explored CD134, which is a receptor specific for HHV-6B, belonging to the TNF receptor superfamily and expressed on activated CD4-positive T cells [41–43].

Human herpesvirus 7, one of the most prevalent viruses in the human population, has also been recognized to target lymphocytes [44]. Furthermore, the activation of infected T lymphocytes leading to the reactivation of HHV-7 has been confirmed [45]. Finally, in HCMV infection, up to 30% of all circulating CD4-positive T lymphocytes become the primary target of the virus in infected elderly individuals. Furthermore, the authors showed that these HCMV-affected T lymphocytes may contribute to significant shifts in the leukocyte composition of peripheral blood and an increase in the number of "effector-memory" T cells [46].

Importantly, the OA synovium has been reported to be a tissue enriched in T cells when compared to the normal synovial membrane [38,39,47–49], and the proportion of CD4-positive T cells and the CD4-positive/CD8-positive ratio found in peripheral blood are recognized as being significantly higher in OA patients when compared to healthy controls [7,50]. Other authors have reported on synovial tissue damage induced by CD4-positive T cells and evidenced, at a later stage of the disease, that activated CD4-positive T cells promote lesions and induce macrophage inflammatory protein-1γ expression and subsequent osteoclast formation in OA patients [51]. Given that the demonstrated overall assessment of CD4-positive T cells is in line with synovial morphological findings, this suggests a clear predominance of OA subjects without histopathologically detectable and low-grade inflammation confirmed in both study groups. In this study, the median number of CD4-positive cells per visual field assessed in the synovial samples of the HHV-7 PCR+ group was significantly higher than that in the HHV-7 PCR- group ($p < 0.0001$). The role of HHV-7 infection in the development and progression of either synovitis or OA remains largely unknown. However, a strong ($r = 0.6629$, $p = 0.0367$) correlation between the number of TNF+ and HHV-7+ lymphocytes has been demonstrated in the samples of the HHV-7 PCR+ group, suggesting the significance of the immune system reaction to a foreign antigen. Furthermore, the vulnerability of vascular endothelial cells, especially in the case of infection reactivation, is shown in the given study. Available serological data suggest that primary herpesvirus infection occurs early in childhood and results in a lifelong infection [24,52–54].

This is consistent with the results of our study. The present study demonstrated the presence of persistent HHV-7 infection in 81.5% of all enrolled OA patients. Similar results were published by Sánchez-Ponce and colleagues conducting studies on beta and gamma human herpesviruses in the case of organ transplantation, and they raised awareness about an increased risk of graft rejection [55].

Our previous studies have pointed out that the eradication of this infection often does not occur, and the virus remains in a latent state [56,57]. Complications associated with virus reactivation involve a wide range of diseases, including joint pathologies; however, the role of HHV-7 has not been completely understood thus far. Other authors have not succeeded in attempts at isolating DNA from herpesviruses in patients with OA, but have showed the presence of DNA from HSV1-2 and VZV in RA and axial spondyloarthritis patients [33]. The strength of our study includes a look at the synovial cellular constituents targeted in the case of latent or active HHV-7 infection. In our study, molecular virology data confirmed that either latent or active HHV-7 infection was coupled to immunohistochemical detection of the viral antigen in the synovial membrane. We observed that HHV-7 latency was characterized by the contribution of inflammatory cells and the presence of CD4-positive cells, establishing a strong, positive correlation with TNF-producers. Simultaneously, we proved that different cellular targets, vascular beds, and their constituents, are more vulnerable and are therefore affected in the case of active HHV-7 infection.

Previous studies have demonstrated that human herpesviruses sustain latency in cells of the hematopoietic lineage, but become reactivated upon immune challenge to cause disease [58]. Synovial macrophages are of great interest in this context since they may act as a reservoir during the period of viral infection latency. This feature has been widely explored, and evidence that even a suppressed viral transcription program exhibits several viral genes that are expressed during latent infection at the protein level has been obtained; many of these have profound effects on the cell and its environment, regulating numerous cellular functions [59,60]. Furthermore, our recent studies provided some insight into the controversial issue related to the chromosomal integration of HHV-7 [61]. In this context, the stimulation of inflammation and oxidative stress are areas of interest when suggesting the contribution of herpesviruses infections to chromosomal telomere attrition [62,63]. Previous studies have proved the role of macrophages in the development of synovial lesions and progression of OA through the production of inflammatory mediators, growth factors, and metalloproteinases, resulting in enhanced cartilage degeneration and osteophyte formation [13]. Furthermore, immunohistochemical studies have produced additional evidence of the presence of TNF, which is the key pro-inflammatory factor released by synovial macrophages, in OA [38,64]. OA synovitis has been recognized as a cytokine-driven disease, especially regarding TNF, even when manifesting with lower levels of pro-inflammatory mediators compared to that in RA [15]. A higher expression of the inflammatory mediators was found in the lining layer, and a lower expression was found in the sublining layer of the lesioned synovium [65,66]. In this study, we found a large number of TNF-labeled synovial lining cells, whereas most of the sublining constituents revealed perivascular localization. Our data are consistent with the results obtained by these authors. Furthermore, more substantial synovial macrophage infiltration demonstrated in patients with early OA, when compared to advanced OA [13], and higher levels of inflammatory cytokines, including IL-6, IL-1, and TNF, were evidenced in early compared to advanced OA [67]. The significance of findings depicting the distribution and functions of synovial macrophages and infiltrating lymphocytes has been pointed out in the given study, without denying other accurate and sensitive tools for visualizing the inflammatory cells in OA [13].

By emphasizing the significance of the immune system reaction to a foreign antigen, one may expect the appearance of system overreaction, causing potentially more harm than the viral agent itself. There is an increasing appreciation of the importance of cellular plasticity on the one hand, and the diversity of strategies and molecular mechanisms for escaping detection by the immune system evolved by HHV-7 on the other [68], suggesting the necessity for further research.

4. Materials and Methods

4.1. Patients' Characteristics

Fifty-four patients that presented with advanced OA and underwent joint replacement surgery for the disease at the Riga East University Hospital Clinic "Gailezers" between March 2019 and January 2020 were enrolled in the study. The inclusion criterion was a primary or previous diagnosis of OA established in the given hospital. All OA subjects fulfilled relevant American College of Rheumatology (ACR) criteria for the disease-affected joints: Hip [69] and knee [70]. All subjects enrolled in the study (mean age 69 (range 35–85 years), standard deviation (SD) ± 12.28 years); 19 (35.2%) males and 35 (64.8%) females) had OA confirmed clinically and radiologically. They did not reveal any objective and subjective evidence of any other inflammatory disease apart from OA. The clinical data of patients included information on the duration, course, and clinical features of the disease at the time of presentation, whereas laboratory analyses employed to monitor OA progress included complete blood count, hemoglobin, and C reactive protein (CPR) data. PCR data were obtained from 48 out of 54 patients. These OA patients were subdivided into two study groups: HHV-7 PCR+ (n = 19) subjects (the first group) and HHV-7 PCR- (n = 29) subjects (the second group), accordingly. The average age of OA subjects of the first group was 68.95 years (SD ± 9.35), whereas that of the second group was

63.93 years (SD ± 12.9). The study was approved by the Ethical Committee of Riga Stradins University (Decisions No. 6-2/7/9 and No. 6-1/01/62) and was conducted according to the Declaration of Helsinki.

4.2. Blood Sample Collection and Detection of TNF and IL-6 Levels

Ethylenediamine tetraacetic acid anti-coagulated peripheral blood samples from OA patients were collected. Plasma samples were separated from peripheral blood by centrifugation. The levels of TNF and IL-6 (pg/mL) were measured by an enzyme-linked immunosorbent assay (ELISA) (TNF-α by Nordic Biosite, Copenhagen, Denmark), according to the manufacturer's guidelines, and analyzed in comparison with the presence or absence of HHV-7 infection markers. The optical density was measured by a microplate reader (Multiscan Ascent, Thermo Electron Corporation, Waltham, MA, USA) at a 450 nm wavelength using Ascent Software, and the results were calculated using Microsoft Excel.

4.3. Nested Polymerase Chain Reaction

A nested polymerase chain reaction (nPCR) was used for the qualitative detection of the viral genomic sequence in DNA isolated from whole blood, synovial membrane tissue samples (a marker for persistent latent infection), and cell-free blood plasma (a marker of active infection). Total DNA was isolated from WPB and synovial membrane tissue samples using the standard phenol-chloroform extraction. The QIA amp DNA Blood Mini Kit (Qiagen, Hilden, Germany) was used to extract DNA from plasma. The concentration of extracted DNA was measured spectrophotometrically (Nanodrop ND-1000 Spectrophotometer, Thermo Fisher Scientific, Waltham, MA, USA). To assure the quality of the whole blood, cell-free blood plasma, and synovial tissue DNA, as well as to exclude the contamination of plasma DNA by cellular DNA debris, a β-globin PCR was carried out using a polymerase chain reaction (PCR) (C1000 Touch Thermal Cycler, BioRad, Hercules, CA, USA). One microgram of whole blood and synovial tissue DNA, as well as 10 μL of plasma DNA, were subjected to nPCR with the HHV-7-specific primer, as described previously [71]. Positive (HHV-7 genomic DNA; ABI, Columbia, MD, USA) and negative controls (DNA obtained from practically healthy HHV-7-negative donors and a reaction without template DNA), as well as water controls, were included in each experiment. In the experiments, the sensitivity of HHV-7-specific primers corresponded to one copy of HHV-7 per reaction [72].

4.4. Light Microscopy and Immunohistochemistry

Synovial membrane tissue specimens (n = 54) were obtained from all OA patients undergoing joint replacement surgery. Two series of histological sections of 4–5 μm were cut from 10% formalin-fixed, paraffin-embedded tissue samples and mounted on SuperFrost Plus slides (Germany Menzel GmbH, Braunschweig, Germany) for histopathological and immunohistochemical evaluation. Before immunostaining, deparaffinization and hydration were conducted in xylene and graded alcohol to distilled water. During hydration, a 5 min blocking process for endogenous peroxidase was conducted with 0.3% (*v/v*) H2O2 in 95% methanol. Heat-induced epitope retrieval was accomplished with the sections immersed in 10 mM sodium citrate buffer, pH 6.0, at 96–98 °C for 5 min in a vapor lock.

Immunohistochemistry was performed conventionally using a monoclonal anti-HHV-7 antibody (Advanced Biotechnologies, Columbia, MD, USA, 1:500) raised against the tegument protein pp85 of HHV-7 [73,74]; the polyclonal rabbit anti-human TNF antibody (Biorbyt, Cambridge, UK, 1:100), which labels a certain peptide of human TNF [75]; monoclonal mouse anti-human CD68 (DacoCytomation, Glostrup, Denmark, clone PG-M1, 1:50), which labels monocytes/macrophages via the recognition of lysosome proteins,; and monoclonal rabbit anti-human CD4 (Cell Marque, Rocklin, CA, USA, SP35, 1:100), which recognizes a 55 kD glycoprotein expressed on the cell surface of T-helper/regulatory T-cells.

The amplification of the primary antibody and visualization of reaction products were performed by applying the HiDef Detection HRP Polymer system and diaminobenzidine tetrahydrochloride substrate kit (Cell Marque, Rocklin, CA, USA). The sections were counterstained with Mayer's hematoxylin, washed, mounted, and covered with coverslips. Immunohistochemical controls included the omission of the primary antibody. Sections were photographed by a Leitz DMRB bright-field microscope using a DFC 450C digital camera or scanned with a Glissando Slide Scanner (Objective Imaging Ltd., Cambridge, UK) with a 10×, 20×, and 40× objective. Reproducible measurements of tissue markers were obtained using the, Aperio ImageScope program v12.2.2.5015, Leica Biosystems Imaging, Vista, CA, USA and images were processed with the ImageJ program (National Institute of Health, Bethesda, MD, USA). Assessment of the histopathology and immunostaining was performed by two independent observers blinded to clinicopathological data.

Cells that were labeled with the anti-HHV-7, anti-TNF, anti-CD68, and anti-CD4 antibody and displayed brown reaction products were considered as immunopositive. The total number of immunopositive cells appearing within the microscopic field, depicting a certain synovial region, was estimated quantitatively in 10 randomly selected visual fields of each sample (magnification 400×).

Additionally, to better visualize the cellular distribution and localization of the HHV-7 antigen, the synovial tissue specimens were processed for fluorescent immunohistochemical staining and confocal microscopy. The sections that immunoreacted with the primary antibody overnight at 4 °C were washed in PBS, followed by incubation in goat anti-mouse IgG-FITC: sc-2010 (Santa Cruz Biotechnology, Inc., Santa Cruz, CA, USA 1:300) as the secondary antibody. Then, sections were counterstained with 4′,6-diamidino-2phenylindole (DAPI) (Thermo Fisher Scientific, Invitrogen, Renfrew, UK, 1:3,000) and mounted in Prolong Gold with DAPI (Thermo Fisher Scientific). Imaging was performed using an Eclipse Ti-E confocal microscope (Nikon, Tokyo, Japan).

4.5. Scoring of Synovitis by Krenn

To define synovitis, involving inflammatory changes of the synovial membrane depicting intra-articular changes of a joint, we graded it using the scoring system introduced by Krenn and Morawietz [76]. Routinely (with hematoxylin and eosin), stained slides were used, and the lesions found in the synovial membrane were assessed. The following histopathological features were evaluated and scored: The cellular hyperplasia of the lining layer; the cellular density of the sublining layer; and the presence of inflammatory infiltration: 0—absent, 1—mild, 2—moderate, and 3—strong. The sum obtained provided the synovitis score, which was interpreted as follows: 0–1, no synovitis; 2–4, low-grade synovitis; and 5–9, high-grade synovitis.

4.6. Statistical Data Analysis

To better interpret molecular virology, serology, histopathology, and immunohistochemistry data, statistical analyses were performed using The GraphPad Prism 8 demo version (GraphPad Software, La Jolla, CA, USA). The D'Agostino and Pearson, Anderson–Darling, and Shapiro–Wilk tests were used to evaluate whether the collected numerical data were normally distributed. If data were not normally distributed, we used nonparametric one-way ANOVA on ranks or Kruskal–Wallis test followed by the two-stage step-up method of Benjamini, Krieger, and Yekutieli as post hoc tests when comparing medians instead of means. The chi-square test was performed for categorical variables. Categorical parameters were expressed as frequencies and percentages. The results of the histopathological assessment of Krenn scores in the synovial membrane samples of the study groups are expressed as violin plots, the median, and the interquartile range (IQR) as dispersion characteristics. To compare numerical values between two groups, the nonparametric two-tailed Mann–Whitney U test was applied. In the case of paired group comparisons, the Wilcoxon matched-pairs signed rank test was used. Correlations between the numbers of immunopositive cells were determined using either parametric Pearson's or nonparametric Spearman's correlation analyses, depending on the data distribution. The correlations were considered as follows: 0.2 to 0.4—weak; 0.4 to 0.7—moderate; and 0.7 to 0.9—strong. A p-value of less than 0.05 ($p < 0.05$) was considered statistically significant.

Author Contributions: Conceptualization and design of research: V.G. and M.T.; formal analysis: V.G.; data curation: V.G., M.T., S.S. (Sofija Semenistaja), Z.N.-K.; and S.S. (Simons Svirskis); writing—original draft preparation: V.G.; writing—review and editing: V.G., M.T., S.S. (Sandra Skuja), Z.N.-K., and M.M.; visualization: V.G., S.S. (Sandra Skuja), M.T., and S.S. (Sofija Semenistaja); prepared figures: V.G., M.T., S.S. (Simons Svirski), and S.S. (Sandra Skuja). All authors have read and agreed to the published version of the manuscript.

Funding: This research received no external funding.

Acknowledgments: This study was supported by the Latvian Council of Science Grant Nr. Izp-2018/1-0149 and the National Research Programme Biomedicine for the Public Health (BIOMEDICINE), project 7.2. The authors would like to thank Anda Kadisa, Rheumatologist at Riga East University Hospital Clinic "Gailezers", Latvia, for advising on the diagnosis and recruitment of osteoarthritis patients.

Conflicts of Interest: The authors declare no conflict of interest.

References

1. Fusco, M.; Skaper, S.D.; Coaccioli, S.; Varrassi, G.; Paladini, A. Degenerative Joint Diseases and Neuroinflammation. *Pain Pract.* **2017**, *17*, 522–532. [CrossRef] [PubMed]
2. Bortoluzzi, A.; Furini, F.; Generali, E.; Silvagni, E.; Luciano, N.; Scirè, C.A. One year in review 2018: Novelties in the treatment of rheumatoid arthritis. *Clin. Exp. Rheumatol.* **2018**, *36*, 347–361. [PubMed]
3. Fu, K.; Robbins, S.; McDougall, J.J. Osteoarthritis: The genesis of pain. *Rheumatology* **2017**, *57*, iv43–iv50. [CrossRef] [PubMed]
4. Bruyère, O.; Cooper, C.; Pelletier, J.-P.; Branco, J.C.; Brandi, M.L.; Guillemin, F.; Hochberg, M.C.; Kanis, J.; Kvien, T.K.; Martel-Pelletier, J.; et al. An algorithm recommendation for the management of knee osteoarthritis in Europe and internationally: A report from a task force of the European Society for Clinical and Economic Aspects of Osteoporosis and Osteoarthritis (ESCEO). *Semin. Arthritis Rheum.* **2014**, *44*, 253–263. [CrossRef]
5. Goldring, M.B.; Otero, M.; Plumb, D.A.; Dragomir, C.; Favero, M.; Hachem, K.E.; Hashimoto, K.; Roach, H.; Olivotto, E.; Borzì, R.; et al. Roles of inflammatory and anabolic cytokines in cartilage metabolism: Signals and multiple effectors converge upon MMP-13 regulation in osteoarthritis. *Eur. Cells Mater.* **2011**, *21*, 202–220. [CrossRef]
6. Rahmati, M.; Mobasheri, A.; Mozafari, M. Inflammatory mediators in osteoarthritis: A critical review of the state-of-the-art, current prospects, and future challenges. *Bone* **2016**, *85*, 81–90. [CrossRef]
7. Li, Y.-S.; Luo, W.; Zhu, S.; Lei, G. T Cells in Osteoarthritis: Alterations and Beyond. *Front. Immunol.* **2017**, *8*, 356. [CrossRef]
8. Griffin, T.M.; Scanzello, C.R. Innate inflammation and synovial macrophages in osteoarthritis pathophysiology. *Clin. Exp. Rheumatol.* **2019**, *37*, 57–63.
9. Berenbaum, F. Osteoarthritis as an inflammatory disease (osteoarthritis is not osteoarthrosis!). *Osteoarthr. Cartil.* **2013**, *21*, 16–21. [CrossRef]
10. Iwanaga, T.; Shikichi, M.; Kitamura, H.; Yanase, H.; Nozawa-Inoue, K. Morphology and Functional Roles of Synoviocytes in the Joint. *Arch. Histol. Cytol.* **2000**, *63*, 17–31. [CrossRef]
11. Shikichi, M.; Kitamura, H.P.; Yanase, H.; Konno, A.; Takahashi-Iwanaga, H.; Iwanaga, T. Three-dimensional Ultrastructure of Synoviocytes in the Horse Joint as Revealed by the Scanning Electron Microscope. *Arch. Histol. Cytol.* **1999**, *62*, 219–229. [CrossRef] [PubMed]
12. Pearson, M.J.; Herndler-Brandstetter, D.; Tariq, M.A.; Nicholson, T.A.; Philp, A.M.; Smith, H.L.; Davis, E.T.; Jones, S.W.; Lord, J.M. IL-6 secretion in osteoarthritis patients is mediated by chondrocyte-synovial fibroblast cross-talk and is enhanced by obesity. *Sci. Rep.* **2017**, *7*, 3451. [CrossRef] [PubMed]
13. Berkelaar, M.H.M.; Korthagen, N.M.; Jansen, G.; van Spil, W.E. Synovial Macrophages: Potential Key Modulators of Cartilage Damage, Osteophyte Formation and Pain in Knee Osteoarthritis. *J. Rheum. Dis. Treat.* **2018**, *4*, 059.
14. Moqbel, S.A.A.; He, Y.; Xu, L.; Ma, C.; Ran, J.; Xu, K.; Wu, L. Rat Chondrocyte Inflammation and Osteoarthritis Are Ameliorated by Madecassoside. *Oxidative Med. Cell Longev.* **2020**, *2020*, 197. [CrossRef] [PubMed]
15. Sutton, S.; Clutterbuck, A.; Harris, P.; Gent, T.C.; Freeman, S.L.; Foster, N.; Barrett-Jolley, R.; Mobasheri, A. The contribution of the synovium, synovial derived inflammatory cytokines and neuropeptides to the pathogenesis of osteoarthritis. *Vet. J.* **2009**, *179*, 10–24. [CrossRef]

16. Zakrzewska, K.; Azzi, A.; de Biasi, E.; Radossi, P.; de Santis, R.; Davoli, P.; Tagariello, G. Persistence of parvovirus B19 DNA in synovium of patients with haemophilic arthritis. *J. Med. Virol.* **2001**, *65*, 402–407. [CrossRef]
17. Mehraein, Y.; Lennerz, C.; Ehlhardt, S.; Venzke, T.; Ojak, A.; Remberger, K.; Zang, K.D. Detection of Parvovirus B19 Capsid Proteins in Lymphocytic Cells in Synovial Tissue of Autoimmune Chronic Arthritis. *Mod. Pathol.* **2003**, *16*, 811–817. [CrossRef]
18. Mehraein, Y.; Lennerz, C.; Ehlhardt, S.; Zang, K.D.; Madry, H. Replicative multivirus infection with cytomegalovirus, herpes simplex virus 1, and parvovirus B19, and latent Epstein–Barr virus infection in the synovial tissue of a psoriatic arthritis patient. *J. Clin. Virol.* **2004**, *31*, 25–31. [CrossRef]
19. Naciute, M.; Mieliauskaite, D.; Rugiene, R.; Nikitenkiene, R.; Jancoriene, L.; Mauricas, M.; Nora-Krūkle, Z.; Murovska, M.; Girkontaite, I. Frequency and significance of parvovirus B19 infection in patients with rheumatoid arthritis. *J. Gen. Virol.* **2016**, *97*, 3302–3312. [CrossRef]
20. Marks, M.; Marks, J.L. Viral arthritis. *Clin. Med.* **2016**, *16*, 129. [CrossRef]
21. Agut, H.; Bonnafous, P.; Gautheret-Dejean, A. Human Herpesviruses 6A, 6B, and 7. *Microbiol. Spectr.* **2016**, *4*, 157–176. [CrossRef] [PubMed]
22. Agut, H.; Bonnafous, P.; Gautheret-Dejean, A. Update on infections with human herpesviruses 6A, 6B, and 7. *Médecine Mal. Infect.* **2017**, *47*, 83–91. [CrossRef] [PubMed]
23. Wołącewicz, M.; Becht, R.; Grywalska, E.; Niedźwiedzka-Rystwej, P. Herpesviruses in Head and Neck Cancers. *Viruses* **2020**, *12*, 172. [CrossRef] [PubMed]
24. Denner, J.; Bigley, T.M.; Phan, T.L.; Zimmermann, C.; Zhou, X.; Kaufer, B.B. Comparative Analysis of Roseoloviruses in Humans, Pigs, Mice, and Other Species. *Viruses* **2019**, *11*, 1108. [CrossRef]
25. Drago, F.; Malaguti, F.; Ranieri, E.; Losi, E.; Rebora, A. Human herpes virus-like particles in pityriasis rosea lesions: An electron microscopy study. *J Cutan. Pathol.* **2002**, *29*, 359–361. [CrossRef]
26. Watanabe, T.; Kawamura, T.; Aquilino, E.A.; Blauvelt, A.; Jacob, S.E.; Orenstein, J.M.; Black, J.B. Pityriasis Rosea is Associated with Systemic Active Infection with Both Human Herpesvirus-7 and Human Herpesvirus-6. *J. Investig. Dermatol.* **2002**, *119*, 793–797. [CrossRef]
27. Broccolo, F.; Drago, F.; Careddu, A.M.; Foglieni, C.; Turbino, L.; Cocuzza, C.E.; Gelmetti, C.; Lusso, P.; Rebora, A.; Malnati, M.S. Additional Evidence that Pityriasis Rosea Is Associated with Reactivation of Human Herpesvirus-6 and -7. *J. Investig. Dermatol.* **2005**, *124*, 1234–1240. [CrossRef]
28. Drago, F.; Ciccarese, G.; Parodi, A. HHV-6 reactivation as a cause of fever in autologous hematopoietic stem cell transplant recipients: A reply. *J. Infect.* **2018**, *76*, 101–102. [CrossRef]
29. Nahidi, Y.; Meibodi, N.T.; Ghazvini, K.; Esmaily, H.; Esmaeelzadeh, M. Association of classic lichen planus with human herpesvirus-7 infection. *Int. J. Dermatol.* **2016**, *56*, 49–53. [CrossRef]
30. Skuja, S.; Zieda, A.; Ravina, K.; Chapenko, S.; Roga, S.; Teteris, O.; Groma, V.; Murovska, M. Structural and Ultrastructural Alterations in Human Olfactory Pathways and Possible Associations with Herpesvirus 6 Infection. *PLoS ONE* **2017**, *12*, e0170071. [CrossRef]
31. Kadiša, A.; Nora-Krūkle, Z.; Kozireva, S.; Svirskis, S.; Studers, P.; Groma, V.; Lejnieks, A.; Murovska, M. Effect of Human Herpesviruses 6 and 7 Infection on the Clinical Course of Rheumatoid Arthritis/Cilvēka Herpesvīrusa 6 un 7 Infekcijas Ietekme uz Reimatoīdā Artrīta Klīnisko Gaitu. *Proc. Latv. Acad. Sci. Sect. B Nat. Exact Appl. Sci.* **2016**, *70*, 165–174. [CrossRef]
32. Kondo, K.; Yamanishi, K. HHV-6A, 6B, and 7: Molecular basis of latency and reactivation. In *Human Herpesviruses: Biology, Therapy, and Immunoprophylaxis*; Cambridge University Press (CUP): Cambridge, UK, 2010; pp. 843–849.
33. Burgos, R.; Ordoñez, G.; Vázquez-Mellado, J.; Pineda, B.; Sotelo, J. Occasional presence of herpes viruses in synovial fluid and blood from patients with rheumatoid arthritis and axial spondyloarthritis. *Clin. Rheumatol.* **2015**, *34*, 1681–1686. [CrossRef] [PubMed]
34. Curtis, J.R.; Xie, F.; Yun, H.; Bernatsky, S.; Winthrop, K.L. Real-world comparative risks of herpes virus infections in tofacitinib and biologic-treated patients with rheumatoid arthritis. *Ann. Rheum. Dis.* **2016**, *75*, 1843–1847. [CrossRef] [PubMed]
35. Siebuhr, A.S.; Bay-Jensen, A.; Jordan, J.; Kjelgaard-Petersen, C.; Christiansen, C.; Abramson, S.; Attur, M.; Berenbaum, F.; Kraus, V.; Karsdal, M.; et al. Inflammation (or synovitis)-driven osteoarthritis: An opportunity for personalizing prognosis and treatment? *Scand J. Rheumatol.* **2015**, *45*, 1–12. [CrossRef]

36. Hussein, M.R.; Fathi, N.A.; El-Din, A.M.E.; Hassan, H.I.; Abdullah, F.; Al-Hakeem, E.; Backer, E.A. Alterations of the CD4+, CD8+ T Cell Subsets, Interleukins-1β, IL-10, IL-17, Tumor Necrosis Factor-α and Soluble Intercellular Adhesion Molecule-1 in Rheumatoid Arthritis and Osteoarthritis: Preliminary Observations. *Pathol. Oncol. Res.* **2008**, *14*, 321–328. [CrossRef]
37. Krenn, V.; Morawietz, L.; Haupl, T.; Neidel, J.; Petersen, I.; König, A. Grading of Chronic Synovitis—A Histopathological Grading System for Molecular and Diagnostic Pathology. *Pathol. Res. Pract.* **2002**, *198*, 317–325. [CrossRef]
38. de Lange-Brokaar, B.J.E.; Ioan-Facsinay, A.; van Osch, G.; Zuurmond, A.-M.; Schoones, J.W.; Toes, R.E.; Huizinga, T.W.; Kloppenburg, M. Synovial inflammation, immune cells and their cytokines in osteoarthritis: A review. *Osteoarthr. Cartil.* **2012**, *20*, 1484–1499. [CrossRef]
39. Riis, R.G.C.; Gudbergsen, H.; Simonsen, O.; Henriksen, M.; Al-Mashkur, N.M.; Eld, M.; Petersen, K.; Kubassova, O.; Bay-Jensen, A.-C.; Damm, J.; et al. The association between histological, macroscopic and magnetic resonance imaging assessed synovitis in end-stage knee osteoarthritis: A cross-sectional study. *Osteoarthr. Cartil.* **2017**, *25*, 272–280. [CrossRef]
40. Mori, Y. Recent topics related to human herpesvirus 6 cell tropism. *Cell Microbiol.* **2009**, *11*, 1001–1006. [CrossRef]
41. Tang, H.; Serada, S.; Kawabata, A.; Ota, M.; Hayashi, E.; Naka, T.; Yamanishi, K.; Mori, Y. CD134 is a cellular receptor specific for human herpesvirus-6B entry. *Proc. Natl. Acad. Sci. USA* **2013**, *110*, 9096–9099. [CrossRef]
42. Tang, H.; Wang, J.; Mahmoud, N.F.; Mori, Y. Detailed Study of the Interaction between Human Herpesvirus 6B Glycoprotein Complex and Its Cellular Receptor, Human CD134. *J. Virol.* **2014**, *88*, 10875–10882. [CrossRef] [PubMed]
43. Tang, H.; Mori, Y. Determinants of Human CD134 Essential for Entry of Human Herpesvirus 6B. *J. Virol.* **2015**, *89*, 10125–10129. [CrossRef] [PubMed]
44. Frenkel, N.; Schirmer, E.C.; Wyatt, L.S.; Katsafanas, G.; Roffman, E.; Danovich, R.M.; June, C.H. Isolation of a new herpesvirus from human CD4+ T cells. *Proc. Natl. Acad. Sci. USA* **1990**, *87*, 748–752. [CrossRef] [PubMed]
45. Caselli, E.; di Luca, D. Molecular biology and clinical associations of Roseoloviruses human herpesvirus 6 and human herpesvirus 7. *Microbiol. Q. J. Microbiol. Sci.* **2007**, *30*, 173–187.
46. Pourgheysari, B.; Khan, N.; Best, D.; Bruton, R.; Nayak, L.; Moss, P. The Cytomegalovirus-Specific CD4+ T-Cell Response Expands with Age and Markedly Alters the CD4+ T-Cell Repertoire. *J. Virol.* **2007**, *81*, 7759–7765. [CrossRef]
47. Pawłowska, J.; Mikosik, A.; Soroczynska-Cybula, M.; Jozwik, A.; Łuczkiewicz, P.; Mazurkiewicz, S.; Lorczyński, A.; Witkowski, J.M.; Bryl, E. Different distribution of CD4 and CD8 T cells in synovial membrane and peripheral blood of rheumatoid arthritis and osteoarthritis patients. *Folia Histochem. Cytobiol.* **2010**, *47*, 627–632. [CrossRef]
48. Yamada, H.; Nakashima, Y.; Okazaki, K.; Mawatari, T.; Fukushi, J.-I.; Oyamada, A.; Fujimura, K.; Iwamoto, Y.; Yoshikai, Y. Preferential Accumulation of Activated Th1 Cells Not Only in Rheumatoid Arthritis but Also in Osteoarthritis Joints. *J. Rheumatol.* **2011**, *38*, 1569–1575. [CrossRef]
49. Moradi, B.; Schnatzer, P.; Hagmann, S.; Rosshirt, N.; Gotterbarm, T.; Kretzer, J.; Thomsen, M.N.; Lorenz, H.-M.; Zeifang, F.; Tretter, T. CD4+CD25+/highCD127low/-regulatory T cells are enriched in rheumatoid arthritis and osteoarthritis joints—Analysis of frequency and phenotype in synovial membrane, synovial fluid and peripheral blood. *Arthritis Res. Ther.* **2014**, *16*, R97. [CrossRef]
50. Zhu, W.; Zhang, X.; Jiang, Y.; Liu, X.; Huang, L.; Wei, Q.; Huang, Y.; Wu, W.; Gu, J. Alterations in peripheral T cell and B cell subsets in patients with osteoarthritis. *Clin. Rheumatol.* **2019**, *39*, 523–532. [CrossRef]
51. Shen, P.-C.; Wu, C.-L.; Jou, I.-M.; Lee, C.-H.; Juan, H.-Y.; Lee, P.-J.; Chen, S.-H.; Hsieh, J.-L. T helper cells promote disease progression of osteoarthritis by inducing macrophage inflammatory protein-1γ. *Osteoarthr. Cartil.* **2011**, *19*, 728–736. [CrossRef]
52. Staheli, J.P.; Dyen, M.R.; Deutsch, G.; Basom, R.S.; FitzGibbon, M.P.; Lewis, P.; Barcy, S. Complete Unique Genome Sequence, Expression Profile, and Salivary Gland Tissue Tropism of the Herpesvirus 7 Homolog in Pigtailed Macaques. *J. Virol.* **2016**, *90*, 6657–6674. [CrossRef] [PubMed]
53. Dowd, J.B.; Bosch, J.A.; Steptoe, A.; Jayabalasingham, B.; Lin, J.; Yolken, R.; Aiello, A.E. Persistent Herpesvirus Infections and Telomere Attrition Over 3 Years in the Whitehall II Cohort. *J. Infect. Dis.* **2017**, *216*, 565–572. [CrossRef] [PubMed]

54. Weidner, M.; Kruminis-Kaszkiel, E.; Savanagouder, M. Herpesviral Latency—Common Themes. *Pathogens* **2020**, *9*, 125. [CrossRef] [PubMed]
55. Sánchez-Ponce, Y.; Varela-Fascinetto, G.; Romo-Vázquez, J.C.; Martínez, B.L.; Sánchez-Huerta, J.L.; Parra-Ortega, I.; Fuentes-Pananá, E.M.; Sánchez, A.M. Simultaneous Detection of Beta and Gamma Human Herpesviruses by Multiplex qPCR Reveals Simple Infection and Coinfection Episodes Increasing Risk for Graft Rejection in Solid Organ Transplantation. *Viruses* **2018**, *10*, 730. [CrossRef]
56. Kakurina, N.; Kadisa, A.; Lejnieks, A.; Mikazane, H.; Kozireva, S.; Murovska, M. Use of exploratory factor analysis to ascertain the correlation between the activities of rheumatoid arthritis and infection by human parvovirus B19. *Medicina* **2015**, *51*, 18–24. [CrossRef]
57. Kadiša, A.; Nora-Krūkle, Z.; Švirskis, S.; Studers, P.; Girkontaite, I.; Lejnieks, A.; Murovska, M. Cytokines and MMP-9 Levels in Rheumatoid Arthritis and Osteoarthritis Patients with Persistent Parvovirus B19, HHV-6 and HHV-7 Infection. *Proc. Latv. Acad. Sci.* **2019**, *73*, 278–287. [CrossRef]
58. Humby, M.S.; O'Connor, C.M. Human Cytomegalovirus US28 Is Important for Latent Infection of Hematopoietic Progenitor Cells. *J. Virol.* **2015**, *90*, 2959–2970. [CrossRef]
59. Poole, E.; Sinclair, J. Sleepless latency of human cytomegalovirus. *Med. Microbiol. Immunol.* **2015**, *204*, 421–429. [CrossRef]
60. Wills, M.; Poole, E.; Lau, B.; Krishna, B.; Sinclair, J.H. The immunology of human cytomegalovirus latency: Could latent infection be cleared by novel immunotherapeutic strategies? *Cell Mol. Immunol.* **2014**, *12*, 128–138. [CrossRef]
61. Prusty, B.K.; Gulve, N.; Rasa, S.; Murovska, M.; Hernandez, P.C.; Ablashi, D.V. Possible chromosomal and germline integration of human herpesvirus 7. *J. Gen Virol.* **2017**, *98*, 266–274. [CrossRef]
62. O'Donovan, A.; Pantell, M.S.; Puterman, E.; Dhabhar, F.S.; Blackburn, E.H.; Yaffe, K.; Cawthon, R.M.; Opresko, P.; Hsueh, W.-C.; Satterfield, S.; et al. Cumulative Inflammatory Load Is Associated with Short Leukocyte Telomere Length in the Health, Aging and Body Composition Study. *PLoS ONE* **2011**, *6*, e19687. [CrossRef] [PubMed]
63. Wong, J.; de Vivo, I.; Lin, X.; Fang, S.C.; Christiani, D C. The Relationship between Inflammatory Biomarkers and Telomere Length in an Occupational Prospective Cohort Study. *PLoS ONE* **2014**, *9*, e87348. [CrossRef] [PubMed]
64. Wei, Y.; Bai, L. Recent advances in the understanding of molecular mechanisms of cartilage degeneration, synovitis and subchondral bone changes in osteoarthritis. *Connect. Tissue Res.* **2016**, *57*, 1–17. [CrossRef] [PubMed]
65. Haynes, M.K.; Hume, E.L.; Smith, J.B. Phenotypic Characterization of Inflammatory Cells from Osteoarthritic Synovium and Synovial Fluids. *Clin. Immunol.* **2002**, *105*, 315–325. [CrossRef] [PubMed]
66. Brenner, S.S.; Klotz, U.; Alscher, D.M.; Mais, A.; Lauer, G.; Schweer, H.; Seyberth, H.W.; Fritz, P.; Bierbach, U.; Alscher, M.D. Osteoarthritis of the knee–clinical assessments and inflammatory markers. *Osteoarthr. Cartil.* **2004**, *12*, 469–475. [CrossRef]
67. Benito, M.J.; Veale, D.J.; Fitzgerald, O.; Berg, W.B.V.D.; Bresnihan, B. Synovial tissue inflammation in early and late osteoarthritis. *Ann. Rheum. Dis.* **2005**, *64*, 1263–1267. [CrossRef]
68. May, N.A.; Glosson, N.L.; Hudson, A.W. Human Herpesvirus 7 U21 Downregulates Classical and Nonclassical Class I Major Histocompatibility Complex Molecules from the Cell Surface. *J. Virol.* **2010**, *84*, 3738–3751. [CrossRef]
69. Altman, R.; Alarcon, G.; Appelrouth, D.; Bloch, D.; Borenstein, D.; Brandt, K.; Brown, C.; Cooke, T.D.; Daniel, W.; Feldman, D.; et al. The American College of Rheumatology criteria for the classification and reporting of osteoarthritis of the hip. *Arthritis Rheum.* **1991**, *34*, 505–514. [CrossRef]
70. Altman, R.; Asch, E.; Bloch, D.; Bole, G.; Borenstein, D.; Brandt, K.; Christy, W.; Cooke, T.D.; Greenwald, R.; Hochberg, M.; et al. Development of criteria for the classification and reporting of osteoarthritis: Classification of osteoarthritis of the knee. *Arthritis Rheum.* **1986**, *29*, 1039–1049. [CrossRef]
71. Berneman, Z.N.; Ablashi, D.V.; Li, G.; Eger-Fletcher, M.; Reitz, M.S.; Hung, C.L.; Brus, I.; Komaroff, A.L.; Gallo, R.C. Human herpesvirus 7 is a T-lymphotropic virus and is related to, but significantly different from, human herpesvirus 6 and human cytomegalovirus. *Proc. Natl. Acad. Sci. USA* **1992**, *89*, 10552–10556. [CrossRef]

72. Kozireva, S.; Užameckis, D.; Bariševs, M.; Murovska, M. Sensitivity and Reproducibility of Polymerase Chain Reaction Assays for Detection of Human Herpesviruses 6 and 7. *Proc. Latv. Acad. Sci. Sect. B Nat. Exact Appl. Sci.* **2009**, *63*, 180–185. [CrossRef]
73. Kempf, W.; Adams, V.; Mirandola, P.; Menotti, L.; di Luca, D.; Wey, N.; Müller, B.; Campadelli-Fiume, G. Persistence of human herpesvirus 7 in normal tissues detected by expression of a structural antigen. *J. Infect. Dis.* **1998**, *178*, 841–845. [CrossRef] [PubMed]
74. Latchney, L.R.; Fallon, M.A.; Culp, D.J.; Gelbard, H.A.; Dewhurst, S. Immunohistochemical Assessment of Fractalkine, Inflammatory Cells, and Human Herpesvirus 7 in Human Salivary Glands. *J. Histochem. Cytochem.* **2004**, *52*, 671–681. [CrossRef] [PubMed]
75. Liu, X.; Shi, F.; Li, Y.; Yu, X.; Peng, S.; Li, W.; Luo, X.; Cao, Y. Post-translational modifications as key regulators of TNF-induced necroptosis. *Cell Death Dis.* **2016**, *7*, e2293. [CrossRef] [PubMed]
76. Krenn, V.; Morawietz, L.; Burmester, G.-R.; Kinne, R.W.; Müller, B.; Häupl, T.; Mueller-Ladner, U. Synovitis score: Discrimination between chronic low-grade and high-grade synovitis. *Histopathology* **2006**, *49*, 358–364. [CrossRef] [PubMed]

International Journal of
Molecular Sciences

MDPI

Article

Association of Electronegative LDL with Macrophage Foam Cell Formation and CD11c Expression in Rheumatoid Arthritis Patients

Ching-Kun Chang [1,2], Po-Ku Chen [1,2,3], Joung-Liang Lan [2,3,4], Shih-Hsin Chang [2,3,5], Tsu-Yi Hsieh [6], Pei-Jyuan Liao [1,2], Chu-Huang Chen [7,8] and Der-Yuan Chen [1,2,3,5,*]

1 Rheumatology and Immunology Center, China Medical University Hospital, Taichung 404, Taiwan; kun80445@gmail.com (C.-K.C.); pago99999@gmail.com (P.-K.C.); pagey06@yahoo.com.tw (P.-J.L.)
2 Translational Medicine Laboratory, China Medical University Hospital, Taichung 404, Taiwan; jounglan@me.com (J.-L.L.); sherry61976@hotmail.com (S.-H.C.)
3 College of Medicine, China Medical University, Taichung 404, Taiwan
4 Rheumatic Diseases Research Center, China Medical University Hospital, Taichung 404, Taiwan
5 Ph.D. Program in Translational Medicine and Rong Hsing Research Center for Translational Medicine, National Chung Hsing University, Taichung 402, Taiwan
6 Department of Medical Education and Research, Taichung Veterans General Hospital, Taichung 407, Taiwan; zuyihsieh@gmail.com
7 Vascular and Medicinal Research, Texas Heart Institute, Houston, TX 6770, USA; cchen@texasheart.org
8 Institute for Biomedical Sciences, Shinshu University, Nagano 390-8621, Japan
* Correspondence: dychen1957@gmail.com; Tel.: +886-4-22052121 (ext. 4628); Fax: +886-4-22073812

Received: 20 July 2020; Accepted: 14 August 2020; Published: 16 August 2020

Abstract: L5, the most negatively charged subfraction of low-density lipoprotein (LDL), is implicated in atherogenesis, but the pathogenic association is relatively unexplored in patients with rheumatoid arthritis (RA). We examined the role of L5 LDL in macrophage foam cell formation and the association of L5 with CD11c expression in THP-1 cells and RA patients. Using quantitative real-time PCR, we determined mRNA expression levels of *ITGAX*, the gene for CD11c, a marker associated with vascular plaque formation and M1 macrophages in atherogenesis, in 93 RA patients. We also examined CD11c expression on THP-1 cells treated with L5 by flow cytometry analysis and the plasma levels of inflammatory mediators using a magnetic bead array. We found a dose-dependent upregulation of foam cell formation of macrophages after L5 treatment (mean ± SEM, 12.05 ± 2.35% in L5 (10 μg/mL); 50.13 ± 3.9% in L5 (25 μg/mL); 90.69 ± 1.82% in L5 (50 μg/mL), $p < 0.01$). Significantly higher levels of CD11c expression were observed in 30 patients with a high percentage of L5 in LDL (L5%) (0.0752 ± 0.0139-fold) compared to 63 patients with normal L5% (0.0446 ± 0.0054-fold, $p < 0.05$). CD11c expression levels were increased in the L5-treated group (30.00 ± 3.13% in L5 (10 μg/mL); 41.46 ± 2.77% in L5 (50 μg/mL), $p < 0.05$) and were positively correlated with plasma levels of interleukin (IL)-6 and IL-8. L5 augmented the expression of IL-6, IL-8, and tumor necrosis factor-α (TNF-α) on monocytes and macrophages. Our findings suggest that L5 may promote atherogenesis by augmenting macrophage foam cell formation, upregulating CD11c expression, and enhancing the expression levels of atherosclerosis-related mediators.

Keywords: L5; macrophage foam cell; CD11c expression; atherosclerosis; rheumatoid arthritis (RA)

1. Introduction

Atherosclerosis, a chronic inflammatory process, is characterized by atheromatous plaque buildup and associated with increased cardiovascular disease (CVD) risk [1]. One of the first events in atherosclerosis is the formation of macrophage foam cells caused by the oxidative modification of low-density lipoprotein (LDL) [2]. Rheumatoid arthritis (RA) is an inflammatory articular disease [3] complicated by accelerated atherosclerosis and elevated CVD risk [4,5]. The high CVD burden in RA patients would be explained by traditional CV risk factors and systemic inflammation in this disease [6,7]. Therefore, inflammatory mediators such as interleukin (IL)-6, IL-8, and tumor necrosis factor-α (TNF-α) are commonly involved in the pathogenesis of RA-related atherosclerosis [8–12].

Because RA patients have low low-density lipoprotein cholesterol (LDL-C) levels combined with an elevated CVD risk (a lipid paradox) [13], LDL-C probably contains critical atherogenic components not reflected in the absolute LDL-C concentration. Anion-cation exchange can be used to divide LDL-C into L1-L5 subfractions, of which L5 is the most negatively charged. Increasing evidence indicates a vital role for L5 in the pathogenesis of atherosclerosis [14]. We recently reported that an elevated the percentage of L5 in LDL (L5%) is associated with an increased CVD risk in patients with RA or systemic lupus erythematosus [15,16]. Therefore, it is important to study the role of L5 in foam cell formation in macrophages.

Accumulating evidence indicates that variants in genes such as *ABCA1* (ATP-binding cassette, sub-family A, member 1) and *NPC1* (Niemann-Pick disease, type C1) are related to CVD risk [17–20]. CD11c, a membrane protein that is associated with β2 integrins, is encoded by the gene *ITGAX (Integrin Subunit Alpha X)* located on chromosome 16p11.2. Previous studies revealed a higher expression of CD11c on circulating monocytes from RA patients than on monocytes from healthy control (HC) subjects [21]. CD11c is a cell surface protein that participates in cell adhesion [22], and knocking out its gene (*ITGAX)* in mice decreased vascular plaque formation [23]. These observations suggest a pathogenic role of CD11c expression in atherogenesis. However, the relationship between electronegative L5 and CD11c expression in the development of atherogenesis in RA is not clear.

In this pilot study, we aimed to investigate the role of LDL-L5 in macrophage foam cell formation and the association of L5 with CD11c expression in THP-1 cells and in RA patients. We also evaluated the correlation between CD11c expression and plasma levels of inflammatory mediators and validated L5's pathogenic role in this process in an in vitro cell-based assay.

2. Results

2.1. Clinical Characteristics of RA Patients

Of the 93 RA patients, 66 (71.0%) tested positive for rheumatoid factor (RF) and 63 (67.7%) for anti-citrullinated peptide antibodies (ACPA). Significantly higher levels of C-reactive protein were observed in RA patients with high L5% compared to those with normal L5% ($p < 0.05$) (Table 1). We found no significant differences between RA patients with high L5% and normal L5% in demographic variables, clinical characteristics, the proportion of positivity for RF or ACPA, disease activity scores, the proportion of comorbidities, or medication use.

Table 1. Demographic and laboratory data in rheumatoid arthritis (RA) patients with high percentage of L5 in low-density lipoprotein (LDL) (L5%) and with normal L5% [a].

	RA with High L5% ($n = 30$)	RA with Normal L5% ($n = 63$)
Age at entry, years	60.4 ± 10.9	58.4 ± 12.1
Women proportion	25 (83.3%)	50 (79.4%)
RA duration, months	68.9 ± 22.6	74.9 ± 28.4
BMI, kg/m^2	23.7 ± 2.2	23.0 ± 2.3
RF positivity	20 (66.7%)	46 (73.0%)
ACPA positivity	18 (60.0%)	45 (71.4%)
ESR, mm/1st hour	24.9 ± 12.2	20.4 ± 15.6
CRP, mg/dl	1.08 ± 1.07 [b]	0.61 ± 0.69

Table 1. *Cont.*

	RA with High L5% (n = 30)	RA with Normal L5% (n = 63)
DAS28 at study entry	4.25 ± 1.27	3.78 ± 1.07
Daily steroid dose (mg)	4.8 ± 1.7	4.2 ± 2.0
csDMARDs alone at entry	8 (26.7%)	15 (23.8%)
Biologics used at entry		
TNF-α inhibitors	11 (36.7%)	19 (30.2%)
IL-6R inhibitor	9 (30.0%)	17 (27.0%)
Rituximab	2 (6.7%)	2 (3.2%)
Hypertension	12 (40.0%)	20 (31.7%)
Diabetes mellitus	5 (16.7%)	6 (9.5%)
Current smoker	2 (6.7%)	5 (7.9%)
TC, mg/dl	207 (164-236)	211 (176–244)
HDL-C, mg/dl	59.5 (44.5–74.8)	59.6 (49.4–75.0)
Triglyceride, mg/dl	114 (77–151)	100 (67–138)
LDL-C, mg/dl	129 (87–154)	129 (105–154)
Atherogenic index	3.4 (2.5–4.4)	3.3 (2.7–4.3)
QRISK-2 score	8.7 (5.8–14.5) [c]	5.7 (2.7–9.1)
CVD events	6 (20.0%) [d]	4 (6.3%) [e]

[a] Data are presented as median (interquartile range, IQR), mean ± standard deviation (SD), or number (%). High L5% is defined as plasma L5 proportion above 1.8%. [b] $p < 0.05$ and [c] $p < 0.01$ vs. patients with normal L5%, as determined by using the Mann–Whitney U test. [d] Included two patients with acute ST-segment elevation myocardial infarction and four with ischemic stroke; [e] included two patients with acute ST-segment elevation myocardial infarction and two with ischemic stroke; BMI: Body mass index; ACPA: Anti-citrullinated peptide antibodies; ESR: Erythrocyte sedimentation rate; CRP: C-reactive protein; DAS28: Disease activity score for 28-joints; csDMARDs: Conventional synthetic disease-modifying anti-rheumatic drugs; TNF-α: Tumor necrosis factor-α; IL-6: Interleukin-6; TC: Total cholesterol; HDL-C: High-density lipoprotein cholesterol; LDL-C: Low-density lipoprotein cholesterol; atherogenic index is the ratio of TC/HDL-C; CVD: Cerebrovascular/cardiovascular disease.

2.2. Comparison of Lipid Profiles, QRISK-2 Scores, and CVD Events between RA Patients with High L5% and Normal L5%

As illustrated in Table 1, RA patients with high L5% had significantly greater QRISK-2 scores, a global 10-year CVD risk score, than in those with normal L5% ($p < 0.01$). During the two-year follow-up period, a higher rate of CVD events was observed in RA patients with high L5% (6/30, 20.0%) compared to those with normal L5% (4/63, 6.3%, $p = 0.071$). However, there were no significant differences in lipid profile including total cholesterol (TC), high-density lipoprotein-cholesterol (HDL-C), triglyceride, or low-density lipoprotein-cholesterol (LDL-C) between RA patients with high L5% and with normal L5%.

2.3. The Effects of L5 on Macrophage Foam Cell Formation

To investigate the potential effects of L5 on macrophage foam cell formation, we treated THP-1 cells with 10 ng/ml phorbol myristate acetate (PMA) for 48 h to stimulate differentiation into macrophages. Then, the monocyte-derived macrophages were stimulated with different doses of L5 (10, 25, or 50 μg/mL) or L1 (10, 25, or 50 μg/mL) at 37 °C for 48 h. As illustrated in Figure 1, the L5 induced foam cell formation, and a dose-dependent upregulation of foam cell formation of macrophages after L5 treatment (mean ± standard error of mean (SEM), 12.05 ± 2.35% in L5 (10 μg/mL); 50.13 ± 3.9% in L5 (25 μg/mL); 90.69 ± 1.82% in L5 (50 μg/mL), $p < 0.05$). The high-dose L5 also induced significantly more foam cell formation than high-dose L1 (11.00 ± 2.59%, $p < 0.05$).

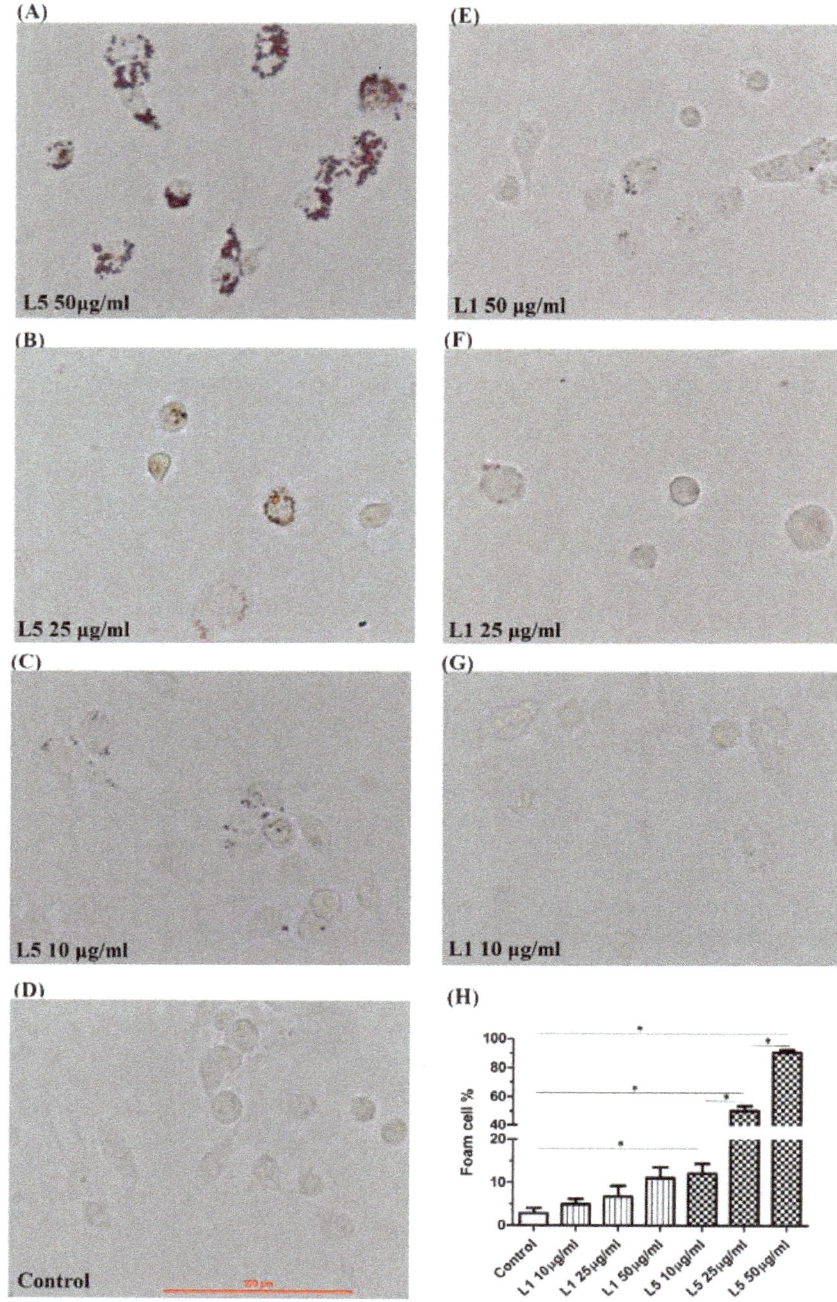

Figure 1. Effects of L5 on macrophage foam cell formation. THP-1 cells were incubated with (**A**) high-dose L5 (50 μg/mL), (**B**) midden-dose L5 (25 μg/mL), (**C**) low-dose L5 (10 μg/mL), (**D**) control (phosphate buffered saline, (**E**) high-dose L1 (50 μg/mL), (**F**) midden-dose L1 (25 μg/mL), and (**G**) low-dose L1 (10 μg/mL) for 48 h. (**H**) Difference in the proportion of macrophage foam cell formation among the different groups. Data are presented as the mean ± SEM for three independent experiments. * $p < 0.05$, determined by one-way ANOVA.

2.4. Comparison of CD11c mRNA Expression Levels between RA Patients with High L5% and Normal L5%

To identify the genes potentially involved in RA-related atherosclerosis, we examined the mRNA expression of 20 candidate genes. The results showed 10 differentially expressed genes in RA patients compared to healthy controls (Figure S1). Given the augmented effects of L5 on macrophage foam cell formation, we identified the candidate genes involved in L5-related atherosclerosis in RA patients by quantitative real-time polymerase chain reaction (qRT-PCR) assay. The results showed a significant difference in the expression levels of 10 candidate genes: *ABCA1, ACTR2, AFF4, CD11c, NPC1, PPFIA1, SMARCA2, WSB1, ZFAND6,* and *ZNF652*, between RA patients and healthy controls (Figure S1). Then, we examined the difference in the expression levels of these 10 genes between RA patients with high L5% and normal L5%. The results indicated a significant difference in the mRNA expression levels of only one gene, *ITGAX* (for CD11c), between the two groups (Figure S2).

In enrolled participants, we examined the difference in CD11c mRNA expression levels between RA patients (n = 93) and healthy controls (n = 41). The results showed significantly higher levels of CD11c expression in RA patients (relative of actin expression, mean ± SEM, 0.0545 ± 0.0059 folds) compared to healthy controls (0.0126 ± 0.0037 folds, $p < 0.01$, Figure 2A). Moreover, significantly higher levels of CD11c expression were observed in RA patients with high L5% (0.0752 ± 0.0139 folds) than in those with normal L5% (0.0446 ± 0.0054 folds, $p < 0.05$, Figure 2B). After exclusion of patients with cardiovascular events, we still revealed a significant difference in the CD11c expression levels between patients with high L5% (mean ± SEM, 0.0617 ± 0.0093 folds) and normal L5% (0.0404 ± 0.0051 folds, $p < 0.05$).

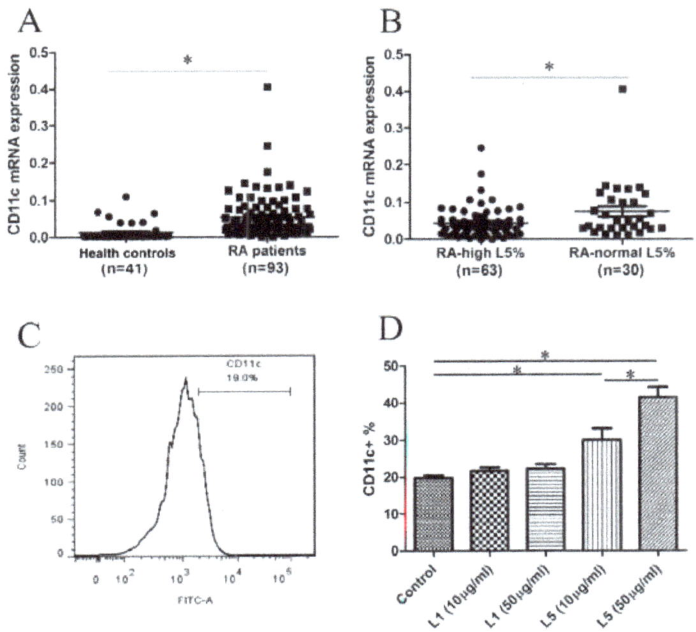

Figure 2. Comparison of CD11c (*ITGAX*) mRNA expression (**A**) between rheumatoid arthritis (RA) patients and healthy controls (HC), and (**B**) between RA patients with high L5% and normal L5%. (**C**) Representative histogram of the flow cytometric analysis of CD11c expression on THP-1 cells. (**D**) Bar graph showing the percent CD11c expression levels on THP-1 cells treated with different doses of L1 or L5 and fetal bovine serum (FBS)-treated control cells. Data are the mean ± SEM for three independent experiments. * $p < 0.05$.

2.5. The Effects of L5 on CD11c Expression in THP-1 Cell

Given the higher levels of CD11c expression in patients with high L5% compared to those with normal L5%, we examined whether L5 could induce CD11c expression on THP-1 cells. After a 48-h stimulation with different doses of L5 or L1, we analyzed CD11c expression by flow cytometry analysis (Figure 2C). CD11c expression levels were increased in L5-treated cells (mean ± SEM, 30.00 ± 3.13% in L5 10 μg/mL; 41.46 ± 2.77% in L5 50 μg/mL, $p < 0.05$); the increases were significantly higher than those in L1-treated (21.77 ± 0.83% in L1 10 μg/mL; 22.20 ± 1.28% in L1 50 μg/mL, both $p < 0.05$) or untreated cells (19.82 ± 0.57%, $p < 0.05$, Figure 2D).

2.6. Correlation between CD11c Expression Levels and Plasma Levels of Inflammatory Mediators in RA Patients

Because CD11c is a marker for classically activated macrophages (M1 macrophages) [24,25], which produce proinflammatory cytokines [26], we examined the correlation between CD11c expression and plasma levels of inflammatory mediators in RA patients. As shown in Figure S3, CD11c expression levels were positively correlated with plasma levels of IL-6 ($r = 0.2928$, $p = 0.0352$) or IL-8 ($r = 0.2917$, $p = 0.0359$). There was no significant correlation between CD11c expression levels and other inflammatory mediators.

2.7. The Effects of L5 on Cytokine Expression in THP-1 Cells

Because of the significant association of L5 with the expression of CD11c, which affects secretion of inflammatory mediators, we examined whether L5 had an effect on the expression of proinflammatory cytokines, such as IL-6, IL-8, and TNF-α, in THP-1 cells and THP-1 cell-derived macrophages. The results showed that L5 upregulated the expression of IL-6, IL-8, and TNF-α in both monocytes and macrophages (Figure 3A–F). Moreover, the levels of IL-6 and IL-8 were significantly higher in monocytes or macrophages treated with high-dose L5 (relative of control group, mean ± SEM, 13.6 ± 2.5 folds, 81.1 ± 7.6 folds; and 365.9 ± 73.5 folds, 9.9 ± 1.6 folds, respectively) than in those treated with high-dose L1 (1.4 ± 0.2 folds, 2.1 ± 0.6 folds; and 0.9 ± 0.4 folds, 2.4 ± 1.1 folds, respectively, all $p < 0.05$, Figure 3A,B,D,E). Monocytes and macrophages treated with high-dose L5 (relative of control group, mean ± SEM, 6.82 ± 0.82 folds, 19.45 ± 3.93 folds) also induced significantly higher TNF-α expression than that seen in untreated cells (all $p < 0.05$, Figure 3C,F).

2.8. Proposed Model for the Potential Role of L5 in RA-Related Atherogenesis

L5 induces the expression of CD11c, which has been reported to be associated with vascular plaque formation [23,27] and as a marker of M1 macrophages with secretion of inflammatory cytokines [26]. L5 also upregulates the expression of IL-6 and IL-8 on both monocytes and macrophages. We have previously shown that L5 induces the expression of lectin-like oxidized LDL receptor-1 (LOX-1) [15], a receptor that is involved in a variety of atherogenic responses including foam cell formation [16]. The combination of foam cell accumulation and increased cytokine activity in the microenvironment synergistically promotes plaque formation (Figure 4).

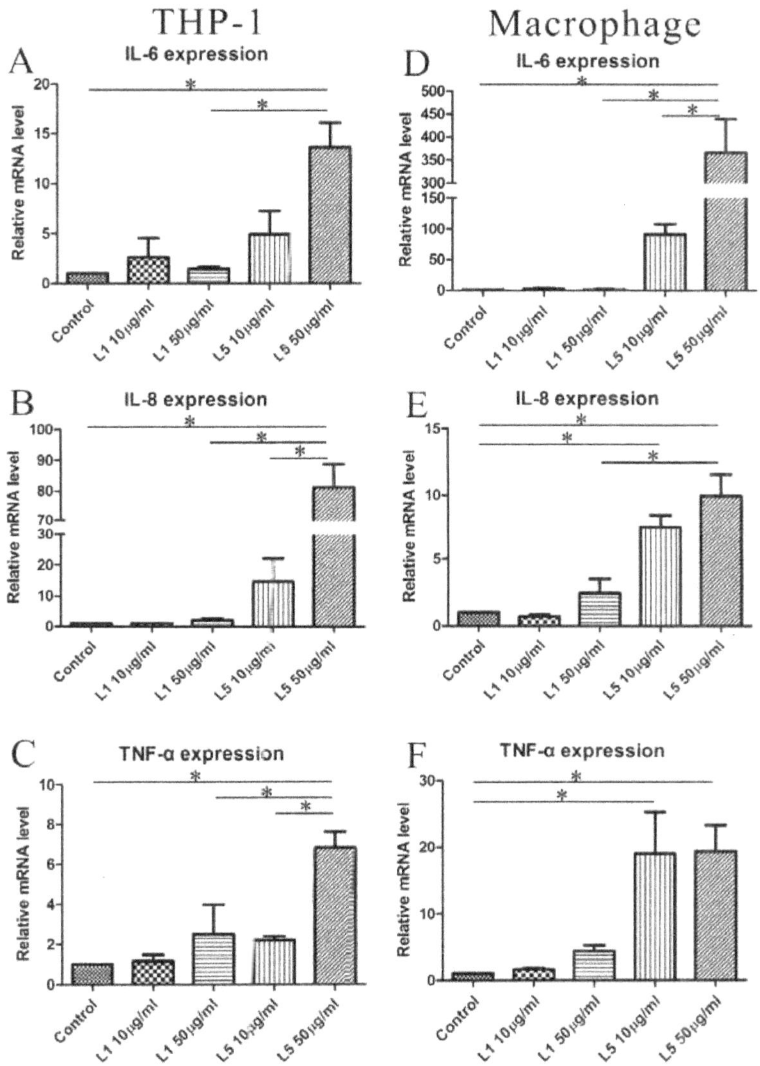

Figure 3. Effects of L5 on the expression of cytokines in monocytes and macrophages. The differences in the mRNA expression levels are shown for IL-6 (**A**), IL-8 (**B**), and (**C**) tumor necrosis factor-α (TNF-α) in THP-1 cells (human monocytic cell line) treated with different doses of L1 and L5. The differences in the mRNA expression levels are shown for IL-6 (**D**), IL-8 (**E**), and (**F**) TNF-α in THP-1 cells-derived macrophages treated with different doses of L1 and L5. Data are the mean ± SEM for three independent experiments. * $p < 0.05$.

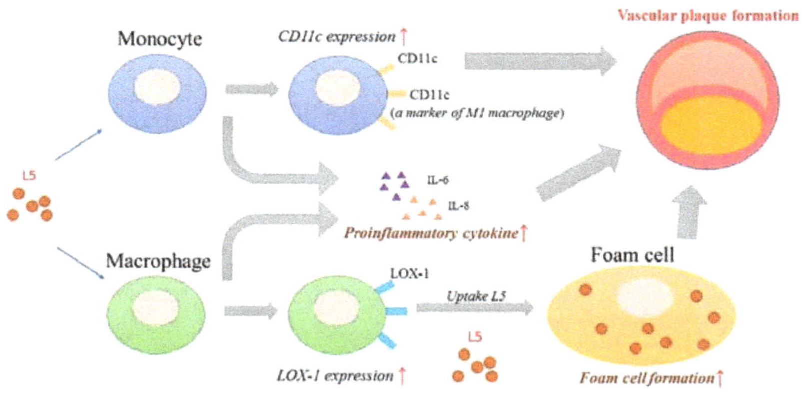

Figure 4. Proposed model for the potential role of L5 in RA-related atherogenesis. L5 induces the expression of CD11c, which is associated with vascular plaque formation [23,27] and is a marker for M1 macrophages that secrete proinflammatory cytokines [26]. L5 also upregulates the expression of inflammatory cytokines, interleukin (IL)-6 and IL-8, in both monocytes and macrophages. In addition, L5 induces LOX-1 expression and promotes foam cell formation by uptake of L5. The elevated levels of inflammatory cytokines and macrophage foam cell formation may contribute to vascular plaque formation in RA-related atherogenesis.

3. Discussion

The association between plasma L5 and the increased CVD risk in RA provides a new explanation for the paradoxically normal plasma LDL levels seen in these patients [15]. The present study was designed to explore the underlying molecular mechanisms of this unique clinical phenomenon. Here, we have shown that treatment with L5 upregulated foam cell formation in THP-1-derived-macrophages, whereas L1, even at high doses, exerted no effect. To identify the genetic variants attributable to L5-related atherosclerosis, we compared expression levels of candidate genes in RA patients with high L5% and normal L5%. We found a significant difference in the expression of *ITGAX*, the gene that encodes the integrin CD11c, which plays a pivotal role in vascular plaque formation [23]. L5 induced CD11c expression in THP-1 cells. Moreover, CD11c expression levels were positively correlated with plasma levels of IL-6 and IL-8. L5 also upregulated the expression of IL-6, IL-8, and TNF-α in in vitro assays. These findings suggest that L5 may contribute to atherogenesis by promoting foam cell formation, upregulating CD11c expression, and inducing the secretion of atherosclerosis-related mediators (Figure 4).

Dyslipidemia is a well-established traditional risk factor for atherosclerosis [6,7], and foam cell formation occurs in the early stage of atherogenesis in RA patients [28,29]. In the present study, we are the first to show significant enhancement of foam cell formation in macrophages treated with L5, which may be related to higher QRISK-2 scores in our patients with high L5% compared to those with normal L5%. Recent studies reveal that L5 promotes the differentiation of monocytes into macrophages in a dose-dependent manner [30], and L5 containing glycosylated apolipoprotein(apo) E may contribute to atherogenicity [31]. In addition, L5 containing apoCIII has been reported to induce monocytes adhesion with endothelial cells to contribute atherogenesis [32]. These findings support the finding that plasma L5% was significantly higher in RA patients with subclinical atherosclerosis than in those without [15], and support the link between L5 and the CVD risk [15,33,34]; L5 promotes foam cell formation.

The increased CVD risk in RA patients results from the intricate interactions among traditional CV risk factors, systemic inflammation, and genetic components [6,7,28,35]. In accordance with the findings that L5 is closely related to an increased CVD risk in autoimmune diseases [15,16], RA patients with high L5% in the current study had significantly higher levels of CD11c mRNA expression compared to those with normal L5%. To validate L5's association with CD11c expression, we examined the effects of L5 on CD11c expression in THP-1 cells using flow cytometry analysis. The results showed that L5 enhanced CD11c expression, whereas L1 had no effect. The different effects may be related to the varied composition of apolipoprotein(apo) in L1, and L5:L1 contains apoB100, while L5 contains apoAI, apoE, and apoCIII [36]. Given the significant association of CD11c expression with vascular plaque formation in atherosclerosis in mice [23] or patients [27], this finding strongly supports the atherogenic role of L5 in RA and possibly other autoimmune diseases.

CD11c is a probable marker of proinflammatory M1 macrophages, which have the propensity to secrete inflammatory mediators [26,37] and thus promote atherogenesis [24,27]. Both IL-6 and IL-8 are well-established mediators of RA-related atherosclerosis [8–10], and we found that CD11c expression was positively correlated with increasing levels of IL-6 and IL-8. This prompted us to examine the effects of L5 on the expression of atherosclerosis-related mediators in monocytes and macrophages. Our finding that L5 upregulated the expression levels of IL-6, IL-8, and TNF-α in monocytes and macrophages further substantiated L5's atherogenic role through a mechanism mediated by CD11c.

Despite the novel findings in this pilot study, there were still some limitations. First, the sample size of RA patients in whom we could observe the emergence of CVD was small, which may reduce the statistical power. The effects of other medications, such as corticosteroids and disease-modifying anti-rheumatic drugs (DMARDs), should be considered because they may affect plasma levels of lipids and inflammatory mediators [38]. Finally, none of the enrolled patients in our study were in the early RA stage, which may limit the generalizability of these results to the whole population.

4. Materials and Methods

4.1. Study Population

In this prospective study, we enrolled 93 patients who met the 2010 revised criteria of the American College of Rheumatology for RA [39] and who had an active disease status. Disease activity was assessed by using the 28-joint disease activity score (DAS28) [40], and active status was defined as DAS28 $\geq$ 3.2. Each patient had previously received corticosteroids, nonsteroidal anti-inflammatory drugs, and at least one conventional synthetic disease-modifying anti-rheumatic drug (csDMARD). Patients with a recent history (i.e., within one year before enrollment) of coronary artery disease or ischemic stroke were excluded. Follow-up for the emergence of CVD, which included acute myocardial infarction and ischemic stroke, was done for at least two years. The healthy control (HC) group comprised 41 sex- and age-matched healthy volunteers with no rheumatic disease. The Institutional Review Board of our hospital approved this study (CMUH107-REC2-038, approval date 19 March 2018), and each participant's written consent was obtained according to the Declaration of Helsinki.

4.2. Determination of Plasma Lipid Profiles and Atherogenic Index (AI)

All blood samples were collected from patients in the early morning after an overnight fast for 12 h. Plasma levels of TC, triglyceride, HDL-C, and LDL-C were measured by using enzymatic methods with a chemistry analyzer (Hitachi 7600, Hitachi, Tokyo, Japan) according to the manufacturer's instructions. The AI (i.e., the ratio of TC /HDL-C) was calculated

4.3. Measurement of 10-Year Risk of CVD Including QRISK-2 Score

Global 10-year risk for a heart attack or stroke was estimated by calculating the QRISK-2 scores [41] on the website: https://www.qrisk.org. Briefly, factors including age, sex, ethnicity, physical characteristics, total cholesterol/HDL-C ratio, self-reported smoking status, diabetic status, the presence of chronic kidney disease, and family history of heart disease were considered in determining the QRISK-2 score.

4.4. Isolation and Fractionation of LDL-C

Lipoproteins were isolated with sequential potassium bromide density ultracentrifugation as described [42]. The plasma was obtained from freshly collected whole blood samples, and 1% antibiotics (penicillin/streptomycin stock solution, Gibco), 0.5 mM EDTA (Thermo Fisher Scientific, Waltham, MA, USA), and a protease inhibitor cocktail (cOmplete, Roche, Sigma-Aldrich, St. Louis, MO, USA) were added to avoid ex vivo oxidation and degradation. LDL-C particles were isolated by using sequential potassium bromide density ultracentrifugation. Purified LDL-C was dialyzed against a degassed solution of 20 mM Tris-HCl and 0.5 mM EDTA at 4 °C with five buffer changes (once/day).

4.5. Anion-Exchange Chromatography Purification of LDL-C Subfractions

LDL subfractions were separated by using UnoQ12 anion-exchange columns (Bio-Rad Laboratories, Inc., Hercules, CA, USA) with an NGC Quest 10 chromatography system (Bio-Rad). The columns were pre-equilibrated with buffer A (0.02 M Tris-HCl (pH 8.0) and 0.5 mM EDTA) in a 4 °C cold room. After dialysis with buffer A, 100 mg of LDL in 10 mL was injected onto a UnoQ12 column and eluted at a flow rate of 2 mL/min with a multistep gradient of buffer B (1 M NaCl in buffer A). Five LDL fractions were eluted with a multistep gradient of buffer B according to electronegativity. L1 was the effluent collected between fractions 11 to 14 (18–28 min); L2, fractions 15 to 16 (28–32 min); L3, fractions 17 to 24 (32–48 min); L4, fractions 25 to 30 (48–60 min); and L5, fractions 31 to 40 (60–80 min). Protein concentrations were determined by using the bicinchoninic acid method. The respective fractions were then concentrated with Centriprep filters (YM-30, MilliporeSigma, Burlington, MA, USA) and sterilized by passage through 0.22 μm syringe filters.

4.6. Examination of Foam Cells Formation in Monocyte-Derived Macrophages Treated with L1 or L5

To induce differentiation of human monocytes into macrophages, THP-1 cells (1×10^5 cells/mL) were grown in media and treated with 10 ng/mL PMA (MilliporeSigma, Temecula, CA, USA) for 48 h. The culture medium was subsequently changed to RPMI and 1% lipid-depleted fetal bovine serum (FBS) from differential ultracentrifugation as described previously [43]. Then, the macrophages were treated with different doses of L1 or L5 (10, 25, or 50 μg/mL) at 37 °C for 48 h. Foam cell formation in macrophages was examined by using Oil red O staining [44]. The images for foam cell formation were observed in an ECLIPSE 50i microscope (Nikon, Tokyo, Japan) and captured at 100× with NIS-Elements software (Nikon, Tokyo, Japan). The percentage of foam cell formation was quantitated by dividing the number of Oil red O staining macrophages by the total number of macrophages in 2 random microscopic fields.

4.7. Database Search, RNA Extraction, and Quantitative Real-Time PCR for Their mRNA Expression Levels

To identify the potential genes involved in the pathogenesis of atherosclerosis in RA patients, we searched the NCBI Gene Expression Omnibus (GEO) database. In group 1, which includes genes associated with hyperlipidemia or CVD, we download 250 genes with the highest (>2) fold change from GSE6054 (Monocytes of patients with familial hypercholesterolemia show alterations in cholesterol metabolism) and GSE62646 (Altered gene expression pattern in peripheral blood mononuclear cells in patients with acute myocardial infarction) through the analysis tool GE02R. In group 2, which includes differentially expressed genes from RA patients compared to healthy controls, we download 250 genes with the highest (>2) fold change from GSE56649 (Expression data from active rheumatoid arthritis patients and healthy control), GSE64707 (Gene expression of human peripheral blood cells of patients with rheumatoid arthritis), and GSE93777 (Multi-omics monitoring of drug response in rheumatoid arthritis). After an integrated analysis, we identified 20 overlapping genes from both groups as target genes for examining mRNA expression using qRT-PCR. The primer sequences of the selected genes were searched from PrimerBank-MGH-PGA (https://pga.mgh.harvard.edu/primerbank/) and are listed in Table S1. Primers were designed and synthesized by Tri-I Biotech (Taipei, Taiwan).

PBMCs were isolated using the Ficoll-Paque™ PLUS (GE Healthcare Biosciences, Uppsala, Sweden) density gradient centrifugation. Total RNAs from PBMCs were extracted by TRI Reagent (Sigma-Aldrich, Missouri, USA) according to the manufacturer's instructions. A High-Capacity cDNA Reverse Transcriptase Kit (Thermo Fisher Scientific) was used to reverse-transcribe 2 μg RNA into cDNA used for qRT-PCR analyses. The qRT-PCR reactions were performed on the CFX96 Real-time PCR system (Bio-Rad) with IQ™ SYBR Green Supermix reagent (Bio-Rad). Quantitative real-time PCR using 10 ng cDNA was performed with one cycle of preincubation at 95 °C for 3 min, 45 cycles of amplification (95 °C for 15 s, 60 °C for 1 min), and the melt curve detection program from 55 °C to 95 °C. The difference in expression in the target gene relative to the averaged internal control gene was calculated by $2^{-\Delta Ct}$, $\Delta Ct = Ct_{targeted\ genes} - Ct_{Actin}$.

We observed a significant difference in the mRNA expression levels of 10 targeted genes between RA patients and healthy controls. Subsequently, we evaluated the difference in mRNA expression levels in the 10 candidate genes between RA patients with a high L5% and with normal L5%. The results showed a significant difference in the mRNA expression levels of one gene, *ITGAX*, between the two groups. Then, we examined the mRNA expression levels of CD11c in 93 RA patients and 41 healthy controls. The primer sequences are as follows: For CD11c (*ITGAX*), 5′-CTGCAA GGGTTTACATACACGG-3′ (forward) and 5′-GAATTTTGGCGGCATCCCTAC-3′ (reverse); and for the housekeeping gene, *Actin*, 5′-ATTGCCGACAGGATGCAGA-3′ (forward) and 5′-GAGTACTTGCGCTCAGGAGGA-3′ (reverse). To standardize mRNA expression levels of CD11c, the mRNA levels of actin were also determined in parallel for each sample. The mRNA expression levels of CD11c were calculated using the comparative threshold cycle (Ct) method and evaluated by $2^{-\Delta Ct}$, $\Delta Ct = Ct_{CD11c} - Ct_{Actin}$.

4.8. Determination of CD11c Expression in THP-1 Cells Treated with Different Doses of L5 by Flow Cytometry Analysis

The human monocytic cell line, THP-1 cells (ATCC TIB-202; American Type Culture Collection, Manassas, VA, USA), was grown in RPMI 1640 (Thermo Fisher Scientific, Taichung, Taiwan) supplemented with 10% FBS and 1% penicillin/streptomycin antibiotics in an incubator (Thermo Fisher Scientific GmbH, Dreieich, Germany) containing 5% CO_2 at 37 °C. At the beginning of the lipid treatment experiment, the medium was changed to RPMI with 1% lipid-depleted FBS. THP-1 cells, at a density of 1×10^5 cells/mL, were treated with L5 (10 or 50 μg/mL) at 37 °C for 2 days. The cells were harvested and washed with phosphate-buffered saline (PBS) and then blocked with TruStain FcX (BioLegend, San Diego, CA, USA) at room temperature for 10 min. The CD11c levels of THP-1 samples were quantified by using FITC (fluorescein isothiocyanate)-conjugated anti-CD11c antibody (BD Biosciences Pharmingen, San Diego, CA, USA) and flow cytometry FACSCelesta™ (BD Biosciences) according to the manufacturer's protocol and the described technique [45]. FITC-conjugated IgG isotype antibody (BD Biosciences) (4 °C, 30 min) served as isotype controls. We analyzed at least 10,000 cells/condition in duplicate. Data analysis was performed with FlowJo software (BD Biosciences). We gain major cell populations (named G1) with dot plots (FSC:SSC) by using an unstained control. Data were expressed as the frequency of CD11c in the gated cell population

4.9. Measurement of Plasma Levels of Inflammatory Mediators

Plasma levels of IL-6, IL-8, TNF-α, interferon gamma-induced protein 10 (IP-10), monocyte chemoattractant protein-1 (MCP-1), granulocyte-macrophage colony-stimulating factor (GM-CSF), IL-10, IL-12p40, soluble CD40 ligand (sCD40L), IL-1Ra, and IL-1β were determined using the HCYTOMAG-60K Cytokine/Chemokine Panel assay according to the manufacturer's instruction (MilliporeSigma, Waltham, MA, USA). Data were analyzed with five-parameter logistic regression by using the MILLIPLEX®Analyst (MilliporeSigma, Burlington, NJ, USA). The overall intra-assay and inter-assay coefficients of variability were calculated (<5% and 20%, respectively).

4.10. Measurement of mRNA Expression Levels of Inflammatory Mediators

To investigate the cytokines mRNA expression of L5-treated monocyte/macrophage, we extracted RNA by the TRI Reagent method (Sigma-Aldrich). The High-Capacity cDNA Reverse Transcriptase Kit (ThermoFisher) was used to reverse-transcribe 1 μg RNA into cDNA using for qRT-PCR analyses. The expression levels of each gene were determined by the CFX96 Real-time PCR system (BioRad, Hercules, USA) with IQ SYBR Green Supermix reagent (BioRad). PCR using 10 ng cDNA was performed with one cycle of preincubation at 95 °C for 3 min, 45 cycles of amplification (95 °C for 15 s, 60 °C for 1 min), and the melt curve detection program from 55 °C to 95 °C. The primer sequences are as follows: IL-6, 5′-AGACAGCCACTCACCTCTTCAG-3′ (forward) and 5′-TTCTGCCAGTGCCTCTTTGCTG-3′ (reverse); IL-8, 5′-GAGAGTGATTGAGAGTGGACCAC-3′ (forward) and 5′-CACAACCCTCTGC ACCCAGTTT-3′ (reverse); TNF-α, 5′-CCACTTCGAAACCTGGGATTC-3′ (forward) and 5′-TTAGTGGTTGCCAGCACTTCA-3′ (reverse). The mRNA expression levels of cytokines were calculated using the comparative threshold cycle (Ct) method and were evaluated by $2^{-\Delta Ct}$, $\Delta Ct = Ct_{Target\ gene} - Ct_{Actin}$. The results were normalized to the levels of actin mRNA and were expressed relative to the levels in control cells (relative value = 1).

4.11. Statistical Analysis

The results are presented as the mean ± standard deviation (SD), the standard error of mean (SEM), or the median (interquartile range). The nonparametric Mann−Whitney U test was used for between-group comparisons of plasma levels of lipid profile, AI, and QRISK-2 scores. The comparison of mRNA expression levels between RA patients and healthy controls or between RA patients with high L5% and normal L5% was analyzed by the Student's t-test. The comparison of CD11c expression or cytokine mRNA expression levels in THP-1 cells or macrophages treated with different doses of L1 and L5 was analyzed by one-way ANOVA. The correlation coefficient was calculated using the nonparametric Spearman's rank correlation test. A two-sided p-value < 0.05 was considered statistically significant.

5. Conclusions

L5 may contribute to atherosclerosis by augmenting macrophage foam cell formation, upregulating CD11c expression, or enhancing the expression of inflammatory mediators, such as IL-6, IL-8, and TNF-α. These findings provide new insight into the pathogenesis of increased CVD risk in RA that cannot be explained by conventional risk factors.

Supplementary Materials: Supplementary materials can be found at http://www.mdpi.com/1422-0067/21/16/5883/s1.

Author Contributions: C.-K.C. conceived and designed the study, performed the data analysis, drafting and revising of the manuscript. P.-K.C. conceived the study, acquired the data, and performed the data analysis. J.-L.L., S.-H.C. and T.-Y.H. performed the clinical assessment, obtained clinical data, and carried out statistical analysis. P.-J.L. conceived the study and collected clinical data. C.-H.C. generated the original hypothesis and revised the manuscript. D.-Y.C. conceived and designed the study, generated the original hypothesis, acquired the clinical data, performed the data analysis, and revised the manuscript. All authors have read and agreed to the published version of the manuscript.

Funding: This work was supported by a grant from China Medical University Hospital (DMR-108-184), and by a grant (MOST 107-2314-B-039-053-MY3) from the Ministry of Science and Technology, Taiwan.

Acknowledgments: The authors thank Shiow-Jiuan Wey, of Chung Shan Medical University Hospital, Taiwan, and Rebecca Bartow, of the Texas Heart Institute, Houston, USA, for editorial assistance. The microscope image was performed in the Medical Research Core Facilities, Office of Research & Development at China medical University, Taiwan.

Conflicts of Interest: The authors declare no conflict of interest.

Abbreviations

ABCA1	ATP-binding cassette, sub-family A, member 1
ACPA	Anti-citrullinated peptide antibodies
AI	Atherogenic index
Apo	Apolipoprotein
CRP	C-reactive protein
csDMARD	conventional synthetic disease-modifying anti-rheumatic drug
CVD	Cardiovascular/cerebrovascular disease
DAS28	28-joint disease activity score
GEO	Gene Expression Omnibus
GM-CSF	Granulocyte-macrophage colony-stimulating factor
HC	Healthy controls
HDL-C	High-density lipoprotein cholesterol
IL	Interleukin
IP-10	Interferon gamma-induced protein 10
ITGAX	Integrin Subunit Alpha X
L5%	Percentage of L5 in LDL
LDL	Low-density lipoprotein
LDL-C	Low-density lipoprotein cholesterol
MCP-1	Monocyte chemoattractant protein-1
NPC1	Niemann-Pick disease, type C1
PMA	Phorbol myristate acetate
qRT-PCR	Quantitative real-time polymerase chain reaction
RA	Rheumatoid arthritis
RF	Rheumatoid factor
sCD40L	Soluble CD40 ligand
SD	Standard deviation
SEM	Standard error of mean
SLE	Systemic lupus erythematosus
TC	Total cholesterol
TNF-α	Tumor necrosis factor-α

References

1. Libby, P. Inflammation in atherosclerosis. *Arter. Thromb. Vasc. Biol.* **2012**, *32*, 2045–2051. [CrossRef] [PubMed]
2. Cvetkovic, J.T.; Wallberg-Jonsson, S.; Ahmed, E.; Rantapaa-Dahlqvist, S.; Lefvert, A.K. Increased levels of autoantibodies against copper-oxidized low density lipoprotein, malondialdehyde-modified low density lipoprotein and cardiolipin in patients with rheumatoid arthritis. *Rheumatology* **2002**, *41*, 988–995. [CrossRef] [PubMed]
3. Choy, E.H.; Panayi, G.S. Cytokine pathways and joint inflammation in rheumatoid arthritis. *N. Engl. J. Med.* **2001**, *344*, 907–916. [CrossRef] [PubMed]
4. Avina-Zubieta, J.A.; Thomas, J.; Sadatsafavi, M.; Lehman, A.J.; Lacaille, D. Risk of incident cardiovascular events in patients with rheumatoid arthritis: A meta-analysis of observational studies. *Ann. Rheum. Dis.* **2012**, *71*, 1524–1529. [CrossRef] [PubMed]
5. Symmons, D.P.; Gabriel, S.E. Epidemiology of CVD in rheumatic disease, with a focus on RA and SLE. *Nat. Rev. Rheumatol.* **2011**, *7*, 399–408. [CrossRef]
6. Im, C.H.; Kim, N.R.; Kang, J.W.; Kim, J.H.; Kang, J.Y.; Bae, G.B.; Nam, E.J.; Kang, Y.M. Inflammatory burden interacts with conventional cardiovascular risk factors for carotid plaque formation in rheumatoid arthritis. *Rheumatology* **2015**, *54*, 808–815. [CrossRef]
7. Choy, E.; Ganeshalingam, K.; Semb, A.G.; Szekanecz, Z.; Nurmohamed, M. Cardiovascular risk in rheumatoid arthritis: Recent advances in the understanding of the pivotal role of inflammation, risk predictors and the impact of treatment. *Rheumatology* **2014**, *53*, 2143–2154. [CrossRef]

8. Bacchiega, B.C.; Bacchiega, A.B.; Usnayo, M.J.; Bedirian, R.; Singh, G.; Pinheiro, G.D. Interleukin 6 Inhibition and Coronary Artery Disease in a High-Risk Population: A Prospective Community-Based Clinical Study. *J. Am. Heart Assoc.* **2017**, *6*, e005038. [CrossRef]
9. Rho, Y.H.; Chung, C.P.; Oeser, A.; Solus, J.; Asanuma, Y.; Sokka, T.; Pincus, T.; Raggi, P.; Gebretsadik, T.; Shintani, A.; et al. Inflammatory mediators and premature coronary atherosclerosis in rheumatoid arthritis. *Arthritis Rheum.* **2009**, *61*, 1580–1585. [CrossRef]
10. Boisvert, W.A.; Curtiss, L.K.; Terkeltaub, R.A. Interleukin-8 and its receptor CXCR2 in atherosclerosis. *Immunol. Res.* **2000**, *21*, 129–137. [CrossRef]
11. Barnabe, C.; Martin, B.J.; Ghali, W.A. Systematic review and meta-analysis: Anti-tumor necrosis factor alpha therapy and cardiovascular events in rheumatoid arthritis. *Arthritis Care Res.* **2011**, *63*, 522–529. [CrossRef] [PubMed]
12. Gonzalez-Juanatey, C.; Vazquez-Rodriguez, T.R.; Miranda-Filloy, J.A.; Gomez-Acebo, I.; Testa, A.; Garcia-Porrua, C.; Sanchez-Andrade, A.; Llorca, J.; Gonzalez-Gay, M.A. Anti-TNF-alpha-adalimumab therapy is associated with persistent improvement of endothelial function without progression of carotid intima-media wall thickness in patients with rheumatoid arthritis refractory to conventional therapy. *Mediat. Inflamm.* **2012**, *2012*, 674265. [CrossRef] [PubMed]
13. Myasoedova, E.; Crowson, C.S.; Kremers, H.M.; Roger, V.L.; Fitz-Gibbon, P.D.; Therneau, T.M.; Gabriel, S.E. Lipid paradox in rheumatoid arthritis: The impact of serum lipid measures and systemic inflammation on the risk of cardiovascular disease. *Ann. Rheum. Dis.* **2011**, *70*, 482–487. [CrossRef] [PubMed]
14. Niccoli, G.; Baca, M.; De Spirito, M.; Parasassi, T.; Cosentino, N.; Greco, G.; Conte, M.; Montone, R.A.; Arcovito, G.; Crea, F. Impact of electronegative low-density lipoprotein on angiographic coronary atherosclerotic burden. *Atherosclerosis* **2012**, *223*, 166–170. [CrossRef]
15. Chang, C.Y.; Chen, C.H.; Chen, Y.M.; Hsieh, T.Y.; Li, J.P.; Shen, M.Y.; Lan, J.L.; Chen, D.Y. Association between Negatively Charged Low-Density Lipoprotein L5 and Subclinical Atherosclerosis in Rheumatoid Arthritis Patients. *J. Clin. Med.* **2019**, *8*, 177. [CrossRef]
16. Chan, H.C.; Chan, H.C.; Liang, C.J.; Lee, H.C.; Su, H.; Lee, A.S.; Shiea, J.; Tsai, W.C.; Ou, T.T.; Wu, C.C.; et al. Role of Low-Density Lipoprotein in Early Vascular Aging Associated with Systemic Lupus Erythematosus. *Arthritis Rheumatol.* **2020**, *72*, 972–984. [CrossRef]
17. Kathiresan, S.; Srivastava, D. Genetics of human cardiovascular disease. *Cell* **2012**, *148*, 1242–1257. [CrossRef]
18. Abbate, R.; Sticchi, E.; Fatini, C. Genetics of cardiovascular disease. *Clin. Cases Min. Bone Metab.* **2008**, *5*, 63–66.
19. Chistiakov, D.A.; Melnichenko, A.A.; Myasoedova, V.A.; Grechko, A.V.; Orekhov, A.N. Mechanisms of foam cell formation in atherosclerosis. *J. Mol. Med.* **2017**, *95*, 1153–1165. [CrossRef]
20. Yu, X.H.; Jiang, N.; Yao, P.B.; Zheng, X.L.; Cayabyab, F.S.; Tang, C.K. NPC1, intracellular cholesterol trafficking and atherosclerosis. *Clin. Chim. Acta* **2014**, *429*, 69–75. [CrossRef]
21. Kurohori, Y.; Sato, K.; Suzuki, S.; Kashiwazaki, S. Adhesion molecule expression on peripheral blood mononuclear cells in rheumatoid arthritis: Positive correlation between the proportion of L-selectin and disease activity. *Clin. Rheumatol.* **1995**, *14*, 335–341. [CrossRef] [PubMed]
22. Sandor, N.; Lukacsi, S.; Ungai-Salanki, R.; Orgovan, N.; Szabo, B.; Horvath, R.; Erdei, A.; Bajtay, Z. CD11c/CD18 Dominates Adhesion of Human Monocytes, Macrophages and Dendritic Cells over CD11b/CD18. *PLoS ONE* **2016**, *11*, e0163120. [CrossRef] [PubMed]
23. Wu, H.; Gower, R.M.; Wang, H.; Perrard, X.Y.; Ma, R.; Bullard, D.C.; Burns, A.R.; Paul, A.; Smith, C.W.; Simon, S.I.; et al. Functional role of CD11c+ monocytes in atherogenesis associated with hypercholesterolemia. *Circulation* **2009**, *119*, 2708–2717. [CrossRef] [PubMed]
24. Vianello, E.; Dozio, E.; Arnaboldi, F.; Marazzi, M.G.; Martinelli, C.; Lamont, J.; Tacchini, L.; Sigruner, A.; Schmitz, G.; Corsi Romanelli, M.M. Epicardial adipocyte hypertrophy: Association with M1-polarization and toll-like receptor pathways in coronary artery disease patients. *Nutr. Metab. Cardiovasc. Dis.* **2016**, *26*, 246–253. [CrossRef]
25. Shu, Q.H.; Ge, Y.S.; Ma, H.X.; Gao, X.Q.; Pan, J.J.; Liu, D.; Xu, G.L.; Ma, J.L.; Jia, W.D. Prognostic value of polarized macrophages in patients with hepatocellular carcinoma after curative resection. *J. Cell. Mol. Med.* **2016**, *20*, 1024–1035. [CrossRef]

26. Shapouri-Moghaddam, A.; Mohammadian, S.; Vazini, H.; Taghadosi, M.; Esmaeili, S.A.; Mardani, F.; Seifi, B.; Mohammadi, A.; Afshari, J.T.; Sahebkar, A. Macrophage plasticity, polarization, and function in health and disease. *J. Cell. Physiol.* **2018**, *233*, 6425–6440. [CrossRef]
27. Cho, K.Y.; Miyoshi, H.; Kuroda, S.; Yasuda, H.; Kamiyama, K.; Nakagawara, J.; Takigami, M.; Kondo, T.; Atsumi, T. The phenotype of infiltrating macrophages influences arteriosclerotic plaque vulnerability in the carotid artery. *J. Stroke Cereb. Dis.* **2013**, *22*, 910–918. [CrossRef]
28. Mahmoudi, M.; Aslani, S.; Fadaei, R.; Jamshidi, A.R. New insights to the mechanisms underlying atherosclerosis in rheumatoid arthritis. *Int. J. Rheum. Dis.* **2017**, *20*, 287–297. [CrossRef]
29. Wen, W.; He, M.; Liang, X.; Gao, S.S.; Zhou, J.; Yuan, Z.Y. Accelerated transformation of macrophage-derived foam cells in the presence of collagen-induced arthritis mice serum is associated with dyslipidemia. *Autoimmunity* **2016**, *49*, 115–123. [CrossRef]
30. Lee, A.S.; Wang, Y.C.; Chang, S.S.; Lo, P.H.; Chang, C.M.; Lu, J.; Burns, A.R.; Chen, C.H.; Kakino, A.; Sawamura, T.; et al. Detection of a High Ratio of Soluble to Membrane-Bound LOX-1 in Aspirated Coronary Thrombi From Patients With ST-Segment-Elevation Myocardial Infarction. *J. Am. Heart Assoc.* **2020**, *9*, e014008. [CrossRef]
31. Ke, L.Y.; Chan, H.C.; Chen, C.C.; Chang, C.F.; Lu, P.L.; Chu, C.S.; Lai, W.T.; Shin, S.J.; Liu, F.T.; Chen, C.H. Increased APOE glycosylation plays a key role in the atherogenicity of L5 low-density lipoprotein. *FASEB J.* **2020**, *34*, 9802–9813. [CrossRef] [PubMed]
32. Kawakami, A.; Aikawa, M.; Libby, P.; Alcaide, P.; Luscinskas, F.W.; Sacks, F.M. Apolipoprotein CIII in apolipoprotein B lipoproteins enhances the adhesion of human monocytic cells to endothelial cells. *Circulation* **2006**, *113*, 691–700. [CrossRef] [PubMed]
33. Chu, C.S.; Chan, H.C.; Tsai, M.H.; Stancel, N.; Lee, H.C.; Cheng, K.H.; Tung, Y.C.; Chan, H.C.; Wang, C.Y.; Shin, S.J.; et al. Range of L5 LDL levels in healthy adults and L5's predictive power in patients with hyperlipidemia or coronary artery disease. *Sci. Rep.* **2018**, *8*, 11866. [CrossRef] [PubMed]
34. Shen, M.Y.; Chen, F.Y.; Hsu, J.F.; Fu, R.H.; Chang, C.M.; Chang, C.T.; Liu, C.H.; Wu, J.R.; Lee, A.S.; Chan, H.C.; et al. Plasma L5 levels are elevated in ischemic stroke patients and enhance platelet aggregation. *Blood* **2016**, *127*, 1336–1345. [CrossRef]
35. Arida, A.; Protogerou, A.D.; Kitas, G.D.; Sfikakis, P.P. Systemic Inflammatory Response and Atherosclerosis: The Paradigm of Chronic Inflammatory Rheumatic Diseases. *Int. J. Mol. Sci.* **2018**, *19*, 1890. [CrossRef]
36. Bancells, C.; Canals, F.; Benitez, S.; Colome, N.; Julve, J.; Ordonez-Llanos, J.; Sanchez-Quesada, J.L. Proteomic analysis of electronegative low-density lipoprotein. *J. Lipid. Res.* **2010**, *51*, 3508–3515. [CrossRef]
37. Chistiakov, D.A.; Bobryshev, Y.V.; Orekhov, A.N. Changes in transcriptome of macrophages in atherosclerosis. *J. Cell. Mol. Med.* **2015**, *19*, 1163–1173. [CrossRef]
38. Charles-Schoeman, C.; Gonzalez-Gay, M.A.; Kaplan, I.; Boy, M.; Geier, J.; Luo, Z.; Zuckerman, A.; Riese, R. Effects of tofacitinib and other DMARDs on lipid profiles in rheumatoid arthritis: Implications for the rheumatologist. *Semin. Arthritis Rheum.* **2016**, *46*, 71–80. [CrossRef]
39. Aletaha, D.; Neogi, T.; Silman, A.J.; Funovits, J.; Felson, D.T.; Bingham, C.O., 3rd; Birnbaum, N.S.; Burmester, G.R.; Bykerk, V.P.; Cohen, M.D.; et al. Rheumatoid arthritis classification criteria: An American College of Rheumatology/European League Against Rheumatism collaborative initiative. *Ann. Rheum. Dis.* **2010**, *69*, 1580–1588. [CrossRef]
40. Prevoo, M.L.; Van 't Hof, M.A.; Kuper, H.H.; Van Leeuwen, M.A.; Van de Putte, L.B.; Van Riel, P.L. Modified disease activity scores that include twenty-eight-joint counts. Development and validation in a prospective longitudinal study of patients with rheumatoid arthritis. *Arthritis Rheum.* **1995**, *38*, 44–48. [CrossRef]
41. Hippisley-Cox, J.; Coupland, C.; Vinogradova, Y.; Robson, J.; Minhas, R.; Sheikh, A.; Brindle, P. Predicting cardiovascular risk in England and Wales: Prospective derivation and validation of QRISK2. *BMJ* **2008**, *336*, 1475–1482. [CrossRef] [PubMed]
42. Ke, L.Y.; Chan, H.C.; Chan, H.C.; Kalu, F.C.U.; Lee, H.C.; Lin, I.L.; Jhuo, S.J.; Lai, W.T.; Tsao, C.R.; Sawamura, T.; et al. Electronegative Low-Density Lipoprotein L5 Induces Adipose Tissue Inflammation Associated With Metabolic Syndrome. *J. Clin. Endocrinol. Metab.* **2017**, *102*, 4615–4625. [CrossRef] [PubMed]
43. Havel, R.J.; Eder, H.A.; Bragdon, J.H. The distribution and chemical composition of ultracentrifugally separated lipoproteins in human serum. *J. Clin. Investig.* **1955**, *34*, 1345–1353. [CrossRef] [PubMed]

44. Halvorsen, B.; Waehre, T.; Scholz, H.; Clausen, O.P.; Von der Thusen, J.H.; Muller, F.; Heimli, H.; Tonstad, S.; Hall, C.; Froland, S.S.; et al. Interleukin-10 enhances the oxidized LDL-induced foam cell formation of macrophages by antiapoptotic mechanisms. *J. Lipid. Res.* **2005**, *46*, 211–219. [CrossRef] [PubMed]
45. Scott, C.S.; Richards, S.J.; Master, P.S.; Kendall, J.; Limbert, H.J.; Roberts, B.E. Flow cytometric analysis of membrane CD11b, CD11c and CD14 expression in acute myeloid leukaemia: Relationships with monocytic subtypes and the concept of relative antigen expression. *Eur. J. Haematol.* **1990**, *44*, 24–29. [CrossRef]

International Journal of
Molecular Sciences

MDPI

Article

The Essential Role of Peptidylarginine Deiminases 2 for Cytokines Secretion, Apoptosis, and Cell Adhesion in Macrophage

Hui-Chun Yu [1], Chien-Hsueh Tung [1,2], Kuang-Yung Huang [1,2], Hsien-Bin Huang [3] and Ming-Chi Lu [1,2,*]

1 Division of Allergy, Immunology and Rheumatology, Dalin Tzu Chi Hospital, Buddhist Tzu Chi Medical Foundation, Dalin, Chiayi 62130, Taiwan; unvsusagi@gmail.com (H.-C.Y.); dr5188@yahoo.com.tw (C.-H.T.); hky0919@yahoo.com.tw (K.-Y.H.)

2 School of Medicine, Tzu Chi University, Hualien City 97071, Taiwan

3 Department of Life Science and Institute of Molecular Biology, National Chung Cheng University, Minxiong, Chiayi 62130, Taiwan; biohbh@ccu.edu.tw

* Correspondence: e360187@yahoo.com.tw; Tel.: +886-5-2648000 (ext. 3205); Fax: +886-5-2648006

Received: 14 July 2020; Accepted: 8 August 2020; Published: 10 August 2020

Abstract: Objective: The study aims to investigate the functional roles of peptidylarginine deiminase 2 (PADI2) in macrophages. Methods: The clustered regularly interspaced short palindromic repeats (CRISPR)–CRISPR-associated protein-9 nuclease (Cas9) system was used to knockout PADI2 in U937 cells. U937 cells were introduced to differentiate macrophages and were stimulated with lipopolysaccharides (LPS). The protein expression of PADI2, PADI4, and citrullinated proteins were analyzed by Western blotting. The mRNA and protein levels of interleukin 1 beta (*IL-1β*), *IL-6*, and tumor necrosis factor-alpha (*TNF-α*) were analyzed using RT-PCR and ELISA, respectively. Cell apoptosis was analyzed using flow cytometry. Cell adhesion assay was performed using a commercially available fibrinogen-coated plate. Results: PADI2 knockout could markedly suppress the PADI2 protein expression, but not the PADI4 protein expression. PADI2 knockout decreased the protein levels of citrullinated nuclear factor κB (NF-κB) p65, but not those of citrullinated histone 3, resulting in the decreased mRNA expression levels of *IL-1β* and *TNF-α* in the U937 cells and *IL-1β* and *IL-6* in the differentiated macrophages and the macrophages stimulated with LPS. The cytokines levels of IL-1β, IL-6, and TNF-α were all dramatically decreased in the PADI2 knockout group compared with in the controls. PADI2 knockout prevented macrophages apoptosis via the decreased caspase-3, caspase-2, and caspase-9 activation. PADI2 knockout also impaired macrophages adhesion capacity through the decreased protein levels of focal adhesion kinase (FAK), phospho-FAK, paxillin, phospho-paxillin, and p21-activated kinase 1. Conclusion: This study showed that PADI2 could promote IL-1β, IL-6, and TNF-α production in macrophages, promote macrophage apoptosis through caspase-3, caspase-2, and caspase-9 activation and enhance cell adhesion via FAK, paxillin, and PAK1. Therefore, targeting PADI2 could be used as a novel strategy for controlling inflammation caused by macrophages.

Keywords: citrullination; macrophages; PADI2; inflammatory cytokines; adhesion; apoptosis

1. Introduction

Peptidylarginine deiminases (PADIs) are a group of enzyme that converts peptidyl-arginine to peptidyl-citrulline, also called protein citrullination, in the presence of Ca^{2+} [1]. There are five members in the human PADI family, and each member has its own tissue distribution and substrate specificity [2]. PADIs and protein citrullination is known not only to contribute to the pathogenesis of several autoimmune diseases, such as rheumatoid arthritis (RA) and multiple sclerosis [1,3,4], but they were also recently found to facilitate cancer invasion and metastasis [5,6]. In human leukocytes, PADI2 and PADI4 are highly expressed [1]. Our previous study showed that the expression of PADI2 and PADI4 was remarkably increased during macrophage differentiation whereas the addition of lipopolysaccharides (LPS) increased the levels of citrullinated proteins. We further provided the evidence that PADI2 might play a critical role in the inflammatory response using plasmid-encoding short hairpin RNA-targeting PADI2 [7]. This result is consistent with that reported by Bawadekar et al., which demonstrated that PADI2-deficient mice showed a reduced joint inflammation in murine tumor necrosis factor-alpha (TNF-α)-induced arthritis [8].

Recently, clustered regularly interspaced short palindromic repeats (CRISPR) and the CRISPR-associated protein-9 nuclease (Cas9) system (CRISPR–Cas9 system), an effective way to edit genome [9], has become a powerful tool for investigating the biologic function of a specific gene [10]. We hypothesized that PADI2 is required for multiple domains of macrophage functions. Therefore, we used the CRISPR–Cas9 system to knockout PADI2 in macrophages and to evaluate the effects of PADI2 knockout on various functions of macrophages, including inflammation, cell survival, and adhesion capacity.

2. Results

2.1. Validation and Characterization of PADI2 Knockout U937 Cells

We confirmed the protein expression of PADI2 was dramatically decreased after gene knockout using the CRISPR–Cas system (Figure 1A). PADI2 and PADI4 are homologous in their structures and amino acid sequences in human [2]. We found that the protein expression of PADI4 did not change in the U937 cells after PADI2 knockout compared with those in the controls (Figure 1A). Next, we analyzed the protein levels for cit-H3. In the U397 cells, the differentiated macrophages, and the macrophages stimulated with LPS, the protein levels of cit-H3 were not different between the PADI2 knockout group and the controls (Figure 1B). Sun et al. reported that PADI4 could citrullinate nuclear factor κB (NF-κB) p65 and enhance its nuclear translocation and transcriptional activity [11]. We found that the protein levels of the citrullinated p65 were decreased in the nuclear extract of macrophages stimulated with LPS in the PADI2 knockout group compared with in the controls (Figure 1C,D).

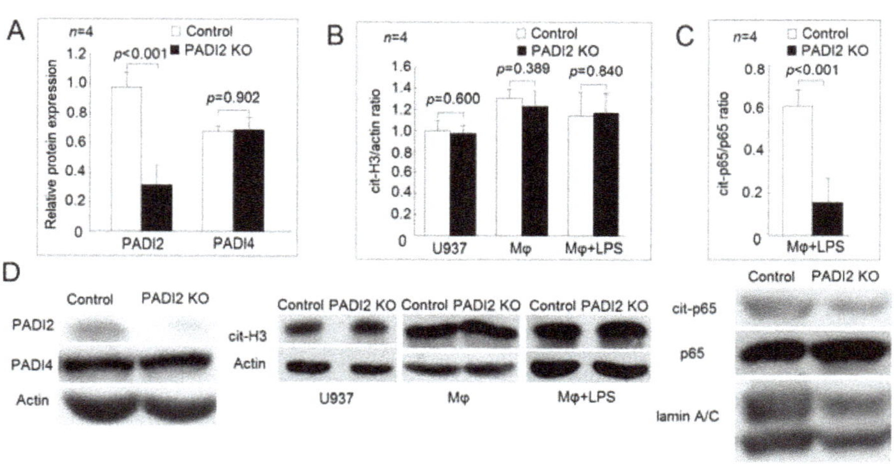

Figure 1. Validation of peptidylarginine deiminase 2 (PADI2) knockout U937 cells and their effects on histone H3 and nuclear factor kappa B (NF-κB) p65 citrullination. (**A**) Comparison of the relative protein expression levels of PADI2 and PADI4 with those of the control. The U937 cells were transfected with CRISPR–Cas9 plasmids containing gRNA that targets PADI2 or control CRISPR-Cas9 plasmids as

the control group. The protein expression levels of PADI2 decreased dramatically, but those of PADI4 did not changed after PADI2 gene knockout (PADI2 knockout group). (**B**) Comparison of the citrullinated histone H3 (cit-H3)/actin ratios of the U937 cells, the differentiated macrophages, and the macrophages stimulated with 20 ng/mL lipopolysaccharides (LPS). The protein level of cit-H3 did not change in the U937 cells, the differentiated macrophages, and the macrophages stimulated with 20 ng/mL LPS for 24 h in the PADI2 knockout group. (**C**) Comparison of the citrullinated p65 subunit of NF-κB (cit-p65) ratios of the LPS-stimulated macrophages. The citrullinated protein was obtained from the nuclear extract of LPS-stimulated macrophages by immunoprecipitation using ACPAs-conjugated protein G Sepharose beads. The protein expression of the cit-p65 in the immunoprecipitates was then analyzed by Western blotting using anti-p65 antibodies as a probe. (**D**) Representative images showing the relative protein expression levels of PADI2 and PADI4; citrullinated histone H3 of the U937 cells, the differentiated macrophages, and the macrophages stimulated with LPS and cit-p65 in the immunoprecipitates of the LPS-stimulated macrophages in the PADI2 knockout group and the control group.

2.2. Effects of PADI2 Knockout on Proinflammatory Cytokines Expression and Secretion

In Figure 2A, we found that the gene expression levels of *IL-1β*, *IL-6*, and *TNF-α* were increased in the differentiated macrophages compared with in the U937 cells in both the PADI2 knockout group and the control group. The addition of LPS further increased the mRNA expression levels of *IL-1β* (23.9 ± 0.2 vs. 23.3 ± 0.3; $p = 0.017$) and *IL-6* (17.2 ± 0.2 vs. 15.5 ± 0.1; $p < 0.001$), but not those of *TNF-α* (19.1 ± 0.5 vs. 19.6 ± 0.3; $p = 0.135$) in the control group. The addition of LPS did not affected the mRNA expression levels of f *IL-1β*, *IL-6*, and *TNF-α* in the PADI2 knockout group.

In the U937 cells, the PADI2 knockout decreased the gene expression levels of *IL-1β* and *TNF-α* compared with those in the controls. In the differentiated macrophages and the macrophages stimulated with LPS, the PADI2 knockout decreased the gene expression levels of *IL-1β* and *IL-6* compared with those in the controls.

In the U937 cells, the secretion levels of IL-1β, IL-6, and TNF-α were very low in both the PADI2 knockout group and the control group (Figure 2B). In both groups, the differentiated macrophages secreted the increased levels of IL-1β, IL-6, and TNF-α compared with the U937 cells. The addition of LPS further increased the secretion levels of IL-1β, IL-6, and TNF-α in both groups.

In the differentiated macrophages and the macrophages stimulated with LPS, PADI2 knockout significantly decreased the cytokine secretion levels of IL-1β, IL-6, and TNF-α compared with in the controls.

2.3. Effects of PADI2 Knockout on Cell Apoptosis and Adhesion

As expected, the apoptotic rate was significantly elevated in the differentiated macrophages compared with in the U937 cells. The addition of LPS further increased the apoptotic rate of the macrophages in both the PADI2 knockout group and the control group (Figure 3A,B). The PADI2 knockout group significantly decreased the apoptotic rates in the U937 cells, the differentiated macrophages, and the macrophages stimulated with LPS compared with the control group. We also noticed that the PADI2 knockout macrophages were more easily detached during trypsinization compared with the controls. Stefanelli et al. showed that protein citrullination could alter focal adhesion stability [12]. Therefore, we speculated that PADI2 knockout might also impair the macrophage adhesion. Using a commercially available fibrinogen-coated plate, we found that the PADI2 knockout group had impaired cell adhesion ability compared with the control group (Figure 3C).

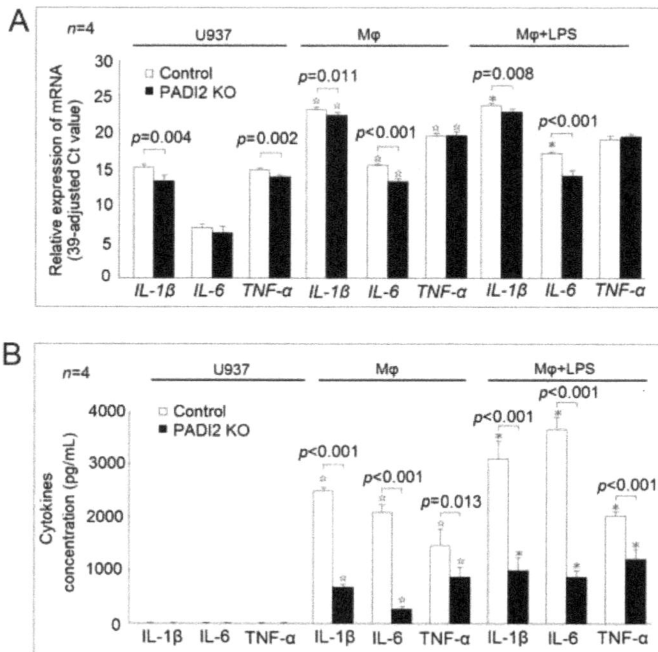

Figure 2. Effects of PADI2 knockout on inflammatory cytokines expression and secretion. (**A**) The mRNA expression levels of *IL-1β*, *IL-6*, and tumor necrosis factor-alpha (*TNF-α*) in the U937 cells, the differentiated macrophages, and the macrophages stimulated with LPS in the PADI2 knockout group compared with those in the controls. (**B**) The cytokines secretion levels of IL-1β, IL-6, and TNF-α in the U937 cells, the differentiated macrophages, and the macrophages stimulated with LPS transfected in the PADI2 knockout group compared with those in the control group. ☆ $p < 0.05$ compared with the U937 cells; * $p < 0.05$ compared with the differentiated macrophages.

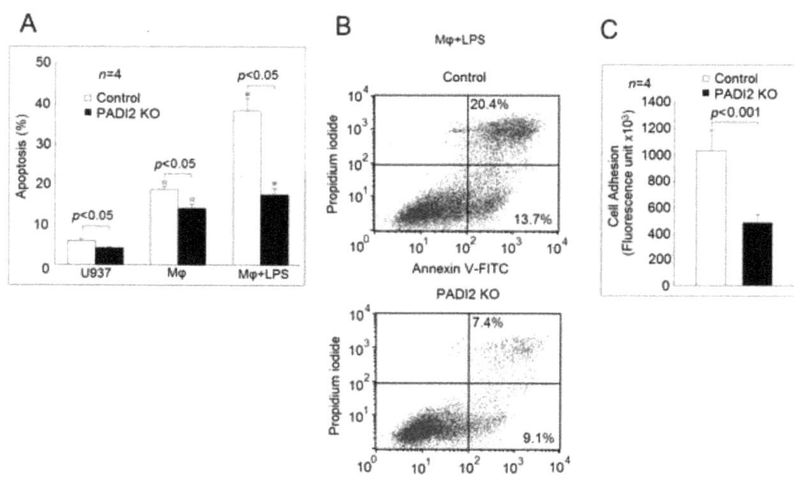

Figure 3. Effects of PADI2 knockout on macrophages apoptosis and adhesion. (**A**) The apoptosis rates of the U937 cells, the differentiated macrophages, and the macrophages stimulated with LPS for 24 h

in the PADI2 knockout and control groups. The apoptotic rates of these cells were measured using flow cytometry analysis. The cells apoptosis was defined as % of annexin V staining. (**B**) Comparison of cell apoptosis in the macrophages stimulated with LPS in the PADI2 knockout group and the control group. It was shown than cell apoptosis in the macrophages stimulated with LPS in the PADI2 knockout group was decreased compared with in the control group. (**C**) The adhesion ability in the differentiated macrophages from the PADI2 knockout group and the control group using a fibrinogen-coated plate. ☆ $p < 0.05$ compared with the U937 cells; * $p < 0.05$ compared with the differentiated macrophages.

2.4. Effecst of PADI2 Knockout on the Protein Expression of Caspases

We further investigated the effects of PADI2 knockout on the activation of different caspases. In the macrophages stimulated with LPS, we found that the protein levels of the cleaved caspase-3, but not those of the intact caspase-3, were decreased in the PADI2 knockout group compared with in the controls. Among the initiator caspases [13], we found that the protein levels of the cleaved caspase-2 and the cleaved caspase-9, but not those of the intact caspase-2 and the intact caspase-9, were also significantly decreased in the PADI2 knockout group compared with in the controls (Figure 4). In contrast, the protein levels of the cleaved caspase-8, but not those of the intact caspase-8, were significantly elevated in the PADI2 knockout group compared with in the controls.

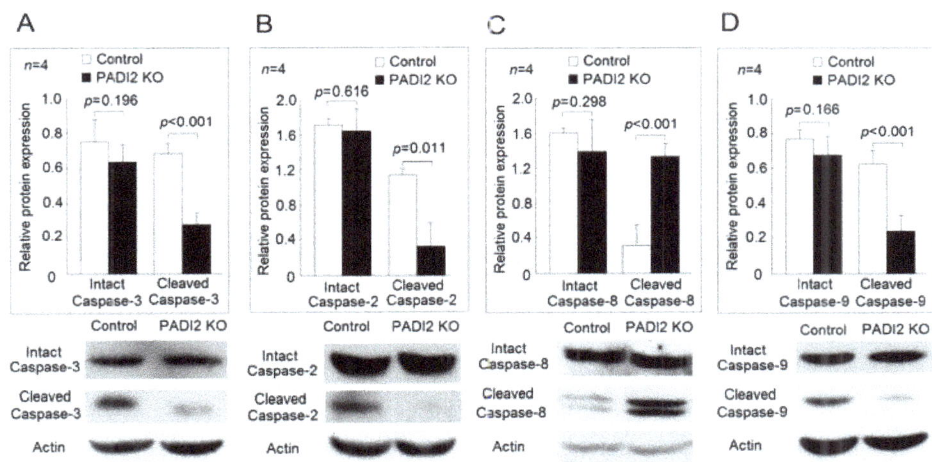

Figure 4. Effects of PADI2 knockout on the relative expression levels of the activated caspase-3, -2, -8, and -9. In the differentiated macrophages stimulated with LPS, the protein expression levels of the intact caspases and the cleaved caspases were performed by Western blotting in the PADI2 knockout group and the control group. The relative protein expression was defined as the ratio of intact caspases or cleaved caspases to the actin band intensity: (**A**) caspase-3; (**B**) caspase-2; (**C**) caspase-8; (**D**) caspase-9.

2.5. Effecst of PADI2 Knockout on the Protein and mRNA Expression of Adhesion-Related Genes

In the U937 cells and the differentiated macrophages, we found that the protein expression levels of phospho-FAK, FAK, phospho-paxillin, paxillin, and PAK1 were all decreased in the PADI2 knockout group compared with in the control group (Figures 5 and 6). For the gene expression of the adhesion-related proteins, we found that there were no statistically significant differences in the mRNA expression of *FAK*, *paxillin*, or *PAK1* between the PADI2 knockout group and the control group in the U937 cells and the differentiated macrophages.

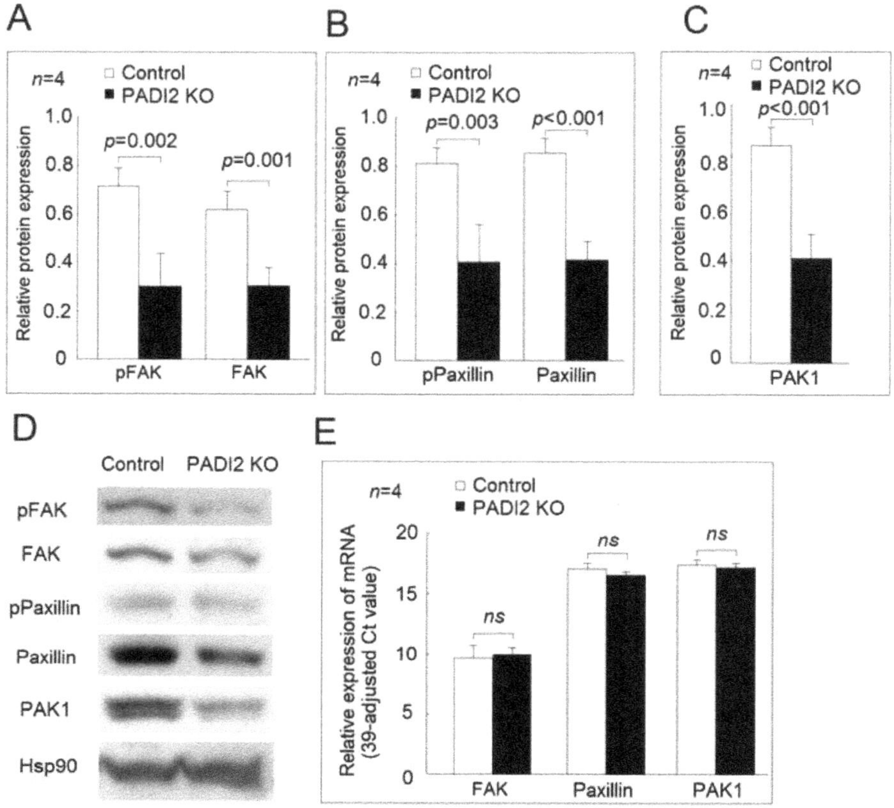

Figure 5. Effects of PADI2 knockout in the protein and mRNA expression of focal adhesion kinase (*FAK*), *paxillin*, and *PAK1* in the U937 cells: (**A**) comparison of the relative protein expression levels of FAK and phospho-FAK in the PADI2 knockout group and the control group; (**B**) comparison of the relative protein expression levels of paxillin and phospho-paxillin in the PADI2 knockout group and the control group; (**C**) comparison of the relative protein expression levels of PAK1 in the PADI2 knockout group and the control group; and (**D**) Representative images showing the relative protein expression levels of FAK, paxillin, and PAK1 in the PADI2 knockout group and the control group; (**E**) the relative mRNA expression levels of *FAK*, *paxillin*, and *PAK1* in the U937 cells. In the U937 cells, the protein expression levels of the cell adhesion-related proteins, including FAK, phospho-FAK, paxillin, phospho-paxillin, and PAK1, were performed by Western blotting in the PADI2 knockout group and the control group. The relative protein expression was defined as the ratio of specific protein/hsp90 band intensity.

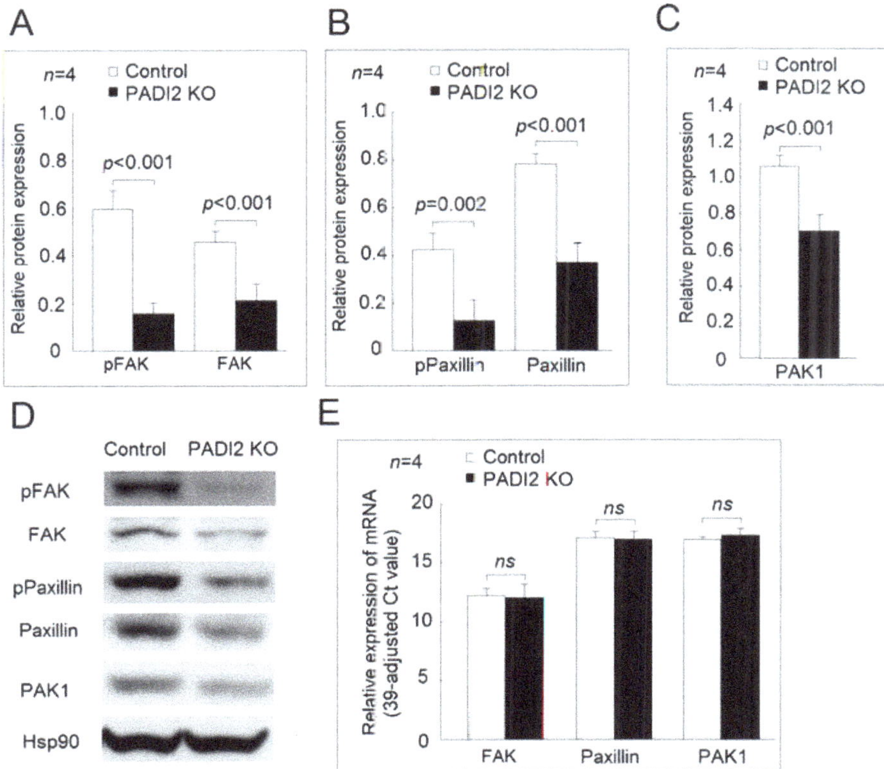

Figure 6. Effects of PADI2 knockout in the protein and mRNA expression of *FAK*, *paxillin*, and *PAK1* in the differentiated macrophages: (**A**) comparison of the relative protein expression levels of FAK and phospho-FAK in the PADI2 knockout group and the control group; (**B**) comparison of the relative protein expression levels of paxillin and phospho-paxillin in the PADI2 knockout group and the control group; (**C**) comparison of the relative protein expression levels of PAK1 in the PADI2 knockout group and the control group; and (**D**) Representative images showing the relative protein expression levels of FAK, paxillin, and PAK1 in the PADI2 knockout group and the control group; (**E**) the relative mRNA expression levels of *FAK*, *paxillin*, and *PAK1*. In differentiated macrophages, the protein expression levels of the cell adhesion-related proteins including FAK, phospho-FAK, paxillin, phospho-paxillin, and PAK1 were performed by Western blotting in the PADI2 knockout group and the control group. The relative protein expression was defined as the ratio of a specific protein/hsp90 band intensity.

3. Discussion

Vossenaar et al. [14], Hojo-Nakashima et al. [15], and our previous study [7] have shown that PADI2 protein levels increased during the macrophage differentiation, resulting in increasing protein citrullination. In the current study, we demonstrated that PADI2 is essential for macrophage proinflammatory cytokine secretion, cell adhesion, and apoptosis using CRISPR/Cas9-mediated knockout of PADI2. As for the target proteins of PADI2, we found the histone H3 citrullination did not change in the U937 cells, the differentiated macrophages, or the macrophages stimulated with LPS in the PADI2 knockout group compared with in the control group. Darrah et al. reported that histone H3 was prone to be citrullinated by PADI4, which might explain our finding [16]. Different antibodies used in diffident studies might detect different epitopes, which could affect the results of histone H3 citrullination. However, we demonstrated that the protein level of citrullinated NF-κB p65 was decreased in the PADI2 knockout group compared with in the controls. Sun et al. showed that the citrullination of NF-κB p65 could enhance *IL-1β* and *TNF-α* expression [11]. Our result also showed that the expression levels of *IL-1β* and *TNF-α* were indeed decreased in the U937 cells after PADI2 knockout. The differentiation of macrophage and further stimulation with LPS could decrease the *IL-1β* and *IL-6* expression in the PADI2 knockout group compared with in the controls. Most importantly, we found that the IL-1β, IL-6, and TNF-α concentrations in the culture soup were dramatically decreased in the PADI2 knockout group compared with in the controls. In addition, Sun et al. showed citrullinated NF-κB p65 was mediated by PADI4 using HeLa cells and neutrophils, which expressed high levels of PADI4 compared with those of monocytes and lymphocytes [6]. In the current study, we used U937 cells, a representative cell line for human monocytes. We demonstrated that PADI2 was also required to citrullinated NF-κB p65 in macrophages upon LPS stimulation. Lee et al. showed that PADI2 could interact with an inhibitor of nuclear factor kappa-B kinase subunit gamma (IKKγ) to suppress NF-κB activity using a murine cell line [17]. However, our results suggested that NF-κB activity decreased in PADI2 knockout U937 cells from a decreased expression of proinflammatory cytokines. Different cell lines used in different studies might explain these variations. Mishra et al. demonstrated that PADI2 and PADI4 activity in macrophages were required for inflammasome assembly and IL-1β release in a murine model [18], which is consistent with our findings. Since proinflammatory cytokines including IL-1β, IL-6, and TNF-α play a critical role in the immunopathogenesis of RA [19,20] and increased PADIs activities have been documented in patients with RA [21], targeting PADIs would be a novel strategy for RA treatment.

We found that PADI2 knockout significantly decreased the apoptotic rates in the U937 cells, the differentiated macrophages, and the macrophages stimulated with LPS. Liu et al. demonstrated the overexpression of PADI4-induced cell apoptosis in human leukemia (HL)-60 cells and human acute T leukemia Jurkat cells [22]. These findings suggested that both PADI2 and PADI4 could promote apoptosis. For the detail mechanism of cell apoptosis, Liu et al. found that PADI4 induced apoptosis mainly through cell cycle arrest and a mitochondria-mediated pathway [22]. Our study showed that PADI2 could activate caspase-2 and -9, leading to the activation of capases-3. Further studies are needed to clarify their molecular mechanisms.

We noted that the inhibition of PADI2 impaired the protein expression of phospho-FAK, FAK, phospho-paxillin, paxillin, and PAK1, resulting in impaired cell adhesion ability in macrophages. We could not detect the phosphorylation of PAK1, which was also not detected in macrophages in a previous study [23]. PAK1 belongs to one of the members of the PAKs family, which plays an important role in cell motility [24], and the phosphorylation of PAK1 is critical for cell migration instead of adhesion [25]. We noted that the protein levels, but not mRNA expression levels of FAK, paxillin, and PAK1, were decreased in the PADI2 knockout group compared with in the controls. We speculated that the citrullination of proteins might accelerate their degradation by changing their binding affinity to proteasome [7,26] or altered protein structure [27], and further studies are needed.

In conclusion, our study showed that PADI2 is essential for the multiple functions of macrophages in enhancing inflammatory cytokines production through the citrullination of NF-κB p65, promoting cell apoptosis with capase-2, -3, and -9 activation, and facilitating cell adhesion via FAK, paxillin, and PAK1.Targeting PADI2 could be a novel strategy for controlling inflammation triggers by macrophages.

4. Material and Methods

4.1. Purification of Anticitrullinated Protein Antibodies (ACPA) from Pooled ACPA(+) Sera in Patients with RA

The study protocol was approved by the institutional review board of Dalin Tzu Chi Hospital, Buddhist Tzu Chi Medical Foundation (No. B10902001, 1 April 2020). The study was performed in accordance with the Declaration of Helsinki. Serum samples from ACPA-positive RA patients with high concentration of ACPAs (>340 IU/mL) and aged 20 years and above, which fulfilled the

2010 American College of Rheumatology (ACR)/European League Against Rheumatism (EULAR) criteria [28], were detected using an ELISA kit (Pharmacia Diagnostics AB, Uppsala, Sweden), collected and pooled. ACPAs were purified according to the method described previously [29]. In brief, the pooled sera containing high concentration of ACPAs from patients with RA were purified by affinity chromatography using an ÄKTA purifier 10 (GE Healthcare, Little Chalfont, UK) with UV detection at 280 nm for the collection of the desired fractions.

4.2. Preparation of PADI2 Knockout U937 Cells

U937 cells were purchased from the European Collection of Cell Cultures (Salisbury, UK) and electroporated with control CRISPR–Cas9 plasmids or CRISPR–Cas9 plasmids containing gRNA that targeted PADI2 (Santa Cruz biotechnology, Dallas, TX, USA) using the Gene Pulser MXcell electroporation system (Bio-Rad Laboratories, Hercules, CA, USA) under the condition of voltage 210 V and capacitance 960 μF. The cells were then cultured in Iscove's Modified Dulbecco's medium (IMDM) (Invitrogen, Carlsbad, CA, USA) with 10% fetal bovine serum (Invitrogen, Carlsbad, CA, USA) with 0.3 μg/mL puromycin (Sigma-Aldrich, St. Louis, MO, USA). After drug selection, the surviving cells were isolated and validated by Western blotting. The U937 cells was then introduced to differentiate with "differentiated macrophages" by coculturation with 500 ng/mL phorbol 12-myristate 13-acetate (PMA, Sigma-Aldrich, St. Louis, MO, USA) at 37 °C in a humidified atmosphere containing 5% CO_2 for 48 h. The differentiated macrophages were cocultured with LPS (20 ng/mL, Sigma-Aldrich, St. Louis, MO, USA) for 24 h at 37 °C in a humidified atmosphere containing 5% CO_2. The culture supernatants were then collected and stored at −80 °C for ELISA.

4.3. ELISA

The concentrations of cytokines in the culture supernatants were determined using the respective ELISA kits (BD Biosciences, Franklin Lakes, NJ, USA) according to the manufacturer's specification.

4.4. Flow Cytometry Analysis

Cell apoptosis was determined by double staining with the FITC-annexin V and propidium iodide (PI) kit (BD Biosciences, Franklin Lakes, NJ, USA) in cells analyzed by flow cytometry (FACScan, Becton Dickinson, Franklin Lakes, NJ, USA) using Lysis II software.

4.5. Cell Adhesion Assay

Cell adhesion assay was performed using a CytoSelect™ Cell Adhesion Assay Kit (Cell Biolabs, San Diego, CA, USA), which used a fibrinogen-coated plate, according to the manufacturer's protocol with modifications. U937 cells cocultured with 500 ng/mL PMA for 24 h (7.5×10^4 per well) were added and incubated with 500 ng/mL PMA at 37 °C for 24 h in a humidified atmosphere containing 5% CO_2. Lysis buffer/CyQuant® GR dyes (200 μL) were added and incubated for 20 min at room temperature with shaking. Finally, the mixture was transferred to a 96-well plate and analyzed using an ELISA microplate reader (Anthos Zenyth 3100, Cambridge, UK) with two separate readings (480 and 520 nm).

4.6. Preparation of the Cell Nuclear Protein Extract

Cells were lysed with 1% NP-40 (Sigma-Aldrich, St. Louis, MO, USA) in the presence of a proteinase inhibitor cocktail (Sigma-Aldrich, St. Louis, MO, USA) and a phosphatase inhibitor cocktail (Thermo Fisher Scientific, Waltham, MA, USA). A nuclear extract was prepared using a Nuclear Extract Kit (Active Motif, Carlsbad, CA, USA) according to the manufacturer's protocol. The protein concentrations of these samples were measured using the Bradford method. The culture supernatants were collected and stored at −80 °C for further analysis.

4.7. Immunoprecipitation of Citrullinated Protein

The nuclear extract from macrophages stimulated by LPS was immunoprecipited by ACPAs-conjugated protein G Sepharose beads (Protein G Immunoprecipitaton kits, Sigma-Aldrich, St. Louis, MO, USA) according to the manufacturer's instruction. Then, protein molecules in the supernatant (immunoprecipitates) were then analyzed by Western blotting using anti-p65 antibodies as a probe.

4.8. Western Blotting Analysis

Cell lysate was electrophoresed and transferred to a polyvinyllidene difluoride (PVDF) sheet (Sigma-Aldrich, St. Louis, MO, USA). The membranes were nonspecifically blocked in a 1% skim milk solution and incubated with primary antibodies for PADI2 (ab56928), PADI4 (ab128086), and citrullinated histone 3 (cit-H3; ab5103), caspase-2 (ab179520) (Abcam, Cambridge, UK), caspase-3 (9662), cleaved caspase-3 (9661), caspase-8 (9746), cleaved caspase-8 (9496), caspase-9 (9502), cleaved caspase-9 (7237), p21-activated kinase 1 (PAK1) (2602), focal adhesion kinase (FAK) (3285), phospho-FAK(8556), paxillin (12065), phospho-paxillin (2541), p65 (8242), and heat shock protein 90 (hsp90) (4874) (Cell Signaling Technology, Danvers, MA, USA) followed by the respective HRP-conjugated secondary antibodies (Jackson ImmunoResearch Laboratories, West Grove, PA, USA). Blotting was visualized by chemiluminescence reaction (ECL; GE Healthcare, Little Chalfont, UK). The respective band intensities were measured using ImageJ (version 1.42; http://rsb.info.nih.gov/ij).

4.9. Measurement of Cytokine Expression Levels by RT-PCR

Total RNA was extracted using a Quick-RNA MiniPrep kit (Zymo Research, Irvine, CA, USA) according to the manufacturer's protocol. RNA concentrations were quantified using a spectrophotometer (NanoDrop 1000, Thermo Fisher Scientific, Waltham, MA, USA). The mRNA expression levels of interleukin 1 beta (*IL-1β*), *TNF-α*, *IL-6*, *FAK*, *paxillin*, and *PAK1* were quantified by RT-PCR by a one-step RT-PCR kit (TaKaRa, Shiga, Japan) with an ABI Prism 7500 Fast Real-Time PCR system (Applied Biosystems, Waltham, MA, USA) as previously described [30]. The relative expression levels of mRNA were defined by the following equation: (39—threshold cycle (Ct) after being adjusted by the expression of 18S ribosomal RNA).

4.10. Statistical Analysis

Data were expressed as mean ± standard deviation. Statistical significance was assessed by the Mann-Whitney U test. All statistical analyses were performed using Stata/SE version 8.0 for Windows (StataCorp, College Station, TX, USA). Two-tailed P values less than 0.05 were considered significant. The datasets analyzed during the current study are available from the corresponding author on reasonable request.

Author Contributions: H.-C.Y., C.-H.T., K.-Y.H., H.-B.H. and M.-C.L. conceived and designed the study. H.-C.Y. and H.B.H. performed the experiment. C.-H.T., K.-Y.H. and M.-C.L. analyzed and interpreted the data. M.-C.L. wrote the paper. All authors revised the manuscript critically for the important intellectual content. All authors have read and agreed to the published version of the manuscript.

Funding: This work was supported by grants from the Ministry of Science and Technology (MOST 107-2314-B-303-020-MY3) and Buddhist Tzu Chi Medical Foundation (TCMF-A 108-05(109)), Taiwan.

Acknowledgments: We thank Malcolm Koo for his writing assistance and statistical advice.

Conflicts of Interest: The authors declare no conflicts of interest.

Abbreviations

PADI	peptidylarginine deiminases
IL	interleukin
TNF-α	tumor necrosis factor-alpha

ACPAs	anticitrullinated protein antibodies
PMA	phorbol 12-myristate 13-acetate
LPS	lipopolysaccharides
CRISPR	clustered regularly interspaced short palindromic repeats
Cas9	CRISPR-associated protein-9 nuclease
RT-PCR	real-time reverse transcription-polymerase chain reaction
ELISA	enzyme-linked immunosorbent assay
NF-κB	nuclear factor kappa-light-chain-enhancer of activated B cells
PAK1	p21-activated kinase 1
FAK	focal adhesion kinase
SDS-PAGE	sodium dodecyl sulfate polyacrylamide gel electrophoresis
HRP	horseradish peroxidase

References

1. Wang, S.; Wang, Y. Peptidylarginine deiminases in citrullination, gene regulation, health and pathogenesis. *Biochim. Biophys. Acta BBA Bioenergy* **2013**, *1829*, 1126–1135. [CrossRef] [PubMed]
2. Alghamdi, M.; Al Ghamdi, K.A.; Khan, R.H.; Uversky, V.; Redwan, E.M. An interplay of structure and intrinsic disorder in the functionality of peptidylarginine deiminases, A family of key autoimmunity-related enzymes. *Cell. Mol. Life Sci.* **2019**, *76*, 4635–4662. [CrossRef] [PubMed]
3. Lu, M.-C.; Yu, H.-C. The roles of anti-citrullinated protein antibodies in the immunopathogenesis of rheumatoid arthritis. *Tzu Chi Med. J.* **2019**, *31*, 5–10. [CrossRef] [PubMed]
4. Curran, A.M.; Naik, P.; Giles, J.T.; Darrah, E. PAD enzymes in rheumatoid arthritis: Pathogenic effectors and autoimmune targets. *Nat. Rev. Rheumatol.* **2020**, *16*, 301–315. [CrossRef] [PubMed]
5. Beato, M.; Sharma, P. Peptidyl Arginine Deiminase 2 (PADI2)-Mediated Arginine Citrullination Modulates Transcription in Cancer. *Int. J. Mol. Sci.* **2020**, *21*, 1351. [CrossRef]
6. Yuzhalin, A.E.; Gordon-Weeks, A.N.; Tognoli, M.L.; Jones, K.; Markelc, B.; Konietzny, R.; Fischer, R.; Muth, A.; O'Neill, E.; Thompson, P.R.; et al. Colorectal cancer liver metastatic growth depends on PAD4-driven citrullination of the extracellular matrix. *Nat. Commun.* **2018**, *9*, 4783. [CrossRef]
7. Lai, N.-S.; Yu, H.-C.; Tung, C.-H.; Huang, K.-Y.; Huang, H.-B.; Lu, M.-C. Increased peptidylarginine deiminases expression during the macrophage differentiation and participated inflammatory responses. *Arthritis Res.* **2019**, *21*, 108. [CrossRef]
8. Bawadekar, M.; Shim, D.; Johnson, C.J.; Warner, T.F.; Rebernick, R.; Damgaard, D.; Nielsen, C.H.; Pruijn, G.J.M.; Nett, J.E.; Shelef, M.A. Peptidylarginine deiminase 2 is required for tumor necrosis factor alpha-induced citrullination and arthritis, but not neutrophil extracellular trap formation. *J. Autoimmun.* **2017**, *80*, 39–47. [CrossRef]
9. Ran, F.A.; Hsu, P.; Lin, C.-Y.; Gootenberg, J.; Konermann, S.; Trevino, A.E.; Scott, D.A.; Inoue, A.; Matoba, S.; Zhang, Y.; et al. Double nicking by RNA-guided CRISPR Cas9 for enhanced genome editing specificity. *Cell* **2013**, *154*, 1380–1389. [CrossRef]
10. Shalem, O.; Sanjana, N.E.; Zhang, F. High-Throughput functional genomics using CRISPR–Cas9. *Nat. Rev. Genet.* **2015**, *16*, 299–311. [CrossRef]
11. Sun, B.; Dwivedi, N.; Bechtel, T.J.; Paulsen, J.L.; Muth, A.; Bawadekar, M.; Li, G.; Thompson, P.R.; Shelef, M.A.; Schiffer, C.A.; et al. Citrullination of NF-κB p65 promotes its nuclear localization and TLR-induced expression of IL-1β and TNFα. *Sci. Immunol.* **2017**, *2*, eaal3062. [CrossRef] [PubMed]
12. Stefanelli, V.L.; Choudhury, S.; Hu, P.; Liu, Y.; Schwenzer, A.; Yeh, C.-R.; Chambers, D.M.; Pesson, K.; Li, W.; Segura, T.; et al. Citrullination of fibronectin alters integrin clustering and focal adhesion stability promoting stromal cell invasion. *Matrix Boil.* **2019**, *82*, 86–104. [CrossRef] [PubMed]
13. Green, D.R.; Llambi, F. Cell death signaling. *Cold Spring Harb. Perspect. Biol.* **2015**, *7*, a006080. [CrossRef] [PubMed]
14. Vossenaar, E.R.; Radstake, T.; Van Der Heijden, A.; Mansum, M.A.M.V.; Dieteren, C.; De Rooij, D.-J.; Barrera, P.; Zendman, A.; Van Venrooij, W.J. Expression and activity of citrullinating peptidylarginine deiminase enzymes in monocytes and macrophages. *Ann. Rheum. Dis.* **2004**, *63*, 373–381. [CrossRef] [PubMed]

15. Hojo-Nakashima, I.; Sato, R.; Nakashima, K.; Hagiwara, T.; Yamada, M. Dynamic Expression of Peptidylarginine Deiminase 2 in Human Monocytic Leukaemia THP-1 Cells during Macrophage Differentiation. *J. Biochem.* **2009**, *146*, 471–479. [CrossRef] [PubMed]
16. Darrah, E.; Rosen, A.; Giles, J.T.; Andrade, F. Peptidylarginine deiminase 2, 3 and 4 have distinct specificities against cellular substrates: Novel insights into autoantigen selection in rheumatoid arthritis. *Ann. Rheum. Dis.* **2011**, *71*, 92–98. [CrossRef]
17. Lee, H.J.; Joo, M.; Abdolrasulnia, R.; Young, D.G.; Choi, I.; Ware, L.B. Peptidylarginine deiminase 2 suppresses inhibitory κB kinase activity in lipopolysaccharide-stimulated RAW 264.7 macrophages. *J. Biol. Chem.* **2010**, *285*, 39655–39662. [CrossRef]
18. Mishra, N.; Schwerdtner, L.; Sams, K.; Mondal, S.; Ahmad, F.; Schmidt, R.E. Cutting edge: Protein arginine deiminase 2 and 4 regulate NLRP3 inflammasome-dependent IL-1beta maturation and ASC speck formation in macrophages. *J. Immunol.* **2019**, *203*, 795–800. [CrossRef]
19. McInnes, I.; Schett, G. Pathogenetic insights from the treatment of rheumatoid arthritis. *Lancet* **2017**, *389*, 2328–2337. [CrossRef]
20. Macdonald, I.J.; Liu, S.-C.; Su, C.-M.; Wang, Y.-H.; Tsai, C.-H.; Tang, C.-H. Implications of Angiogenesis Involvement in Arthritis. *Int. J. Mol. Sci.* **2018**, *19*, 2012. [CrossRef]
21. Chang, H.-H.; Liu, G.-Y.; Dwivedi, N.; Sun, B.; Okamoto, Y.; Kinslow, J.D.; Deane, K.D.; Demoruelle, M.K.; Norris, J.M.; Thompson, P.R.; et al. A molecular signature of preclinical rheumatoid arthritis triggered by dysregulated PTPN22. *JCI Insight* **2016**, *1*. [CrossRef] [PubMed]
22. Liu, G.-Y.; Liao, Y.-F.; Chang, W.-H.; Liu, C.-C.; Hsieh, M.-C.; Hsu, P.-C.; Tsay, G.J.; Hung, H.-C. Overexpression of peptidylarginine deiminase IV features in apoptosis of haematopoietic cells. *Apoptosis* **2006**, *11*, 183–196. [CrossRef] [PubMed]
23. Osma-García, I.C.; Punzón, C.; Fresno, M.; Diaz-Munoz, M.D. Dose-Dependent effects of prostaglandin E2 in macrophage adhesion and migration. *Eur. J. Immunol.* **2015**, *46*, 677–688. [CrossRef] [PubMed]
24. Bokoch, G.M. Biology of the p21-Activated Kinases. *Ann. Rev. Biochem.* **2003**, *72*, 743–781. [CrossRef] [PubMed]
25. Rajah, A.; Boudreau, C.G.; Ilie, A.; Wee, T.L.; Tang, K.; Borisov, A.Z. Paxillin S273 phosphorylation regulates adhesion dynamics and cell migration through a common protein complex with PAK1 and betaPIX. *Sci. Rep.* **2019**, *9*, 11430. [CrossRef]
26. Kuzina, E.; Kudriaeva, A.A.; Glagoleva, I.S.; Gabibov, A.G.; Belogurov, A.A.; Knorre, V.D. Deimination of the myelin basic protein decelerates its proteasome-mediated metabolism. *Dokl. Biochem. Biophys.* **2016**, *469*, 277–280. [CrossRef]
27. Cau, L.; Pendaries, V.; Lhuillier, E.; Thompson, P.R.; Serre, G.; Takahara, H.; Méchin, M.-C.; Simon, M. Lowering relative humidity level increases epidermal protein deimination and drives human filaggrin breakdown. *J. Dermatol. Sci.* **2017**, *86*, 106–113. [CrossRef]
28. Aletaha, D.; Neogi, T.; Silman, A.J.; Funovits, J.; Felson, D.T.; Bingham, C.O. 2010 Rheumatoid arthritis classification criteria: An American College of Rheumatology/European League Against Rheumatism collaborative initiative. *Arthritis Rheum.* **2010**, *62*, 2569–2581. [CrossRef]
29. Lu, M.C.; Lai, N.S.; Yin, W.Y.; Yu, H.C.; Huang, H.B.; Tung, C.H. Anti-Citrullinated protein antibodies activated ERK1/2 and JNK mitogen-activated protein kinases via binding to surface-expressed citrullinated GRP78 on mononuclear cells. *J. Clin. Immunol.* **2013**, *33*, 558–566. [CrossRef]
30. Lu, M.; Lai, N.; Chen, H.; Yu, H.; Huang, K.; Tung, C.; Huang, H.-B.; Yu, C.-L. Decreased microRNA(miR)-145 and increased miR-224 expression in T cells from patients with systemic lupus erythematosus involved in lupus immunopathogenesis. *Clin. Exp. Immunol.* **2012**, *171*, 91–99. [CrossRef]

International Journal of *Molecular Sciences*

MDPI

Article

Human Lymph Node Stromal Cells Have the Machinery to Regulate Peripheral Tolerance during Health and Rheumatoid Arthritis

Janine S. Hähnlein [1,2,†], Reza Nadafi [3,4,†], Tineke A. de Jong [1,2], Johanna F. Semmelink [1,2], Ester B. M. Remmerswaal [5], Mary Safy [1], Krijn P. van Lienden [6], Mario Maas [6], Danielle M. Gerlag [1], Paul P. Tak [1,7,8,9], Reina E. Mebius [3], Heidi Wähämaa [10], Anca I. Catrina [10] and Lisa G. M. van Baarsen [1,2,*]

1 Department of Rheumatology & Clinical Immunology and Department of Experimental Immunology, Amsterdam Infection & Immunity Institute, Amsterdam UMC, University of Amsterdam, Meibergdreef 9, 1105 AZ Amsterdam, The Netherlands; jhaehnlein@hotmail.com (J.S.H.); t.a.dejong@amsterdamumc.nl (T.A.d.J.); j.fsemmelink@amsterdamumc.nl (J.F.S.); m.safy@umcutrecht.nl (M.S.); dmgerlag@gmail.com (D.M.G.); tak.paulpeter@gmail.com (P.P.T.)

2 Amsterdam Rheumatology & Immunology Center (ARC), Academic Medical Center, 1105 AZ Amsterdam, The Netherlands

3 Department of Molecular Cell Biology and Immunology, Amsterdam UMC, VU Medical Center, Vrije Universiteit Amsterdam, 1081 HZ Amsterdam, The Netherlands; r.nadafi@amsterdamumc.nl (R.N.); r.mebius@amsterdamumc.nl (R.E.M.)

4 Department of Immunology, Leiden University Medical Center, 2333 ZA Leiden, The Netherlands

5 Renal Transplant Unit, Division of Internal Medicine and Department of Experimental Immunology, Amsterdam Infection & Immunity Institute, Amsterdam UMC, University of Amsterdam, Meibergdreef 9, 1105 AZ Amsterdam, The Netherlands; b.m.remmerswaal@amsterdamumc.nl

6 Department of Radiology, Amsterdam UMC, University of Amsterdam, 1105 AZ Amsterdam, The Netherlands; k.p.vanlienden@amc.uva.nl (K.P.v.L.); m.maas@amc.uva.nl (M.M.)

7 Kintai Therapeutics, Cambridge, MA 02140, USA

8 Internal Medicine, Cambridge University, Cambridge, CB2 1TN, UK

9 Rheumatology, Ghent University, 9000 Ghent, Belgium

10 Rheumatology Unit, Department of Medicine, Karolinska University Hospital and Karolinska Institutet, 17176 Stockholm, Sweden; heidi.wahamaa@ki.se (H.W.); anca.catrina@ki.se (A.I.C.)

* Correspondence: e.g.vanbaarsen@amsterdamumc.nl, Tel.: +31-205668043

† These authors contributed equally to this work.

Received: 15 July 2020; Accepted: 5 August 2020; Published: 9 August 2020

Abstract: Background: In rheumatoid arthritis (RA) the cause for loss of tolerance and anti-citrullinated protein antibody (ACPA) production remains unidentified. Mouse studies showed that lymph node stromal cells (LNSCs) maintain peripheral tolerance through presentation of peripheral tissue antigens (PTAs). We hypothesize that dysregulation of peripheral tolerance mechanisms in human LNSCs might underlie pathogenesis of RA. Method: Lymph node (LN) needle biopsies were obtained from 24 RA patients, 23 individuals positive for RA-associated autoantibodies but without clinical disease (RA-risk individuals), and 14 seronegative healthy individuals. Ex vivo human LNs from non-RA individuals were used to directly analyze stromal cells. Molecules involved in antigen presentation and immune modulation were measured in LNSCs upon interferon γ (IFNγ) stimulation (n = 15). Results: Citrullinated targets of ACPAs were detected in human LN tissue and in cultured LNSCs. Human LNSCs express several PTAs, transcription factors autoimmune regulator (AIRE) and deformed epidermal autoregulatory factor 1 (DEAF1), and molecules involved in citrullination, antigen presentation, and immunomodulation. Overall, no clear differences between donor groups were observed with exception of a slightly lower induction of human leukocyte antigen-DR (HLA-DR) and programmed cell death 1 ligand (PD-L1) molecules in LNSCs from RA patients. Conclusion:

Human LNSCs have the machinery to regulate peripheral tolerance making them an attractive target to exploit in tolerance induction and maintenance.

Keywords: lymph node stromal cells; rheumatoid arthritis; tolerance; autoimmunity

---

1. Introduction

Rheumatoid arthritis (RA) is a debilitating inflammatory autoimmune disease hallmarked by disease-specific autoantibody production against citrullinated proteins, but the underlying etiopathogenesis remains largely unknown [1,2]. Citrullination is a post-translational modification changing arginine side chain residues to citrulline, thereby altering structure and charge of the protein. This process occurs regularly under homeostatic conditions like apoptosis of cells where high levels of calcium activate the peptidylarginine deiminase (PADI) enzymes catalyzing citrullination. PADI activity is also detected in a wide range of inflammatory tissues [3] including RA synovial tissue where high expression levels of PADI2 and PADI4 enzymes have been reported [4]. However, *anti-citrullinated protein antibodies* (ACPAs) can be present years before the actual onset of clinical disease [5], while synovial inflammation seems absent [6,7] during this pre-clinical RA-risk phase [8]. Therefore, breaking of tolerance against citrullinated proteins is probably generated at an extra-articular site like lymphoid organs.

Tolerance by negative selection, anergy, or by generation of regulatory T cells (T_{regs}) is induced during lymphocyte maturation in thymus and maintained in the periphery. Through presentation of peripheral tissue antigens (PTAs) by medullary thymic epithelial cells (mTECs) in the thymus, self-reactive thymocytes are deleted or become unresponsive [9]. Unsurprisingly, loss of expression of these PTAs, which is driven by the transcription factors autoimmune regulator (AIRE), deformed epidermal autoregulatory factor 1 (DEAF1), and FEZ family zinc finger 2 (Fezf2) [10–13], leads to autoimmunity [10,12,14]. In humans, where AIRE expression is observed in the thymus and in dendritic cells (DCs) [15,16], AIRE mutations cause a multi-systemic autoimmune syndrome, known as autoimmune polyendocrinopathy-candidiasis-ectodermal dystrophy (APECED) [17].

Some self-reactive lymphocytes escape the thymic negative selection and are present in healthy individuals [18]. Safeguarding tolerance in the periphery is therefore crucial and studies in mice show that lymph node (LN) stromal cells (LNSCs) have therein a dominant role. LNSCs possess an impressive arsenal to shape T and B cell responses for maintenance of the delicate balance between tolerance and appropriate immune response [19,20]. Several subsets of LNSCs have been described, and although the number of subsets is expanding, six subsets are well defined according to their function, location within the LN, and the expression of surface markers podoplanin (PDPN, gp38) and CD31 (PECAM-1): fibroblastic reticular cells (FRCs: CD31− gp38+), follicular dendritic cells (FDCs: CD31− gp38+/−), marginal reticular cells (MRCs: CD31− gp38+/−), the rather poorly studied double negative cells (DNs: CD31− gp38−), lymphatic endothelial cells (LECs: CD31+ gp38+), and blood endothelial cells (BECs: CD31+ gp38−) [21,22]. Among others, FDCs and LECs serve as antigen libraries since they catch, preserve, and present antigens over longer periods, thereby enhancing T cell memory [23,24]. FRCs and LECs have the ability to limit T cell proliferation during ongoing inflammation by secretion of nitric oxide (NO) and expression of other negative regulators such as indoleamine 2,3-dioxygenase (IDO) to protect LN integrity and to contract immune responses for return to steady state [25,26]. Furthermore, studies have convincingly demonstrated that several LNSC subsets present PTAs on major histocompatibility complex (MHC) class I and induce clonal deletion [10,11,27,28]. Additionally, CD4+ T cells can be tolerized via PTA presentation on MHC class II or by presentation of MHC-II-peptide complexes acquired from DCs [29,30]. Moreover, expression and subsequent presentation of PTAs by LNSC in the context of MHC class II to CD4+ T cells can also lead to maintenance of T_{regs} [31]. Moreover, recently we demonstrated that LNSCs convert naïve autoreactive CD4+ T cells into antigen-specific T_{regs} cells and suppress autoreactive T follicular helper (T_{fh}) and B cells responses [32].

Taking into account the tremendous influence of LNSCs on peripheral tolerance and lymphocyte regulation we hypothesize that malfunctioning of LNSCs might lead to a microenvironment causing loss of tolerance and autoantibody production. In this study we investigated for the first time in humans whether the LN is a potential place where citrullination of RA-related PTAs occurs and whether human LNSCs, like murine LNSCs, exhibit the tools for tolerance induction. Finally, we compared the expression of citrullinated proteins, PTAs, and immunomodulatory molecules on human LNSCs of healthy individuals to LNSCs from RA patients and autoantibody positive individuals at risk of developing RA (RA-risk individuals). Our data reveal that human LNSCs express citrullinated proteins targeted by ACPAs and are well equipped to regulate (RA-related) tolerance.

2. Results

2.1. Citrullinated Antigens Targeted by ACPAs Are Present in Human LN Tissue and in Cultured LNSCs

First we investigated by immunohistochemistry the presence of PADI enzymes required for citrullination in LN tissue and cultured LNSCs of a small cohort of individuals (healthy individuals, RA-risk ACPA− individuals, RA-risk ACPA+ individuals, RA ACPA− patients, and RA ACPA+ patients; for each subgroup $n = 3$, total $n = 15$). Both PADI2 and PADI4 enzymes were abundantly present in LN tissue. In cultured LNSCs, PADI2 and PADI4 enzymes were detected intracellularly with PADI4 showing a nuclear expression pattern as reported before [33] (Figure 1A,B, upper panels). Using unique monoclonal ACPAs isolated from RA patients' synovial fluid, which are cross-reactive to one or more citrullinated antigens [34,35], we next analyzed the presence of RA-associated citrullinated proteins in LN tissues and cultured LNSCs. Staining with monoclonal ACPAs C03 and B09 revealed the presence of ACPA-targets in LN tissue as well as in cultured LNSCs derived from all study groups (Figure 1A,B, lower panels). Overall, each antibody showed a distinct staining pattern with variable intensity between donors tested. C03-binding was only detected in a few donors, while B09 was highly abundant in most donors tested, with expression mainly restricted to nuclei. These data show that citrullinated proteins, targeted by ACPAs, are present in LN tissue and cultured LNSCs, and at similar levels in healthy individuals, RA-risk individuals, and RA patients.

2.2. Cultured Human LNSCs Express the Transcription Factors AIRE and DEAF1

The expression of an abundant number of PTAs is regulated by transcription factor AIRE [17] and DEAF1 [10,11]. In culture expanded LNSCs (all passage 2) DEAF1 mRNA was strongly expressed at similar levels in all donor groups (Figure 2A, healthy individuals $n = 5$, RA-risk individuals $n = 12$, and RA patients $n = 14$). In contrast, AIRE mRNA was very low but detected by qPCR while AIRE protein expression was easily measured by flow cytometry (Figure 2B,C), immunohistochemistry (Figure 2D), and Western blot (Figure 2E). Mean fluorescence intensity (MFI) of AIRE expression (intracellular) in cultured LNSCs (passages 3–5) was comparable between healthy individuals, RA-risk individuals, and RA patients (Figure 2C, healthy individuals $n = 5$, RA-risk individuals $n = 9$ and RA patients $n = 4$). Moreover, comparing intracellular versus intranuclear staining revealed most AIRE protein within the nucleus, which was confirmed by immunohistochemistry (Figure 2D and Figure S1). Additionally, also by Western blot, we observed that AIRE protein was ubiquitously expressed in cultured LNSCs from healthy individuals, RA-risk individuals, and RA patients (Figure 2E) and that the protein band in LNSCs corresponded to the AIRE expression observed in thymus tissue. Overall, these data show that both AIRE and DEAF1 are present in cultured human LNSCs.

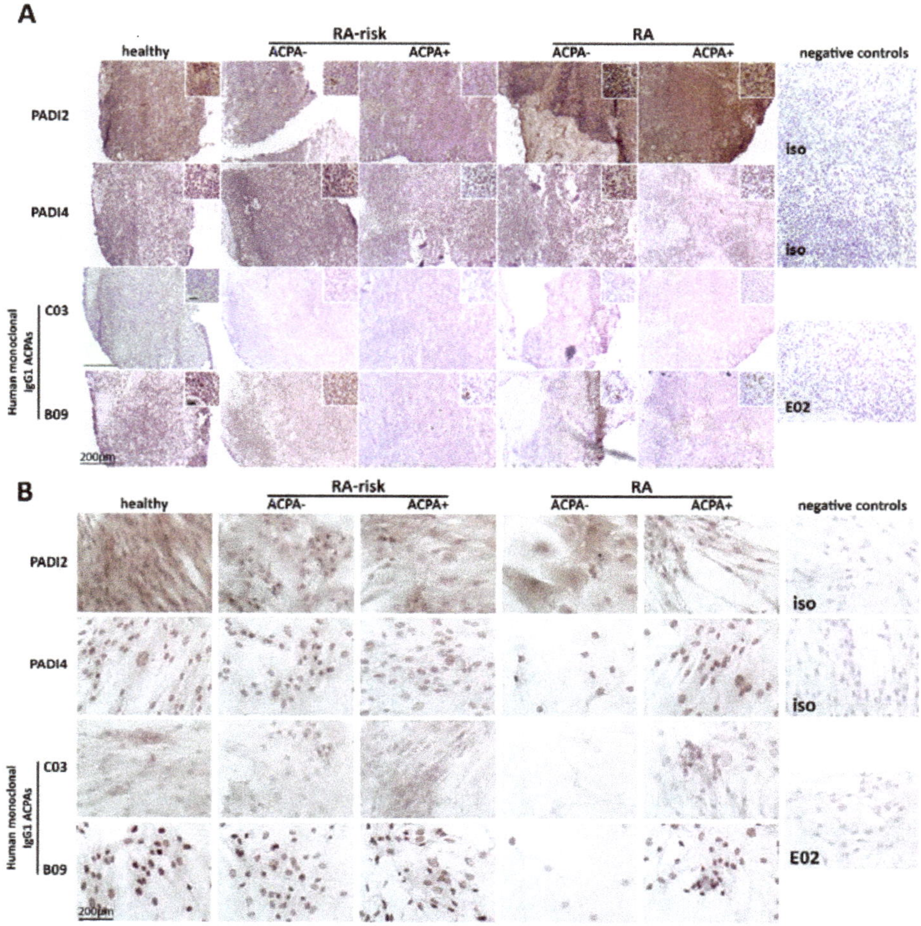

Figure 1. Expression of peptidylarginine deiminases (PADIs) and citrullinated proteins targeted by anti-citrullinated protein antibodies (ACPAs) in lymph node (LN) tissue and cultured lymph node stromal cells (LNSCs). (**A**) LN tissue was stained for PADI2 and PADI4 proteins and citrullinated proteins targeted by ACPAs using human monoclonal antibodies C03 and B09. Staining with isotype control (iso) (healthy LN tissues for PADI2 and PADI4 are represented) or control antibody E02 (rheumatoid arthritis (RA) ACPA+ patients LN tissue is represented) was negative. A representative picture of each donor group of the immunohistochemical analysis in LN tissue is displayed ($n = 3$ per donor group; healthy individuals, RA-risk ACPA− individuals, RA-risk APCA+ individuals, RA ACPA− patients, and RA ACPA+ patients). (**B**) Cultured LNSCs were stained against PADI2 and PADI4 protein and citrullinated proteins targeted by ACPAs using human monoclonal antibodies C03 and B09. Staining with isotype controls (iso; RA-risk ACPA+ individuals LNSCs for PADI2 and healthy individuals LNSCs for PADI4 are represented) and control antibody E02 (RA ACPA+ patients LNSCs is represented) was negative. A representative picture of each donor per group of the immunohistochemical analysis in cultured LNSCs is displayed ($n = 3$ per donor group; healthy individuals, RA-risk ACPA− individuals, RA-risk APCA+ individuals, RA ACPA− patients and RA ACPA+ patients, passages 3–11). The larger bar in the left corner of images represents 200 µm and the smaller bar inside the magnified images in (**A**) represents 20 µm.

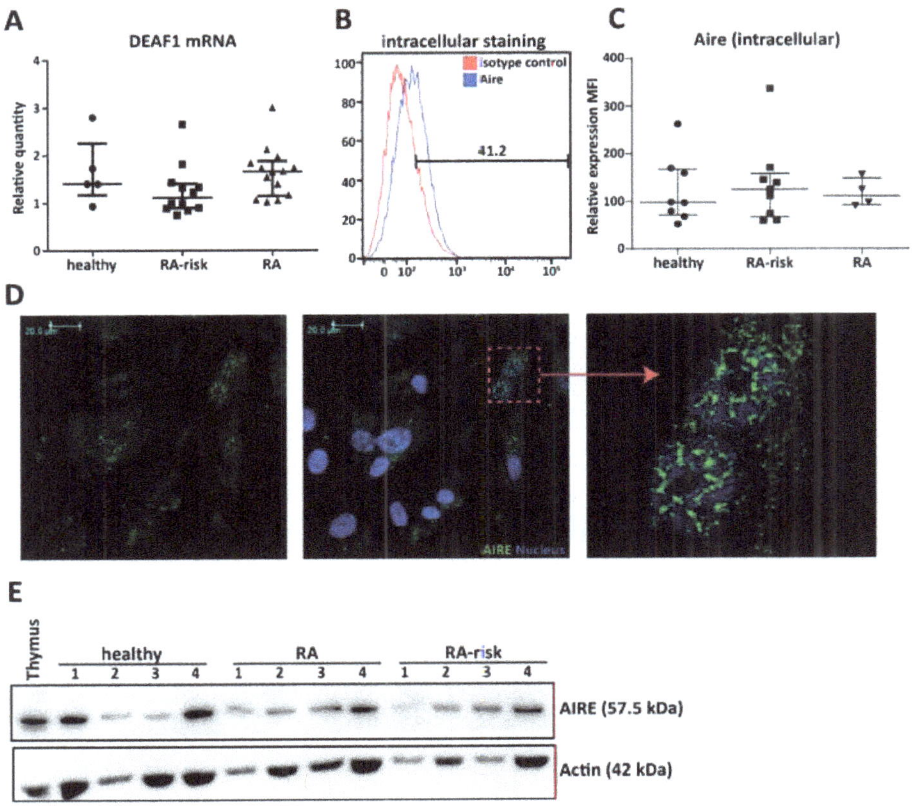

Figure 2. Expression of the peripheral tissue antigen (PTA) driving transcription factors autoimmune regulator (AIRE) and deformed epidermal autoregulatory factor 1 (DEAF1) in human LNSCs. (**A**) Expression of DEAF1 in cultured LNSCs of passage 2 was assessed by qPCR and compared between different donor groups (healthy individuals $n = 5$, RA-risk individuals $n = 12$ and RA patients $n = 14$). Relative quantity is displayed as median and interquartile range. (**B**) Intracellular expression of AIRE protein in cultured LNSCs was measured by flow cytometry. Histograms presenting % of positive cells in comparison to isotype staining. (**C**) The scatter plot represents the mean fluorescence intensity (MFI) of intracellular AIRE expression in cultured human LNSCs (passages 3–5) from individuals in different donor groups (healthy individuals $n = 8$, RA-risk individuals $n = 9$ and RA patients $n = 4$). Relative quantity is presented as median and interquartile range. (**D**) Representative pictures of immunofluorescence staining combined with confocal microscopy displaying AIRE (green) and nucleus (blue) in LNSCs (RA patient; passage 3) cultured on chambers slides. Isotype controls were negative. (**E**) Western blot analysis of AIRE protein expression in cultured LNSCs of 12 donors (passages 4–8) is shown. Actin was used as loading control and thymic tissue was used as positive control for AIRE expression.

2.3. Variable Expression of Disease-Related PTAs in Human LNSCs

Given that we found the presence of the transcription factors potentially driving PTA expression in LNSCs, we next investigated the expression levels of several disease-related PTAs. We selected PTAs previously reported to be expressed by mouse LNSCs [27,28] and involved in human diseases: Ras Related Glycolysis Inhibitor and Calcium Channel Regulator (RRAD), Glutamate Decarboxylase 1 (GAD1), Proteolipid Protein 1 (PLP1), and Alpha Fetoprotein (AFP). RRAD is implicated in several cancers [36] and plays an important role in type II diabetes [37]. GAD1 is a major autoantigen in type I diabetes and highly expressed in brain and pancreas [38]. PLP1 encodes the most abundant myelin protein which is a main target of autoreactive T cells in multiple sclerosis (MS) and is detected in cervical LNs of MS patients [39]. AFP levels serve as diagnostic marker of liver injury such as hepatocellular carcinoma or Hepatitis C infection [40]. With the exception of AFP, all these disease-related PTAs were expressed by human LNSCs (passages 3 and 4) (Figure 3A). While we did not observe a significant difference in PLP1 expression by LNSCs from different donor groups, we interestingly found that GAD1 and RRAD has a variable expression pattern in LNSCs (all passage 2) derived from healthy individuals, RA-risk individuals and RA patients (healthy individuals $n = 14$, RA-risk individuals $n = 23$, and RA patients $n = 24$). RRAD was significantly expressed at a lower level in LNSCs of RA patients ($p = 0.037$), whereas GAD1 was highly expressed in LNSCs of RA-risk individuals ($p = 0.0129$) when compared to healthy individuals (Figure 3B). Furthermore, after stratification according to ACPA status, the difference in PTA expression was especially clear in ACPA negative RA patients with almost no RRAD expression in LNSCs from ACPA negative RA patients (Figure S2). The expression of these PTAs did not correlate with any other clinical parameters such as age, gender, or antibody titers.

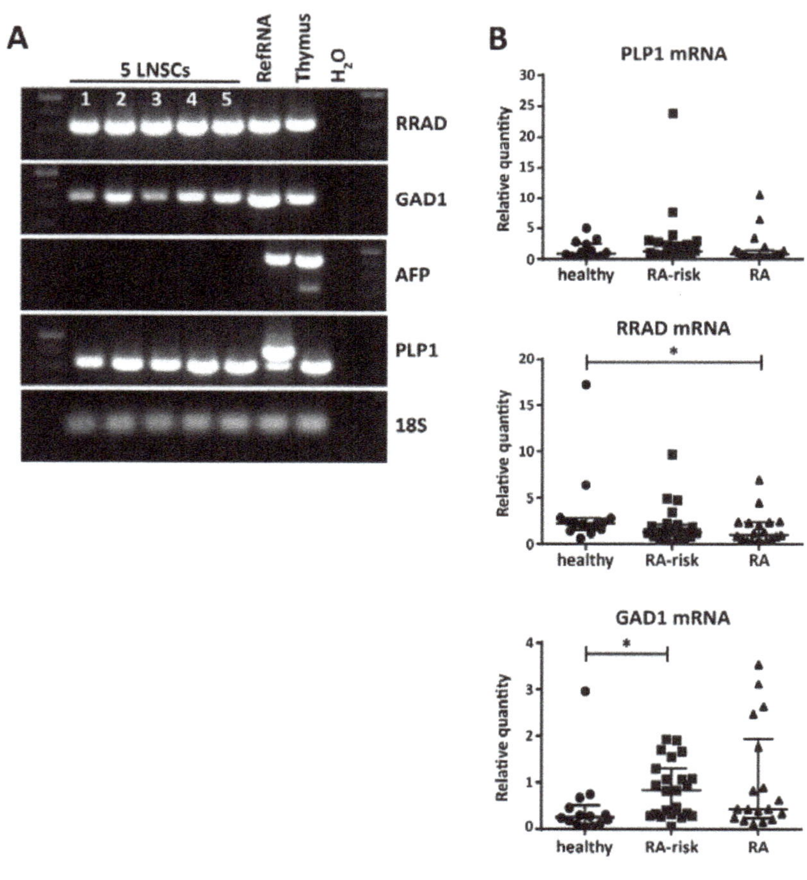

Figure 3. Expression of disease-related PTAs in human LNSCs. (**A**) mRNA expression of Ras Related Glycolysis Inhibitor and Calcium Channel Regulator (RRAD), Glutamate Decarboxylase 1 (GAD1), Proteolipid Protein 1 (PLP1), and Alpha Fetoprotein (AFP) in five LNSC individuals (1: healthy individuals passage 4; 2: RA-risk individuals passage 4; 3: RA patients passage 4; 4: RA patients passage

4; 5: RA patients passage 3) analyzed by PCR and visualized on agarose gel. cDNA prepared from an arbitrary in house-made RNA sample pool containing all human tissues (RefRNA) as well as a human thymus sample served as positive control and H_2O in exchange for cDNA as negative control. (**B**) Expression of PLP1, RRAD, and GAD1 and was assessed by qPCR in different donor groups (healthy individuals n = 14, RA-risk individuals n = 23, and RA patients n = 24, all passage 2). Relative quantity is displayed as median and interquartile range. Differences between donor groups were assessed by Kruskal–Wallis followed by a post Dunn's test. * $p < 0\ 050$.

2.4. MHC Class II Expression by Human LNSC In Vitro

Since direct antigen presentation is very difficult to study in human LNSCs due to MHC restriction and lack of high number of antigen-specific T cells recognizing PTAs, we aimed to study the machinery needed for antigen presentation and lymphocyte modulation in cultured LNSCs. Under homeostatic conditions the human leukocyte antigen-DR (HLA-DR) gene participating in the MHC class II complex, is expressed by cultured human LNSCs (all passage 2) at very low levels in all donor groups tested (Figure 4A). Of interest, a non-significant lower expression of HLA-DR was observed in cultured LNSCs obtained from RA-risk individuals and RA patients. We next used interferon γ (IFNγ) to study regulation of MHC class II as previously reported in mice and humans [26,29]. HLA-DR mRNA was strongly increased after 24 and 48 h of stimulation, when compared to unstimulated (US), with no significant differences between donor groups, though induction was highly variable between donors (Figure 4B, n = 5 per donor group). On protein level, HLA-DR was strongly increased after 72 h of IFNγ stimulation (Figure 4C,D). Interestingly, next to FRCs (Podoplanin+, CD31−) also DNs (Podoplanin−, CD31−) clearly upregulated MHC class II. Podoplanin expression was not influenced by IFNγ stimulation (Figure 4C). Furthermore, the number of FRCs and DNs was similar between donor groups (Figure 4D) and within these two subsets HLA-DR expression was similarly increased in all donor groups although a large inter-donor variation in induction was observed (Figure 4E, healthy individuals n = 5, RA-risk individuals n = 4, and RA patients n = 3). These findings did not correlate with clinical parameters such as age, gender, or antibody titers. Overall, these data suggest that human FRCs as well as DNs are equipped to potentially present antigens to CD4+ T cells.

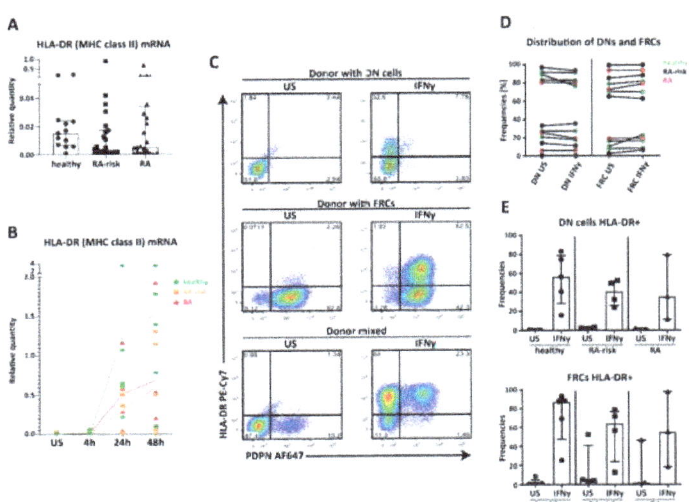

Figure 4. Expression of human leukocyte antigen-DR (HLA-DR) (major histocompatibility complex (MHC) class II) in cultured human LNSCs. (**A**) Expression of HLA-DR mRNA in cultured human LNSCs

(all passage 2) from healthy individuals, RA-risk individuals, and RA patients. (**B**) Induction of HLA-DR was assessed by qPCR after stimulation with interferon γ (IFNγ) at different time points (unstimulated (US), 4, 24, and 48 h, all passage 2). Data are represented as relative quantity in each donor (dot) measured over time, where the line indicates the median expression level within one study group over time. (**C**) Flow cytometry gating strategy used to identify CD45− stromal cells according to their Podoplanin (PDPN) and HLA-DR (MHC class II) expression. Gating was based on negative isotype staining. FACS plots display cultured LNSCs from three representative donors (double negative (DN) cells derived from RA-risk individuals passage 5, fibroblastic reticular cells (FRCs) from RA patients passage 7, and LNSCs from healthy individuals passage 5 containing DN and FRCs) out of 13 individuals tested (healthy individuals $n = 5$, RA-risk individuals $n = 5$, and RA patients $n = 3$). Dot blot shows their expression profile under unstimulated condition versus stimulation for 72 h with IFNγ. Numbers adjacent to the outlined areas indicate percentage of cells in the gated population. (**D**) Frequencies of DNs and FRCs per donor under unstimulated conditions and stimulated for 72 h with IFNγ is shown. (**E**) The frequencies of HLA-DR positive cells after stimulation for 72 h with IFNγ in FRCs (PDPN+) and DN cells (PDPN−) are depicted in two separate graphs. Data are represented as median with interquartile range.

2.5. Potential Immunomodulation by Cultured Human LNSC

Next we analyzed the expression of genes potentially involved in LNSC-mediated T cell modulation, thereby we used IFNγ, which is produced by T cells upon their activation and differentiation, as a stimulus [41]. Genes analyzed in cultured LNSCs of passages 4–9 after 4, 24, and 48 h stimulation included interferon gamma receptor 1 (IFNGR1), co-stimulatory molecules cluster of differentiation 40 (CD40), CD80 and CD86 [27,42], immunosuppressive cytokines interleukin 10 (IL-10) and transforming growth factor beta 1 (TGFB1), which are both involved in T_{reg} cell induction [43,44], and the negative T cell regulators CD274 (programmed cell death 1 ligand (PD-L1)), nitric oxide synthase 2 (NOS2) and indoleamine 2,3-dioxygenase 1 (IDO1) [25,26] (Figure 5A, healthy individuals $n = 5$, RA-risk individuals $n = 5$, and RA patients $n = 5$, passages 4–9). Under homeostatic conditions no differences between donor groups were observed. IFNGR1 was stably expressed, at similar levels in all donor groups and unaffected by stimulation (Figure S3), showing that all donor groups are equally equipped to respond to IFNγ. TGFB1 was strongly expressed under homeostatic conditions and not strongly affected by IFNγ (Figure 5A). In contrast, IL-10 was not detected by qPCR. For the co-stimulatory molecules, we found that CD40 was strongly expressed and slightly induced at 24 h, while expression of CD80 was very low and CD86 was undetectable (Figure 5A). On the other hand, the negative regulators CD274 (PD-L1), NOS2, and IDO1 strongly responded to IFNγ, with CD274 (PD-L1) and NOS2 expression peaking at 4 h and IDO1 at 24 h (Figure 5A). Furthermore, at protein level we could detect CD40 by flow cytometry on cultured human LNSCs and expression was upregulated after 72 h stimulation with IFNγ (Figure 5B) though no significant differences between donor groups were observed (passages 4–9) (Figure 5C). Finally, none of these findings reported here on mRNA or protein level correlated with any clinical parameter such as age, gender, or autoantibody titers. Overall, these data show that human LNSCs have the capacity to modulate the adaptive immunity.

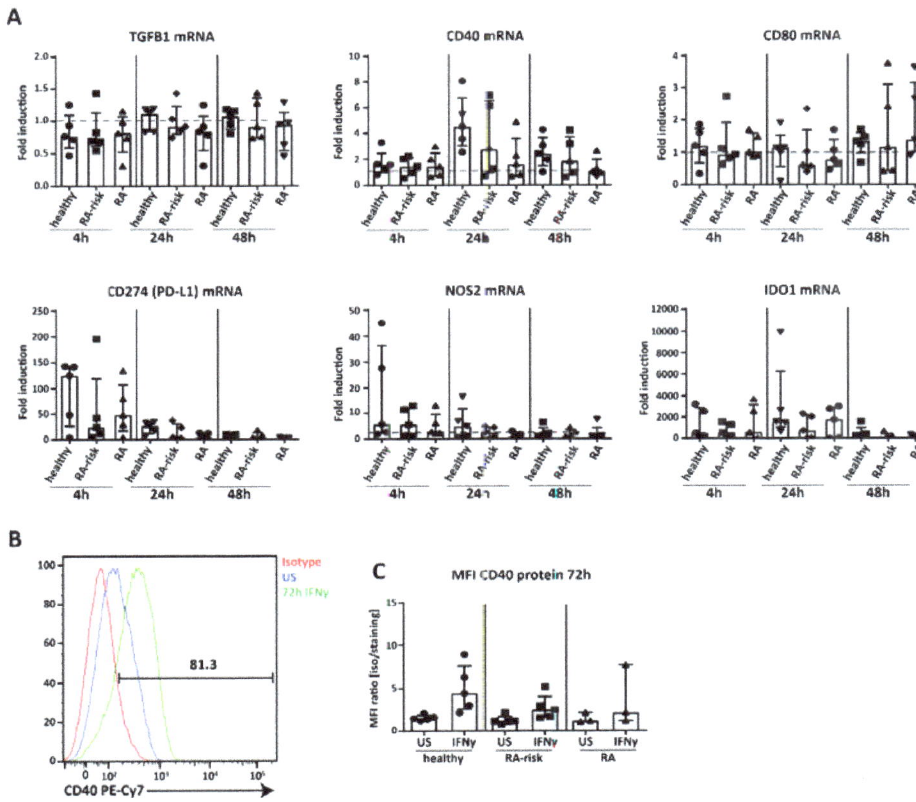

Figure 5. Expression of immunomodulatory molecules in cultured human LNSCs. (**A**) Induction of transforming growth factor beta 1 (TGFB1) CD40, CD80, CD274 (PD-L1; programmed cell death 1 ligand), nitric oxide synthase 2 (NOS2), and indoleamine 2,3-dioxygenase 1 (IDO1) was assessed by qPCR in cultured LNSCs (passages 4–9) after stimulation with IFNγ at different time points (4, 24, and 48 h). Data are represented as fold induction (median with interquartile range) by comparing the mRNA levels in stimulated cells to corresponding unstimulated cells in 15 donors (n = 5 per donor group). The dotted line represents a fold induction of 1. (**B**) CD40 protein expression was measured by flow cytometry in CD45− stromal cells. Histogram depicts the increase in staining between isotype, unstimulated and stimulated for 72 h with IFNγ and is displayed for one representative donor (RA-risk individuals passage 8) out of 13 donors tested. (**C**) Induction of CD40 protein upon stimulation with IFNγ for 72 h is further presented as Mean Fluorescent Intensity (MFI) ratio (isotype/staining) in all donors measured (healthy individuals n = 5, RA-risk individuals n = 5, and RA patients n = 3, passages 4–9).

2.6. Ex Vivo Human LNSCs Express HLA-DR and Low Level of Co-Stimulatory and Co-Inhibitory Molecules

Finally, we acquired larger pieces of human LNs from kidney transplant recipients which enabled the directly ex vivo analysis of HLA-DR, co-stimulatory, and co-inhibitory molecules on human LNSCs in comparison to DCs (live CD45+CD11c+) as classical antigen presenting cells. In line with murine LNs [31,45], the human LN stromal compartment consists of four distinct subsets when gated on live CD45− cells and additional staining for CD31 and PDPN, thereby considering the PDPN+ population as one population containing FRCs, MRCs, as well as FDCs (Figure 6A,B). However, we observed more BECs and DNs in human LNs compared to mice [31,45]. HLA-DR was expressed on all subsets of human LNSCs but at different levels and considerably lower than DCs (Figure 6C,D). The MFI of HLA-DR in FRCs, LECs, and BECs was higher than DNs which is comparable to MHC-II expression described for murine LNSCs (Figure 6C,D) [31]. Similar to cultured human LNSCs (Figure 5A), co-stimulatory ligand CD80 was detected on freshly digested LNs at protein level in which the expression was relatively higher on LECs compared to other subsets. Furthermore, we could detect low levels of CD86 surface expression on different subsets of LNSCs while we were unable to detect the CD86 at mRNA level in cultured stromal cells (Figure 6C,D). CD40 expression was present on all the subsets and at lower levels than DCs (Figure 6C,D). The expression level of PD-L1+ on endothelial cells (LECs and BECs) was equivalent to DCs but lower on FRCs and DNs. These data noticeably show that ex vivo LNSCs possess HLA-DR, co-stimulatory and co-inhibitory molecules.

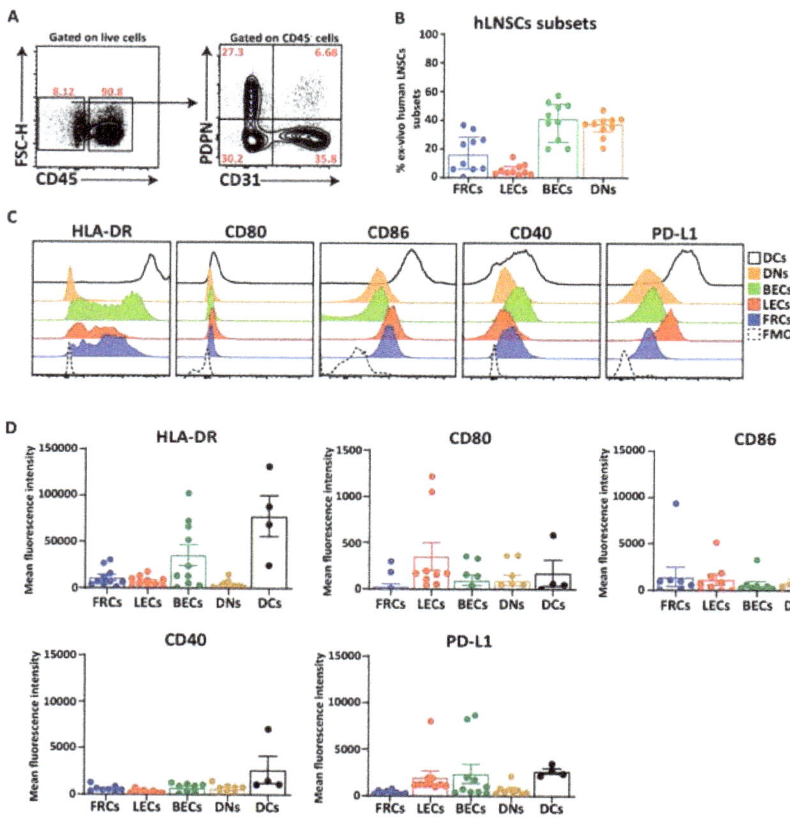

Figure 6. Expression of HLA-DR and co-stimulatory molecules on freshly isolated human LNSCs. (**A**) Human LNs obtained from kidney transplantation recipients were enzymatically digested, and stained for LNSC subsets based on the expression of CD31 and Podoplanin (PDPN) when gated on live CD45− cells. (**B**) Scatter plot represents the frequencies of different subsets of human LNSCs (hLNSCs) directly after digestion. (**C**) Stromal cells were gated as live CD45− cells and expression of co-stimulatory and inhibitory molecules on different subclasses of LNSCs and CD45+CD11c+ dendritic cells (DCs) were assessed using flow cytometry. Histograms show the expression of indicated molecules on different stromal cell subsets and DCs. The fluorescence minus one (FMO) was used as negative control. (**D**) Scatter plots represent mean fluorescence intensity of HLA-DR, CD80, CD86, CD40, and PD-L1 of each subset of LNSCs when gated on live CD45− cells in comparison to DCs. Data are represented as mean with SEM (n = 3–10 kidney recipients).

3. Discussion

Herein we demonstrate for the first time that PADI2 and PADI4 enzymes as well as citrullinated proteins targeted by ACPAs are present in human LN tissue as well as in cultured human LNSCs during health and different phases of RA. Furthermore, we show that human LNSCs express certain PTAs as well as transcription factors AIRE and DEAF1 together with molecules involved in antigen presentation and immunomodulation. Of interest, our data points towards an altered LN microenvironment in RA patients compared to healthy individuals as seen by variable expression levels of some PTAs.

Citrullination occurs during life under homeostatic conditions but increases in many tissues during inflammation [46]. With PADIs and citrullinated proteins observed in healthy individuals, ACPA-negative and ACPA-positive LN tissue, and cultured LNSCs, our data clearly reveals that citrullination is on-going in human LNs and that this process occurs in both healthy individuals and RA patients' LNSCs. However, a deeper conclusion cannot be drawn since the antibodies used are reactive to several citrullinated targets [47] and we only investigated a small number of donors in this explorative study.

In the context of peripheral tolerance by LNSCs we confirm expression of DEAF1 and AIRE, with AIRE protein being localized primarily nuclear [11] with some cytosolic AIRE as reported in other mammalian cells [48]. Furthermore, we observed a differential expression pattern of disease-related PTAs in LNSCs of RA-risk individuals and RA patients. Of interest, these differences were especially pronounced in LNSCs derived from ACPA negative individuals, which form potentially a genetically distinct patient group [49]. Expression of RRAD was found to be significantly lower in LNSCs of RA patients compared to healthy individuals. At first glance there is no link to autoimmunity since RRAD overexpression is associated with type II diabetes [37,50], which is caused by acquired insulin resistance. However, RA is an important risk factor [51] for this type of diabetes, possibly due to RA-driven inflammation [52]. Since it has been shown that murine LNSCs can control the formation of autoreactive T cells by presenting specific PTA in the context of MHC molecules [27,32,53], it is possible to speculate that LNSCs obtained from RA patients are not capable of suppressing RRAD-specific T cells due to lower expression of this PTA. Although the limitation of our study is the low number of PTAs we analyzed. Investigating the expression of various PTAs by LNSCs from RA patients will be of interest in future studies to confirm this observation. Moreover, further experiments showing antigen presentation and tolerance induction by human LNSCs are necessary, though highly challenging to conduct. So far, we lack the knowledge on well-defined PTA presented by human LNSCs and the availability of corresponding autoreactive human T cells. However, recently a multi-tetramer assay has been developed to detect citrulline-specific T cells in both healthy individuals and RA patients [54]. These tetramers might allow us to study tolerance capacity of LNSCs in controlling citrulline-specific T cells using our in vitro model containing expanded human LNSCs.

Our data reveal that both ex vivo and in vitro, human LNSCs might have the potential to present PTAs directly as they strongly express HLA-DR especially after stimulation with IFNγ. Of interest, our study shows that human FRCs, and also DNs have equal capacity to induce HLA-DR, pointing towards potentially similar roles of these two subsets in humans [21]. However, studies in mice diverge on whether LNSCs present directly to CD4+ T cells. Two studies promoted direct presentation [31,55] and shuttling MHC class II-peptide complexes from DCs [29], while another group showed that LNSCs shuttle antigens to DCs and do not induce tolerance themselves [30]. Similarly, in humans, LECs were able to process antigens, but failed to induce allogeneic CD4+ T cell proliferation [26]. Since LNSCs needed several weeks to grow to confluence and did not contain CD45 positive hematopoietic cells such as DCs, we can conclude that human LNSCs express MHC class II themselves. Accordingly, our ex vivo analyses reveal that human LNSCs express low level HLA-DR in comparison to DCs. Furthermore, the antibody L243 used to stain MHC class II molecules detects a conformational epitope on HLA-DR$\alpha\beta$ which depends on the peptide-loading and consequent correct folding of the $\alpha\beta$ heterodimer [56], indicating the presence of functional MHC class II molecules containing peptides on the LNSC cell membrane. Nonetheless, this culture technique for human LNSCs provides a robust basis for applying modern techniques in future research to identify MHC class loaded peptides on LNSCs by mass spectrometry [57] or reverse immunology using bioinformatics [58].

Next to possible antigen presentation by LNSCs, we demonstrated in this study that human LNSCs possess an arsenal of immunomodulatory molecules both in vitro on cultured human LNSCs and ex vivo on freshly isolated human LNSCs. As previously reported, PD-L1 expression is mostly restricted to endothelial cells (LECs and BECs) on freshly isolated human LN [59]. Similarly, our data also showed that PD-L1 protein expression was higher on endothelial cells in comparison to FRCs and DNs. Interestingly, at mRNA level we could detect low level of PD-L1 and HLA-DR in cultured stromal cells and the expression was lower in RA-risk individuals and RA patients compared with healthy individuals, but future studies are needed to confirm this. Moreover, our data reveal very low levels of co-stimulatory molecules CD80, CD86, and CD40 expression on freshly isolated human LNSCs. This is interesting since tolerogenic DCs possess a low level of costimulatory molecules and therefore can control autoreactive T cells. From these observations we can conclude that human LNSCs have the machinery to interact and influence lymphocytes and therefore to potentially regulate tolerance and adaptive immunity.

Overall, our explorative study shows for the first time citrullination in human LNSCs targeted by autoantibodies isolated from RA patients. Further challenging mechanistic studies are required to investigate whether LNSCs from RA (-risk) patients have an altered tolerogenic effect on autoreactive T cells. To study LNSCs immunoregulatory function, in vitro expansion of LNSCs is required, which is a limitation of this study. The difficulty of obtaining LN biopsies from a large number of individuals and the slow growth rate of human LNSCs limits the number of donors analyzed in this study. In addition, the variation between donors is high. However, by revealing that human LNSCs exhibit the tools to induce tolerance as observed in mice, they become an attractive new therapeutic target to exploit in tolerance maintenance and induction.

4. Material and Methods

4.1. Study Individuals and Lymph Node Needle Biopsy Sampling

Individuals with arthralgia and elevated IgM-RF and/or ACPA levels, but without any evidence of arthritis upon examination were included (RA-risk individuals, phase c/d upon examination were included (RA-risk individuals, phase c/d; n= 23 [8]). Median follow up time of RA-risk individuals was 20.3 months (12.9–33.2 (IQR)) and none of the RA-risk individuals developed arthritis during this period. RA-risk individuals were not allowed to have systemic or intra-articular corticosteroid injection less than 28 days before enrolment. In addition, RA patients with established disease based on fulfillment of the American College of Rheumatology and European League Against Rheumatism (ACR/EULAR 2010 [60] criteria and as assessed by the rheumatologist were included (n = 24). Healthy individuals without any joint complaints and without elevated IgM-RF and/or ACPA level and without active viral infection or any history of autoimmunity or malignancy and no present or previous use of disease-modifying antirheumatic drugs (DMARDs), biologicals, or other experimental drugs served as the (voluntary) control group (n = 14). IgM-RF was measured using IgM-RF ELISA (Hycor Biomedical, Indianapolis, IN, USA) (ULN (upper limit of normal) 49 kU/mL)). ACPA was measured using anti-CCP2 ELISA CCPlus (Eurodiagnostica, Nijmegen, The Netherlands (ULN 25 kAU/L)). The study was performed according to the principles of the Declaration of Helsinki, approved by the institutional medical ethical review board of the Academic Medical Center (Ethical permission: NL20951.018.07, date: 25 February 2008 and NL52469.018.15, date: 17 July 2015), and all study individuals gave written informed consent. All study individuals underwent an ultrasound-guided inguinal LN needle core biopsy as previously described [61]. At the day of LN sampling none of the donors showed signs of an infection. Table 1 shows the demographics of the included individuals.

Table 1. Demographic data of study participants.

Variables	Healthy	RA-Risk	RA
Sex (female) (*n*) (%)	9 (64)	20 (87)	17 (70)
Age (years) (median (IQR))	29 (26–37) †	49 (35–57)	56 (44–61)
IgM-RF positive (*n*) (%)	0 (0)	10 (43)	20 (3–107)
IgM-RF level (kU/mL) (median (IQR))	—	20 (3–107)	131 (31–309)
ACPA positive (*n*) (%)	0 (0)	13 (57)	18 (75)
ACPA level (kAU/L) (median (IQR))	—	43 (4–177)	115 (21–924)
IgM-RF and ACPA both positive (*n*) (%)	0 (0)	0 (0)	14 (58)
DAS28 (median (IQR))	—	—	5 (1–10) [a,b]
ESR (mm/h) (median (IQR))	—	7 (2–10)	11 (5–27) [c]
CRP (mg/L) (median (IQR))	0.5 (0.3–1.2) [a]	1.6 (0.9–3.2)	4.6 (1.4–13) [d]
68TJC (median (IQR))	0 (0)	1.5 (0–4.5)	9 (4–20) [e]
68SJC (median (IQR))	0 (0)	0 (0)	5 (1–10) [d]
Treatment (*n*) (%)			9 (39)
Corticoids			6 (26)
NSAID			4 (17) [f]
DMARD			5 (22)
Failed TNF inhibitor therapy			5 (22)

IgM-RF, IgM rheumatoid factor; ACPA, anti-citrullinated protein antibodies; ESR, erythrocyte sedimentation rate; CRP, C-reactive protein; TJC, tender joint count; NSAID, non-steroidal anti-inflammatory drug; DMARD, disease-modifying antirheumatic drugs. [a] levels missing from one individual, [b] levels missing from two individuals, [c] levels missing from six individuals, [d] levels missing from seven individuals, [e] levels missing from five individuals, [f] treatment unknown for five individuals. † Healthy individuals are significantly younger than RA-risk individuals and RA patients ($p < 0.0050$, tested by Kruskal–Wallis followed by a post Dunn's test).

4.2. Lymph Node Collection and Processing from Kidney Transplantation Recipients

LNs were collected from surgical residual material of kidney transplantation recipients ($n = 10$) during implantation of the kidney. Before anastomosing the arteria and vena renalis, the iliac artery and vein were dissected free. The resulting residual tissue that was removed in this procedure often contains LNs. Though all patients were treated with a quadruple immunosuppressive therapy, only the first dose of CD25mAb was administered before the procedure and we have demonstrated that CD25mAb (basiliximab; Novartis Pharma, Amsterdam, The Netherlands) was not detectable in LN cells and that ex vivo CD25 expression on cells could be blocked with CD25mAb [62]. LNs were carefully cleaned of fat and connective tissue, then cut into small pieces (< 0.5 cm) after which a cell suspension was obtained by grinding the material through a flow-through chamber. The remaining tissue stroma was used in this study and digested as described before [45] to isolate and analyze LNSCs directly ex vivo. In summary, LN stroma was digested using the enzymatic mixture of 0.2 mg/mL collagenase *p* (Roche, Woerden, The Netherlands), 0.8 mg/mL Dispase II (Roche, Woerden, The Netherlands), and 0.1 mg/mL DNAse I (Roche, Woerden, The Netherlands) in RPMI medium (Invitrogen, Landsmeer, The Netherlands) without serum. Cell suspensions were filtered through a 70-µm nylon cell strainer and directly stained for flow cytometry.

4.3. Lymph Node Stromal Cell Culture and Stimulation

LNSC culture was performed as previously described [63,64]. In short, after depletion of lymphocytes through a 70 µm cell strainer (BD Falcon, San Jose, CA, USA) the remaining stromal tissue of a freshly collected LN needle core biopsy was plated on a 6-well culture dish (Greiner CELLSTAR®, Sigma Aldrich, Zwijndrecht, The Netherlands) (passage 0; P0). Complete cell culture medium was added which consists of Dulbecco's Modified Eagle Medium (DMEM) low glucose (Gibco, Bleiswijk, The Netherlands) supplemented with 0.1% penicillin (Astellas Pharma Inc, Leiden, The Netherlands), 0.1% streptomycin, 0.05 mg/mL gentamicin, 10 mM HEPES buffer, 2 mM L-glutamine (all Gibco, Bleiswijk, The Netherlands), and 10% fetal calf serum (FCS) (GE Healthcare, Zeist, The Netherlands). To expand cell numbers and for passaging, cultured monolayers of human LNSCs were treated with trypsin (0.05% trypsin/5 mM ethylenediaminetetraacetic acid (Thermo Fisher Scientific, Landsmeer, The Netherlands)) in phosphate buffer saline (PBS, Fresenius Kabi Nederland BV, Zeist, The Netherlands) for 7 min at 37 °C. For harvesting, cells were washed with sterile PBS, trypsinized and the cell suspension was collected and centrifuged for 10 min, 1000 rpm (212 g) at 4 °C. Cells were resuspended in cold complete medium and counted using trypan blue (Sigma Aldrich) in a Bürker-Türk chamber (LO Labor Optik, Lancing, UK). Subsequently, human LNSCs were seeded for different experiments. For flow cytometry LNSCs were plated in a 6-well plate (100,000–200,000/well) and stimulated with 50 ng/mL IFNγ (Affymetrix eBioscience, Landsmeer, The Netherlands). For real-time PCR analysis LNSCs were seeded in a 24-well plate (30,000/well) and stimulated with 10 ng/mL IFNγ. For chamber slides (Thermo Fisher Scientific, Landsmeer, The Netherlands) 5000 LNSCs/well were used. As described previously, this ex vivo LNSC culture model contains a mixture of FRCs and DNs [64].

4.4. Immunohistochemical Analysis and (Confocal) Microscopy

LN needle biopsies were snap frozen in Tissue-Tek OCT (Thermo Fisher Scientific, Landsmeer, The Netherlands), cryostat sectioned (7 µm), and stored at −80 °C till further use. Before staining, sections were fixed for 20 min using 2% formaldehyde (Sigma-Aldrich, Zwijndrecht, The Netherlands). Cultured LNSCs were plated out (5000/well) in chamber slides (Thermo Fisher Scientific, Landsmeer, The Netherlands), rested for 24 h in complete medium, washed, fixed with cold methanol (Sigma Aldrich, Zwijndrecht, The Netherlands) for 10 min, and stored at −80 °C till further use. LNSCs on chamber slides were blocked with 1% H_2O_2 (Sigma Aldrich, Zwijndrecht, The Netherlands) and 20% human serum (Akademiska pharmacy, Stockholm, Sweden). The following antibodies were generated at the Karolinska Institutet as previously described [35]: human biotinylated monoclonal ACPAs (1325:04C03 = C03, 1325:01B09 = B09) are second generation validated ACPAs as described in Steen et al. [35]. A human biotinylated concentration-matched antibody (E02, reactive against tetanus) was used as a non-ACPA control antibody. Furthermore, in this study rabbit polyclonal anti-PADI2 (Cosmo Bio, Tokyo, Japan), mouse monoclonal anti-PADI4 (Abcam, Cambridge, UK) and corresponding isotype controls were used. Slides were incubated overnight in a moist chamber at 4 °C with the primary/detection antibodies. The next day, slides were first blocked with 1% normal goat serum (Dako, Stockholm, Sweden) and then incubated for 30 min with either biotin-conjugated goat anti-mouse secondary antibody (Invitrogen, Stockholm, Sweden) or a biotin anti-rabbit IgG (H + L) (Vector Laboratories, Stockholm, Sweden). Staining was performed using the VECTASTAIN Elite ABC kit (Vector Laboratories, Stockholm, Sweden) and visualized with 3,3-diaminobenzidine (DAB, Vector Laboratories, Stockholm, Sweden). Slides were counterstained with Mayer's hematoxylin (Sigma Aldrich Zwijndrecht, The Netherlands), permanently mounted and viewed by a light microscope (Reichert Polyvar 2 type 302001, Leica Microsystems, Wetzlar, Germany). Sections of LN tissue were scored by two independent researchers with a scale ranging from 0 to 4 with 0 = no signal and 4 = very strong signal. For AIRE staining, LNSCs on chamber slides were blocked and permeabilized with PBS buffer containing 3% bovine serum albumin (BSA) and 0.3% Triton (both Sigma Aldrich, Zwijndrecht, The Netherlands) for 30 min and then incubated overnight at 4 °C with monoclonal mouse IgG1 anti-human AIRE antibody (Santa Cruz, Huissen, The Netherlands) or control mouse IgG1 antibody (Dako, Amstelveen, The Netherlands). Subsequently, secondary anti-mouse IgG1-AlexaFluor488 (Invitrogen, Landsmeer, The Netherlands) was used for labelling and chamber slides were mounted using Vectashield Hardset (Vector Laboratories, Stockholm, Sweden). After hardening overnight staining was analyzed by confocal microscope (TCS SP8, Leica Microsystems, Wetzlar, Germany).

4.5. Flow Cytometry Analysis

Human LNSCs (passages 5–10) were harvested from a 6-well dish using 1 mL TripLE™ Select (Gibco, Bleiswijk, The Netherlands) for 10 min at 37 °C. Subsequently, cells were washed in PBA buffer (PBS containing 0.01% NaN3 and 0.5% BSA (Sigma Aldrich, Zwijndrecht, The Netherlands), and stained for 1 h with rat IgG2a anti-human Podoplanin (clone NZ-1, AngioBio, Huissen, The Netherlands) on ice. Afterwards cells were washed again in PBS buffer, followed by a second incubation for 30 min on ice protected from light using the following directly labelled antibodies: polyclonal goat anti-rat IgG AlexaFluor647 (Invitrogen, Landsmeer, The Netherlands), CD45 FITC (clone HI30, Becton Dickinson (BD) Pharmingen, Vianen, The Netherlands), CD80 PE (clone 2D10.4, eBioscience, Landsmeer, The Netherlands), CD274 (PD-L1) BV421 (clone MIH1, BD Biosciences, Vianen, The Netherlands), HLA-DR PE-Cy7 (clone L243, Sony Biotechnology, Surrey, UK), and CD40 PE-Cy7 (clone 5C3, Sony Biotechnology, Surrey, UK) or with corresponding isotype control antibodies. Staining with HLA-ABC PE-Cy7 (clone G46–2.6, Biolegend, London, UK) served as a positive control and was used to set-up the correct compensation configuration settings. To assess the HLA-DR and co-stimulatory expression on human LNSCs directly ex vivo, freshly isolated cells were stained with eBioscience™ Fixable Viability Dye eFluor™ 780 (Invitrogen, Landsmeer, The Netherlands) for 15 min, followed by 10 min blocking in PBS containing 5% normal human serum and 2% FCS (Biowest) on ice in the dark. The cells were then incubated with CD45 eFlour 450 (MI30, Invitrogen, Landsmeer, The Netherlands), CD11c Alexa 700 (Bu15, Biolegend, London, UK), HLA-DR PE (clone L243, Invitrogen, Landsmeer, The Netherlands), CD80 Pe-Cy7 (clone 2D10, Biolegend, London, UK), CD86 Pe-Cy5 (clone IT2.2, Biolegend, London, UK), CD40 PerCP/Cy5.5 (clone 5C3, Biolegend, London, UK), PD-L1 BV711 (clone 29E.2A3, Biolegend, London, UK) antibodies for 30 min on ice in the dark. For staining of AIRE protein in LNSCs we used the Fixation/Permeabilization Solution Kit (BD Biosciences, Vianen, The Netherlands) to detect intranuclear expression or the Foxp3/Transcription Factor Staining Buffer Set (eBioscience, Landsmeer, The Netherlands) according to the manufacturer's instructions. Cells were stained with AIRE PE (clone 614530, R&D Systems, Minneapolis, MN, USA) and mouse IgG1 isotype control (eBioscience, Landsmeer, The Netherlands) for 30 min at RT. Cells were measured on a FACS CANTO II (BD, Vianen, The Netherlands) or a BD LSRFortessa™ X-20 (BD Biosciences, Vianen, The Netherlands) and analyzed with FlowJo software (TreeStar Inc., Ashland, OR, USA).

4.6. Quantitative Real-Time PCR and Conventional PCR

Total RNA was isolated using the RNeasy Mini kit or RNeasy Micro kit (Qiagen, Venlo, The Netherlands) according to the manufacturer's instructions, including a DNAse step to remove genomic DNA. Subsequently cDNA was prepared using the RevertAid H Minus First Strand cDNA Synthesis kit (Thermo Fisher Scientific, Landsmeer, The Netherlands). Quantitative PCR was performed using either Taqman® Universal PCR master mix combined with Taqman assays or SYBR® Green PCR master mix (all from Applied Biosystems, Life Technologies, Zwijndrecht, The Netherlands) combined with in house designed primers (Thermo Fisher Scientific, Landsmeer, The Netherlands). Taqman assays and primer sequences are described in Table S1. For detection we used a StepOnePlus™ Real-Time PCR System or the QuantStudio 3 (Applied Biosystems, Life Technologies, Zwijndrecht, The Netherlands). Values for each target gene were normalized by the expression level of 18S RNA. An arbitrary calibrator sample was used to correct for inter-plate differences. For calculating the relative quantity (RQ) the delta-delta Ct method was used for Taqman assays and a standard curve method was applied for SYBR green assays. An arbitrary calibrator sample was used to correct for inter-plate differences. The fold induction was calculated using the following formula: (RQ stimulated / RQ unstimulated).

For conventional PCR we used the GoTaq DNA, GoTaq green reaction buffer and dNTPs (Promega, Leiden, The Netherlands), and the Biometra T-gradient Thermoblock (Analytic Jena, Jena, Germany) with the following program: denaturation step 3 min at 95 °C, then cycle of 40 times of 30 s 95 °C followed by 30 s at 61 °C and elongation for 45 s at 72 °C and finally 2 min at 72 °C. As positive controls we used an in house made arbitrary RNA sample containing a mixture of RNA isolated from all human tissues (kindly provided by Dr. Huitinga from The Netherlands Institute for Neuroscience) as well as RNA from human thymus tissue (kindly provided by the Pathology department of the AMC, Amsterdam, The Netherlands). Samples were loaded on a 1.5% agarose gel (Invitrogen, Landsmeer,

The Netherlands) and mRNA expression was visualized using gel imager Gene Flash (Syngene, Amsterdam, the Netherlands).

4.7. Western Blot

Approximately 300,000 LNSCs were collected in 50 μL of radioimmunoprecipitation assay (RIPA) buffer (Bioke, Leiden, The Netherlands) supplemented with leupeptin (1 μL/mL, Sigma Aldrich, Zwijndrecht, The Netherlands), pepstatin A (1 μL/mL, Sigma Aldrich, Zwijndrecht, The Netherlands), and PMSF (phenylmethanesulfonyl fluoride, 4 μL/mL, Sigma Aldrich, Zwijndrecht, The Netherlands) and were stored at −80 °C till further use. After thawing, protein concentration was measured using Pierce BCA protein assay kit (Thermo Fisher Scientific, Landsmeer, The Netherlands). Then, 10 μg of each sample, diluted in NuPAGE reducing agent and NuPAGE LDC buffer (Thermo Fisher Scientific, Landsmeer, The Netherlands) was loaded into a NuPAGE 4–12% gradient gel together with a Protein Molecular Weight Marker (Odyssey® One-Color, LI-COR, Bad Homburg, Germany). Gel was run in MES buffer (Thermo Fisher Scientific, Landsmeer, The Netherlands) for 1 h at 200 V. Subsequently, proteins were transferred onto a PVDF membrane (Immobilon-FL, Merck Millipore, Amsterdam, The Netherlands) for 70 min at 30 V. For washing TBST buffer (50 mM Tris, 150 nM NaCl, 0.1% Tween 20) was used and after blocking of membrane with 5% Blotting-Grade Blocker (Bio-Rad, Veenendaal, The Netherlands), the membrane was incubated with monoclonal mouse IgG1 anti human AIRE (1:500) or polyclonal goat IgG anti human Actin (1:2000) (both Santa Cruz, Huissen, The Netherlands) overnight at 4 °C. The next day the membrane was washed and incubated with anti-mouse or anti-rabbit secondary antibodies conjugated with horseradish peroxidase (HRP) (both 1:2000, both Dako, Stockholm, Sweden) and were visualized using the HRP substrate Lumi-Light Plus (Roche, Woerden, The Netherlands). Blot was analyzed using ImageQuant LAS4000 (GE Healthcare, Zeist, The Netherlands).

4.8. Statistics

Data are presented as median with interquartile range (IQR) or mean with standard deviation when normally distributed. Differences between the study groups were analyzed using Kruskal–Wallis test followed by a post-hoc Dunn's test or a two-way ANOVA test followed by Dunnett's multiple comparison test, where appropriate. GraphPad Prism software (V.7.01, La Jolla, CA, USA) was used for statistical analysis. p-values < 0.05 were considered statistically significant.

Supplementary Materials: The following are available online at http://www.mdpi.com/1422-0067/21/16/5713/s1. Figure S1: Intranuclear staining of Aire protein in cultured human LNSCs; Figure S2: Expression of RRAD and GAD1 stratified according to ACPA status; Figure S3: Induction of IFNGR1 after stimulation with IFNγ in human LNSCs; Table S1: Primers used in this study.

Author Contributions: Conceptualization, D.M.G., P.P.T. and L.G.M.v.B.; methodology, J.S.H., R.N., T.A.d.J. and J.F.S.; validation, J.S.H., R.N. and L.G.M.v.B.; formal analysis, J.S.H., R.N. and T.A.d.J.; data curation, J.S.H., R.N., T.A.d.J. and J.F.S.; writing—original draft preparation, J.S.H. and R.N.; writing—review and editing, J.S.H., R.N., T.A.d.J., J.F.S., E.B.M.R., M.S., K.P.v.L., M.M., R.E.M., H.W., A.I.C. and L.G.M.v.B.; supervision, R.E.M. and L.G.M.v.B.; funding acquisition, R.E.M. and L.G.M.v.B.; All authors have read and agreed to the published version of the manuscript.

Funding: This work was supported by the Innovative Medicines Initiative European Union IMI EU funded project BeTheCure (nr115142), FP7 HEALTH program under the grant agreement FP7-HEALTH-F2-2012-305549 (Euro-TEAM), Dutch Arthritis Foundation grant 11-1-308 and 14-2-403 and The Netherlands Organisation for Health Research and Development (ZonMw) Veni project 91612109 and VIDI project 91718371.

Acknowledgments: We thank the study participants in the study, the radiology department at the AMC for LN sampling, F.J. Bemelman (department of Nephrology, AMC) for the collection of LNs from renal transplantation patients, the flow cytometry facility at the Haematology department at AMC especially J.A. Dobber and the AMC Rheumatology department, especially M.J.H. de Hair and M. Safy for patient recruitment, G. Rikken and D. Drop for sample processing and Y. de Wit for western blot experiment. We thank V. Malmström and L. Klareskog for the design and production of the antibodies used in this study and M. Engström and V. Balasingh of the Karolinska Institutet for their help with experiments and interpretation of data.

Conflicts of Interest: The authors declare no conflict of interest.

References

1. England, B.R.; Thiele, G.M.; Mikuls, T.R. Anticitrullinated protein antibodies: Origin and role in the pathogenesis of rheumatoid arthritis. *Curr. Opin. Rheumatol.* **2017**, *29*, 57–64. [CrossRef] [PubMed]
2. Pollard, L.; Choy, E.H.; Scott, D.L. The consequences of rheumatoid arthritis: Quality of life measures in the individual patient. *Clin. Exp. Rheumatol.* **2005**, *23*, S43–S52. [PubMed]
3. Valesini, G.; Gerardi, M.C.; Iannuccelli, C.; Pacucci, V.A.; Pendolino, M.; Shoenfeld, Y. Citrullination and autoimmunity. *Autoimmun. Rev.* **2015**, *14*, 490–497. [CrossRef] [PubMed]
4. Foulquier, C.; Sebbag, M.; Clavel, C.; Chapuy-Regaud, S.; Al Badine, R.; Mechin, M.C.; Vincent, C.; Nachat, R.; Yamada, M.; Takahara, H.; et al. Peptidyl arginine deiminase type 2 (PAD-2) and PAD-4 but not PAD-1, PAD-3, and PAD-6 are expressed in rheumatoid arthritis synovium in close association with tissue inflammation. *Arthritis Rheum.* **2007**, *56*, 3541–3553. [CrossRef] [PubMed]
5. Nielen, M.M.; van Schaardenburg, D.; Reesink, H.W.; van de Stadt, R.J.; van der Horst-Bruinsma, I.E.; de Koning, M.H.; Habibuw, M.R.; Vandenbroucke, J.P.; Dijkmans, B.A. Specific autoantibodies precede the symptoms of rheumatoid arthritis: A study of serial measurements in blood donors. *Arthritis Rheum.* **2004**, *50*, 380–386. [CrossRef]
6. De Hair, M.J.; van de Sande, M.G.; Ramwadhdoebe, T.H.; Hansson, M.; Landewe, R.; van der Leij, C.; Maas, M.; Serre, G.; van Schaardenburg, D.; Klareskog, L.; et al. Features of the synovium of individuals at risk of developing rheumatoid arthritis: Implications for understanding preclinical rheumatoid arthritis. *Arthritis Rheumatol.* **2014**, *66*, 513–522. [CrossRef]
7. Van de Sande, M.G.; de Hair, M.J.; van der Leij, C.; Klarenbeek, P.L.; Bos, W.H.; Smith, M.D.; Maas, M.; de Vries, N.; van Schaardenburg, D.; Dijkmans, B.A.; et al. Different stages of rheumatoid arthritis: Features of the synovium in the preclinical phase. *Ann. Rheum. Dis.* **2011**, *70*, 772–777. [CrossRef]
8. Gerlag, D.M.; Raza, K.; van Baarsen, L.G.; Brouwer, E.; Buckley, C.D.; Burmester, G.R.; Gabay, C.; Catrina, A.I.; Cope, A.P.; Cornelis, F.; et al. EULAR recommendations for terminology and research in individuals at risk of rheumatoid arthritis: Report from the Study Group for Risk Factors for Rheumatoid Arthritis. *Ann. Rheum. Dis.* **2012**, *71*, 638–641. [CrossRef]
9. Xing, Y.; Hogquist, K.A. T-cell tolerance: Central and peripheral. *Cold Spring Harb. Perspect. Biol.* **2012**, *4*, 6. [CrossRef]
10. Yip, L.; Su, L.; Sheng, D.; Chang, P.; Atkinson, M.; Czesak, M.; Albert, P.R.; Collier, A.R.; Turley, S.J.; Fathman, C.G.; et al. Deaf1 isoforms control the expression of genes encoding peripheral tissue antigens in the pancreatic lymph nodes during type 1 diabetes. *Nat. Immunol.* **2009**, *10*, 1026–1033. [CrossRef]
11. Gardner, J.M.; Devoss, J.J.; Friedman, R.S.; Wong, D.J.; Tan, Y.X.; Zhou, X.; Johannes, K.P.; Su, M.A.; Chang, H.Y.; Krummel, M.F.; et al. Deletional tolerance mediated by extrathymic Aire-expressing cells. *Science* **2008**, *321*, 843–847. [CrossRef] [PubMed]
12. Anderson, M.S.; Venanzi, E.S.; Klein, L.; Chen, Z.; Berzins, S.P.; Turley, S.J.; von Boehmer, H.; Bronson, R.; Dierich, A.; Benoist, C.; et al. Projection of an immunological self shadow within the thymus by the aire protein. *Science* **2002**, *298*, 1395–1401. [CrossRef] [PubMed]
13. Takaba, H.; Morishita, Y.; Tomofuji, Y.; Danks, L.; Nitta, T.; Komatsu, N.; Kodama, T.; Takayanagi, H. Fezf2 Orchestrates a Thymic Program of Self-Antigen Expression for Immune Tolerance. *Cell* **2015**, *163*, 975–987. [CrossRef]
14. Gavanescu, I.; Kessler, B.; Ploegh, H.; Benoist, C.; Mathis, D. Loss of Aire-dependent thymic expression of a peripheral tissue antigen renders it a target of autoimmunity. *Proc. Natl. Acad. Sci. USA* **2007**, *104*, 4583–4587. [CrossRef] [PubMed]
15. Poliani, P.L.; Kisand, K.; Marrella, V.; Ravanini, M.; Notarangelo, L.D.; Villa, A.; Peterson, P.; Facchetti, F. Human peripheral lymphoid tissues contain autoimmune regulator-expressing dendritic cells. *Am. J. Pathol.* **2010**, *176*, 1104–1112. [CrossRef] [PubMed]
16. Zuklys, S.; Balciunaite, G.; Agarwal, A.; Fasler-Kan, E.; Palmer, E.; Hollander, G.A. Normal thymic architecture and negative selection are associated with Aire expression, the gene defective in the autoimmune-polyendocrinopathy-candidiasis-ectodermal dystrophy (APECED). *J. Immunol.* **2000**, *165*, 1976–1983. [CrossRef]
17. Mathis, D.; Benoist, C. Aire. *Annu. Rev. Immunol.* **2009**, *27*, 287–312. [CrossRef]

18. Lohse, A.W.; Dinkelmann, M.; Kimmig, M.; Herkel, J.; Meyer zum Buschenfelde, K.H. Estimation of the frequency of self-reactive T cells in health and inflammatory diseases by limiting dilution analysis and single cell cloning. *J. Autoimmun.* **1996**, *9*, 667–675. [CrossRef]
19. Cremasco, V.; Woodruff, M.C.; Onder, L.; Cupovic, J.; Nieves-Bonilla, J.M.; Schildberg, F.A.; Chang, J.; Cremasco, F.; Harvey, C.J.; Wucherpfennig, K.; et al. B cell homeostasis and follicle confines are governed by fibroblastic reticular cells. *Nat. Immunol.* **2014**, *15*, 973–981. [CrossRef]
20. Brown, F.D.; Turley, S.J. Fibroblastic reticular cells: Organization and regulation of the T lymphocyte life cycle. *J. Immunol.* **2015**, *194*, 1389–1394. [CrossRef]
21. Malhotra, D.; Fletcher, A.L.; Astarita, J.; Lukacs-Kornek, V.; Tayalia, P.; Gonzalez, S.F.; Elpek, K.G.; Chang, S.K.; Knoblich, K.; Hemler, M.E.; et al. Transcriptional profiling of stroma from inflamed and resting lymph nodes defines immunological hallmarks. *Nat. Immunol.* **2012**, *13*, 499–510. [CrossRef] [PubMed]
22. Chang, J.E.; Turley, S.J. Stromal infrastructure of the lymph node and coordination of immunity. *Trends Immunol.* **2015**, *36*, 30–39. [CrossRef]
23. Heesters, B.A.; Myers, R.C.; Carroll, M.C. Follicular dendritic cells: Dynamic antigen libraries. *Nat. Rev. Immunol.* **2014**, *14*, 495–504. [CrossRef] [PubMed]
24. Tamburini, B.A.; Burchill, M.A.; Kedl, R.M. Antigen capture and archiving by lymphatic endothelial cells following vaccination or viral infection. *Nat. Commun.* **2014**, *5*, 3989. [CrossRef]
25. Lukacs-Kornek, V.; Malhotra, D.; Fletcher, A.L.; Acton, S.E.; Elpek, K.G.; Tayalia, P.; Collier, A.R.; Turley, S.J. Regulated release of nitric oxide by nonhematopoietic stroma controls expansion of the activated T cell pool in lymph nodes. *Nat. Immunol.* **2011**, *12*, 1096–1104. [CrossRef]
26. Norder, M.; Gutierrez, M.G.; Zicari, S.; Cervi, E.; Caruso, A.; Guzman, C.A. Lymph node-derived lymphatic endothelial cells express functional costimulatory molecules and impair dendritic cell-induced allogenic T-cell proliferation. *FASEB J.* **2012**, *26*, 2835–2846. [CrossRef]
27. Fletcher, A.L.; Lukacs-Kornek, V.; Reynoso, E.D.; Pinner, S.E.; Bellemare-Pelletier, A.; Curry, M.S.; Collier, A.R.; Boyd, R.L.; Turley, S.J. Lymph node fibroblastic reticular cells directly present peripheral tissue antigen under steady-state and inflammatory conditions. *J. Exp. Med.* **2010**, *207*, 689–697. [CrossRef]
28. Lee, J.W.; Epardaud, M.; Sun, J.; Becker, J.E.; Cheng, A.C.; Yonekura, A.R.; Heath, J.K.; Turley, S.J. Peripheral antigen display by lymph node stroma promotes T cell tolerance to intestinal self. *Nat. Immunol.* **2007**, *8*, 181–190. [CrossRef]
29. Dubrot, J.; Duraes, F.V.; Potin, L.; Capotosti, F.; Brighouse, D.; Suter, T.; LeibundGut-Landmann, S.; Garbi, N.; Reith, W.; Swartz, M.A.; et al. Lymph node stromal cells acquire peptide-MHCII complexes from dendritic cells and induce antigen-specific CD4(+) T cell tolerance. *J. Exp. Med.* **2014**, *211*, 1153–1166. [CrossRef]
30. Rouhani, S.J.; Eccles, J.D.; Riccardi, P.; Peske, J.D.; Tewalt, E.F.; Cohen, J.N.; Liblau, R.; Makinen, T.; Engelhard, V.H. Roles of lymphatic endothelial cells expressing peripheral tissue antigens in CD4 T-cell tolerance induction. *Nat. Commun.* **2015**, *6*, 6771. [CrossRef]
31. Baptista, A.P.; Roozendaal, R.; Reijmers, R.M.; Koning, J.J.; Unger, W.W.; Greuter, M.; Keuning, E.D.; Molenaar, R.; Goverse, G.; Sneeboer, M.M.; et al. Lymph node stromal cells constrain immunity via MHC class II self-antigen presentation. *Elife* **2014**, *3*, e04433. [CrossRef] [PubMed]
32. Nadafi, R.; Gago de Graca, C.; Keuning, E.D.; Koning, J.J.; de Kivit, S.; Konijn, T.; Henri, S.; Borst, J.; Reijmers, R.M.; van Baarsen, L.G.M.; et al. Lymph node stromal cells generate antigen-specific regulatory t cells and control autoreactive T and B cell responses. *Cell Rep.* **2020**, *30*, 4110–4123. [CrossRef] [PubMed]
33. Jones, J.E.; Causey, C.P.; Knuckley, B.; Slack-Noyes, J.L.; Thompson, P.R. Protein arginine deiminase 4 (PAD4): Current understanding and future therapeutic potential. *Curr. Opin. Drug Discov. Devel.* **2009**, *12*, 616–627. [PubMed]
34. Hansson, M.; Mathsson, L.; Schlederer, T.; Israelsson, L.; Matsson, P.; Nogueira, L.; Jakobsson, P.J.; Lundberg, K.; Malmstrom, V.; Serre, G.; et al. Validation of a multiplex chip-based assay for the detection of autoantibodies against citrullinated peptides. *Arthritis Res. Ther.* **2012**, *14*, R201. [CrossRef]
35. Steen, J.; Forsstrom, B.; Sahlstrom, P.; Odowd, V.; Israelsson, L.; Krishnamurthy, A.; Badreh, S.; Mathsson Alm, L.; Compson, J.; Ramskold, D.; et al. Human plasma cell derived monoclonal antibodies to post-translationally modified proteins recognize amino acid motifs rather than specific proteins. *Arthritis Rheumatol.* **2018**. [CrossRef]

36. Shang, R.; Wang, J.; Sun, W.; Dai, B.; Ruan, B.; Zhang, Z.; Yang, X.; Gao, Y.; Qu, S.; Lv, X.; et al. RRAD inhibits aerobic glycolysis, invasion, and migration and is associated with poor prognosis in hepatocellular carcinoma. *Tumor Biol.* **2016**, *37*, 5097–5105. [CrossRef]
37. Ilany, J.; Bilan, P.J.; Kapur, S.; Caldwell, J.S.; Patti, M.E.; Marette, A.; Kahn, C.R. Overexpression of Rad in muscle worsens diet-induced insulin resistance and glucose intolerance and lowers plasma triglyceride level. *Proc. Natl. Acad. Sci. USA* **2006**, *103*, 4481–4486. [CrossRef]
38. Baekkeskov, S.; Aanstoot, H.J.; Christgau, S.; Reetz, A.; Solimena, M.; Cascalho, M.; Folli, F.; Richter-Olesen, H.; De Camilli, P. Identification of the 64K autoantigen in insulin-dependent diabetes as the GABA-synthesizing enzyme glutamic acid decarboxylase. *Nature* **1990**, *347*, 151–156. [CrossRef]
39. Fabriek, B.O.; Zwemmer, J.N.; Teunissen, C.E.; Dijkstra, C.D.; Polman, C.H.; Laman, J.D.; Castelijns, J.A. In vivo detection of myelin proteins in cervical lymph nodes of MS patients using ultrasound-guided fine-needle aspiration cytology. *J. Neuroimmunol.* **2005**, *161*, 190–194. [CrossRef]
40. Tateyama, M.; Yatsuhashi, H.; Taura, N.; Motoyoshi, Y.; Nagaoka, S.; Yanagi, K.; Abiru, S.; Yano, K.; Komori, A.; Migita, K.; et al. Alpha-fetoprotein above normal levels as a risk factor for the development of hepatocellular carcinoma in patients infected with hepatitis C virus. *J. Gastroenterol.* **2011**, *46*, 92–100. [CrossRef]
41. Schoenborn, J.R.; Wilson, C.B. Regulation of interferon-gamma during innate and adaptive immune responses. *Adv. Immunol.* **2007**, *96*, 41–101. [PubMed]
42. Nurieva, R.I.; Liu, X.; Dong, C. Yin-Yang of costimulation: Crucial controls of immune tolerance and function. *Immunol. Rev.* **2009**, *229*, 88–100. [CrossRef]
43. Hsu, P.; Santner-Nanan, B.; Hu, M.; Skarratt, K.; Lee, C.H.; Stormon, M.; Wong, M.; Fuller, S.J.; Nanan, R. IL-10 potentiates differentiation of human induced regulatory T cells via STAT3 and Foxo1. *J. Immunol.* **2015**, *195*, 3665–3674. [CrossRef] [PubMed]
44. Shevach, E.M.; Tran, D.Q.; Davidson, T.S.; Andersson, J. The critical contribution of TGF-beta to the induction of Foxp3 expression and regulatory T cell function. *Eur. J. Immunol.* **2008**, *38*, 915–917. [CrossRef]
45. Fletcher, A.L.; Malhotra, D.; Acton, S.E.; Lukacs-Kornek, V.; Bellemare-Pelletier, A.; Curry, M.; Armant, M.; Turley, S.J. Reproducible isolation of lymph node stromal cells reveals site-dependent differences in fibroblastic reticular cells. *Front. Immunol.* **2011**, *2*, 35. [CrossRef] [PubMed]
46. Makrygiannakis, D.; af Klint, E.; Lundberg, I.E.; Lofberg, R.; Ulfgren, A.K.; Klareskog, L.; Catrina, A.I. Citrullination is an inflammation-dependent process. *Ann. Rheum. Dis.* **2006**, *65*, 1219–1222. [CrossRef] [PubMed]
47. Giorno, R. Immunohistochemical analysis of the distribution of vimentin in human peripheral lymphoid tissues. *Anat. Rec.* **1985**, *211*, 43–47. [CrossRef] [PubMed]
48. Pitkanen, J.; Vahamurto, P.; Krohn, K.; Peterson, P. Subcellular localization of the autoimmune regulator protein. characterization of nuclear targeting and transcriptional activation domain. *J. Biol. Chem.* **2001**, *276*, 19597–19602. [CrossRef]
49. Ohmura, K.; Terao, C.; Maruya, E.; Katayama, M.; Matoba, K.; Shimada, K.; Murasawa, A.; Honjo, S.; Takasugi, K.; Tohma, S.; et al. Anti-citrullinated peptide antibody-negative RA is a genetically distinct subset: A definitive study using only bone-erosive ACPA-negative rheumatoid arthritis. *Rheumatology (Oxford)* **2010**, *49*, 2298–2304. [CrossRef]
50. Reynet, C.; Kahn, C.R. Rad: A member of the Ras family overexpressed in muscle of type II diabetic humans. *Science* **1993**, *262*, 1441–1444. [CrossRef]
51. Su, C.C.; Chen Ie, C.; Young, F.N.; Lian Ie, B. Risk of diabetes in patients with rheumatoid arthritis: A 12-year retrospective cohort study. *J. Rheumatol.* **2013**, *40*, 1513–1518. [CrossRef] [PubMed]
52. Chung, C.P.; Oeser, A.; Solus, J.F.; Gebretsadik, T.; Shintani, A.; Avalos, I.; Sokka, T.; Raggi, P.; Pincus, T.; Stein, C.M. Inflammation-associated insulin resistance: Differential effects in rheumatoid arthritis and systemic lupus erythematosus define potential mechanisms. *Arthritis Rheum.* **2008**, *58*, 2105–2112. [CrossRef] [PubMed]
53. Krishnamurty, A.T.; Turley, S.J. Lymph node stromal cells: Cartographers of the immune system. *Nat. Immunol.* **2020**, *21*, 369–380. [CrossRef] [PubMed]

54. Gerstner, C.; Turcinov, S.; Hensvold, A.H.; Chemin, K.; Uchtenhagen, H.; Ramwadhdoebe, T.H.; Dubnovitsky, A.; Kozhukh, G.; Ronnblom, L.; Kwok, W.W.; et al. Multi-HLA class II tetramer analyses of citrulline-reactive T cells and early treatment response in rheumatoid arthritis. *BMC Immunol.* **2020**, *21*, 27. [CrossRef]
55. Abe, J.; Shichino, S.; Ueha, S.; Hashimoto, S.; Tomura, M.; Inagaki, Y.; Stein, J.V.; Matsushima, K. Lymph node stromal cells negatively regulate antigen-specific CD4+ T cell responses. *J. Immunol.* **2014**, *193*, 1636–1644. [CrossRef]
56. Stern, L.J.; Wiley, D.C. The human class II MHC protein HLA-DR1 assembles as empty alpha beta heterodimers in the absence of antigenic peptide. *Cell* **1992**, *68*, 465–477. [CrossRef]
57. Van Haren, S.D.; Herczenik, E.; ten Brinke, A.; Mertens, K.; Voorberg, J.; Meijer, A.B. HLA-DR-presented peptide repertoires derived from human monocyte-derived dendritic cells pulsed with blood coagulation factor VIII. *Mol. Cell. Proteom.* **2011**, *10*, M110.002246. [CrossRef]
58. Viatte, S.; Alves, P.M.; Romero, P. Reverse immunology approach for the identification of CD8 T-cell-defined antigens: Advantages and hurdles. *Immunol. Cell Biol.* **2006**, *84*, 318–330. [CrossRef]
59. Postigo-Fernandez, J.; Farber, D.L.; Creusot, R.J. Phenotypic alterations in pancreatic lymph node stromal cells from human donors with type 1 diabetes and NOD mice. *Diabetologia* **2019**, *62*, 2040–2051. [CrossRef]
60. Aletaha, D.; Neogi, T.; Silman, A.J.; Funovits, J.; Felson, D.T.; Bingham, C.O.; Birnbaum, N.S., 3rd; Burmester, G.R.; Bykerk, V.P.; Cohen, M.D.; et al. 2010 rheumatoid arthritis classification criteria: An American College of Rheumatology/European League Against Rheumatism collaborative initiative. *Ann. Rheum. Dis.* **2010**, *69*, 1580–1588. [CrossRef]
61. De Hair, M.J.; Zijlstra, I.A.; Boumans, M.J.; van de Sande, M.G.; Maas, M.; Gerlag, D.M.; Tak, P.P. Hunting for the pathogenesis of rheumatoid arthritis: Core-needle biopsy of inguinal lymph nodes as a new research tool. *Ann. Rheum. Dis.* **2012**, *71*, 1911–1912. [CrossRef] [PubMed]
62. Remmerswaal, E.B.; Havenith, S.H.; Idu, M.M.; van Leeuwen, E.M.; van Donselaar, K.A.; Ten Brinke, A.; van der Bom-Baylon, N.; Bemelman, F.J.; van Lier, R.A.; Ten Berge, I.J. Human virus-specific effector-type T cells accumulate in blood but not in lymph nodes. *Blood* **2012**, *119*, 1702–1712. [CrossRef] [PubMed]
63. Hahnlein, J.S.; Ramwadhdoebe, T.H.; Semmelink, J.F.; Choi, I.Y.; Berger, F.H.; Maas, M.; Gerlag, D.M.; Tak, P.P.; Geijtenbeek, T.B.H.; van Baarsen, L.G.M. Distinctive expression of T cell guiding molecules in human autoimmune lymph node stromal cells upon TLR3 triggering. *Sci. Rep.* **2018**, *8*, 1736. [CrossRef] [PubMed]
64. Hahnlein, J.S.; Nadafi, R.; de Jong, T.; Ramwadhdoebe, T.H.; Semmelink, J.F.; Maijer, K.I.; Zijlstra, I.A.; Maas, M.; Gerlag, D.M.; Geijtenbeek, T.B.H.; et al. Impaired lymph node stromal cell function during the earliest phases of rheumatoid arthritis. *Arthritis Res. Ther.* **2018**, *20*, 35. [CrossRef]

International Journal of *Molecular Sciences*

MDPI

Article

Identification of Subclinical Lung Involvement in ACPA-Positive Subjects through Functional Assessment and Serum Biomarkers

Bruno Lucchino [1,†], Marcello Di Paolo [2,†], Chiara Gioia [1], Marta Vomero [1], Davide Diacinti [3], Cristina Mollica [4], Cristiano Alessandri [1], Daniele Diacinti [3], Paolo Palange [2] and Manuela Di Franco [1,*]

1 Dipartimento di Scienze Cliniche, Internistiche, Anestesiologiche e Cardiovascolari- Reumatologia, Sapienza University of Rome, 00161 Roma, Lazio, Italy; bruno.lucchino@uniroma1.it (B.L.); chiara.gioia@uniroma1.it (C.G.); marta.vomero@uniroma1.it (M.V.); cristiano.alessandri@uniroma1.it (C.A.)

2 Dipartimento di Sanità Pubblica e Malattie Infettive, Sapienza University of Rome, 00161 Roma, Lazio, Italy; marcello.dipaolo@uniroma1.it (M.D.P.); paolo.palange@uniroma1.it (P.P.)

3 Dipartimento di Scienze Radiologiche, Oncologia e Anatomia Patologica, Sapienza University of Rome, 00161 Roma, Lazio, Italy; davide.diacinti@uniroma1.it (D.D.); daniele.diacinti@uniroma1.it (D.D.)

4 Dipartimento di Metodi e Modelli per l'Economia, il Territorio e la Finanza, Sapienza University of Rome, 00161 Roma, Lazio, Italy; cristina.mollica@uniroma1.it

* Correspondence: manuela.difranco@uniroma1.it

† These authors contributed equally to this work.

Received: 30 May 2020; Accepted: 16 July 2020; Published: 21 July 2020

Abstract: Lung involvement is related to the natural history of anti-citrullinated proteins antibodies (ACPA)-positive rheumatoid arthritis (RA), both during the pathogenesis of the disease and as a site of disease-related injury. Increasing evidence suggests that there is a subclinical, early lung involvement during the course of the disease, even before the onset of articular manifestations, which can potentially progress to a symptomatic interstitial lung disease. To date, reliable, non-invasive markers of subclinical lung involvement are still lacking in clinical practice. The aim of this study is to evaluate the diagnostic potential of functional assessment and serum biomarkers in the identification of subclinical lung involvement in ACPA-positive subjects. Fifty ACPA-positive subjects with or without confirmed diagnosis of RA (2010 ARC-EULAR criteria) were consecutively enrolled. Each subject underwent clinical evaluation, pulmonary function testing (PFT) with assessment of diffusion lung capacity for carbon monoxide (DL_{CO}), cardiopulmonary exercise testing (CPET), surfactant protein D (SPD) serum levels dosage and high-resolution computed tomography (HRCT) of the chest. The cohort was composed of 21 ACPA-positive subjects without arthritis (ND), 10 early (disease duration < 6 months, treatment-naïve) RA (ERA) and 17 long-standing (disease duration < 36 months, on treatment) RA (LSRA). LSRA patients had a significantly higher frequency of overall HRCT abnormalities compared to the other groups ($p = 0.001$). SPD serum levels were significantly higher in ACPA-positive subjects compared with healthy controls (158.5 ± 132.3 ng/mL vs 61.27 ± 34.11 ng/mL; $p < 0.0001$) and showed an increasing trend from ND subjects to LSRD patients ($p = 0.004$). Patients with HRCT abnormalities showed significantly lower values of DL_{CO} (74.19 ± 13.2% pred. vs 131.7 ± 93% pred.; $p = 0.009$), evidence of ventilatory inefficiency at CPET and significantly higher SPD serum levels compared with subjects with no HRCT abnormalities (213.5 ± 157.2 ng/mL vs 117.7 ± 157.3 ng/mL; $p = 0.018$). Abnormal CPET responses and higher SPD levels were also associated with specific radiological findings. Impaired DL_{CO} and increased SPD serum levels were independently associated with the presence of HRCT abnormalities. Subclinical lung abnormalities occur early in RA-associated autoimmunity. The presence of subclinical HRCT abnormalities is associated with several functional abnormalities and increased SPD serum levels of SPD. Functional evaluation through PFT and CPET, together with SPD assessment, may have a diagnostic potential in ACPA-positive subjects, contributing to the identification of those patients to be referred to HRCT scan.

Keywords: rheumatoid arthritis; interstitial lung disease; subclinical involvement; ACPA; pulmonary function testing; CPET; surfactant protein D; DL_{CO}; HRCT

1. Introduction

Rheumatoid arthritis (RA) is a chronic inflammatory disease, characterized by progressive joint damage and systemic extra-articular involvement [1,2]. Although considered primarily as an inflammatory disease of synovium, extra-articular features are not uncommon and currently represent the leading causes of death among patients with RA, with lung involvement second only to cardiovascular morbidity [3].

In genetically predisposed individuals exposed to various environmental factors, the disease develops progressively following a multistep process, starting with the breaking of tolerance against modified auto-antigens, including citrullinated proteins. This is followed by the appearance of serum autoantibodies in the absence of clinical manifestations. After a variable period of time, the individual at first may develop arthralgia without evidence of synovitis, which eventually evolves into a clinically manifest arthritis, classifiable at last as RA [4]. Mucosal surfaces play an important role in the immune response against foreign and potentially harmful environmental pathogens or toxins. Indeed, several risk factors for RA, such as cigarette smoking or dusts inhalation, act on lung parenchyma and may induce a subtle inflammatory state.

Lung inflammation is associated with an increased citrullination of tissue proteins and with local production of anti-citrullinated proteins antibodies (ACPA) not only in RA, but also in other chronic inflammatory conditions [5–7]. Sputum from RA patients as well as from subjects at risk for RA shows the presence of ACPA. Furthermore, ACPA can be found in sputum even before any evidence of them in serum [8]. Similarly, broncho-alveolar lavage from early, untreated RA is enriched in ACPA compared to serum [9]. This evidence is parallel to the demonstration of several subclinical lung abnormalities at high-resolution computed tomography (HRCT) in more than 70% of subjects positive for serum autoantibodies without arthritis [10].

The lung also represents a site of disease-related injury. RA-associated interstitial lung disease (RA-ILD) is a significant cause of morbidity and mortality among patients with RA [11]. The incidence of RA-ILD is around 10%, but it increases to 58% when subclinical lung abnormalities detected at HRCT are taken into account [12]. Although the clinical meaning of subclinical lung alteration is still unclear, there are reports of a potentially progressive nature up to the development of a clinically manifest RA-ILD [13,14]. Once developed, RA-ILD carries a poor prognosis; hence, early identification of those patients at risk for RA-ILD is of paramount importance, even if it is still unknown whether an immunosuppressive treatment can modify the course of the disease [15–17].

Pulmonary function testing (PFT) is commonly used as the first screening tool for RA-ILD identification. Impairment in pulmonary functional parameters, particularly reduction in diffusion lung capacity for carbon monoxide (DL_{CO}), shows a good sensitivity in subclinical RA-ILD identification, although the clinical applicability of this finding remains unclear [17].

Cardiopulmonary exercise testing (CPET) provides a non-invasive, dynamic and global assessment of cardiopulmonary responses to physical exercise and represents a useful tool to assess the integrity of lung structures [18]. Its clinical utility has been increasingly recognized over the past decades [19]. In rheumatic conditions, CPET is commonly used in scleroderma-associated ILD, in which it has shown accuracy to identify early abnormalities and to provide several prognostic indications [20,21]. However, CPET utility in RA has not been extensively studied, especially regarding subclinical lung abnormalities.

Several serum biomarkers have been investigated for the identification of idiopathic pulmonary fibrosis (IPF). RA-ILD and IPF share several pathological and radiological features so that, predictably, validated IPF biomarkers showed good performance in RA-ILD identification as well. Among these, surfactant protein D (SPD) has been shown to be significantly increased in both clinically evident and subclinical RA-ILD [22]. SPD belongs to the collectin family and is primarily produced in type II pneumocytes and in Clara cells [23]. SPD plays an essential role in pulmonary innate immune defenses, enhancing pathogen clearance and regulating adaptive and innate immune-cell functions [24]. Circulating SPD has been correlated with a variety of pulmonary disorders [25], but has not been evaluated in the early phases of RA-associated lung abnormalities.

We hypothesized that, independently of the development of manifest RA, ACPA-positive subjects feature subclinical lung abnormalities, which could be non-invasively detected by pulmonary functional and SPD serum level assessment. Hence, the purposes of the present study were threefold:

- to evaluate the presence of subclinical lung involvement among ACPA-positive subjects without respiratory complains with and without confirmed diagnosis of RA;
- to assess pulmonary functional impairment at rest and during exercise through PFT and CPET, respectively;
- to evaluate the diagnostic potential of serum autoantibodies and SPD levels, with regard to radiology findings of lung involvement.

2. Results

2.1. Subjects' Characteristics

A total cohort of 50 subjects was enrolled. At HRCT scan, two patients showed a "probable UIP" pattern and were consequently excluded from the study. The remaining 48 subjects, 37 female (77.1%) and 11 males (22.9%) were included in the study. The three study groups were composed by a total of 21, 10 and 17 ACPA-positive subjects without evidence of arthritis (ND), early RA (ERA) and long-standing RA (LSRA), respectively. Patients did not suffer from other significant comorbidities. The demographic, clinical and laboratory characteristics are summarized in Table 1. Within the LSRA group, eight patients (47.1%) were already on treatment with methotrexate (MTX), four patients (23.5%) were taking sulphasalazine and three patients (17.6%) hydroxychloroquine, either as monotherapy or as combination therapy. For the laboratory evaluation, 22 healthy control subjects (HC) were also enrolled, 15 females (68.2%) and 7 males (31.8%), the mean age being 47.3 ± 10.5 years.

Table 1. Demographic, clinical features and autoantibodies of enrolled subjects.

	Overall (n = 48)	ND (n = 21)	ERA (n = 10)	LSRA (n = 17)	HC (n = 22)	p
Age, years	49.8 ± 11	50.38 ± 13.6	48.5 ± 10.8	53.06 ± 7.3	47.3 ± 10.5	0.49
Sex, M/F	11/37	3/18	3/7	5/12	7/15	0.45
BMI, kg/m^2	24.1 ± 4	23.3 ± 3.01	25.5 ± 5.6	25.5 ± 5.6	24.9 ± 2.8	0.28
Smoking, current/former/never	14/12/22	7/1/13	2/5/3	5/6/6	8/4/10	0.1
Disease duration, months	13.78 ± 11.02	-	3.6 ± 1.5	19.97 ± 9.6 †	-	<0.0001
DAS28	3.6 ± 1.5	-	4.21 ± 1.7	3.2 ± 1.45	-	0.2
ACPA, UI/L	321.3 ± 394.9	342 ± 429.6	298.8 ± 202.2	309 ± 450.8	-	0.73
RF, UI/L	139.9 ±179.2	101.2 ± 138.8	182.2 ± 195.4	163 ± 212.5	-	0.46

Data are reported as mean ± SD, unless stated otherwise. p values intended for comparisons between ND, ERA, LSRA and HC (whenever applicable) subgroups of participants. †: post hoc test $p < 0.05$ vs. ERA. Abbreviations: ND, no disease subjects; ERA, early rheumatoid arthritis patients; LSRA, long standing rheumatoid arthritis patients; HC, healthy controls; BMI, body mass index; ACPA, anti-citrullinated proteins antibodies; RF, rheumatoid factor.

2.2. Lung Function and Physiological Responses to Exercise

The results of the main PFT and CPET parameters are shown in Table 2.

Table 2. Selected pulmonary functional responses measured at rest and during exercise testing.

	Overall (n = 48)	ND (n = 21)	ERA (n = 10)	LSRA (n = 17)	p
FEV_1, % pred.	102.6 ± 11.9	104.3 ± 11.0	100.5 ± 14.7	101.9 ± 11.5	0.56
FVC, % pred.	107.8 ± 12.8	108.3 ± 13.8	105.4 ± 9.3	108.7 ± 13.7	0.81
FEV_1/FVC, %	80.2 ± 7.0	81.4 ± 6.9	80.0 ± 7.6	78.8 ± 6.9	0.7
TLC, % pred.	99.3 ± 12.1	98.5 ± 13.5	97.9 ± 11.9	101.3 ± 11.3	0.5
DL_{CO}, % pred.	81.5 ± 16.6	83.7 ± 18.7	82.5 ± 19.4	78.5 ± 13.0	0.76
K_{CO}, % pred.	84.3 ± 17.5	85.8 ± 17.8	90.2 ± 20.4	79.6 ± 15.3	0.21
Reduced DL_{CO}, n (%)	28 (58.3)	12 (57.1)	5 (50.0)	11 (64.7)	0.71
Work rate $_{peak}$, % pred.	76.1 ± 15.4	71.4 ± 14.2	71.1 ± 12.7	84.4 ± 15.4	0.35
$V'O_{2\,peak}$, mL/min/kg	22.7 ± 4.4	23.1 ± 3.9	23.6 ± 5.6	21.8 ± 4.3	0.81
$V'O_{2\,peak}$, % pred.	90.1 ± 15.9	92.6 ± 17.8	90.7 ± 14.5	86.7 ± 14.6	0.63
Reduced exercise tolerance, n (%)	19 (39.6)	7 (33.3)	3 (30.0)	9 (52.9)	0.53
$V'O_2$ at θ_L, % pred. $V'O_{2\,peak}$	52.7 ± 10.6	55.2 ± 9.6	47.3 ± 11.7	53.0 ± 10.6	0.2
$V'E_{peak}$, l/min	57.3 ± 18.9	54.0 ± 10.1	65.0 ± 20.3	56.7 ± 24.9	0.39
$V'E_{peak}$, %eMVV	49.8 ± 12.0	49.3 ± 11.8	54.5 ± 11.9	47.6 ± 12.2	0.63
$SpO_{2\,peak}$, %	97.3 ± 1.4	97.7 ± 1.1	97.6 ± 1.2	96.8 ± 1.7 *	0.017
ΔSpO_2, %	-0.3 ± 1.3	-0.2 ± 1.2	0 ± 0.9	-0.7 ± 1.5	0.26
$V'E/V'CO_2$ at θ_L	30.6 ± 4.6	29.9 ± 5.0	31.6 ± 5.6	30.7 ± 4.6	0.72
$V'E/V'CO_2$ slope	27.8 ± 4.6	27.0 ± 5.0	29.0 ± 3.8	28.0 ± 4.5	0.5
Impaired ventilatory efficiency, n (%)	15 (31.2)	6 (28.6)	2 (20.0)	7 (41.2)	0.5

Data are reported as mean ± SD. P values intended for comparisons between ND, ERA and LSRA subgroups of participants. *: post hoc test $p < 0.05$ vs. ND; Reduced DL_{CO}: DL_{CO} < 80% of predicted value; reduced exercise tolerance: V'O2 peak < 80% of predicted value; impaired ventilatory efficiency: $V'E/V'CO_2$ a $\theta_L > 34$ and/or $V'E/V'CO_2$ slope > 30. Abbreviations: ND, no disease subjects; ERA, early rheumatoid arthritis patients; LSRA, long standing rheumatoid arthritis patients; FEV_1, forced expiratory volume; FVC, forced vital capacity; TLC, total lung capacity; DL_{CO}, diffusing lung capacity for carbon monoxide; K_{CO}, transfer coefficient of the lung; $V'O_2$, oxygen uptake; $V'CO_2$, carbon dioxide output; V'E, minute ventilation; θ_L, lactate threshold; eMVV, estimated maximal voluntary ventilation; SpO_2, peripheral capillary oxygen saturation; ΔSpO_2, peak-rest change in peripheral capillary oxygen saturation.

Reduced DL_{CO} (i.e., <80% predicted value) was observed in 57.1%, 50% and 64.7% of ND, ERA and LSRA subjects, respectively ($p = 0.747$). There were no significant differences between groups in the examined PFT parameters, even after correction for smoking status. FEV_1, when expressed as percentage of predicted value, was significantly lower in patients who were current or former smokers compared to non-smokers ($p = 0.018$). DL_{CO} values in current and former smokers were not different from those of never smoker subjects.

All patients achieved maximal effort during CPET. Mean work rate at peak exercise was 105 ± 32.5 W (76.1 ± 15.4% predicted value). Reduced exercise tolerance, defined as $V'O_{2\,peak}$ < 80% predicted value, was found in 19 out of 48 (39.6%) patients. Even if not significantly different, ND and ERA subjects showed lower rates of exercise intolerance than LSRA. Anticipated θ_L (i.e., $V'O_2$ at θ_L < 40% predicted $V'O_{2\,peak}$), indicating impaired aerobic fitness, was observed in six (12.5%) subjects, with no difference among subgroups. No abnormalities in cardiovascular responses were found, neither within the whole group nor among each subgroup.

Overall, there was no sign of ventilatory limitation, average $V'E_{peak}$ being 49.8 ± 12% eMVV. In this regard, none of the recruited patients showed $V'E_{peak}$ values > 85% eMVV. Mean V_T was 1.8 ± 0.5 L at peak exercise, corresponding to 50.0 ± 10.0% of FVC, confirming the absence of ventilatory constraints during exercise. Apparently, no differences in breathing patterns were observed between subgroups.

Peak SpO_2 fell within normal values for all groups, although a significant trend in progressive reduction was found between groups (97.7 ± 1.1% vs 97.6 ± 1.2% vs 96.8 ± 1.7% among ND, ERA and LSRA patients, respectively; $p = 0.008$). Significant haemoglobin desaturation (peak—rest change in SpO_2 > 4%) was found only in one patient with LSRA.

Impaired ventilatory efficiency, defined as $V'E/V'CO_2$ at $\theta_L > 34$ and/or $V'E/V'CO_2$ slope > 30, was found in about one third of the study group. The highest frequency was registered among LSRA patients (41.2%); however, no significant differences were observed in the rate of reduced ventilatory efficiency among the three subgroups.

2.3. Laboratory Results

There were no significant differences in ACPA and RF levels between the groups. Significantly higher values of RF were registered among subjects from all the three groups with reduced exercise tolerance (263.8 ± 216.5 IU/L vs 119.4 ± 171.71 IU/ L; $p = 0.019$) and with impaired ventilatory efficiency (326.6 ± 282.9 IU/ L vs 90.8 ± 98.6 IU/ L; $p = 0.015$). No further relations were observed between ACPA and RF levels and pulmonary function at rest and during exercise.

SPD serum levels were significantly higher among study group subjects compared with HC (158.5 ± 132.3 ng/mL vs. 61.27 ± 34.11 ng/mL; $p < 0.0001$). Similarly, subgroup analysis revealed higher SPD levels within the ND (132.1 ± 125.1 ng/mL; $p = 0.023$), ERA (181.1 ± 151.3 ng/mL; $p = 0.003$) and LSRA subgroups (176.1 ± 131.8 ng/mL; $p < 0.0001$) compared with HC (61.2 ± 34.1 ng/mL) (Figure 1). No difference was observed between patient groups; nonetheless, a significant trend in increasing levels of SPD was noticed from ND to LSRA ($p = 0.004$). There were no differences in SPD levels based on smoking history (i.e., current, former or never smoker). However, significantly higher levels of SPD were present in ACPA-positive never smokers (ND+ERA+LSRA) compared with healthy controls (142.2 ± 94.1 ng/mL vs 61.2 ± 34.1 ng/mL; $p < 0.0001$). In the LSRA group, no difference was found in SPD serum levels concerning treatment with MTX.

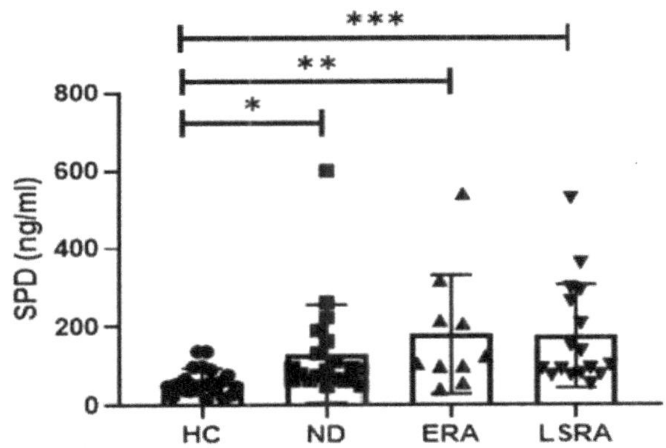

Figure 1. Comparison of SPD serum levels between ACPA-positive subjects and healthy controls. *: $p < 0.05$; **: $p < 0.005$; ***: $p < 0.0005$. Abbreviations: SPD, surfactant protein D; HC, healthy controls; ND, no disease subjects; ERA, early rheumatoid arthritis patients; LSRA, long standing rheumatoid arthritis patients.

SPD levels were inversely related to $V'O_{2\ peak}$ (expressed as percentage of predicted value; $p = 0.024$; rho = −0.32), $V'O_2$ at θ_L (percentage of predicted $V'O_{2\ peak}$; $p = 0.013$; rho = −0.36) and peak SpO2 ($p = 0.008$; rho = −0.38). As observed for RF, SPD levels were also shown to be significantly higher among patients with reduced exercise ventilatory efficiency ($V'E/V'CO_2$ a $\theta_L > 34$) (250.8 ± 155.3 ng/mL vs. 141.2 ± 121.9 ng/mL; $p = 0.007$). A similar result was also observed when limiting the analysis to ND patients (351.15 ± 219 ng/mL vs 93.5 ± 44.9 ng/mL; $p = 0.01$).

2.4. HRCT Abnormalities

Of the entire cohort, 62.5% had HRCT abnormalities. The most frequently detected abnormality was the presence of nodules, followed by evidence of fibrosis. The less frequent abnormality was the presence of air trapping. There were no differences in the frequency of the various HRCT abnormalities according to smoking status or, among LSRA patients, to treatment with methotrexate (MTX). The frequencies of HRCT abnormalities are shown in Table 3.

Table 3. Frequencies of total and selected lung abnormalities at high-resolution computed tomography (HRCT) scan.

	Overall (n = 48)	ND (n = 21)	ERA (n = 10)	LSRA (n = 17)	p
Total, %	62.5	38	60	94.1 *,†	0.001
Parenchymal, %	62.5	38	60	94.1 *,†	0.001
Airways, %	16.6	14.3	10	23.5	0.98
Emphysema, %	16.6	-	30 *	29.4 *	0.02
Fibrosis, %	29.1	14.3	10	58.8 *,†	0.003
Ground glass, %	6.25	-	-	17.6	0.054
Consolidations, %	10.4	4.7	10	17.6	0.43
Nodules, %	50	28	60	76.4 *	0.004
Bronchiectasis, %	12.5	4.7	20	17.6	0.43
Airways thickening, %	16.6	14.3	10	23.5	0.61
Air trapping, %	8.3	-	10	11.8	0.14

Data are reported as percentage of the total. P values intended for comparisons between ND, ERA and LSRA subgroups of participants. *: post hoc test $p < 0.05$ vs. ND; †: post hoc test $p < 0.05$ vs. ERA. Abbreviations: ND, no disease subjects; ERA, early rheumatoid arthritis patients; LSRA, long standing rheumatoid arthritis patients.

Subgroup analysis revealed significantly higher rates of overall HRCT abnormalities, nodules, emphysema and fibrosis among LSRA patients compared with the other subgroups ($p = 0.001$, $p = 0.004$, $p = 0.02$ and $p = 0.003$, respectively). The same differences in HRCT total abnormalities and nodules were also observed when limiting the analysis to those patients who never smoked ($p = 0.049$ and $p = 0.016$, respectively). Current and former smokers showed a significantly higher frequency of fibrosis compared with subjects who never smoked ($p = 0.03$), with a relative risk of 2.77 (CI 95% 1.054–8.359). Of note, no difference in fibrosis prevalence was found based on MTX treatment.

2.5. Relations between Functional and Laboratory Data and the Presence of HRCT Abnormalities

There were no differences in both dynamic and static lung volumes in patients with or without HRCT abnormalities. On the contrary, a significant reduction in DL_{CO} (74.19 ± 13.2% pred. vs. 131.7 ± 93% pred.; $p = 0.009$) and K_{CO} (77.5 ± 15.8% pred. vs 138.92 ± 97% pred.; $p = 0.01$) was found among patients with HRCT abnormalities compared with patients with normal HRCT scans. Impaired DL_{CO} was present only among patients with HRCT abnormalities who had already developed the disease (ERA and LSRA), but not in the ND group ($p = 0.042$). In the former group, the presence of a reduced DL_{CO} had a positive likelihood ratio for the presence of HRCT abnormalities ($LR = 4.7$). Reduction in DL_{CO} (73.8 ± 14.2% pred. vs 91.7 ± 18.5% pred.; $p = 0.002$) and K_{CO} (75.9 ± 16.6%pred. vs 96.1 ± 19% pred.; $p = 0.003$) was also present in patients with nodules at HRCT.

Patients with signs of ventilatory inefficiency at CPET also had an increased frequency of HRCT abnormalities. In particular, patients with increased $V'E/V'CO_2$ at θ_L (i.e., >34) showed a higher frequency of overall HRCT abnormalities ($p = 0.029$) and specifically bronchiectasis ($p = 0.009$) and airways thickening ($p = 0.035$), while patients with an abnormal $V'E/V'CO_2$ slope (i.e., >30) had an increased frequency of emphysema ($p = 0.007$). A significant difference in the rate of HRCT abnormalities according to $V'E/V'CO_2$ at θ_L values persisted also when limiting the analysis to the ND group alone ($p = 0.022$).

SPD serum levels were significantly higher in subjects with HRCT abnormalities compared to subjects without abnormalities (213.5 ± 157.2 ng/mL vs 117.7 ± 157.3 ng/mL; $p = 0.018$) (Figure 2). Considering only patients who already had arthritis (ERA+LSRA groups), significantly higher levels of SPD were observed in subjects who had airways abnormalities ($p = 0.023$), but not in those who showed parenchymal abnormalities. There was a significant negative correlation in subjects with HRCT abnormalities between SPD serum levels and FVC % pred. ($p = 0.039$; rho = −0.465), FEV1/FVC % pred. ($p = 0.005$; rho = −0.599) and peak SpO_2 ($p = 0.033$; rho = −0.477). In the same subjects,

ACPA levels correlated with $V'O_2$ at θ_L expressed both as absolute value ($p < 0.001$; rho = −0.726) and as percentage of predicted $V'O_{2\,peak}$ ($p = 0.021$; rho = −0.508).

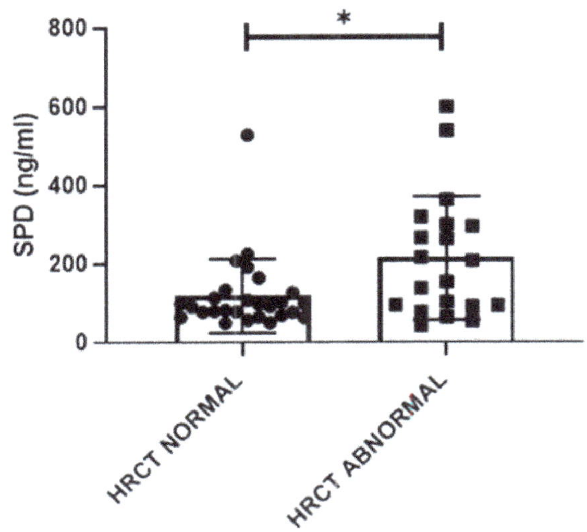

Figure 2. SPD serum levels in subjects with normal and abnormal HRCT. *: $p < 0.05$.

In order to evaluate the diagnostic performance of SPD serum levels with regard to the detection of HRCT abnormalities, ROC analysis was performed (Figure 3). The AUC value was 0.77 (95% CI: 0.65–0.9). The optimal cut-off point of diagnostic performance was 90.78 ng/mL, with a sensitivity of 80% and a specificity of 62% for HRCT abnormalities detection.

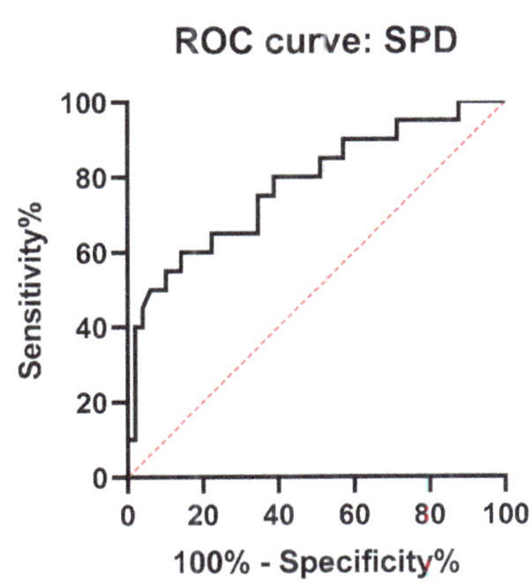

Figure 3. Receiver operating characteristic (ROC) curve of diagnostic performance of SPD serum levels in the identification of HRCT abnormalities.

Finally, in order to further evaluate the diagnostic potential of serum and functional biomarkers, a logistic regression model to find independent predictors of the presence of HRCT abnormalities was performed. This model found that an abnormal DL_{CO} (beta coefficient −2.9) and SPD (beta coefficient 0.009) stepped into the final model and retained statistically significant association with HRCT abnormalities, suggesting that normal DL_{CO} and increased SPD serum levels related to a decreased and increased likelihood of HRCT abnormalities (sensitivity 56.3%, specificity 86.4%), respectively (Table 4).

Table 4. Logistic regression model for predictors associated to the presence of HRCT abnormalities.

Dependent Variable	Predictors	B	SE	OR	95% CI	p	R^2
HRCT Abnormal (Yes)	SPD	0.009	0.05	1.009	1.000–1.018	0.041	
	Reduced DL_{CO} (No)	−2.94	1.26	0.053	0.04–0.63	0.02	
	ACPA	0.001	0.001	1.001	0.998–1.003	0.44	
	$V'E/V'CO_2$ at θ_L Impaired (No)	−0.65	1.32	0.52	0.039–6.9	0.62	
	Constant	−0.629	1.477	0.53		0.67	
							0.506

Variables included in the model: SPD, reduced DL_{CO} (i.e., <80% of predicted value), ACPA, impaired $V'E/V'CO_2$ at θ_L. (i.e., >34). Abbreviations: SPD, surfactant protein D; DL_{CO}, diffusing capacity for carbon monoxide; ACPA, anti-citrullinated proteins antibodies.

3. Discussion

The occurrence of subclinical lung abnormalities in the natural history of RA is frequent and largely dependent on the serological status. As mentioned above, Demoruelle et al. demonstrated the presence of subclinical lung abnormalities at HRCT in more than 70% of ACPA-positive subjects without evidence of arthritis [10]. The most frequent abnormalities were airways alterations, such as bronchial wall thickening and air trapping, with a minority of parenchymal alterations [10]. In a different cohort, Fisher et al. reported a prevalence of 54% of airways abnormalities, 14% of RA-ILD and 26% of a combination of both in ACPA-positive subjects without arthritis and with respiratory complaints [26]. Further evidence derives from the ancillary studies performed on the Multi-Ethnic Study of Atherosclerosis (MESA) cohort, a large, multi-centric cohort of healthy subjects undergoing CT scans for subclinical cardiovascular disease investigation. Within this cohort, the presence of high attenuation areas (HAA), a marker of subclinical ILD, was associated with the presence of RA-related autoantibodies [27]. Our results show that the transition from a systemic autoimmunity to the development of the disease is associated with a progressive increase in the prevalence of subclinical HRCT abnormalities, which are also frequently present before the onset of the arthritis. This increased frequency is already evident in the first years of the disease, considering that LSRA patients had a maximum disease duration of 3 years. This is in line with the finding of HRCT abnormalities in 68% of RA patients with a median disease duration shorter than 6 months described by Reynisdottir et al. [28]. Moreover, in up to one third of the cases, the diagnosis of symptomatic ILD is established between 1 year prior to and 1 year after the diagnosis of RA [29]. Globally, there is an increasing amount of evidence suggesting that the occurrence of HRCT abnormalities is an early event in the natural history of the disease, occurring in a parallel manner to joint involvement. In our study, the most frequently detected abnormalities were nodules. Although MTX treatment has been traditionally associated with accelerated nodulosis in RA [30], our study does not support the evidence of an increased prevalence of lung nodules in patients treated with MTX. Accordingly, a recent study on a large cohort of newly diagnosed RA confirmed that MTX treatment is not associated with the incidence of any kind of RA-ILD [31]. Conversely, our results confirm the association between smoking habit and pulmonary fibrosis risk in RA, as largely reported in the literature [32].

Several reasons may justify the importance of subclinical HRCT abnormalities detection in ACPA-positive subjects. Previous studies demonstrated a progressive nature of subclinical HRCT abnormalities, potentially evolving into clinical manifest ILD over a 2 year period [14]. Moreover, some evidence suggests that treatment of subclinical HRCT lung abnormalities that show a tendency to progress to ILD may stabilize the HRCT alterations [13]. The presence of subclinical lung abnormalities may also influence the decision regarding treatment options. In fact, there are several reports of new-onset ILD as well as worsening of pre-existing ILD for all available anti-TNF agents. However, the potential harm related to anti-TNF treatment is still not clear, with some studies reporting, on the contrary, a stabilization of lung function [33]. Indeed, specific manifestations of inflammatory lung involvement, such as bronchiectasis, may increase the risk of severe complications of biologic treatment [34]. To date, there are no specific recommendations about the diagnosis and treatment of RA-ILD, although a diagnostic algorithm has been proposed [35]. PFTs are informative in case of suspected RA-ILD. Previous studies reported a reduced DL_{CO} as a valuable marker of RA-ILD as well as of preclinical ILD in RA patients [14,36]. Our study confirms that subjects with subclinical HRCT abnormalities had subtle but statistically significant reductions in DL_{CO} compared with subjects without these alterations and that a reduced DL_{CO}, expressed as percentage of predicted value, increased the likelihood of HRCT abnormalities. Notably, these associations were more evident in patients who already had developed manifest RA, not achieving statistical significance in the ND group.

Several studies investigated the diagnostic role of CPET in preclinical, non-rheumatologic conditions. In the MESA cohort, a ventilatory limitation to exercise was present in subjects with subclinical HAA at HRCT compared to subjects without HAA [37]. In a cohort of preclinical familial pulmonary fibrosis, CPET revealed that the percentage of reduction in dead space ventilation at peak exercise was significantly lower in subjects with asymptomatic ILD compared with subjects with normal HRCT scans [38,39]. We detected several CPET abnormalities in our patients, which could be associated with the early involvement of lung parenchyma. Indeed, the presence of a difference in SpO_2 reached at peak exercise between groups may be related to the frequency of the subclinical HRCT abnormalities detected. In subjects with HRCT abnormalities, CPET showed a significant impairment in $V'E/V'CO_2$ at θ_L and $V'E/V'CO_2$ slope, suggesting a ventilation/perfusion mismatch. In our study, an abnormal $V'E/V'CO_2$ relationship was associated with HRCT abnormalities involving both airways and lung parenchyma. This is in line with what has already been described across a wide spectrum of lung diseases, including emphysema and cystic fibrosis [40–42]. CPET may thus have a diagnostic value in RA patients, non-invasively suggesting the presence of HRCT abnormalities. Furthermore, the evidence of a similar association even among ND subjects suggests a possible utility of CPET for early identification of ACPA-positive subjects without arthritis who may be candidates for HRCT, for diagnostic or research purposes.

SPD is increasingly gaining attention for its potential role as a serum biomarker of RA-ILD. Within our study population, the fact that SPD was found to be significantly higher than healthy controls and the progressive increase in SPD serum levels from ND to LSRA groups is in agreement with the current knowledge of an early, subclinical lung involvement in the natural history of RA. Moreover, SPD may have a diagnostic role in HRCT abnormalities identifications, showing a good discriminative ability. Clara cells in small airways are one of the main sources of SPD [23]. The pulmonary expression of SPD increases to protect the lung against pathogens and to regulate the inflammatory response in the airways, as observed in chronic bronchitis exacerbations [43]. Accordingly, the negative correlation found between SPD and FVC % pred., FEV1/FVC % pred. and peak SpO_2, as well as the finding of increased SPD serum levels among patients with airways involvement at HRCT, further suggests that SPD may be a selective marker of airway disease. Considering the difference in SPD serum levels between healthy controls and never smoker ACPA-positive subjects, the higher levels of SPD found in the latter may be directly related to the inflammatory process in the airways specifically associated with early phases of RA. Despite the presence of autoantibodies having been associated with an increased prevalence of subclinical ILD [27], we did not find any association between ACPA or RF levels and the presence of HRCT abnormalities. Anyway, all our patients were ACPA-positive, suggesting that the association with subclinical lung abnormalities depends on the serological positivity status for autoantibodies rather than the autoantibodies titer. RF levels showed a negative correlation with several CPET parameters of ventilatory efficiency, suggesting a higher lung involvement with increasing levels of autoantibodies. This observation may be related to a more significant functional pulmonary impairment with increasing levels of autoantibodies or, alternatively, may indicate the airways as a site of autoantibodies production as a consequence of harmful environmental stimuli [44,45].

This study presents several limitations. First, some of our results may be underpowered by the small sample size of this study. Larger cohorts could in fact reveal associations between the non-invasive markers and the various specific lung manifestations of the disease, which can be only supposed by the present study. Indeed, reliable markers of the most severe lung manifestations, such as fibrosis, may be relevant in clinical practice. A second limitation is represented by the cross-sectional nature of the study. The modification of the various functional and serum parameters during the evolution of the disease is currently unknown, limiting the prognostic potential of non-invasive assessment. Prospective cohorts are needed to address this issue, especially in the case of ACPA-positive subjects without arthritis. Finally, despite the observation of an abnormal ventilatory efficiency in 31.2% of the enrolled patients, a proper interpretation of ventilatory efficiency in our study group is limited by the absence of data concerning arterial CO_2 partial pressure during exercise. This data is indeed essential in order to define how inappropriate the ventilatory response of the lung is to the amount of carbon dioxide produced during the effort [46]. Whether this phenomenon actually stems from uneven lung ventilation or from a reset of arterial CO_2 set-point should be investigated with properly designed studies.

4. Materials and Methods

4.1. Study Subjects

ACPA-positive subjects referred to the Early Arthritis Clinic of Policlinico Umberto I Hospital/ "Sapienza" University of Rome were consecutively enrolled. Participants were divided into three groups. The first group included ACPA-positive subjects without clinical evidence of arthritis (no disease subjects, ND). The second group included ACPA-positive Early Rheumatoid Arthritis (ERA) patients, diagnosed according to the 2010 American College of Rheumatology (ACR)/European League Against Rheumatism (EULAR) criteria, naïve to treatment and with a disease duration shorter than 6 months. The third group included established, ACPA-positive Rheumatoid Arthritis patients (long-standing Rheumatoid Arthritis, LSRA), with a disease duration shorter than 36 months, on treatment with disease-modifying antirheumatic drugs (DMARDs). Subjects of both sexes and aged between 18 and 65 years were included in the study. Exclusion criteria were: any persistent respiratory complains, personal history of any kind of lung disease (e.g., asthma, chronic obstructive pulmonary disease) chronic heart failure NHYA class II-III-IV, overlap autoimmune syndromes, ongoing treatment with glucocorticoids, presumed or established pregnancy. Finding of Usual Interstitial Pneumonia (UIP) patterns at HRCT was also considered an exclusion criterion (see below).

Each subject underwent clinical and clinimetric, laboratory, functional and imaging evaluation. Age- and sex-matched healthy controls (HC) were also enrolled for comparison concerning laboratory assessment. Written informed consent was obtained from all patients and the study was approved by the local Ethics Committee (Comitato Etico Policlinico Umberto I, Sapienza Università di Roma, study reference number 815/13).

4.2. Clinic and Clinimetric Evaluation

Detailed medical history was taken for each subject. Every ACPA-positive subject without evidence of arthritis was evaluated to assess the absence of current or previous arthritis. General and musculoskeletal physical examination was performed, and counts of involved joints were registered for all participants.

Clinimetric scales were administered at the time of enrolment to evaluate global disease activity (i.e., Visual Analog Scale, VAS) and to calculate the composite index of disease activity (i.e., Disease Activity Score 28, DAS28). Moreover, disease onset and laboratory data regarding erythrocyte sedimentation rate (ESR), C-reactive protein (CRP), rheumatoid factor (RF) and ACPA levels were collected for each subject.

4.3. Laboratory Evaluation

A 15 mL venous blood sample was collected from each enrolled patient and from HC subjects. Serum was separated from blood samples and stored at −20 °C. After samples were defrosted, SPD serum levels were evaluated through a commercial ELISA kit (Biovendor, Modrice, Czech Republic), following the manufacturer's guidelines. Each sample from the same patient has been evaluated in duplicate, with a variation coefficient of 3.9%. The analytic limit for SPD detection was 0.01 ng/mL.

4.4. Functional Evaluation

Spirometry and nitrogen wash-out for measurement of dynamic and static lung volumes, respectively, as well as single-breath determination of DL_{CO}, were performed for each patient through an automated lung function testing system (Quark PFT, Cosmed, Rome, Italy) according to the standards recommended by the American Thoracic Society (ATS)/European Respiratory Society (ERS) [47,48]. All measurements were recorded as raw value and percentage of predicted value [49,50].

On the same day of PFT, incremental symptom-limited CPET was performed for every participant on an electronically braked cycle ergometer through an automated testing system (OMNIA, Cosmed, Rome, Italy), in accordance with international recommendations [19,51]. A fixed work rate increment of 10 W min^{-1} was used. The test was continued until the point of symptom limitation (peak of exercise).

Oxygen uptake ($V'O_2$), carbon dioxide output ($V'CO_2$), minute ventilation (V'E), tidal volume (V_T) and respiratory frequency (f_R) were analysed breath-by-breath during the test. Heart rate (HR), ECG and haemoglobin saturation by pulse oximetry (SpO_2) were continuously monitored whilst blood pressure was measured every two minutes from rest to peak of exercise. All measured and derived parameters [e.g., ventilatory equivalents for O_2 and CO_2 ($V'E/V'O_2$ and $V'E/V'CO_2$, respectively), end-tidal O_2 and CO_2 partial pressures ($P_{ET}O_2$ and $P_{ET}CO_2$, respectively)] were recorded and averaged every ten seconds. Lactate threshold (θ_L) was non-invasively estimated by the use of the dual methods approach (V-slope and ventilatory equivalents methods) [52].

$V'O_2$ at peak exercise ($V'O_{2\ peak}$) was normalized for body weight and expressed also as percentage of predicted value. Peak V'E response ($V'E_{peak}$) was expressed as a raw value and relative to estimated maximal voluntary ventilation (eMVV), which was defined as forced expiratory volume in the 1st second (FEV_1) × 40 [19].

Ventilatory efficiency was evaluated through the analysis of the relationship between V'E (*y* axis) and $V'CO_2$. The linear phase of the $V'E/V'CO_2$ relationship was detected on the V'E (*y* axis) on $V'CO_2$ (*x* axis) plot, between the beginning of loaded exercise and the end of the isocapnic buffering period, which was identified when $V'E/V'CO_2$ increased and $P_{ET}CO_2$ decreased. Linear regression was then applied and the $V'E/V'CO_2$ slope and its intercept on the *y* axis were calculated. $V'E/V'CO_2$ raw value at θ_L was also recorded.

The subject's effort was considered maximal either if the respiratory exchange ratio reached ≥1.10 or if HR achieved ≥85% of maximal predicted value at peak exercise (f). CPET parameters were compared with the predicted normal values [53].

All PFT and CPET were executed and analyzed by two physicians blinded to patients' clinical and laboratory features.

4.5. Imaging Evaluation

All ACPA-positive participants underwent HRCT of the chest by the use of a multidetector scanner (Somatom Definition Siemens, Erlangen, Germany) with helical supine inspiratory contiguous acquisition (5 mm); images were reconstructed at 0.6 mm every 20 mm with high-resolution algorithms. HRCT images were reviewed by 2 radiologists who were blinded to each subject with regard to disease status, in order to evaluate the presence of subclinical parenchymal abnormalities (i.e., emphysema, fibrosis, ground-glass opacities, consolidations, nodules) and/or airways abnormalities (bronchiectasis, airways thickening, air trapping) as described previously [10]. The occurrence of "definite UIP" or "probable UIP" pattern was considered an exclusion criterion [54].

4.6. Statistical Analysis

Continuous variables are shown as mean ± SD or as median (range) for normally and non-normally distributed data, respectively. Categorical variables are presented as frequencies. Comparisons of continuous variables between two groups were performed using an independent samples T test or Mann–Whitney U test, whilst comparisons between more than two groups were tested through the ANOVA (with Bonferroni's correction for post hoc adjustment) or Kruskal–Wallis test, according to data distribution. Chi-squared analysis tested the differences between categorical variables. Logistic regression analysis was performed to assess the strength of association between HRCT abnormalities and clinical, laboratory and functional features of interest. The predictive capacity of SPD serum levels for the presence of HRCT abnormalities was analyzed using ROC curves. Cut-offs with sensitivity and specificity to discriminate subjects with HRCT abnormalities from subjects without them were calculated. The significance of the correlations was evaluated with Spearman's rank correlation coefficient.

All statistical analyses were performed using the SPSS Statistics version 24.0 software package (SPSS Inc., Chicago, IL, USA), and a two-sided p value < 0.05 was considered statistically significant.

5. Conclusions

The role of the lung in RA is dual: a site of autoimmunity generation and of disease-related injury. The identification of subclinical lung abnormalities can be relevant in the management of the disease, but a reliable biomarker that can easily identify lung involvement in RA patients is still lacking in clinical practice. HRCT is the gold standard for the evaluation of lung parenchyma but entails a significant exposure to ionizing radiations. Stratifying the risk for lung abnormalities in the individual patients may help to identify who needs to be referred early to a HRCT scan.

This study shows that PFR and CPET may help to identify RA patients who have an increased likelihood of HRCT abnormalities, and provide information about the kind of lung involvement that may have an impact on the clinical management and the therapeutic decision. SPD shows a good accuracy in identifying HRCT abnormalities in ACPA-positive subjects, confirming its role as a biomarker of lung involvement. The combination of serum biomarkers and PFT may provide a safe and harmless tool to identify subjects who require further investigations. SPD and functional parameters, especially DL_{CO}, also have a potential application among individuals in the preclinical phase of the disease, contributing to identifying ACPA-positive subjects who likely have subclinical lung abnormalities, for research and clinical purposes. However, larger studies are needed to validate the potential role of PFR, CPET and SPD in ACPA-positive subjects.

Author Contributions: Conceptualization, B.L. and M.D.F.; Data curation, B.L., M.D.P., C.G. and C.M.; Formal analysis, B.L., M.D.P. and C.M.; Investigation, B.L., M.D.P. and C.G.; Methodology, B.L., M.D.P., C.G., M.V., D.D. (Diacinti Davide) and D.D. (Diacinti Daniele); Project administration M.D.F.; Supervision, C.A., P.P. and M.D.F.; Validation, B.L., M.D.P., P.P. and M.D.F.; Writing—original draft, B.L.; Writing—review & editing, B.L., M.D.P. and M.D.F. All authors have read and agreed to the published version of the manuscript.

Funding: This research received no external funding.

Conflicts of Interest: The authors declare no conflict of interest.

References

1. Scott, D.L.; Wolfe, F.; Huizinga, T.W. Rheumatoid arthritis. *Lancet* **2010**, *376*, 1094–1108. [CrossRef]
2. Smolen, J.S.; Aletaha, D.; McInnes, I.B. Rheumatoid arthritis. *Lancet* **2016**, *388*, 2023–2038. [CrossRef]
3. Young, A.; Koduri, G.; Batley, M.; Kulinskaya, E.; Gough, A.; Norton, S.; Dixey, J. Mortality in rheumatoid arthritis. Increased in the early course of disease, in ischaemic heart disease and in pulmonary fibrosis. *Rheumatology* **2006**, *46*, 350–357. [CrossRef] [PubMed]

4. Van Steenbergen, H.W.; Aletaha, D.; Beaart-Van De Voorde, L.J.J.; Brouwer, E.; Codreanu, C.; Combe, B.; Fonseca, J.E.; Hetland, M.L.; Humby, F.; Kvien, T.K. EULAR definition of arthralgia suspicious for progression to rheumatoid arthritis. *Ann. Rheum. Dis.* **2017**, *76*, 491–496. [CrossRef] [PubMed]

5. Klareskog, L.; Malmström, V.; Lundberg, K.; Padyukov, L.; Alfredsson, L. Smoking, citrullination and genetic variability in the immunopathogenesis of rheumatoid arthritis. *Semin. Immunol.* **2011**, *23*, 92–98. [CrossRef]

6. Lucchino, B.; Spinelli, F.R.; Iannuccelli, C.; Guzzo, M.P.; Conti, F.; Di Franco, M. Mucosa–Environment Interactions in the Pathogenesis of Rheumatoid Arthritis. *Cells* **2019**, *8*, 700. [CrossRef] [PubMed]

7. Gerardi, M.C.; Luca, N.D.; Alessandri, C.; Iannuccelli, C.; Valesini, G.; Di Franco, M. Frequency of antibodies to mutated citrullinated vimentin in chronic obstructive pulmonary disease: Comment on the article by Demoruelle et al. *Arthritis Rheum.* **2013**, *65*, 1672–1673. [CrossRef]

8. Willis, V.C.; Demoruelle, M.K.; Derber, L.A.; Chartier-Logan, C.J.; Parish, M.C.; Pedraza, I.F.; Weisman, M.H.; Norris, J.M.; Holers, V.M.; Deane, K.D. Sputum autoantibodies in patients with established rheumatoid arthritis and subjects at risk of future clinically apparent disease. *Arthritis Rheum.* **2013**, *65*, 2545–2554. [PubMed]

9. Reynisdottir, G.; Karimi, R.; Joshua, V.; Olsen, H.; Hensvold, A.H.; Harju, A.; Engström, M.; Grunewald, J.; Nyren, S.; Eklund, A. Structural changes and antibody enrichment in the lungs are early features of anti–citrullinated protein antibody–positive rheumatoid arthritis. *Arthritis Rheumatol.* **2014**, *66*, 31–39. [CrossRef] [PubMed]

10. Demoruelle, M.K.; Weisman, M.H.; Simonian, P.L.; Lynch, D.A.; Sachs, P.B.; Pedraza, I.F.; Harrington, A.R.; Kolfenbach, J.R.; Striebich, C.C.; Pham, Q.N. Brief Report: Airways abnormalities and rheumatoid arthritis–related autoantibodies in subjects without arthritis: Early injury or initiating site of autoimmunity? *Arthritis Rheum.* **2012**, *64*, 1756–1761. [CrossRef]

11. Shaw, M.; Collins, B.F.; Ho, L.A.; Raghu, G. Rheumatoid arthritis-associated lung disease. *Eur. Respir. Rev.* **2015**, *24*, 1–16. [CrossRef] [PubMed]

12. Ha, Y.-J.; Lee, Y.J.; Kang, E.H. Lung involvements in rheumatic diseases: Update on the epidemiology, pathogenesis, clinical features, and treatment. *BioMed Res. Int.* **2018**, *2018*, 19. [CrossRef]

13. Yamasaki, M. Long-Term Follow up of Subclinical Interstitial Lung Disease in Rheumatoid Arthritis. In Proceedings of the 2018 American College Rheumatology/Association of Rheumatology Professionals Annual Meeting, Chicago, IL, USA, 19–24 October 2018.

14. Gochuico, B.R.; Avila, N.A.; Chow, C.K.; Novero, L.J.; Wu, H.-P.; Ren, P.; MacDonald, S.D.; Travis, W.D.; Stylianou, M.P.; Rosas, I.O. Progressive preclinical interstitial lung disease in rheumatoid arthritis. *Arch. Intern. Med.* **2008**, *168*, 159–166. [CrossRef]

15. Solomon, J.J.; Chung, J.H.; Cosgrove, G.P.; Demoruelle, M.K.; Fernandez-Perez, E.R.; Fischer, A.; Frankel, S.K.; Hobbs, S.B.; Huie, T.J.; Ketzer, J. Predictors of mortality in rheumatoid arthritis-associated interstitial lung disease. *Eur. Respir. J.* **2016**, *47*, 588–596. [CrossRef]

16. Yang, J.A.; Lee, J.S.; Park, J.K.; Lee, E.B.; Song, Y.W.; Lee, E.Y. Clinical characteristics associated with occurrence and poor prognosis of interstitial lung disease in rheumatoid arthritis. *Korean J. Intern. Med.* **2019**, *34*, 434. [CrossRef] [PubMed]

17. Chen, J.; Shi, Y.; Wang, X.; Huang, H.; Ascherman, D. Asymptomatic preclinical rheumatoid arthritis-associated interstitial lung disease. *Clin. Dev. Immunol.* **2013**, *2013*. [CrossRef] [PubMed]

18. Guazzi, M.; Bandera, F.; Ozemek, C.; Systrom, D.; Arena, R. Cardiopulmonary exercise testing: What is its value? *J. Am. Coll. Cardiol.* **2017**, *70*, 1618–1636. [CrossRef] [PubMed]

19. Palange, P.; Ward, S.A.; Carlsen, K.H.; Casaburi, R.; Gallagher, C.G.; Gosselink, R.; O'Donnell, D.E.; Puente-Maestu, L.; Schols, A.M.; Singh, S. Recommendations on the use of exercise testing in clinical practice. *Eur. Respir. J.* **2007**, *29*, 185–209. [CrossRef]

20. Tzilas, V.; Bouros, D. Cardiopulmonary Exercise Testing in Systemic Sclerosis: 'Ars longa, vita brevis'. *Respiration* **2016**, *91*, 202–203. [CrossRef]

21. Rosato, E.; Romaniello, A.; Magrì, D.; Bonini, M.; Sardo, L.; Gigante, A.; Quarta, S.; Digiulio, M.A.; Viola, G.; Di Paolo, M. Exercise tolerance in systemic sclerosis patients without pulmonary impairment: Correlation with clinical variables. *Clin. Exp. Rheumatol.* **2014**, *32*, 103–108.

22. Doyle, T.J.; Patel, A.S.; Hatabu, H.; Nishino, M.; Wu, G.; Osorio, J.C.; Golzarri, M.F.; Traslosheros, A.; Chu, S.G.; Frits, M.L. Detection of rheumatoid arthritis–interstitial lung disease is enhanced by serum biomarkers. *Am. J. Respir. Crit. Care Med.* **2015**, *191*, 1403–1412. [CrossRef]

23. Madsen, J.; Kliem, A.; Tornøe, I.; Skjødt, K.; Koch, C.; Holmskov, U. Localization of lung surfactant protein D on mucosal surfaces in human tissues. *J. Immunol.* **2000**, *164*, 5866–5870. [CrossRef] [PubMed]
24. Wright, J.R. Immunoregulatory functions of surfactant proteins. *Nat. Rev. Immunol.* **2005**, *5*, 58–68. [CrossRef] [PubMed]
25. Sorensen, G.L.; Husby, S.; Holmskov, U. Surfactant protein A and surfactant protein D variation in pulmonary disease. *Immunobiology* **2007**, *212*, 381–416. [CrossRef] [PubMed]
26. Fischer, A.; Solomon, J.J.; du Bois, R.M.; Deane, K.D.; Olson, A.L.; Fernandez-Perez, E.R.; Huie, T.J.; Stevens, A.D.; Gill, M.B.; Rabinovitch, A.M. Lung disease with anti-CCP antibodies but not rheumatoid arthritis or connective tissue disease. *Respir. Med.* **2012**, *106*, 1040–1047. [CrossRef]
27. Bernstein, E.J.; Barr, R.G.; Austin, J.H.M.; Kawut, S.M.; Raghu, G.; Sell, J.L.; Hoffman, E.A.; Newell, J.D.; Watts, J.R.; Nath, P.H. Rheumatoid arthritis-associated autoantibodies and subclinical interstitial lung disease: The Multi-Ethnic Study of Atherosclerosis. *Thorax* **2016**, *71*, 1082–1090. [CrossRef] [PubMed]
28. Reynisdottir, G.; Olsen, H.; Joshua, V.; Engström, M.; Forsslund, H.; Karimi, R.; Sköld, C.M.; Nyren, S.; Eklund, A.; Grunewald, J. Signs of immune activation and local inflammation are present in the bronchial tissue of patients with untreated early rheumatoid arthritis. *Ann. Rheum. Dis.* **2016**, *75*, 1722–1727. [CrossRef] [PubMed]
29. Hyldgaard, C.; Hilberg, O.; Pedersen, A.B.; Ulrichsen, S.P.; Løkke, A.; Bendstrup, E.; Ellingsen, T. A population-based cohort study of rheumatoid arthritis-associated interstitial lung disease: Comorbidity and mortality. *Ann. Rheum. Dis.* **2017**, *76*, 1700–1706. [CrossRef]
30. Patatanian, E.; Thompson, D.F. A review of methotrexate-induced accelerated nodulosis. *Pharmacother. J. Hum. Pharmacol. Drug Ther.* **2002**, *22*, 1157–1162. [CrossRef]
31. Kiely, P.; Busby, A.D.; Nikiphorou, E.; Sullivan, K.; Walsh, D.A.; Creamer, P.; Dixey, J.; Young, A. Is incident rheumatoid arthritis interstitial lung disease associated with methotrexate treatment? Results from a multivariate analysis in the ERAS and ERAN inception cohorts. *BMJ Open* **2019**, *9*, e028466. [CrossRef] [PubMed]
32. Kelly, C.A.; Saravanan, V.; Nisar, M.; Arthanari, S.; Woodhead, F.A.; Price-Forbes, A.N.; Dawson, J.; Sathi, N.; Ahmad, Y.; Koduri, G. Rheumatoid arthritis-related interstitial lung disease: Associations, prognostic factors and physiological and radiological characteristics—A large multicentre UK study. *Rheumatology* **2014**, *53*, 1676–1682. [CrossRef] [PubMed]
33. Roubille, C.; Haraoui, B. Interstitial lung diseases induced or exacerbated by DMARDS and biologic agents in rheumatoid arthritis: A systematic literature review. *Semin. Arthritis Rheum.* **2014**, *43*, 613–626. [CrossRef] [PubMed]
34. Geri, G.; Dadoun, S.; Bui, T.; Pinol, N.D.C.; Paternotte, S.; Dougados, M.; Gossec, L. Risk of infections in bronchiectasis during disease-modifying treatment and biologics for rheumatic diseases. *BMC Infect. Dis.* **2011**, *11*, 1–8. [CrossRef]
35. Hamblin, M.J.; Horton, M.R. Rheumatoid arthritis-associated interstitial lung disease: Diagnostic dilemma. *Pulm. Med.* **2011**, *2011*, 12. [CrossRef]
36. Wang, T.; Zheng, X.-J.; Liang, B.-M.; Liang, Z.-A. Clinical features of rheumatoid arthritis-associated interstitial lung disease. *Sci. Rep.* **2015**, *5*, 14897. [CrossRef] [PubMed]
37. Podolanczuk, A.J.; Oelsner, E.C.; Barr, R.G.; Hoffman, E.A.; Armstrong, H.F.; Austin, J.H.M.; Basner, R.C.; Bartels, M.N.; Christie, J.D.; Enright, P.L. High attenuation areas on chest computed tomography in community-dwelling adults: The MESA study. *Eur. Respir. J.* **2016**, *48*, 1442–1452. [CrossRef] [PubMed]
38. Doyle, T.J.; Hunninghake, G.M.; Rosas, I.O. Subclinical interstitial lung disease: Why you should care. *Am. J. Respire. Crit. Care Med.* **2012**, *185*, 1147–1153. [CrossRef]
39. Rosas, I.O.; Ren, P.; Avila, N.A.; Chow, C.K.; Franks, T.J.; Travis, W.D.; McCoy, J.P., Jr.; May, R.M.; Wu, H.-P.; Nguyen, D.M. Early interstitial lung disease in familial pulmonary fibrosis. *Am. J. Respir. Crit. Care Med.* **2007**, *176*, 698–705. [CrossRef]
40. Crisafulli, E.; Alfieri, V.; Silva, M.; Aiello, M.; Tzani, P.; Milanese, G.; Bertorelli, G.; Sverzellati, N.; Chetta, A. Relationships between emphysema and airways metrics at high-resolution computed tomography (HRCT) and ventilatory response to exercise in mild to moderate COPD patients. *Respir. Med.* **2016**, *117*, 207–214. [CrossRef]

41. Paoletti, P.; De Filippis, F.; Fraioli, F.; Cinquanta, A.; Valli, G.; Laveneziana, P.; Vaccaro, F.; Martolini, D.; Palange, P. Cardiopulmonary exercise testing (CPET) in pulmonary emphysema. *Respir. Physiol. Neurobiol.* **2011**, *179*, 167–173. [CrossRef]
42. Crisafulli, E.; Teopompi, E.; Luceri, S.; Longo, F.; Tzani, P.; Pagano, P.; Ielpo, A.; Longo, C.; Di Paolo, M.; Sverzellati, N. The value of high-resolution computed tomography (HRCT) to determine exercise ventilatory inefficiency and dynamic hyperinflation in adult patients with cystic fibrosis. *Respir. Res.* **2019**, *20*, 78. [CrossRef]
43. Ju, C.-R.; Liu, W.; Chen, R.-C. Serum surfactant protein D: Biomarker of chronic obstructive pulmonary disease. *Dis. Markers* **2012**, *32*, 281–287. [CrossRef] [PubMed]
44. Giles, J.T.; Danoff, S.K.; Sokolove, J.; Wagner, C.A.; Winchester, R.; Pappas, D.A.; Siegelman, S.; Connors, G.; Robinson, W.H.; Bathon, J.M. Association of fine specificity and repertoire expansion of anticitrullinated peptide antibodies with rheumatoid arthritis associated interstitial lung disease. *Ann. Rheum. Dis.* **2014**, *73*, 1487–1494. [CrossRef] [PubMed]
45. Demoruelle, M.K.; Harrall, K.K.; Ho, L.; Purmalek, M.M.; Seto, N.L.; Rothfuss, H.M.; Weisman, M.H.; Solomon, J.J.; Fischer, A.; Okamoto, Y. Anti–citrullinated protein antibodies are associated with neutrophil extracellular traps in the sputum in relatives of rheumatoid arthritis patients. *Arthritis Rheumatol.* **2017**, *69*, 1165–1175. [CrossRef]
46. Weatherald, J.; Sattler, C.; Garcia, G.; Laveneziana, P. Ventilatory response to exercise in cardiopulmonary disease: The role of chemosensitivity and dead space. *Eur. Respir. J.* **2018**, *51*, 1700860. [CrossRef] [PubMed]
47. Miller, M.R.; Hankinson, J.; Brusasco, V.; Burgos, F.; Casaburi, R.; Coates, A.; Crapo, R.; Enright, P.; Van Der Grinten, C.P.M.; Gustafsson, P. Standardisation of spirometry. *Eur. Respir. J.* **2005**, *26*, 319–338. [CrossRef]
48. Wanger, J.; Clausen, J.L.; Coates, A.; Pedersen, O.F.; Brusasco, V.; Burgos, F.; Casaburi, R.; Crapo, R.; Enright, P.; Van Der Grinten, C.P.M. Standardisation of the measurement of lung volumes. *Eur. Respir. J.* **2005**, *26*, 511–522. [CrossRef]
49. Quanjer, P.H.; Tammeling, G.J.; Cotes, J.E.; Pedersen, O.F.; Peslin, R.; Yernault, J.C. Lung volumes and forced ventilatory flows. *Eur. Respir. Soc.* **1993**, *6*, 5–40. [CrossRef]
50. Cotes, J.E.; Chinn, D.J.; Quanjer, P.H.; Roca, J.; Yernault, J.C. Standardization of the measurement of transfer factor (diffusing capacity). *Eur. Respir. Soc.* **1993**, *6*, 41–52. [CrossRef] [PubMed]
51. American Thoracic, S. ATS/ACCP statement on cardiopulmonary exercise testing. *Am. J. Respir. Crit. Care Med.* **2003**, *167*, 211–277.
52. Wasserman, K.; Hansen, J.; Sue, D.; Stringer, W.; Whipp, B. *Principles of Exercise Testing and Interpretation*, 5th ed.; Lippincott Williams & Wilkins: Philadelphia, PA, USA, 2011.
53. Koch, B.; Schäper, C.; Ittermann, T.; Spielhagen, T.; Dörr, M.; Völzke, H.; Opitz, C.F.; Ewert, R.; Gläser, S. Reference values for cardiopulmonary exercise testing in healthy volunteers: The SHIP study. *Eur. Respir. J.* **2009**, *33*, 389–397. [CrossRef] [PubMed]
54. Raghu, G.; Remy-Jardin, M.; Myers, J.L.; Richeldi, L.; Ryerson, C.J.; Lederer, D.J.; Behr, J.; Cottin, V.; Danoff, S.K.; Morell, F. Diagnosis of idiopathic pulmonary fibrosis. An official ATS/ERS/JRS/ALAT clinical practice guideline. *Am. J. Respir. Crit. Care Med.* **2018**, *198*, e44–e68. [CrossRef] [PubMed]

International Journal of *Molecular Sciences*

MDPI

Article

Upregulation of miR-941 in Circulating CD14+ Monocytes Enhances Osteoclast Activation via WNT16 Inhibition in Patients with Psoriatic Arthritis

Shang-Hung Lin [1,2,3], Ji-Chen Ho [1], Sung-Chou Li [4], Yu-Wen Cheng [1], Yi-Chien Yang [1], Jia-Feng Chen [5], Chung-Yuan Hsu [5], Toshiaki Nakano [2,6], Feng-Sheng Wang [7], Ming-Yu Yang [2,8], Chih-Hung Lee [1,*] and Chang-Chun Hsiao [2,9,*]

1 Department of Dermatology, Kaohsiung Chang Gung Memorial Hospital and Chang Gung University College of Medicine, Kaohsiung 83301, Taiwan; hong51@cgmh.org.tw (S.-H.L.); jichenho@cgmh.org.tw (J.-C.H.); yuwen@cgmh.org.tw (Y.-W.C.); yichienyang@gmail.com (Y.-C.Y.)
2 Graduate Institute of Clinical Medical Sciences, College of Medicine, Chang Gung University, Taoyuan 33302, Taiwan; toshi.nakano@msa.hinet.net (T.N.); yangmy@mail.cgu.edu.tw (M.-Y.Y.)
3 Chang Gung University of Science and Technology—Chiayi Campus, Chiayi 61363, Taiwan
4 Genomics and Proteomics Core Laboratory, Kaohsiung Chang Gung Memorial Hospital, Chang Gung University College of Medicine, Kaohsiung 83301, Taiwan; raymond.pinus@gmail.com
5 Division of Rheumatology, Allergy and Immunology, Department of Internal Medicine, Kaohsiung Chang Gung Memorial Hospital and Chang Gung University College of Medicine, Kaohsiung 83301, Taiwan; uporchid@cgmh.org.tw (J.-F.C.); chungyuango@gmail.com (C.-Y.H.)
6 Department of Surgery, Kaohsiung Chang Gung Memorial Hospital, Kaohsiung 83301, Taiwan
7 Department of Medical Research, Kaohsiung Chang Gung Memorial Hospital and Chang Gung University College of Medicine, Kaohsiung 83301, Taiwan; wangfs@ms33.hinet.net
8 Department of Otolaryngology, Kaohsiung Chang Gung Memorial Hospital and Chang Gung University College of Medicine, Kaohsiung 83301, Taiwan
9 Center for Shockwave Medicine and Tissue Engineering, Kaohsiung Chang Gung Memorial Hospital, Kaohsiung 83301, Taiwan
* Correspondence: zieben@cgmh.org.tw or dermlee@gmail.com (C.-H.L.); cchsiao@mail.cgu.edu.tw (C.-C.H.); Tel.: +886-7-7317123 (ext. 2424) (C.-H.L.); +886-7-7317123 (ext. 8979) (C.-C.H.)

Received: 11 May 2020; Accepted: 11 June 2020; Published: 17 June 2020

Abstract: Psoriatic arthritis (PsA) is a destructive joint disease mediated by osteoclasts. MicroRNAs (miRNAs) regulate several important pathways in osteoclastogenesis. We profiled the expression of miRNAs in CD14+ monocytes from PsA patients and investigated how candidate microRNAs regulate the pathophysiology in osteoclastogenesis. The RNA from circulatory CD14+ monocytes was isolated from PsA patients, psoriasis patients without arthritis (PsO), and healthy controls (HCs). The miRNAs were initially profiled by next-generation sequencing (NGS). The candidate miRNAs revealed by NGS were validated by PCR in 40 PsA patients, 40 PsO patients, and 40 HCs. The osteoclast differentiation and its functional resorption activity were measured with or without RNA interference against the candidate miRNA. The microRNA-941 was selectively upregulated in CD14+ monocytes from PsA patients. Osteoclast development and resorption ability were increased in CD14+ monocytes from PsA patients. Inhibition of miR-941 abrogated the osteoclast development and function while increased the expression of WNT16. After successful treatment, the increased miR-941 expression in CD14+ monocytes from PsA patients was revoked. The expression of miR-941 in CD14+ monocytes is associated with PsA disease activity. MiR-941 enhances osteoclastogenesis in PsA via WNT16 repression. The miR-941 could be a potential biomarker and treatment target for PsA.

Keywords: psoriatic arthritis; osteoclastogenesis; miR-941; WNT16

1. Introduction

Psoriatic arthritis (PsA) is a chronic and indolent inflammatory disease involving progressive arthropathy in approximately 30% of patients with psoriasis. Skin manifestations usually precede the onset of PsA by an average of 10 years. [1]. The diagnosis of PsA is based on the recognition of clinical and imaging features [2]. The most widely used diagnostic criteria for PsA is the Classification Criteria for Psoriatic Arthritis (CASPAR) [3]. PsA is easily overlooked and missed with incorrect diagnosis or messed up with delayed diagnosis, both of which could lead to poor radiographic and devastating functional outcome [4]. In fact, Haroon et al. reported that a diagnostic delay of more than six months contributes to poor radiographic and functional outcome in PsA [5].

PsA is featured with bone erosions mediated by activated osteoclasts. Osteoclasts, the multinucleated giant cells with a monocyte/macrophage lineage, are the main cells responsible for bone resorption [6,7]. It was reported that numbers of osteoclast precursors are increased in PsA patients as compared with those from healthy controls [8]. Consistently, we have demonstrated that circulating CD14+ monocytes from patients with PsA have active osteoclastogenesis and active resorption activity.

MicroRNAs (miRNAs) are a class of small noncoding RNAs that negatively regulate the expression of protein-coding genes. Emerging evidence suggests that miRNA-mediated regulation represents a fundamental layer of epigenetic control over diverse physiological and pathological processes [9,10].

With a hypothesis-driven approach, we previously investigated the role of three common osteoclast activation microRNAs (miR-146a/b and miR-155) in CD14+ monocytes in PsA. We demonstrated miR-146a-5p in CD14+ monocytes from PsA patients correlates with its disease severity in vivo and active bone resorption in vitro [11]. However, in that study, only three microRNAs are investigated in osteoclasts of PsA patients. A general expression profile of various miRNAs in PsA is required to investigate whether there were other important miRNAs critical in the pathogenesis of PsA.

Next-generation sequencing (NGS) provides a high-throughput sequencing platform that performs much better than the traditional Sanger sequencing. NGS facilitates the discovery of genes and regulatory elements associated with disease [12] so that we could determine miRNA expression profile of the pooled RNA libraries from osteoclasts of PsA patients, psoriasis patients without arthritis (PsO), and healthy controls (HC). We adopted MiSeq platform (Illumina) for large scale profiling. The RNA libraries are first prepared with TruSeq Small RNA Sample Preparation protocol (Illumina) followed by sequencing with MiSeq platform. The generated NGS data is further analyzed with miRSeq for evaluating sequencing quality and determining miRNA expression profile.

Circulating monocytes in the blood are appropriate and readily accessible for bone-related studies and are a good source of osteoclast precursors to study [13,14]. Therefore, in this study, we utilized circulating monocytes to investigate the functional activation osteoclasts in individual subjects. In addition, the overall expression of miRNAs from osteoclast precursors, the CD14+ monocytes, has not been profiled independently. The present study aimed to identify whether specific miRNAs (through NGS) from CD14+ monocytes could serve as diagnostic biomarkers and treatment targets for PsA (through clinical subject categories). This study also addressed the mechanisms by which specific miRNAs contribute to active osteoclastogenesis and functional activity in PsA (through RNA interference and bone resorption assay).

2. Results

2.1. Subject Demographics

Forty patients with PsA (Female/Male: 12/28, average age: 47.6 years old), 40 PsO patients (Female/Male: 9/31, average: 43.8 years old), and 40 HCs (Female/male: 11/29, average age: 44.1 years old) were recruited (Table 1). Most PsA patients had severe psoriasis (average PASI of 14.2), and all of them had peripheral arthritis, including 35% with axial arthritis, 35% with dactylitis, and 45% with enthesitis.

Table 1. Demographics of psoriatic arthritis patients (PsA), psoriatic patients without arthritis (PsO), and healthy controls (HCs).

	PsA (n = 40)	PsO (n = 40)	HC (n = 40)
Age (years)	47.6 ± 12.2	43.8 ± 13.3	44.1 ± 12.4
Female/Male	12/28	9/31	11/29
Weight (kg)	72.4 ± 15.5	73.1 ± 14.1	70.0 ± 10.0
Psoriasis duration (years)	14.9 ± 7.4	15.8 ± 7.4	
Psoriatic arthritis duration (years)	7.9 ± 7.2		
Skin PASI *	14.2 ± 9.1	15.9 ± 5.3	
Peripheral arthritis no. (%)	40 (100)		
Peripheral and axil arthritis no. (%)	14 (35)		
Dactylitis no. (%)	14 (35)		
Enthesitis no. (%)	18 (45)		
No. of tender-joints (78 joints)	7.5 ± 7.0		
No. of swollen-joint (76 joints)	6.7 ± 6.9		
Uveitis no. (%)	2 (5)		
Previous drug usage: Anti-TNF, anti-IL12/23 or anti-IL17 biologics. no. (%)	4 (10)	4 (10)	
Methotrexate no. (%)	31 (77.5)	33 (82.5)	
Leflunomide no. (%)	10 (25)	0	
NSAID no. (%)	38 (95)	0	

* PASI: Psoriasis Area and Severity Index.

2.2. *Upregulation of miR-941 in CD14+ Monocytes from PsA Patients by qRT-PCR, with Support Vector Machine Learning, Identified miR-941 as an Early Predictor for PsA*

In order to screen specific miRNA expressions in patients with PsA, we first profiled the miRNA expression from two pooled samples from HCs (from two males and one female, respectively), two pooled samples from PsA patients (from two males and one female, respectively) and one pooled sample from PsO patients (from two males). We collected approximately 32.0 million raw reads in total, and each sample yielded 6.4 million reads on average. Twelve miRNAs with transcripts per million (TPM) values higher than 1000 in at least one sample and with average expression ratios relative to HCs > 1.5 were identified. The overall expression levels of these 12 miRNAs from PsO, PsA, and HC monocytes are presented in Figure 1A,B. Notably, expression of miR-941 and miR-146b-5p were 1.5-fold greater in the PsA group compared to that in both HC and PsO group. To validate the results revealed by NGS, the expression of miR-941 and miR-146b-5p were measured by quantitative real-time reverse transcription polymerase chain reaction (qRT-PCR) in CD14+ monocytes from 40 PsA, 40 PsO, and 40 HC subjects. While expression level of miR-146b-5p was similar among groups (Figure 1C), miR-941 expression was significantly greater in PsA patients than that in both PsO patients and HCs (Figure 1D). MiR-941 expression was significantly higher in CD14+ monocytes derived from PsA patients compared to PsO (ORs: 2.87 (95% CI: 1.62–5.06), $p < 0.001$) or HCs (ORs: 3.85 (95% CI: 2.12–6.98), $p < 0.001$). Therefore, miR-941 could be a potential biomarker able to identify PsA patients from PsO or HCs. To address this, we used support vector machine (SVM) learning [15,16] to calculate the discrimination power of miR-941 with an SVM model. The result showed the area under the receiver operating curve (auROC) was 0.79 (Figure 1E), confirming that miR-941 expression alone is able to distinguish PsA patients from PsO or HCs.

A

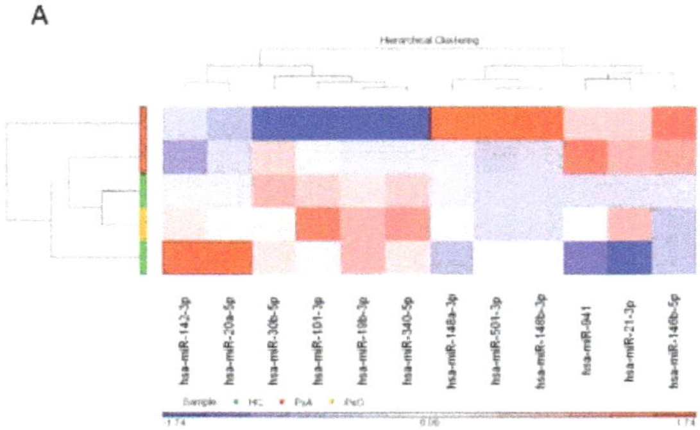

B

miR_ID	HC-M	PsA-M	HC-F	PsA-F	PsO-M
hsa-miR-941	1808.4	4024.4	1048.4	3160.4	2280.4
hsa-miR-148b-3p	4651.1	5917.1	9504.1	24585.1	4934.1
hsa-miR-501-3p	417.1	269.1	959.1	2497.1	319.1
hsa-miR-148a-3p	6327.1	6491.1	5111.1	12029.1	6778.1
hsa-miR-21-3p	6016.1	8318.1	4129.1	7879.1	8101.1
hsa-miR-146b-5p	3759.1	5421.1	3615.1	5810.1	3483.1
hsa-miR-101-3p	4366.2	3236.2	3340.2	1568.2	5110.2
hsa-miR-30b-5p	1752.1	1547.1	1459.1	402.1	1394.1
hsa-miR-19b-3p	1323.2	1064.2	1452.2	608.2	1522.2
hsa-miR-142-3p	1175.1	853.1	2056.1	1046.1	1467.1
hsa-miR-340-5p	5377.1	4091.1	5263.1	2123.1	6084.1
hsa-miR-20a-5p	1203.1	1087.1	2315.1	944.1	1266.1

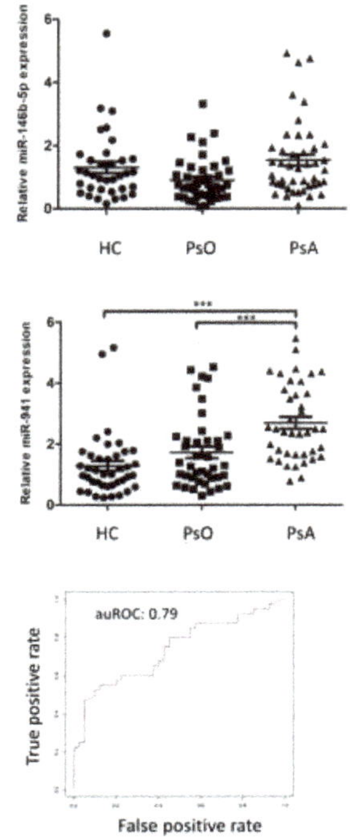

Figure 1. High expression of miR-941 in CD14+ monocytes from PsA patients. (**A**) The RNA samples were analyzed from (1) the healthy control group (HC), including two pooled samples from two males and one female, respectively; (2) the psoriasis group (PsO), including one pooled sample from two males; and (3) the psoriasis arthritis group (PsA), including two samples from two males and one female, respectively. MicroRNAs (miRNAs) with transcript per million (TPM) values more than 1000 in at least one sample and with average expression ratio (normal to disease or disease to normal) more than 1.5 are plotted on the heat map. (**B**) The microRNA expression level was presented in the unit of TPM. (**C**,**D**) The expression levels of miR-146b-5p and miR-941 were measured in HCs (n = 40), PsO patients (n = 40) and PsA patients (n = 40) by quantitative real-time reverse transcription polymerase chain reaction (qRT-PCR). Patients with PsA showed increased expression of miR-941 in CD14+ monocytes. (**E**) We set training model from miR-941 expression of CD14+ monocytes from patients with PsA, PsO, and HCs using a Support Vector Machine (SVM) learning algorithm. To distinguish PsA from PsO and HC, the value of auROC was 0.79, indicating that miR-941 expression can distinguish PsA patients from PsO and HCs with high accuracy. *** $p < 0.001$.

2.3. Enhanced Osteoclast Activation and Bone Resorption in PsA Patients with Increased miR-941 Expression

Given that miR-941 expression is elevated in CD14+ monocytes from PsA patients, we first examined whether these cells exhibited enhanced capacity to differentiate into osteoclasts and demonstrated enhanced resorption activity. The result showed that osteoclast formation was higher in CD14+ monocytes from PsA patients than that from PsO patients or HCs (12.7 ± 1.2, 6.3 ± 0.8, and 5.5 ± 0.9/per HPF from 10 PsA patients, 10 PsO patients, and 10 HCs, respectively, $p < 0.001$; Figure 2A,C). Regarding the bone resorption, the average percent area of resorption pits in dentine slices was also significantly higher in the differentiated osteoclasts from PsA patients than that from PsO patients or HCs (7.2 ± 2.0%, 2.9 ± 2.1%, 1.8 ± 1.8%/per HPF from average of 10 PsA samples, 10 PsO samples and 10 HC samples, respectively, $p < 0.001$; Figure 2B,D), indicating the enhanced osteoclast formation and active resorption activity from monocytes in PsA patients. To examine if miR-941 is important for osteoclastogenesis in PsA, we measured the expression of miR-941 in osteoclast from CD14+ monocytes of PsA, PsO patients and HCs. The expression of miR-941 in monocytes and osteoclasts from PsA patients are both higher than that from PsO patients ($p < 0.05$) or HCs ($p < 0.05$) (Figure 2E). These results suggest that miR-941 upregulation is in parallel with the elevated osteoclast differentiation potential in PsA patients.

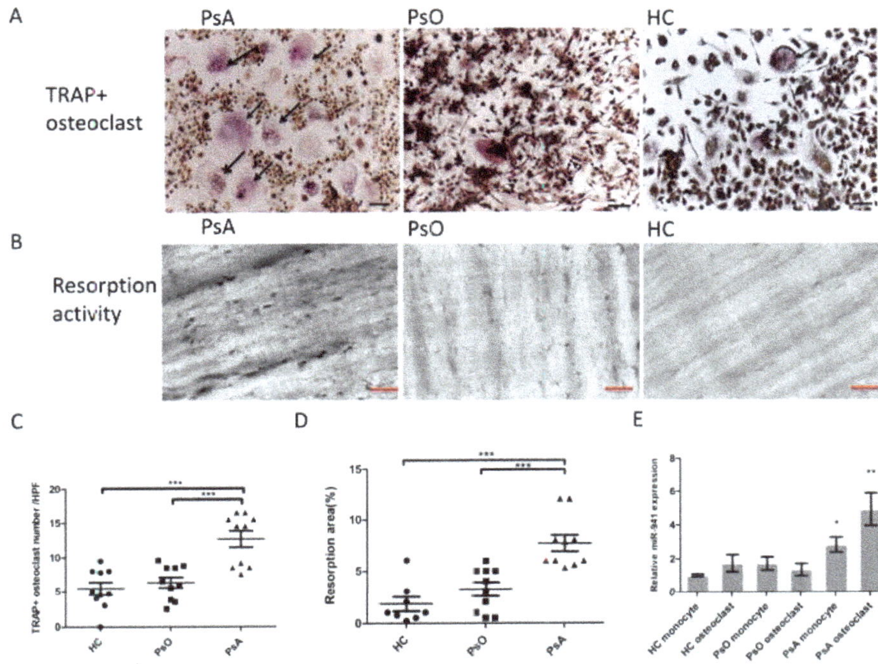

Figure 2. PsA patients with higher miR-941 expression demonstrated increased osteoclast differentiation potential and resorption activity derived from CD14+ monocytes. CD14+ monocytes from PsA patients, PsO patients, and HCs were cultured with macrophage colony-stimulating factor (M-CSF) 20 ng/mL for three days, followed by nine days in 100 ng/mL receptor activator of nuclear factor-κB ligand (RANKL) and 100 ng/mL tumor necrosis factor-α (TNF-α) for osteoclast differentiation. For evaluation of resorption activity, the osteoclasts were cultured on dentine slices. (**A**) At day 13, cells were stained with tartrate-resistant acid phosphatase (TRAP) to calculate the number of CD14+ monocyte-derived osteoclasts from PsA patients and NCs. Scale bar: 50 μm. (**B**) At day 13, resorption pits made by osteoclasts from psoriatic patients and NCs were recorded under a bright field microscope. Scale bar: 50 μm. (**C**) Osteoclast formation from CD14+ monocytes was compared between 10 HCs, 10 PsO patients, and 10 PsA patients. The number of osteoclasts was quantified among the three groups. (**D**) The eroded surface area on the dentine slices from PsA patients ($n = 10$), PsO patients ($n = 10$), and HCs ($n = 10$) were quantified using ImageJ and expressed as % of total dentine slice area. (**E**) The expression of miR-941 in monocytes and osteoclasts from PsA patients are higher than that from HCs and PsO patients using qRT-PCR. * $p < 0.05$; ** $p < 0.01$ and *** $p < 0.001$.

2.4. *miR-941 Inhibition Abolished the Osteoclast Activation and Functional Resportion in PsA Patients*

To address the direct involvement of miR-941 in the enhanced activation and functional resorption of osteoclasts derived from PsA patients, we examined whether miR-941 inhibition could reverse these effects. Peripheral CD14+ monocytes were obtained from 10 PsA patients and treated with M-CSF for 72 h. Cells were then divided into three treatment groups—one transfected with a control microRNA inhibitor (mock transfection control), one with a miR-941 inhibitor, and one without transfection.

After transfection, cultures were treated with TNF-α and RANKL every three days for nine days to induce osteoclast formation. At day 13, the number of osteoclasts formed was significantly lower in the miR-941 inhibitor group (3.0 ± 1.1/HPF) than that in the non-transfected and mock transfected control groups (12.1 ± 3.4/HPF and 11.4 ± 2.2/HPF, respectively; $p < 0.01$) (Figure 3A,B). Similarly, resorption activity was significantly lower in the group transfected with miR-941 inhibitor (2.8 ± 1.2%) than that in the non-transfected and mock transfected control groups (7.2% ± 2.0% and 7.4% ± 2.0%, respectively; $p < 0.01$) (Figure 3A,C). The miR-941 inhibition abrogated the osteoclast development in PsA. The result also showed that microRNA-941 expression was reduced to 50% of baseline in the miR-941 inhibitor group as compared to that in the non-transfected and mock-transfected control miRNA groups (Figure 3B,C). These results indicated that the miR-941 inhibitor in CD14+ monocytes may reverse the active osteoclastogenesis and resorption activity in PsA patients.

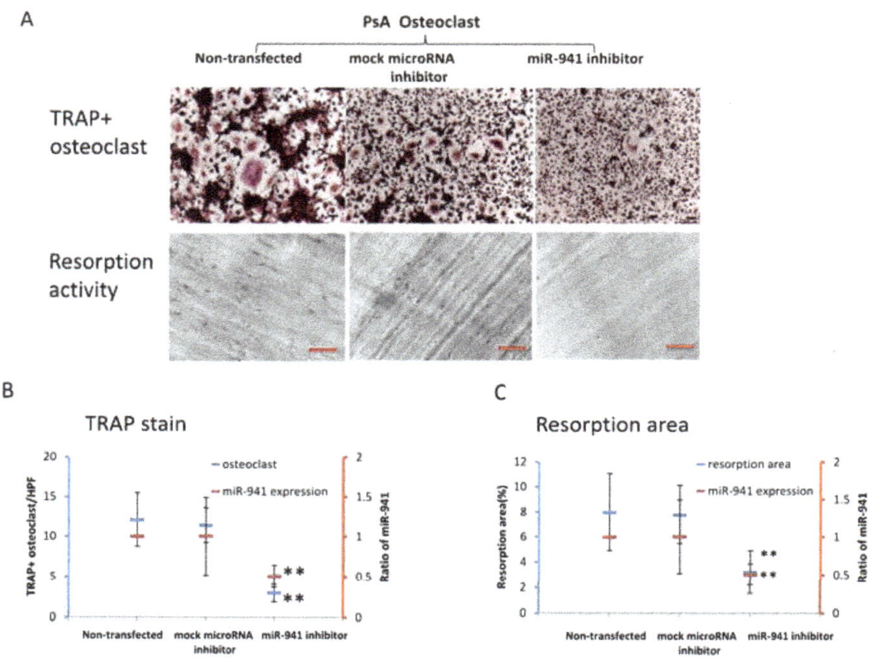

Figure 3. miR-941 inhibitor reversed osteoclast differentiation and bone resorption activity in patients with PsA. The CD14+ monocytes were obtained from eight PsA patients and were subsequently activated into osteoclasts with treatment of M-CSF for 72 h. Cells were either nontransfected or transfected with the control-microRNA inhibitor or miR-941 inhibitor followed by TNF-α and RANKL very three days for nine days to study their ability to form osteoclasts and their activity of bone resorption. At day 13, the number of osteoclast formations and percentage of resorption pits were measured. (**A**) The cells were stained with TRAP to calculate the number of osteoclasts among non-transection, negative control miRNA and miR-941 inhibitor transfection groups, Scale bar: 50 μm. For the evaluation of resorption activity, the resorption pits were recorded by a bright field microscope, Scale bar: 50 μm. (**B**) The number of osteoclasts was quantified among the three groups (blue). The relative expression of miR-941, as standardized to the level of non-transfected osteoclasts, was depicted as orange color. (**C**) The eroded surface areas on the dentine slice were quantified using ImageJ software as percentage of expressions in total areas (blue line). The expressions of miR-941 in the osteoclasts were measured by qRT-PCR to evaluate the effect of miR-941 inhibitors transfection. The relative expression of miR-941, as standardized to the level of non-transfected osteoclasts, was depicted as orange color. ** $p < 0.01$.

2.5. MicroRNA-941 Inhibits WNT16 Expression in CD14+ Monocyte, and then Contributes to Active Osteoclastogenesis Independent of miR-146a-5p

Our previous study demonstrated that higher expression of miR-146a-5p in CD14+ monocytes of psoriatic arthritis than that in HCs. We then asked whether miR-941 and miR-146a-5p interact to activate osteoclastogenesis. Peripheral CD14+ monocytes were obtained from five PsA patients. Some cells were cultured with medium only while other cells were treated with M-CSF for 72 h. We then asked whether miR-941 regulated miR-146a-5p expression or vice versa. Therefore, four treatment groups were designed—one transfected with a control microRNA inhibitor (mock transfection control), one with a miR-941 inhibitor, one with miR-146a-5p inhibitor, and one without transfection. After transfection, cultures were treated with TNF-α and RANKL every three days for nine days to induce osteoclast formation. At day 13, expressions of miR-941 and miR-146a-5p in monocytes and monocyte-derived osteoclasts were measured. As anticipated, the results showed that the expressions of miR-941 and miR-146a-5p increased after osteoclastogenesis (Figure 4A,B). However, blocking miR-941 did not alter the expressions of miR-146a-5p. Conversely, blocking of miR-146a-5p did not alter the expressions of miR-941, either (Figure 4A,B). The results indicated that the two miRNA pathways may not directly interact with each other in the osteoclastogenesis of PsA. We next asked what regulatory pathways mediate the miR-941-induced osteoclastogenesis and bone resorption. Both hedgehog-signaling and insulin-signaling pathways were reported as the potential target genes of miR-941, including *SMO, SUFU, GLI, WNT16, IRS1, mTOR*, and *PPP1CA* [17]. Notably, specifically in the process of osteoclastrogenesis, Movérare-Skrtic et al. reported that WNT16 represses human osteoclastogenesis and prevents cortical bone fragility fractures through direct effects on osteoclast progenitors [18]. Hence, we examined whether miR-941 could negatively regulate WNT16 expression, leading to active osteoclastogenesis. To address that, we investigated if miR-941 inhibition could reverse the expression of WNT16 in CD14+ monocytes of PsA patients, PsO patients, and HCs. In addition, we also measured the expression of mTOR as an internal control in the same experimental setting. The result showed that WNT16 expression was significantly lower in monocytes, monocytes derived osteoclasts with/without mock microRNA transfection of PsA patients compared to those from PsO patients or HCs ($p < 0.05$). The expression of WNT16 in osteoclast with miR-941 inhibitor from PsA patients is similar to that from PsO patients or HCs (Figure 4C). In contrast, the expression of mTOR did not change with or without miR-941 inhibition (Figure 4D).

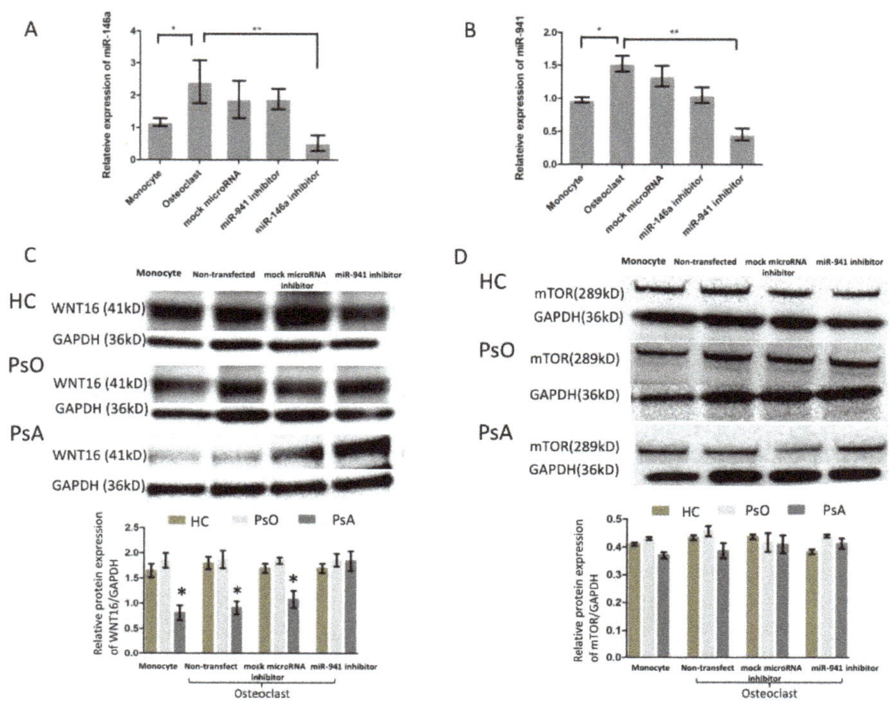

Figure 4. miR-941 inhibits osteoclastogenesis and negatively regulates WNT16 independent of miR-146a-5p. The CD14+ monocytes obtained from five PsA patients, five PsO patients, and five HCs were treated with medium only or subsequently activated into osteoclasts with treatment of M-CSF for 72 h. The cells with M-CSF treatment were either nontransfected or transfected with the control-microRNA inhibitor, miR-941 inhibitor or miR-146a-5p followed by TNF-α and RANKL every three days for nine days to study their ability to form osteoclasts and their activity of bone resorption. (**A**,**B**) At day 13, the expressions of miR-941 and miR-146a-5p in the monocytes and osteoclasts were measured by qRTPCR to evaluate the effect of miR-941 and miR-146a-5p inhibitors transfection. (**C**,**D**) The protein expression of WNT16 and mTOR, the target genes of miR-941, were measured by western blot. * $p < 0.05$ and ** $p < 0.01$.

2.6. The Enhanced miR-941 Expression was Reduced in CD14+ Cells from PsA Patients after Successful Biologics Treatment

To address whether the expression of miR-941 from circulating monocytes might serve as a potential biomarker, we examined whether the increased miR-941 expression in CD14+ monocytes from PsA patients was reduced after successful treatment. Among the 12 PsA patients that met the ACR20 achievement after 28 weeks of biologics treatment (etanercept, adalimumab, secukinumab, or ustekinumab) (Figure 5A), the enhanced expression of miR-941 in CD14+ monocytes returned to the level of NCs (Figure 5B).

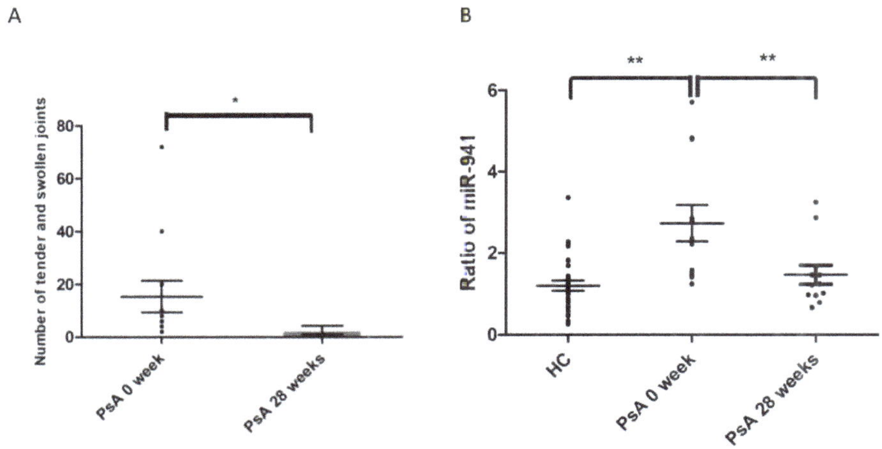

Figure 5. Reduced miR-941 expression in CD14+ monocytes from PsA patients after successful biologics treatment. The expression levels of miR-941 were measured in CD14+ monocytes from HCs and PsA patients before and after successful biologic treatment. (**A**) The total number of tender and swollen joints in PsA patients were measured before and 28 weeks after biologics treatment. (**B**) The expression levels of miR-941 were measured in CD14+ monocytes from 31 NCs and 12 PsA patients before and after 28 weeks of biologics treatment using qRT-PCR. * $p < 0.05$; ** $p < 0.01$.

3. Discussion

Our study investigated the overall expression of miRNAs from CD14+ monocytes of PsA patients. Expression of miR-941 was higher in CD14+ monocytes from PsA patients than that from PsO patients and HCs, and CD14+ monocytes from PsA patients tend to exhibit enhanced osteoclast differentiation potential and resorption activity. Further, miR-941 inhibition resumed the elevated osteoclast formation potential and resorption activity of PsA monocytes with a reciprocal upregulation of WNT16. The expression of miR-941 in CD14+ monocytes of PsA patients correlated with disease severity.

Pathological bone resorption in PsA results from increased numbers of osteoclast precursors [8]. Early diagnosis of PsA has been hindered by the lack of reliable biomarkers. Our study identifies miRNA-941 in CD14+ monocytes as an easily accessible marker for prompt computer-aided diagnosis of PsA (with an auROC value 0.79 by SVM model). In addition, we demonstrate that the increased miR-941 expression in CD14+ monocytes from PsA patients enhances osteoclast formation potential and active resorption activity. Our previous study reported that miR-146a-5p expression in CD14+ monocytes of PsA patients correlates with clinical efficacy and inducts osteoclast activation and bone resorption [11]. In this study, the overall microRNAs were measured using NGS study. The result showed that the increased expression of miR-941 from CD14+ monocytes could be used for detection of PsA. In addition, miR-941 and miR-146a-5p did not interact to activate osteoclastogenesis. In other disease, miR-941 has been indicated to be a severity marker. For example, in acute coronary syndrome, miR-941 expression was reported to be increased in the plasma of the patients [19]. Duttagupta et al. identify that miR-941 is associated with ulcerative colitis [20].

The pro-inflammatory cytokines, including TNF-α, IL-17, IL-33, and osteopontin, through activation of RANKL, induce osteoclast differentiation and activation in PsA [21–24]. Biologics selectively targeting these specific cytokines (TNF-α, IL-17 and IL-12/23) and/or intracellular signaling pathways effectively inhibit osteoclastogenesis. However, more than 40% of PsA patients show only a partial response or fail to respond to current biologics [25]. On the other hand, both enhanced osteoclast differentiation and bone resorption could be reversed by miR-941 inhibition in CD14+ monocytes from PsA patients in this study (n = 10), indicating that miR-941 may serve as both a potential biomarker and treatment target for PsA.

WNT16 is a strong anti-resorptive soluble factor acting on osteoclast precursors [26]. It can significantly inhibit RANKL-induced osteoclastogenesis of human CD14+ peripheral blood monocytes, indicating a direct action of WNT16 on osteoclast precursors. Reduced osteoclast formation by WNT16 was associated with a time- and dose-dependent blunted mRNA expression of osteoclast functional genes [18,27]. Our results provide miR-941 inhibitor increased the expression of WNT16 and inhibit osteoclastogenesis, indicating the potential involvement of miR-941-WNT in the active osteoclastogenesis in patients with PsA.

This study has several limitations. First, the case number was small. The results may be validated by large-scale studies to identify potential confounders. Second, the PsA patients recruited may have different intrinsic co-morbidities that also alter miRNA expression (e.g., diabetes mellitus, cerebrovascular disease, hypertension, etc.), making these confounders could potentially interfere the results. Third, the expression level of miR-941 in CD14+ monocytes from PsA patients before and after conventional synthetic disease-modifying antirheumatic drugs was not investigated. Fourth, although there was a reciprocal change of miR-941 and WNT16 expression in this study, whether WNT16 could be a direct target for miR-941 may require a luciferase assay.

In conclusion, the elevated expression of miR-941 in CD14+ monocytes from PsA patients enhances osteoclast activation and bone resorption activity through WNT16 repression. The activation of miR-941 and reciprocal changes of WNT16 in osteoclasts contribute to bone destruction in PsA.

4. Materials and Methods

4.1. Study Subjects

This study was conducted in accordance with the Declaration of Helsinki and was approved by the institutional review board of Chang-Gung Memorial Hospital, Taiwan (104-9618A3, 01/08/2016). Signed informed consent was obtained from all patients. 40 PsA patients and 40 PsO patients were diagnosed by both dermatologists and rheumatologists. All patients of the PsA group fulfilled the CASPAR criteria. 40 healthy adults were included as a control group (HC). The absence of psoriatic lesions and inflammatory joint were examined thoroughly in HC group. The Psoriasis Area and Severity Index (PASI) score, comorbidities of arthritis, presence of uveitis and treatment regimens were recorded. Peripheral blood from all participants was acquired at baseline and from patients after 28 weeks of standard biologics treatment (etanercept, adalimumab, secukinumab, or ustekinumab).

4.2. Isolation and Culture of Peripheral Monocytes

Monocytes were isolated directly from PBMCs using CD14+ MicroBeads (Miltenyi Biotec, Auburn, CA, USA) according to the manufacturer's instructions. The purity of the CD14+ cells after the selection is above 95% using flow cytometry showed according to our previous study [28].

4.3. MicroRNA Expression Profiling in CD14+ Monocytes by Next-Generation Sequencing (NGS)

RNA of CD14+ monocytes was extracted using Direct-zol™ RNA Kits (Zymo Research, Irvine, CA, USA) according to the manufacturer's protocol and measured quantitatively using Agilent Bioanalyzer 2100 O (Agilent, Santa Clara, CA, USA). Only samples with RNA integrity number (RIN) $\geq$ 8.0 were then used for the TruSeq Small RNA Preparation protocol (Illumina, San Diego, CA, USA). The prepared amplicons were sequenced with a V3 150-cycle sequencing reagent on the MiSeq system (Illumina, San Diego, CA, USA) to generate 51-nt single-end reads. The generated NGS data were first analyzed with miRSeq [29], a toolkit for sequencing quality evaluation and miRNA quantification (in transcripts per million, TPM).

4.4. Osteoclast Formation

Then, 3 × 10^5 purified human CD14+ monocytes were seeded in 24-well plates containing a-MEM with FBS (10%, *v/v*; Invitrogen, Waltham, MA, USA) and M-CSF (20 ng/mL; PeproTech, Rocky Hill, NJ, USA) for three days. RANKL (100 ng/mL; PeproTech, Rocky Hill, NJ, USA) and TNF-α (100 ng/mL; PeproTech, Rocky Hill, NJ, USA) were added to induce osteoclast differentiation [11]. The osteoclasts were stained with tartrate-resistant acid phosphatase (TRAP) at day 13 using the Acid Phosphate Leukocyte Kit (Sigma, St. Louis, MO, USA) according to the manufacturer's instructions. TRAP-stained cells containing three or more nuclei were defined as osteoclasts [30]. We measured the number of osteoclasts from four randomly selected higher power fields (HPF) (200×) per quadrant of the well. Four HPF were chosen from each quadrant. The number of osteoclasts was counted from the average value from 16 HPFs.

4.5. Bone Resorption Assay

Here, 5 × 10^4 purified human CD14+ monocytes were seeded on dentine slices (IDS, Gaithersburg, MD, USA) in 96-well plates containing a-MEM with 10% FBS and M-CSF (20 ng/mL) for 72 h. The cells were subsequently incubated with RANKL (100 ng/mL) and TNF-α (100 ng/mL) to induce osteoclast differentiation. At day 13, dentine slices were imaged using a bright filed microscope (Leica DM2500, Wetzlar, Germany). The Bone resorption pits were calculated using ImageJ software (NIH, Bethesda, MD, USA) from four randomly selected HPFs.

4.6. Transient Transfection of miR-941 Inhibitors

Isolated CD14+ monocyte was cultured in a-MEM with 10% FBS and M-CSF for 72 h in 96-well plates on dentine slices. Cells were then transfected with 10 nM hsa-miR-941 hairpin inhibitor or 10 nM miRNA hairpin inhibitor as a negative control (Dharmacon, Lafayette, CO, USA) using lipofectamine 3000 for 6 h based on manufacturer's instructions (Invitrogen, Carlsbad, CA, USA). The sequences of miR-941 inhibitor and negative control miRNA are GUGGGCCGACACACGUGUACACG and UCACAACCUCCUAGAAAGAGUAGA. The transfection efficiency was measured by qRT-PCR.

4.7. Quantitative Real-Time Reverse Transcription Polymerase Chain Reaction (qRT-PCR) Analysis

The complementary DNAs (cDNAs) were obtained from RNA samples (100 ng per run) using a TaqMan MicroRNA Reverse Transcription kit (Applied Biosystems; Thermo Fisher Scientific, Inc, Carlsbad, CA, USA) according to the manufacturer's protocol. Expressions of miR-941 (Assay ID. 002183) and miR-146b-5p (Assay ID. 001097) were examined using TaqMan microRNA assays (Applied Biosystems; Thermo Fisher Scientific, Inc, Carlsbad, CA, USA). The following primers of miRNAs were used: hsa-miR-941, UGAGAACUGAAUUCCAUGGGUU and hsa-miR-146b-5p, UGAGAACUGAAUUCCAUAGGCU. Quantitative RT-PCR was performed on an Applied Biosystems QuantStudio 7 Flex system. Target gene expression levels were normalized to U6 (Assay ID. 4427975). We quantified the PCR values using a 2-ΔΔCt method with U6 as an internal control by adopting the method from a previous study [31].

4.8. Western Blot Analysis

Total proteins from monocytes and monocytes-derived osteoclasts from patients with PsA were separated on a 10% SDS polyacrylamide gel and the proteins transferred to a PVDF membrane (Merck Millipore, Darmstadt, Germany). Non-specific binding sites were blocked with 5% BSA for one hour at room temperature. Membranes were subsequently incubated overnight at 4 °C with rabbit anti-WNT16 (Invitrogen, Carlsbad, CA, USA), rabbit anti-mTOR (Invitrogen, Carlsbad, CA, USA), and mouse anti-GAPDH (Merck Millipore, Darmstadt, Germany) antibodies conjugated with horseradish peroxidase. Band densities were quantified using ImageJ software (NIH, Bethesda, MD, USA).

4.9. Statistical Analysis

Age, sex, PASI score, number of tender or swollen joints, disease duration, treatment regimen, miRNA expression level, number of osteoclasts formation, and resorption area were compared among groups by chi-square, *t*-test, One-way ANOVA, or logistic regression based on the data normality. Receiver-operator characteristic analysis (ROC) and area under the curve (AUC) were used to assess whether expressions of miRNAs in CD14+ monocytes, could distinguish between PsA samples and PsO samples or healthy controls. A *p*-value less than 0.05 was considered statistically significant for all tests.

Author Contributions: S.-H.L. designed the study, conducted the experiments, analyzed the results, and wrote the manuscript. C.-H.L. and C.-C.H. contributed to study design, analyzed the results, and critically revised the paper. S.-C.L. contributed to data analysis. J.-C.H., Y.-W.C., Y.-C.Y., J.-F.C., C.-Y.H., T.N., F.-S.W., and M.-Y.Y. contributed to data acquisition. All authors have read and agreed to the published version of the manuscript.

Funding: The authors received grants from Ministry of Science and Technology of Taiwan (MOST 105-2628-B-182A-004-MY3 and MOST 108-2314-B-182A-105-MY3) and the Chang-Gung Memorial Foundation (CMRPG8J0411).

Acknowledgments: We thank the Genomics & Proteomics Core Laboratory, Department of Medical Research, Kaohsiung Chang-Gung Memorial Hospital for technical support. Kaohsiung, Taiwan.

Conflicts of Interest: The authors declare that they have no competing interests.

References

1. Gladman, D.D.; Antoni, C.; Mease, P.; Clegg, D.; Nash, P. Psoriatic arthritis: Epidemiology, clinical features, course, and outcome. *Ann. Rheum. Dis.* **2005**, *64*, ii14–ii17. [CrossRef] [PubMed]
2. Anandarajah, A.P.; Ritchlin, C.T. The diagnosis and treatment of early psoriatic arthritis. *Nat. Rev. Rheumatol.* **2009**, *5*, 634–641. [CrossRef]
3. Taylor, W.J.; Gladman, D.; Helliwell, P.; Marchesoni, A.; Mease, P.; Mielants, H.; CASPAR Study Group. Classification criteria for psoriatic arthritis: Development of new criteria from a large international study. *Arthritis Rheum.* **2006**, *54*, 2665–2673. [PubMed]
4. Bosch, F.V.D.; Coates, L. Clinical management of psoriatic arthritis. *Lancet* **2018**, *391*, 2285–2294. [PubMed]
5. Haroon, M.; Gallagher, P.; Fitzgerald, O. Diagnostic delay of more than 6 months contributes to poor radiographic and functional outcome in psoriatic arthritis. *Ann. Rheum. Dis.* **2014**, *74*, 1045–1050. [CrossRef]
6. Teitelbaum, S. Bone Resorption by Osteoclasts. *Science* **2000**, *289*, 1504–1508. [CrossRef]
7. Massey, D.B.; Flanagan, A.M. Human osteoclasts derive from CD14-positive monocytes. *Br. J. Haematol.* **1999**, *106*, 167–170. [CrossRef]
8. Ritchlin, C.T.; Haas-Smith, S.A.; Li, P.; Hicks, D.G.; Schwarz, E.M. Mechanisms of TNF-alpha- and RANKL-mediated osteoclastogenesis and bone resorption in psoriatic arthritis. *J. Clin. Investig.* **2003**, *111*, 821–831. [CrossRef]
9. Paek, S.Y.; Han, L.; Weiland, M.; Lu, C.; McKinnon, K.; Zhou, L.; Lim, H.W.; Elder, J.T.; Mi, Q.-S. Emerging biomarkers in psoriatic arthritis. *IUBMB Life* **2015**, *67*, 923–927. [CrossRef]
10. Mehta, A.; Baltimore, D. MicroRNAs as regulatory elements in immune system logic. *Nat. Rev. Immunol.* **2016**, *16*, 279–294. [CrossRef]
11. Lin, S.-H.; Ho, J.; Li, S.-C.; Chen, J.-F.; Hsiao, C.-C.; Lee, C.-H. MiR-146a-5p Expression in Peripheral CD14+ Monocytes from Patients with Psoriatic Arthritis Induces Osteoclast Activation, Bone Resorption, and Correlates with Clinical Response. *J. Clin. Med.* **2019**, *8*, 110. [CrossRef] [PubMed]
12. Grada, A.; Weinbrecht, K. Next-Generation Sequencing: Methodology and Application. *J. Investig. Dermatol.* **2013**, *133*, 11. [CrossRef] [PubMed]
13. Hemingway, F.; Cheng, X.; Knowles, H.; Estrada, F.M.; Gordon, S.; Athanasou, N. In Vitro Generation of Mature Human Osteoclasts. *Calcif. Tissue Int.* **2011**, *89*, 389–395. [CrossRef] [PubMed]
14. Zhou, Y.; Deng, H.; Shen, H. Circulating monocytes: An appropriate model for bone-related study. *Osteoporos. Int.* **2015**, *26*, 2561–2572. [CrossRef] [PubMed]
15. Kvon, E.; Kazmar, T.; Stampfel, G.; Yáñez-Cuna, J.O.; Pagani, M.; Schernhuber, K.; Dickson, B.J.; Stark, A. Genome-scale functional characterization of Drosophila developmental enhancers in vivo. *Nature* **2014**, *512*, 91–95. [CrossRef]

16. Kuo, H.-C.; Hsieh, K.-S.; Guo, M.M.-H.; Weng, K.-P.; Ger, L.-P.; Chan, W.-C.; Li, S.-C. Next-generation sequencing identifies micro-RNA–based biomarker panel for Kawasaki disease. *J. Allergy Clin. Immunol.* **2016**, *138*, 1227–1230. [CrossRef]
17. Hu, H.; He, L.; Fominykh, K.; Yan, Z.; Guo, S.; Zhang, X.; Taylor, M.S.; Tang, L.; Li, J.; Liu, J.; et al. Evolution of the human-specific microRNA miR-941. *Nat. Commun.* **2012**, *3*, 1145. [CrossRef] [PubMed]
18. Movérare-Skrtic, S.; Henning, P.; Liu, X.; Nagano, K.; Saito, H.; Börjesson, A.E.; Sjögren, K.; Windahl, S.H.; Farman, H.; Kindlund, B.; et al. Osteoblast-derived WNT16 represses osteoclastogenesis and prevents cortical bone fragility fractures. *Nat. Med.* **2014**, *20*, 1279–1288. [CrossRef]
19. Bai, R.; Yang, Q.; Xi, R.; Li, L.-Z.; Shi, D.; Chen, K. miR-941 as a promising biomarker for acute coronary syndrome. *BMC Cardiovasc. Disord.* **2017**, *17*, 227. [CrossRef]
20. Duttagupta, R.; DiRienzo, S.; Jiang, R.; Bowers, J.; Gollub, J.; Kao, J.; Kearney, K.; Rudolph, D.; Dawany, N.B.; Showe, M.K.; et al. Genome-Wide Maps of Circulating miRNA Biomarkers for Ulcerative Colitis. *PLoS ONE* **2012**, *7*, e31241. [CrossRef]
21. Mun, S.H.; Ko, N.Y.; Kim, H.S.; Kim, J.W.; Kim, K.; Kim, A.-R.; Lee, S.H.; Kim, Y.-G.; Lee, C.K.; Lee, S.H.; et al. Interleukin-33 stimulates formation of functional osteoclasts from human CD14+ monocytes. *Cell. Mol. Life Sci.* **2010**, *67*, 3883–3892. [CrossRef] [PubMed]
22. Lacey, D.; Timms, E.; Tan, H.-L.; Kelley, M.; Dunstan, C.; Burgess, T.; Elliott, R.; Colombero, A.; Elliott, G.; Scully, S.; et al. Osteoprotegerin Ligand Is a Cytokine that Regulates Osteoclast Differentiation and Activation. *Cell* **1998**, *93*, 165–176. [CrossRef]
23. Yago, T.; Nanke, Y.; Ichikawa, N.; Kobashigawa, T; Mogi, M.; Kamatani, N.; Kotake, S. IL-17 induces osteoclastogenesis from human monocytes alone in the absence of osteoblasts, which is potently inhibited by anti-TNF-α antibody: A novel mechanism of osteoclastogenesis by IL-17. *J. Cell. Biochem.* **2009**, *108*, 947–955. [CrossRef] [PubMed]
24. Lam, J.; Takeshita, S.; Barker, J.E.; Kanagawa, O.; Ross, F.P.; Teitelbaum, S.L. TNF-α induces osteoclastogenesis by direct stimulation of macrophages exposed to permissive levels of RANK ligand. *J. Clin. Investig.* **2000**, *106*, 1481–1488. [CrossRef]
25. Veale, D.J.; Fearon, U. The pathogenesis of psoriatic arthritis. *Lancet* **2018**, *391*, 2273–2284. [CrossRef]
26. Gori, F.; Lerner, U.; Ohlsson, C.; Baron, R. A new WNT on the bone: WNT16, cortical bone thickness, porosity and fractures. *BoneKEy Rep.* **2015**, *4*, 669. [CrossRef]
27. Kobayashi, Y.; Thirukonda, G.J.; Nakamura, Y.; Koide, M.; Yamashita, T.; Uehara, S.; Kato, H.; Udagawa, N.; Takahashi, N. Wnt16 regulates osteoclast differentiation in conjunction with Wnt5a. *Biochem. Biophys. Res. Commun.* **2015**, *463*, 1278–1283. [CrossRef]
28. Lin, S.-H.; Chuang, H.-Y.; Ho, J.; Lee, C.-H.; Hsiao, C.-C. Treatment with TNF-α inhibitor rectifies M1 macrophage polarization from blood CD14+ monocytes in patients with psoriasis independent of STAT1 and IRF-1 activation. *J. Dermatol. Sci.* **2018**, *91*, 276–284. [CrossRef]
29. Pan, C.-T.; Tsai, K.-W.; Hung, T.-M.; Lin, W.-C.; Pan, C.-Y.; Yu, H.-R.; Li, S.-C. miRSeq: A User-Friendly Standalone Toolkit for Sequencing Quality Evaluation and miRNA Profiling. *BioMed Res. Int.* **2014**, 1–8. [CrossRef]
30. Kurihara, N.; Suda, T.; Miura, Y.; Nakauchi, H.; Kodama, H.; Hiura, K.; Hakeda, Y.; Kumegawa, M. Generation of osteoclasts from isolated hematopoietic progenitor cells. *Blood* **1989**, *74*, 1295–1302. [CrossRef]
31. Tseng, H.-W.; Li, S.-C.; Tsai, K.-W. Metformin Treatment Suppresses Melanoma Cell Growth and Motility through Modulation of microRNA Expression. *Cancers* **2019**, *11*, 209. [CrossRef] [PubMed]

International Journal of
Molecular Sciences

MDPI

Article

Effect of Angiotensin II on Bone Erosion and Systemic Bone Loss in Mice with Tumor Necrosis Factor-Mediated Arthritis

Takahiko Akagi [1], Tomoyuki Mukai [1,*], Takafumi Mito [1], Kyoko Kawahara [1], Shoko Tsuji [1], Shunichi Fujita [1], Haruhito A. Uchida [2] and Yoshitaka Morita [1]

1 Department of Rheumatology, Kawasaki Medical School, Kurashiki, Okayama 701-0192, Japan; akagitahiko@gmail.com (T.A.); mito.tac@gmail.com (T.M.); kyoko.k0925@gmail.com (K.K.); shoko7.05.13@gmail.com (S.T.); shunic117@gmail.com (S.F.); morita@med.kawasaki-m.ac.jp (Y.M.)

2 Department of Chronic Kidney Disease and Cardiovascular Disease, Okayama University Graduate School of Medicine, Dentistry and Pharmaceutical Sciences, Okayama 700-0914, Japan; hauchida@okayama-u.ac.jp

* Correspondence: mukait@med.kawasaki-m.ac.jp; Tel.: +81-86-462-1111

Received: 24 April 2020; Accepted: 7 June 2020; Published: 10 June 2020

Abstract: Angiotensin II (Ang II) is the main effector peptide of the renin-angiotensin system (RAS), which regulates the cardiovascular system. The RAS is reportedly also involved in bone metabolism. The upregulation of RAS components has been shown in arthritic synovial tissues, suggesting the potential involvement of Ang II in arthritis. Accordingly, in the present study, we investigated the role of Ang II in bone erosion and systemic bone loss in arthritis. Ang II was infused by osmotic pumps in tumor necrosis factor-transgenic (TNFtg) mice. Ang II infusion did not significantly affect the severity of clinical and histological inflammation, whereas bone erosion in the inflamed joints was significantly augmented. Ang II administration did not affect the bone mass of the tibia or vertebra. To suppress endogenous Ang II, Ang II type 1 receptor (AT1R)-deficient mice were crossed with TNFtg mice. Genetic deletion of AT1R did not significantly affect inflammation, bone erosion, or systemic bone loss. These results suggest that excessive systemic activation of the RAS can be a risk factor for progressive joint destruction. Our findings indicate an important implication for the pathogenesis of inflammatory bone destruction and for the clinical use of RAS inhibitors in patients with rheumatoid arthritis.

Keywords: angiotensin II; arthritis; bone erosion; inflammation; tumor necrosis factor; renin-angiotensin system; angiotensin II type 1 receptor

1. Introduction

Rheumatoid arthritis is a chronic inflammatory disorder that can cause painful swelling and bone erosion in the inflamed joints [1]. The accumulation of joint damage results in long-lasting pain and deformity of the affected joints [2]. Persistent systemic inflammation in rheumatoid arthritis can also cause tissue damage in organs such as the lungs, heart, eyes, and bone [3]. Increased inflammatory cytokines affect bone metabolism throughout the body and decrease bone mass and strength, leading to increased risks of osteoporosis and fracture [4]. Joint deformities impair activities of daily life and thus exacerbate osteoporosis in patients with rheumatoid arthritis. This highlights the importance of resolving joint damage and systemic bone loss issues in these patients.

Angiotensin II (Ang II) is the main effector peptide of the renin-angiotensin system (RAS), which causes vasoconstriction and an increase in blood pressure [5,6]. The RAS is one of the most important systems in cardiovascular control [5]. Ang II is generated from its precursor angiotensinogen through serial enzymatic processes mediated by renin and angiotensin-converting enzyme (ACE). Ang II is converted mainly in the kidneys and lungs. Recent studies have shown that Ang II is generated locally in various tissues such as the brain, vascular wall, and reproductive tract [5,7]. Locally produced Ang II plays a role in many physiological and pathological processes such as hypertension, inflammation, tissue fibrosis, and oxidative stress [8], and it fulfills a key function in bone metabolism [6,9]. Animal studies have revealed that Ang II and Ang II type1 receptor (AT1R) are expressed locally within bone tissue and regulate bone mass [6,9,10]. Additionally, studies using mouse models have indicated that the local RAS is involved in the pathogenesis of several bone diseases, such as postmenopausal [11], age-related [12], and glucocorticoid-induced osteoporosis [13].

Components of the RAS are expressed at elevated levels in the synovium of patients with rheumatoid arthritis compared to those in the non-inflamed synovium [9,14,15]. However, the role of the RAS in the mechanisms underlying bone erosion and inflammation-mediated bone loss in arthritic conditions remains unclear. In the present study, we investigated the in vivo effects of Ang II on bone erosion and systemic bone loss in a tumor necrosis factor (TNF)-induced arthritis model. We also aimed to assess whether the deletion of AT1R ameliorates the bone erosion and systemic bone loss caused by arthritis.

2. Results

2.1. Increased AT1R Expression in the Joint Tissue of Tumor Necrosis Factor-Transgenic (TNFtg) Mice

As a first step to explore the effect of Ang II on arthritis, the expression of *Agtr1a*, encoding AT1R, in the joints was assessed by quantitative polymerase chain reaction (qPCR). *Agtr1a* mRNA was detected in the joint tissues from both wild-type (WT) and TNFtg mice, and the expression levels were 2.5-fold elevated in the tissues of the TNFtg mice compared with those in the WT mice (Figure 1A). Increased AT1R protein expression was also shown in arthritic joint tissues by Western blotting (Figure A1A). Immunohistochemical stain of the arthritic joints revealed AT1R expression in the tissues, including proliferated synovial cells (Figure A2B).

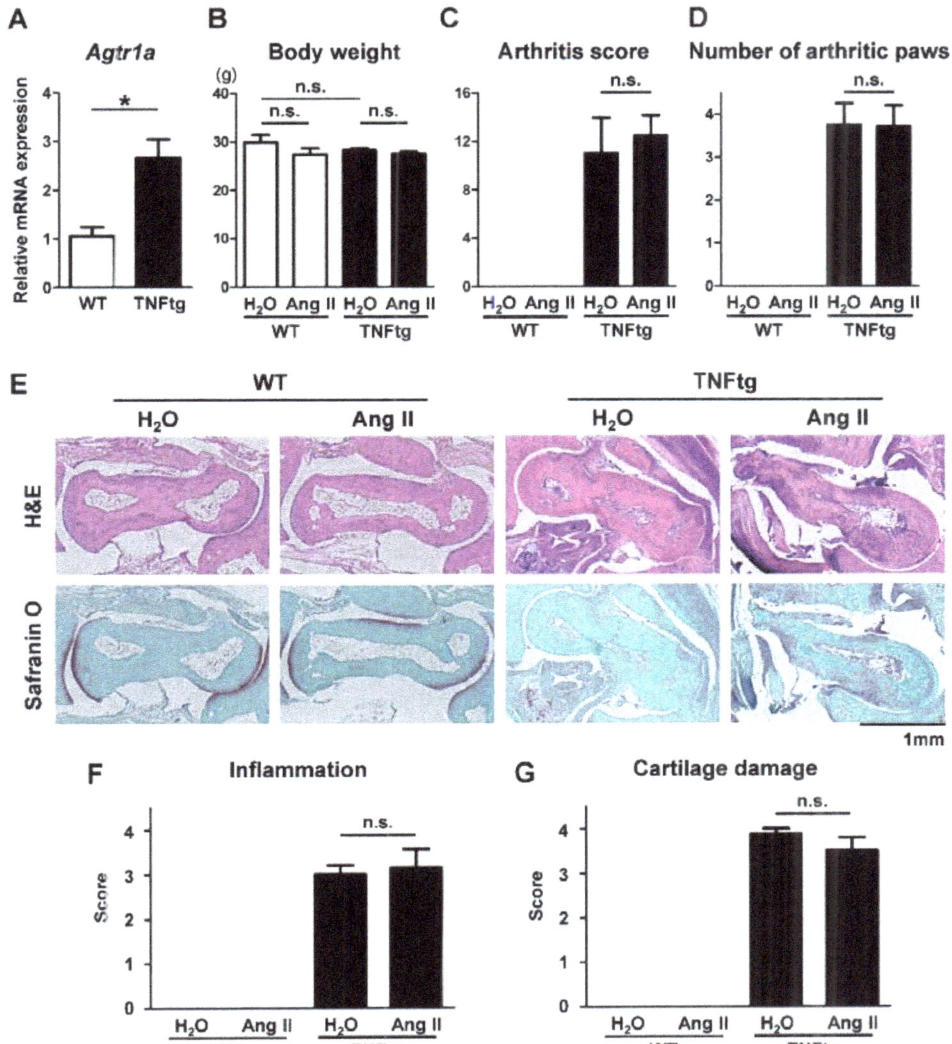

Figure 1. No significant effect of angiotensin II (Ang II) administration on the severity of inflammatory cell infiltration and cartilage damage in tumor necrosis factor-transgenic (TNFtg) mice. Ang II was administered by osmotic pumps to wild-type (WT; $n = 6$) and TNFtg ($n = 7$) male mice from 12 to 16 weeks of age. Water (H_2O) was administered by osmotic pumps to WT ($n = 6$) and TNFtg ($n = 4$) male mice as controls. (**A**) Quantitative real-time PCR analysis. *Agtr1a* mRNA expression levels in the right ankle joint tissue were determined. (**B**) Body weight at the age of 16 weeks. (**C**) Arthritis scores at the age of 16 weeks. (**D**) The numbers of arthritic paws with an arthritis score of 2 or higher. (**E**) Representative images of stained sections around the talus bones of indicated mice; sections were stained with hematoxylin and eosin (H&E) and Safranin O; original magnification ×40. (**F**,**G**) Histological scores of inflammation (**F**) and cartilage damage (**G**). Values are the mean ± SEM. n.s., not significant. *, $p < 0.05$.

2.2. No Significant Effect of Ang II Administration on the Severity of Inflammatory Cell Infiltration in TNFtg Mice

To assess the effect of Ang II on arthritis, exogenous Ang II (1.44 mg/kg/day) or water (H_2O) was administered by osmotic pumps to the WT and TNFtg mice for 4 weeks. The treatment with Ang II did not significantly alter body weight (Figure 1B), but did induce hypertension (Figure A2). We monitored the severity of paw swelling in each limb during the experimental period. We found that the TNFtg mice exhibited severe swelling of the paws and that the severity of clinical arthritis was not affected by the Ang II infusion. The arthritis score and number of arthritic limbs at the age of 16 weeks are presented in Figure 1C,D.

To analyze the inflamed joints histologically, we performed hematoxylin and eosin (H&E) and Safranin O staining to determine the inflammatory cell infiltration and cartilage damage. In WT mice, Ang II administration did not cause any detectable histological changes (Figure 1E,F). TNFtg mice exhibited massive inflammatory cell infiltration, and Ang II administration did not affect the severity of inflammation in these mice, which is consistent with the arthritis score results (Figure 1C). Additionally, the severity of cartilage damage, represented by decreased staining of the cartilage matrix, was not affected by the administration of Ang II (Figure 1E,G).

2.3. Exacerbation of Bone Erosion by Ang II Administration in TNFtg Mice

We then examined the impact of Ang II on the erosive bone changes of the ankle. Bone erosion around the talus was quantified using micro-computed tomography (CT) and 3D image analysis software. The micro-CT analysis revealed that the destructive bone change was significantly more severe in the Ang II-infused TNFtg mice than in the H_2O-infused TNFtg mice (Figure 2A). This aggravated bone erosion was revealed by the following quantitative analyses: the bone volume (BV) of the talus, the reduction rate of BV, and the eroded volume per repaired volume (Ev/Rpv) of the talus (Figure 2B–D). Tartrate-resistant acid phosphatase (TRAP)-stained images showed slightly increased osteoclast formation in the joints of the Ang II-infused TNFtg mice compared to those in the H_2O-infused TNFtg mice (Figure 2E). Quantitative histological analyses also revealed increased bone erosion and slightly enhanced osteoclast formation around the talus (Figure 2F,G). These findings suggest that Ang II, imported to the joints from circulation, served as an osteoclast-activating factor in the arthritic joint, resulting in enhanced bone erosion without affecting the clinical severity of arthritis.

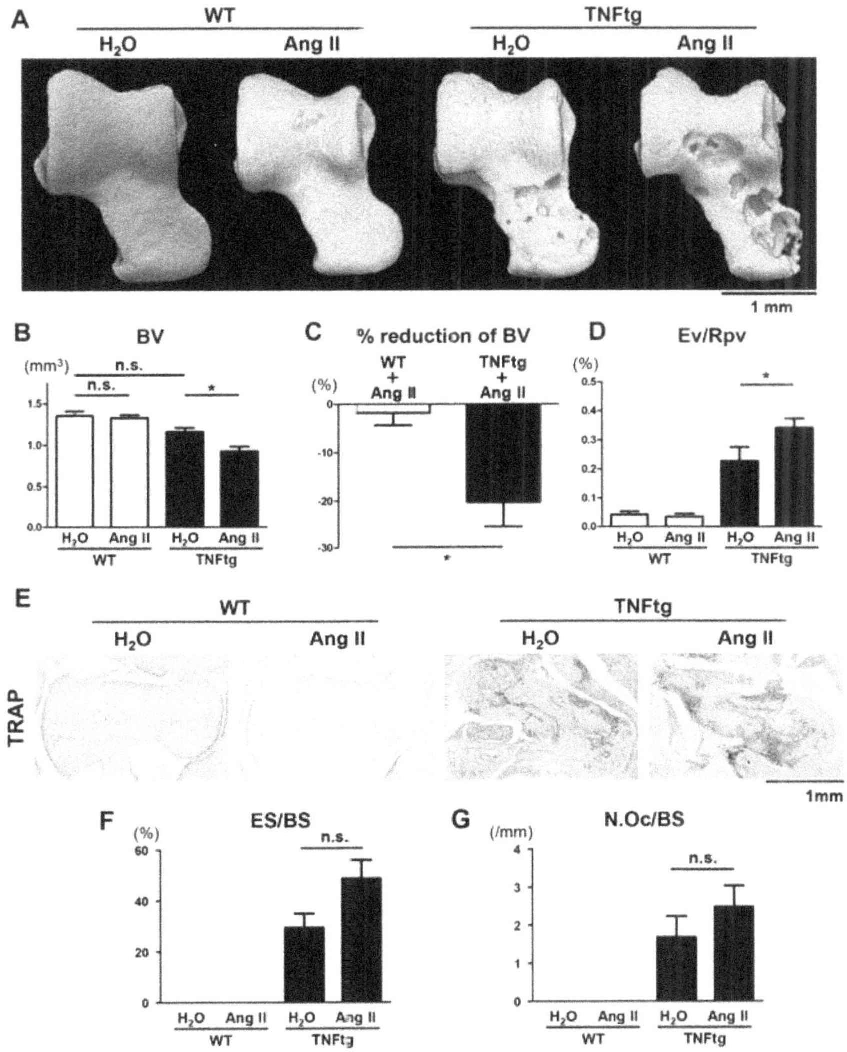

Figure 2. Exacerbation of bone erosion by angiotensin II (Ang II) administration in tumor necrosis factor-transgenic (TNFtg) mice. Ang II was administered by osmotic pumps to WT (n = 6) and TNFtg (n = 7) male mice from 12 to 16 weeks of age. Water (H_2O) was administered by osmotic pumps to WT (n = 6) and TNFtg (n = 4) male mice as controls. (**A**) Representative 3D micro-computed tomography (CT) images of the talus. (**B**) Bone volume (BV) of the talus. (**C**) Rates of reduction in BV of Ang II-infused WT and TNFtg mice relative to H_2O-infused control mice of each genotype. (**D**) Eroded volume per repaired volume (Ev/Rpv) of the talus. (**E**) Representative images of tartrate-resistant acid phosphatase (TRAP) staining around the talus bones of indicated mice; original magnification ×40. (**F**) Eroded surface per bone surface (ES/BS) around the taluses. (**G**) The number of osteoclasts per bone surface (N.Oc/BS) around the taluses. Values are the mean ± SEM. n.s., not significant. *, $p < 0.05$.

2.4. No Detectable Changes in the Trabecular and Cortical Bone Parameters with Ang II Administration

Since both systemic inflammation and excess of Ang II have been reported to decrease the mass of systemic bones [4,11], we examined the bone properties of the tibia and vertebra and determined whether

Ang II could synergistically enhance inflammation-mediated bone loss in the Ang II-administered arthritic mice. We assessed the tibia trabecular bone (secondary spongiosa, Figure 3A), the tibia cortical bone (midshaft of the tibia, Figure 3B), and the trabecular bone of the spine (fifth lumbar vertebra, Figure 3C) using micro-CT. The tibia trabecular bone tended to be decreased in the arthritic mice compared to that in the WT mice, although the difference was not statistically significant in the current set of experiments. The bone reduction rates with Ang II infusion were comparable between WT and TNFtg mice at approximately 30% (Figure 3D), indicating that the synergistic effect of inflammation and Ang II on osteopenia was not noticeable. In the tibia cortical bone, the presence of arthritis significantly increased bone loss, but the reduction rates with Ang II infusion were comparable between WT and TNFtg mice (Figure 3E). In the vertebral trabecular bone, the presence of arthritis did not significantly affect the bone volume (Figure 3F). Ang II administration tended to decrease bone volume by approximately 10%, but there was no significant difference in the reduction rates between WT and TNFtg mice (Figure 3F). The other analyzed parameters of the trabecular and cortical bones also indicated no significant effect of Ang II administration on bone properties (Figure A3). Collectively, these findings suggest that both inflammation and Ang II tended to decrease bone mass, but there was no apparent synergistic effect on the osteopenic phenotype.

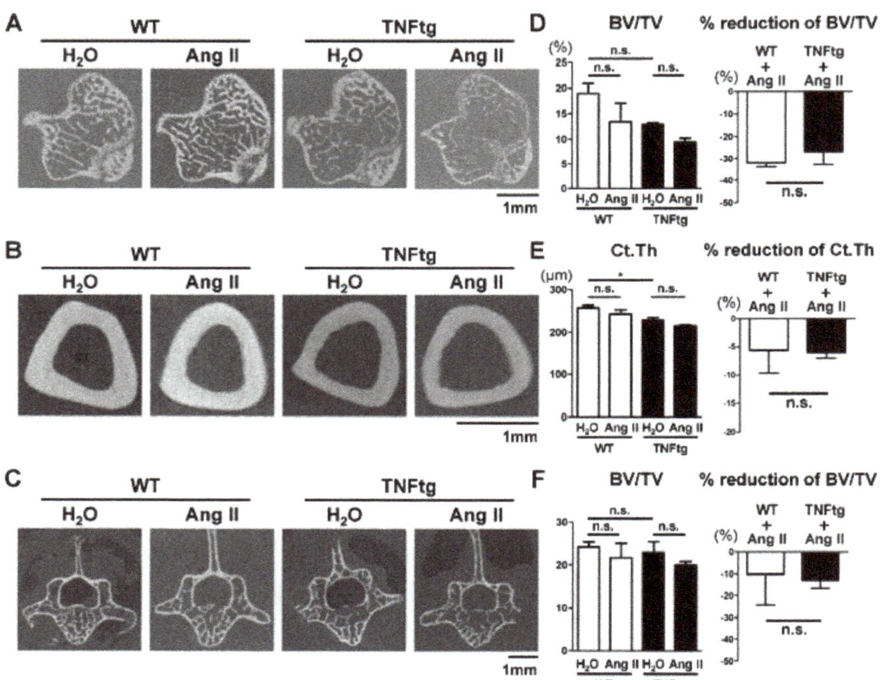

Figure 3. No detectable changes in the trabecular and cortical bone parameters with Ang II administration. Angiotensin II (Ang II) was administered by osmotic pumps to WT (n = 6) and tumor necrosis factor-transgenic (TNFtg; n = 7) male mice from 12 to 16 weeks old. Water (H_2O) was administered by osmotic pumps to WT (n = 6) and TNFtg (n = 4) male mice as controls. (**A–C**) Representative 2D micro-CT images of the tibia trabecular bone (**A**), the tibia cortical bone (**B**), and the trabecular bone of the spine (the fifth lumbar vertebra) (**C**). (**D**) Bone volume per total volume (BV/TV) and reduction rate of the tibia trabecular bone. (**E**) Cortical thickness (Ct.Th) and reduction rate of the tibia midshaft. (**F**) Bone volume per total volume (BV/TV) and reduction rate of the fifth lumbar vertebral trabecular bone. Values are the mean ± SEM. n.s., not significant. *, $p < 0.05$.

2.5. Effect of AT1R Deficiency on the Severity of Inflammatory Cell Infiltration in TNFtg Mice

Since an excess of exogenous Ang II accelerated inflammatory bone destruction (Figure 2A), we investigated whether endogenous Ang II could play a role in bone destruction using AT1R-deficient arthritic mice generated by crossing TNFtg mice with AT1R-knockout (AT1R$^{-/-}$) mice. AT1R deficiency did not significantly alter body weight (Figure 4A). We found that the severity of clinical arthritis (Figure 4B,C) and the extent of inflammatory cell infiltration (Figure 4D,E) were comparable between TNFtg and TNFtg/AT1R$^{-/-}$ mice. In addition, the severity of cartilage damage was not affected by AT1R deficiency (Figure 4D,F).

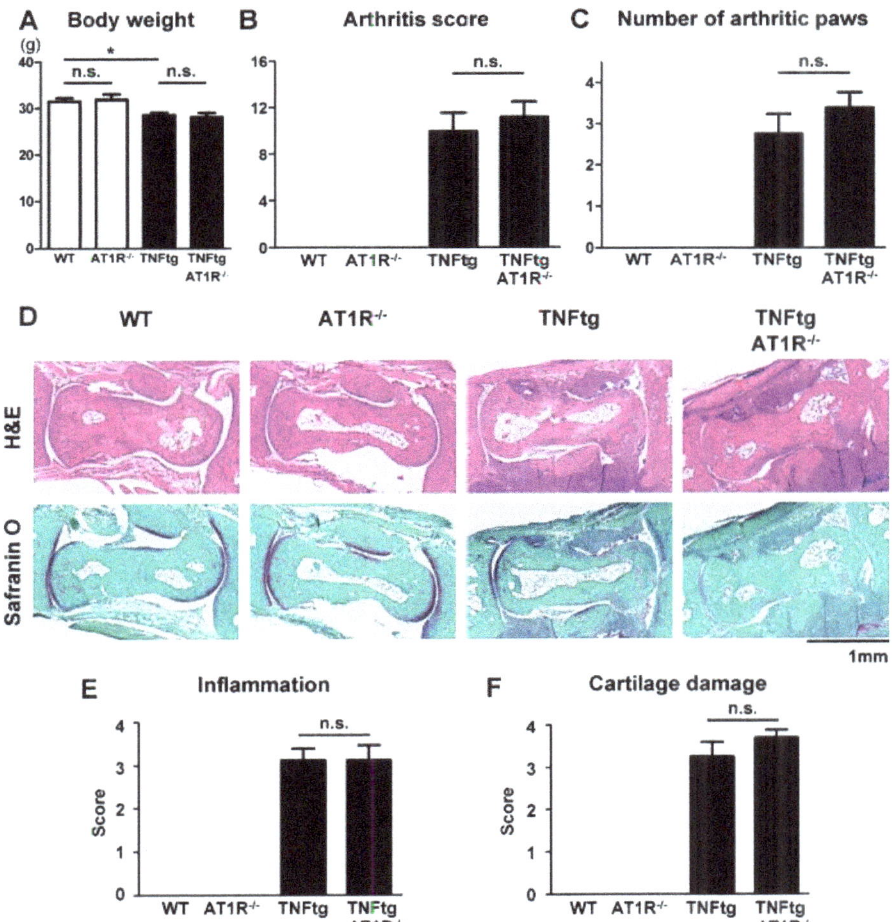

Figure 4. Effect of angiotensin II type 1 receptor (AT1R) deficiency on the severity of inflammatory cell infiltration in tumor necrosis factor-transgenic (TNFtg) mice. TNFtg mice were crossed with AT1R-deficient (AT1R$^{-/-}$) mice. WT (n = 9), AT1R$^{-/-}$ (n = 7), TNFtg (n = 12), and TNFtg AT1R$^{-/-}$ (n = 8) male mice were analyzed at the age of 16 weeks. (**A**) Body weight at the age of 16 weeks. (**B**) Arthritis score at the age of 16 weeks. (**C**) The number of arthritic paws with an arthritis score of 2 or higher. (**D**) Representative images of stained sections around the talus bones of indicated mice; sections were stained with hematoxylin and eosin (H&E) and Safranin O; original magnification ×40. (**E**,**F**) Histological scores of inflammation (**E**) and cartilage damage (**F**). Values are the mean ± SEM. n.s., not significant. *, $p < 0.05$.

2.6. Influence of AT1R Depletion on Bone Erosion in TNFtg Mice

We next examined whether the deletion of AT1R could reduce bone destruction in the arthritic mice. Micro-CT analysis of the ankle joints revealed that TNFtg/AT1R$^{-/-}$ mice exhibited the same extent of severe bone loss as TNFtg mice (Figure 5A,B). Additionally, the BV reduction rate and the erosive volume (Ev/Rpv) of the talus in the TNFtg/AT1R$^{-/-}$ mice were comparable to those in the TNFtg mice (Figure 5C,D). These findings indicate that AT1R deficiency did not alleviate the destructive bone changes in the inflammatory joints of the arthritic mice. Histological analyses revealed that the extents of bone erosion and osteoclast formation were comparable between TNFtg and TNFtg/AT1R$^{-/-}$ mice (Figure 5E–G).

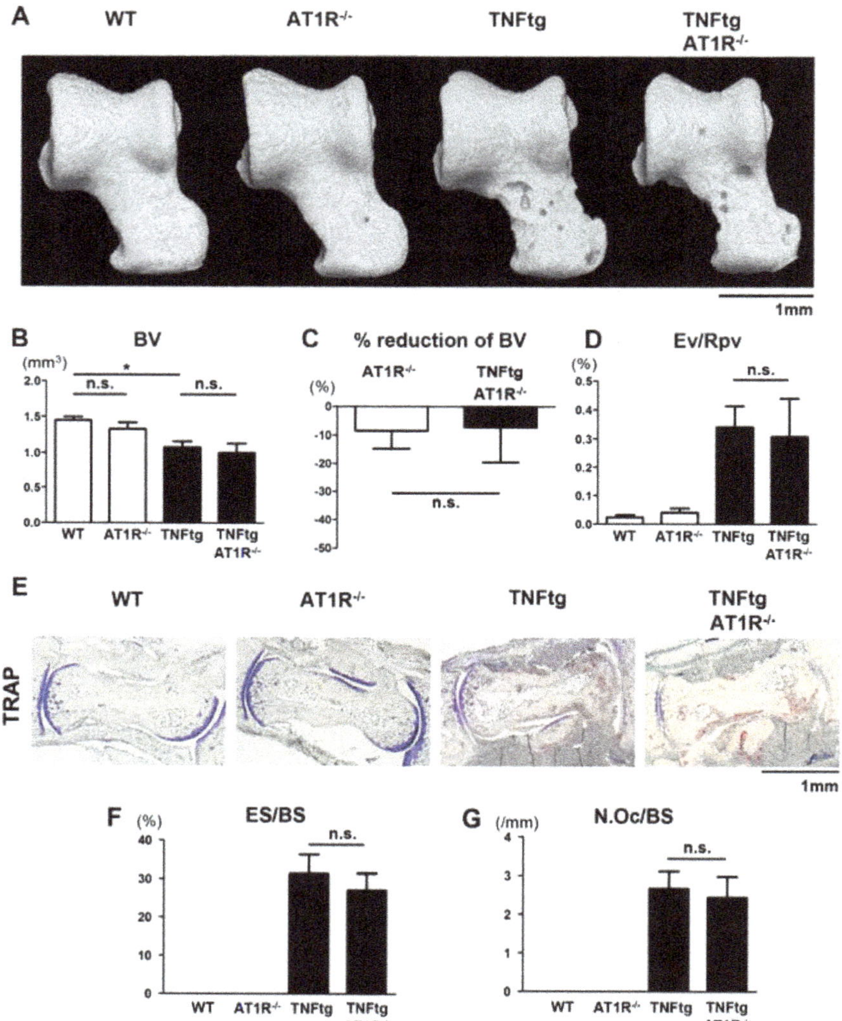

Figure 5. Influence of AT1R depletion on bone erosion in tumor necrosis factor-transgenic (TNFtg) mice. TNFtg mice were crossed with AT1R-deficient (AT1R$^{-/-}$) mice. WT (n = 9), AT1R$^{-/-}$ (n = 7), TNFtg (n = 12), and TNFtg AT1R$^{-/-}$ (n = 8) male mice were analyzed at the age of 16 weeks. (**A**) Representative 3D micro-CT images of the talus. (**B**) Bone volume (BV) of the talus. (**C**) Rate of reduction in BV by

AT1R deficiency relative to that in the control mice of each genotype. (**D**) Eroded volume per repaired volume (Ev/Rpv) of the talus. (**E**) Representative images of tartrate-resistant acid phosphatase (TRAP) staining around the talus bones of indicated mice; original magnification ×40. (**F**) Eroded surface per bone surface (ES/BS) around the taluses. (**G**) The number of osteoclasts per bone surface (N.Oc/BS) around the taluses. Values are the mean ± SEM. n.s., not significant. *, $p < 0.05$.

2.7. Effect of AT1R Deficiency on Bone Properties of the Trabecular and Cortical Bones in TNFtg Mice

AT1R$^{-/-}$ mice were previously reported to exhibit an increased trabecular BV and increased trabecular number and connectivity [16]. To examine the effect of AT1R deficiency on the bone volume of systemic bones in the arthritic condition, we analyzed the bone properties of the tibia and vertebra of the TNFtg arthritic mice using micro-CT (Figure 6A–C). The TNFtg mice exhibited a significant reduction in BV/TV of the tibia and the AT1R deficiency modestly alleviated the bone loss caused by arthritis, even though the difference between TNFtg and TNFtg/AT1R$^{-/-}$ mice was not statistically significant (Figure 6D). A similar insignificant tendency was observed in the vertebral trabecular bone (Figure 6F). In the tibia cortical bone, AT1R deficiency did not show any protective effect on bone loss (Figure 6E). The other analyzed parameters of the trabecular and cortical bones also indicated no significant effect of AT1R deficiency on bone properties (Figure A4). These findings suggest that the inhibition of endogenous Ang II has a limited protective effect on bone loss in arthritic mice.

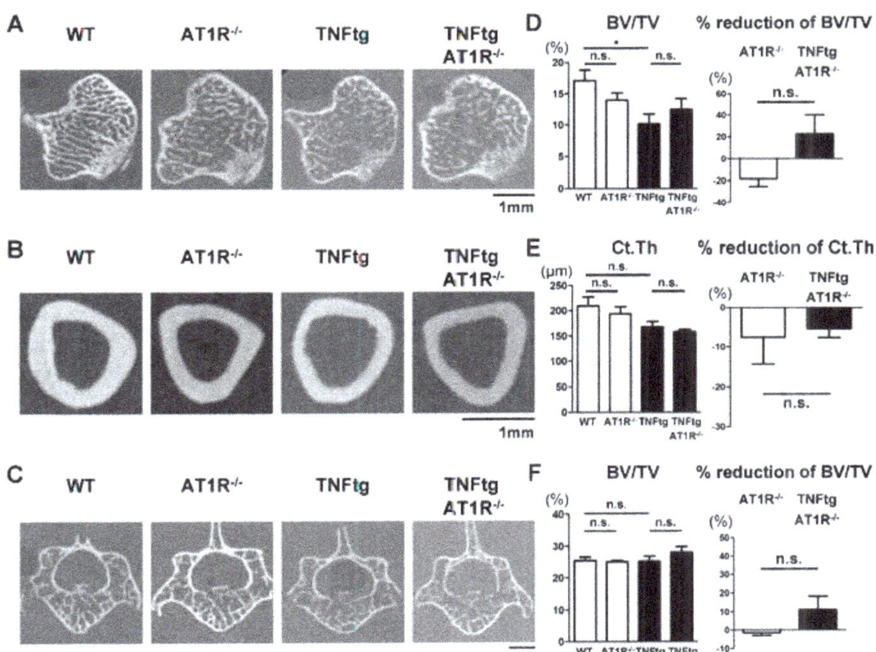

Figure 6. Effect of AT1R deficiency on bone properties of the trabecular and cortical bones in tumor necrosis factor-transgenic (TNFtg) mice. TNFtg mice were crossed with AT1R-deficient (AT1R$^{-/-}$) mice. WT (n = 9), AT1R$^{-/-}$ (n = 7), TNFtg (n = 12), and TNFtg AT1R$^{-/-}$ (n = 8) male mice were analyzed at the age of 16 weeks. Representative 2D micro-CT images of the tibia trabecular bone (**A**), the tibia cortical bone (**B**), and the trabecular bone of the spine (fifth lumbar vertebra) (**C**). (**D**) Bone volume per total volume (BV/TV) and reduction rate of the tibia trabecula bone. (**E**) Cortical thickness (Ct.Th) and reduction rate of the tibia midshaft. (**F**) Bone volume per total volume (BV/TV) and reduction rate of the fifth lumbar vertebral trabecular bone. Values are the mean ± SEM. n.s., not significant. *, $p < 0.05$.

3. Discussion

In this study, we sought to clarify the impact of excessive Ang II and inhibition of the endogenous RAS on bone erosion and systemic bone loss in a TNF-mediated arthritic condition. We found that the administration of Ang II enhanced destructive bone changes in inflammatory joints without affecting the severity of inflammation. There was no noticeable synergistic effect of Ang II administration and inflammation on osteopenia of the tibia and vertebra in mice. Further, we found that AT1R deficiency had a minimal protective effect on bone erosion and systemic bone loss in the arthritis model.

Interestingly, we observed that the administration of Ang II aggravated joint destruction in the arthritic mice. Ang II has been reported to enhance systemic bone loss in murine osteoporosis models [11,17]. Ang II induces RANKL expression in osteoblasts and subsequently enhances osteoclastogenesis, resulting in systemic bone loss [6,11]. However, no previous studies have explored the role of the RAS in the development of bone erosion in an arthritis model. In rheumatoid arthritis, inflammatory cytokines such as TNF increase RANKL expression in synoviocytes and subsequently promote osteoclastic differentiation and activation, resulting in erosive bone changes in joints [2]. Our results demonstrate that excessive Ang II could exacerbate the TNF-induced inflammatory joint destruction associated with increased osteoclast formation.

The current study has important clinical implications for the management of rheumatoid arthritis. Our findings suggest that in patients in whom the local effect of Ang II is upregulated via increased imported Ang II from circulation, joint destruction can be promoted as a consequence of systemic RAS activation. Systemic activation of the RAS can be observed in several pathological conditions, such as renal artery stenosis, congestive heart failure, cardiac hypertrophy, chronic kidney disease, and obesity [18,19]. Such pathological conditions could be risk factors for progressive joint destruction in inflammatory arthropathies.

Although Ang II appeared to promote bone erosion in inflamed joints, its effects on systemic bones, represented by the tibia and vertebra, were found to be very limited. There are several possible explanations for this. Firstly, in the arthritic joints of mice, other inflammatory cytokines such as IL-1 and IL-6 are highly produced [2,20]. In addition to TNF, these other osteoclast-activating factors might play important synergistic roles in the Ang II-promoted bone erosion in joints. Secondly, the expression of AT1R was significantly increased in the arthritic joints (Figure 1A). This could contribute to hyper-responsiveness to Ang II, resulting in increased osteoclastic bone destruction in the joints. Thirdly, the exposure period to Ang II (4 weeks in this study) might be too short for this effector to exert an osteopenic effect on systemic bones. Indeed, a previous study showed a significant osteopenic effect of excessive RAS activation in 6-month-old Tsukuba hypertensive mice that were continuously exposed to excessive Ang II via transgenes encoding human renin and human angiotensinogen [17].

Since the expression of AT1R was increased in the arthritic joints of the TNFtg mice (Figure 1A), we assumed that AT1R deficiency would ameliorate bone erosion in this arthritis model. Contrary to our expectation, AT1R deficiency did not significantly improve the erosive bone changes in the TNFtg mice. These data indicate a limited role of the local RAS during the process of joint destruction in this arthritic model. The RAS might modulate bone mass only under pathological conditions with excessive systemic activation. Analyses of AT1R-deficient arthritic mice with excessive Ang II would be needed to verify this concept.

The limitation of our study is that the precise mechanisms through which Ang II enhances bone erosion are unclear. We have tested the effect of Ang II on osteoclast differentiation in murine primary bone marrow-derived macrophage cultures. Ang II stimulation did not promote osteoclast formation in the mono-culture of bone marrow-derived macrophage (Figure A5A,B), whereas Ang II enhanced osteoclast formation in the co-culture system with osteoblasts (Figure A5C,D). These data suggest that Ang II promotes osteoclast formation indirectly via stromal cells. In support of this notion, Ang II has been previously reported to induce RANKL expression in stromal cells [17]. Various cells can express RANKL in arthritic joints, synovial cells, osteoblasts, or osteocytes, which might be attributed to the

Ang II-mediated bone erosion. Other possibilities are that Ang II regulates angiogenesis in arthritic joints or that Ang II modulates cellular functions via the Ang II type 2 receptor, which reportedly regulates inflammation in the arthritic synovium [21]. Further research will be required to clarify the underlying mechanisms.

Another possible limitation of this study is the relatively small sample sizes which may have insufficient statistical power to detect a small difference in some comparisons. For instance, a statistically significant difference was not detected in the trabecular BV/TV of the tibia between H_2O-treated WT ($n = 6$) and H_2O-treated TNFtg ($n = 4$) mice (Figure 3D), although there is a statistically significant difference between WT ($n = 9$) and TNFtg ($n = 12$) mice in the AT1R$^{-/-}$ strain (Figure 6D). Post-hoc power analyses have shown that a larger sample size would be needed to detect a substantial difference in Figure 3D. Therefore, future studies with larger sample sizes would be necessary to detect a small but significant difference.

We previously reported that the RAS is involved in vascular damage and that AT1R blockers have potent vascular protective effects in an arthritis model [22]. Therefore, in patients with rheumatoid arthritis complicated by RAS-dependent hypertension, the blockade of the RAS might be beneficial not only to reduce blood pressure and vascular damage but also to prevent bone erosion.

In conclusion, this study provides novel insights into the pathophysiological function of Ang II in the regulation of inflammatory bone destruction. In patients with rheumatoid arthritis, the systemically activated RAS in concurrent pathological conditions could be involved in the progression of joint destruction in conjunction with increased local expression of AT1R. The effects of pharmacological inhibition of the Ang II-mediated pathway on bone erosion remain unclear but warrant further clinical examination.

4. Materials and Methods

4.1. Mice

Human TNFtg mice (C57BL/6 background) were obtained (#1006; Taconic Biosciences, Hudson, NY, USA). The TNFtg heterozygous mice spontaneously develop arthritis on the fore and hind paws at approximately 8 weeks of age, and arthritis progresses with age [23]. AT1R-knockout mice (AT1R$^{-/-}$; C57BL/6 background) were obtained (#002682; The Jackson Laboratory, Bar Harbor, ME, USA) [24] and crossed with TNFtg mice to generate AT1R-deficient arthritic mice. Age- and sex-matched littermates were used as control mice. All mutant mice were maintained in the animal facility of Kawasaki Medical School (Okayama, Japan) and were housed in a group (2–5 mice per cage) and maintained at 22 °C under 12 h light/12 h dark cycles with free access to water and standard laboratory food. All animal experiments were approved by the Institutional Safety Committee for Recombinant DNA Experiments (Nos. 14–40, 14–41, and 19–27, which are approved on 3/13/2015, 3/13/2015, and 10/17/2019, respectively) and the Institutional Animal Care and Use Committee of Kawasaki Medical School (Nos. 17–129, 18–057, and 18–130, which are approved on 2/1/2018, 4/1/2018, and 2/1/2019, respectively). All experimental procedures were conducted in accordance with institutional and NIH guidelines for the humane use of animals.

4.2. Ang II Infusion Model

Twelve-week-old WT and TNFtg male mice were randomly divided into two groups that were infused with either water (H_2O) or Ang II, which was dissolved in H_2O. Ang II was administered by osmotic pumps to WT ($n = 6$) and TNFtg mice ($n = 7$) from 12 to 16 weeks of age. H_2O was administered by osmotic pumps to WT ($n = 6$) and TNFtg mice ($n = 4$) as controls. The mice were anesthetized, and an osmotic pump containing 100 μL of either H_2O or Ang II (Sigma-Aldrich, St. Louis, MO, USA) was implanted subcutaneously as previously described [22,25]. Ang II was continuously infused at a dose of 1.44 mg/kg/day from 12 to 16 weeks of age. Arterial blood pressure was measured by the tail-cuff method with a pulse transducer (BP98-A; Softron, Tokyo, Japan), as reported [26]. Mice were monitored for signs of arthritis in a blinded manner, and each limb was individually scored on a scale of 0–4. Scores were assigned based on the extent of erythema or swelling present in each limb, assigning a maximum score of 16 per mouse, as described previously [27,28]. Mice were monitored until the age of 16 weeks, and then serum, hind limb, and spine (the fifth lumbar vertebra) samples were collected.

4.3. Micro-Computed Tomography (CT) Analysis

Bone samples were fixed in 4% paraformaldehyde (PFA) in phosphate-buffered saline for 2 days, and PFA-fixed bone samples were immersed in 70% ethanol. Three-dimensional microarchitecture of the talus, tibia, and spine was evaluated by using a micro-CT system (Ele Scan mini; Nittetsu Elex, Tokyo, Japan) with an X-ray energy of 45 kVP (145 μA), as described previously [29,30]. The voxel resolution of all bone images was 15 μm. The bone properties of the tibia and the fifth lumbar vertebra, and bone erosion of the ankle (talus bones) were analyzed using analysis software (TRI/3D-BON; Ratoc System Engineering Co. Ltd., Tokyo, Japan). The analyzed region of the tibia trabecular bone comprised 67 slices of secondary spongiosa adjacent to the primary spongiosa (starting 0.5 mm from the distal border of the growth plate), that of the vertebra comprised the entire fifth lumbar vertebral body area (approximately 140 slices), and that of the tibia cortical bone comprised 33 slices of the midshaft (1 mm proximal region from the tibiofibular junction). The micro-CT parameters of the tibia and spine were described according to international guidelines [31]. The talus bones were evaluated using BV and Ev/Rpv for quantitative measurements of bone erosion [32]. Ev/Rpv on the whole talus was calculated automatically with the software according to the software program (TRI/3D-BON). We set the concave surface search range up to 0.15 mm, and the absorption surface extraction radius of curvature was 960 μm or less as described previously [33].

4.4. Histological Analysis

The hind limbs were decalcified in 10% EDTA (pH 7.2) at 4 °C for 4 weeks and subsequently embedded in paraffin. Sections (3 μm) were stained with hematoxylin and eosin (H&E) and Safranin O. The severity of inflammation and cartilage damage around the talus bone was scored on a scale of 0–4 under blinded conditions as described previously [27,28]. TRAP staining was performed to visualize osteoclast formation, and the sections were counterstained with methyl green. Histological analyses were performed using a BZ-X analyzer (Keyence, Osaka, Japan). The eroded surface per bone surface (ES/BS) and the number of osteoclasts per bone surface (N.Oc/BS) around the taluses were determined.

4.5. Real-Time Quantitative Polymerase Chain Reaction (qPCR)

qPCR was performed as described previously [30,34]. Total RNA was extracted from the right ankle joint using RNAiso Plus (Takara Bio, Shiga, Japan) and solubilized in ribonuclease (RNase)-free water. Complementary DNA (cDNA) was synthesized using the Prime Script RT reagent Kit (Takara Bio). qPCR reactions were performed using SYBR Green PCR Master Mix (Takara Bio) with the StepOnePlus Real-Time PCR System (Thermo Fisher Scientific, Waltham, MA, USA). Gene expression levels relative to *Gapdh* were calculated by the $\Delta\Delta$Ct method and normalized to control samples obtained from the WT mice. The qPCR analysis used the following primers: 5′-taccagctctgcggctct-3′ and 5′-gccagccatttt ataccaatct-3′ for *Agtr1a* (AT1R); 5′-atcaagaaggtggtgaagca-3′ and 5′-gacaacctggtcctcagtgt-3′ for *Gapdh*. All qPCR reactions yielded products with single peak dissociation curves.

4.6. Statistical Analysis

All values are given as the mean ± standard error of the mean (SEM). A two-tailed unpaired Student's *t*-test was used to compare two groups, and a one-way analysis of variance (ANOVA) followed by Tukey's post-hoc test was used to compare three or more groups by using GraphPad Prism 5 (GraphPad Software, San Diego, CA, USA). p values lower than 0.05 were considered statistically significant.

4.7. Supplementary Methods

Additional Supporting Information can be found online in the Supplementary Materials tab for this article.

Supplementary Materials: Supplementary materials can be found at http://www.mdpi.com/1422-0067/21/11/4145/s1.

Author Contributions: Conceptualization, T.A., T.M. (Tomoyuki Mukai), and Y.M.; formal analysis, T.A., T.M. (Tomoyuki Mukai), and T.M. (Takafumi Mito); funding acquisition, T.M. (Tomoyuki Mukai) and Y.M.; investigation, T.M. (Tomoyuki Mukai); methodology, T.A. and T.M. (Tomoyuki Mukai); project administration, T.M. (Tomoyuki Mukai); software, T.A.; supervision, T.M. (Tomoyuki Mukai) and Y.M.; validation, T.A., T.M. (Tomoyuki Mukai), K.K., S.T., S.F., H.A.U., and Y.M.; writing—original draft, T.A., T.M. (Tomoyuki Mukai), and Y.M.; writing—review and editing, T.A., T.M. (Tomoyuki Mukai), T.M (Takafumi Mito), K.K., S.T., S.F., H.A.U., and Y.M. All authors have read and agreed to the published version of the manuscript.

Funding: This work was supported by grants from JSPS KAKENHI (20K08814 and 17K09991 to Y.M.), Kawasaki Medical School (Research Project Grants; R01-060 and 30-051 to Y.M.), and UCB Japan (T.M., Tomoyuki Mukai).

Acknowledgments: We would like to thank M. Sato and H. Nagasu (Department of Nephrology and Hypertension, Kawasaki Medical School), Y. Jyu (Department of Health and Sports Sciences, Kawasaki University of Medical Welfare), and T. Sone (Department of Nuclear Medicine, Kawasaki Medical School) for technical assistance and critical suggestions; Y. Mino, M. Yoshimoto, K. Maitani, A. Kusumoto, H. Nakashima, N. Takemasa, and N. Obara for their technical assistance; and N. Nango (Ratoc System Engineering Co., Ltd.) for his kind instruction regarding the micro-CT analysis software. We are also indebted to N. Iwachidou and the staff at the Research Center of Kawasaki Medical School. We are especially grateful to David A. Fox (University of Michigan, Ann Arbor, MI) for critically reading the manuscript.

Conflicts of Interest: T.A., T.M. (Tomoyuki Mukai), T.M. (Takafumi Mito), K.K., S.T., S.F., and Y.M. received scholarship donations from Takeda Pharmaceutical Co., Astellas Pharma Inc., Merck & Co., Daiichi Sankyo Inc., Shionogi & Co., Chugai Pharmaceutical Co., and AYUMI Pharmaceutical Co. H.A.U. belongs to the Department of Chronic Kidney Disease and Cardiovascular Disease, which is endowed by Kawanishi Holdings, Chugai pharmaceutical Co., Boehringer Ingelheim GmbH, and Terumo Co. The funders had no role in the design of the study; the collection, analyses, or interpretation of data; the writing of the manuscript; or in the decision to publish the results.

Abbreviations

Ang II	Angiotensin II
TNF	Tumor necrosis factor
TNFtg	Tumor necrosis factor-transgenic
AT1R	Angiotensin II type 1 receptor
WT	Wild-type

Appendix A

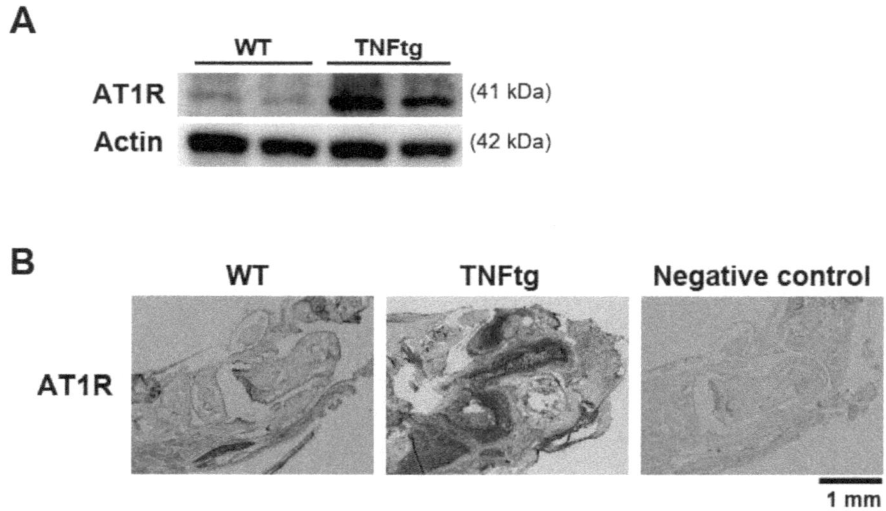

Figure A1. The protein expression of angiotensin II type 1 receptor (AT1R) in the joint tissues was increased in tumor necrosis factor-transgenic (TNFtg) mice. (**A**) Western blot analysis of AT1R expression in the fore paw tissues. The fore paw samples were obtained from 16-week-old wild-type (WT) and TNFtg mice. (**B**) Immunohistochemistry staining images of AT1R. The expression of AT1R in the left ankle joint specimens was determined. Original magnification ×40. A tissue specimen processed without the primary antibody is presented as a negative control. Detailed methods are described in the Supporting Information.

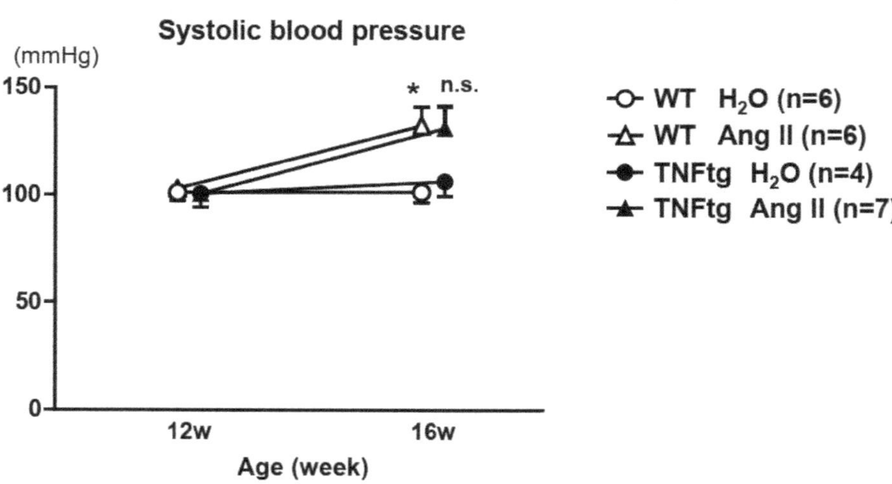

Figure A2. Systolic blood pressure in wild-type (WT) and tumor necrosis factor-transgenic (TNFtg) mice administered angiotensin II (Ang II) and water (H_2O). Ang II was administered by osmotic pumps to WT and TNFtg mice from 12 to 16 weeks of age. Values are the mean ± SEM. *, $p < 0.05$ (WT (Ang II) vs. WT (H_2O)). n.s., not significant (TNFtg (Ang II) vs. TNFtg (H_2O)).

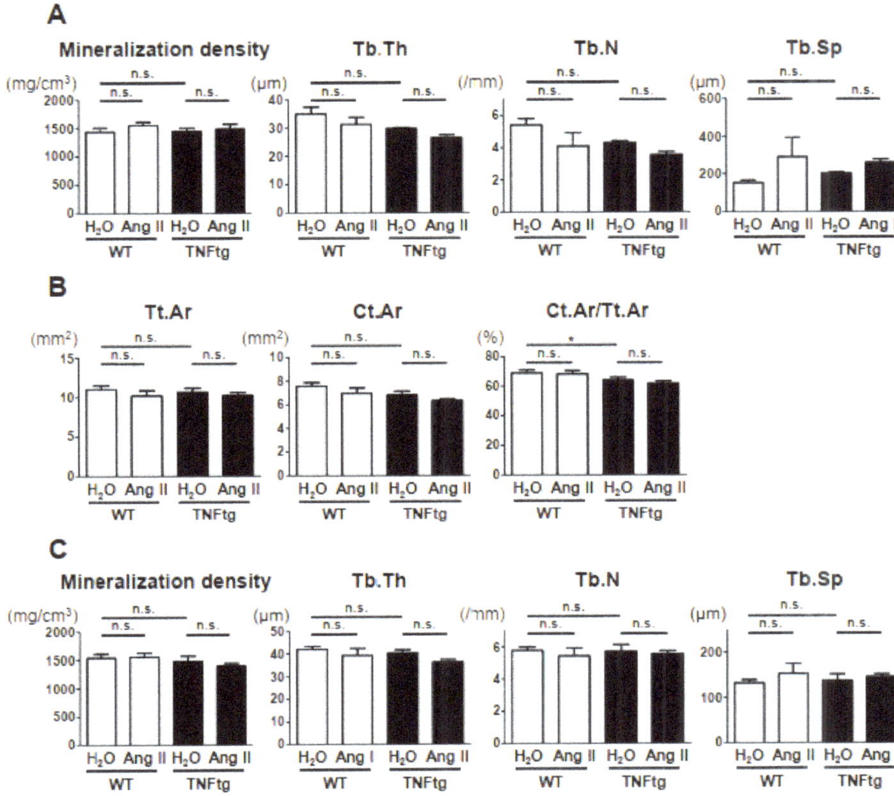

Figure A3. Trabecular and cortical bone parameters in wild-type (WT) and tumor necrosis factor-transgenic (TNFtg) mice administered angiotensin II (Ang II) and water (H_2O). Ang II was administered by osmotic pumps to WT (n = 6) and TNFtg (n = 7) male mice from 12 to 16 weeks of age. H_2O was administered by osmotic pumps to WT (n = 6) and TNFtg (n = 4) male mice as controls. (**A**) Trabecular bone parameters of the tibia. (**B**) Cortical bone parameters of the tibia midshaft. (**C**) Trabecular bone parameters of the spine (fifth lumbar vertebra). Tb.Th, trabecular thickness; Tb.N, trabecular number; Tb.Sp, trabecular separation; Tt.Ar, total cross-sectional area inside the periosteal envelope; Ct.Ar, cortical cross-sectional area. Values are the mean ± SEM. n.s., not significant. *, $p < 0.05$.

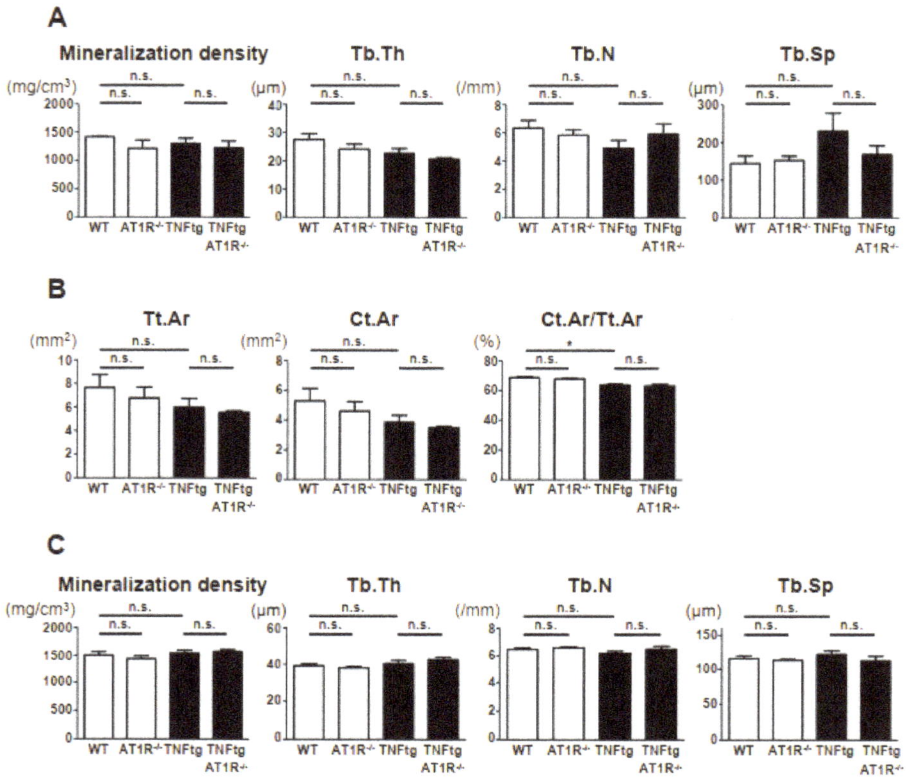

Figure A4. Trabecular and cortical bone parameters of the tibia and spine. Tumor necrosis factor-transgenic (TNFtg) mice were crossed with AT1R-deficient (AT1R$^{-/-}$) mice. Wild-type (WT; $n = 9$), AT1R$^{-/-}$ ($n = 7$), TNFtg ($n = 12$), and TNFtg AT1R$^{-/-}$ ($n = 8$) male mice were analyzed at the age of 16 weeks. (**A**) Trabecular bone parameters of the tibia. (**B**) Cortical bone parameters of the tibia midshaft. (**C**) Trabecular bone parameters of the spine (fifth lumbar vertebra). Tb.Th, trabecular thickness; Tb.N, trabecular number; Tb.Sp, trabecular separation; Tt.Ar, total cross-sectional area inside the periosteal envelope; Ct.Ar, cortical cross-sectional area. Values are the mean ± SEM. n.s., not significant. *, $p < 0.05$.

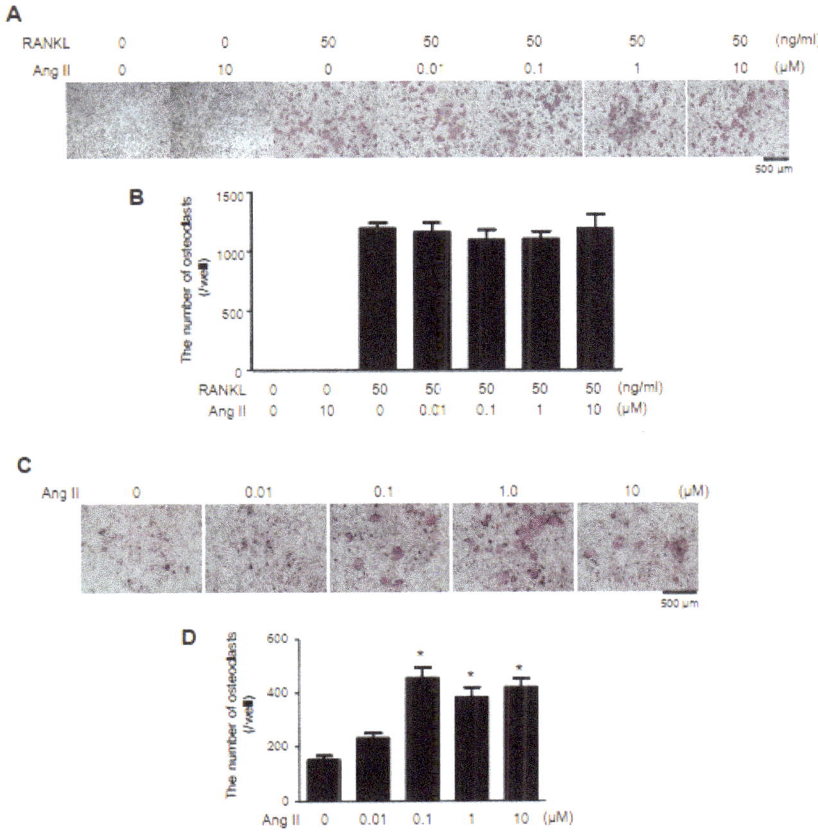

Figure A5. Effect of angiotensin (Ang II) on osteoclast differentiation. Primary mouse bone marrow cells were isolated from the long bones of 10-week-old wild-type mice. Non-adherent bone marrow cells were seeded on 48-well plates and incubated for 2 days with macrophage colony-stimulating factor (M-CSF; 25 ng/mL). After pre-culture for 2 days, yielded bone marrow-derived macrophages were stimulated with RANKL (50 ng/mL) and Ang II at the indicated concentrations for an additional 3 days in the presence of M-CSF. The formation of tartrate-resistant acid phosphatase (TRAP)-positive multinucleated cells (TRAP + MNCs) was visualized by TRAP staining. (**A**) Representative TRAP staining images. (**B**) The number of osteoclasts. TRAP + MNCs with three or more nuclei were counted as osteoclasts. Bone marrow-derived macrophages were co-cultured with neonatal calvarial osteoblasts in the presence of 10 nM 1α, 25-dihydroxyvitamin D3, and 1 μM prostaglandin E2. The cells were stimulated with Ang II (0.01–10 μM) for 7 days. TRAP + MNCs were visualized by TRAP staining. (**C**) Representative TRAP staining images. (**D**) The number of osteoclasts. Values are the mean ± SEM. n.s., not significant. *, $p < 0.05$ vs. non-treated control. Detailed methods are described in the Supporting Information.

References

1. Aletaha, D.; Smolen, J.S. Diagnosis and Management of Rheumatoid Arthritis: A Review. *JAMA* **2018**, *320*, 1360–1372. [CrossRef] [PubMed]
2. Smolen, J.S.; Aletaha, D.; Barton, A.; Burmester, G.R.; Emery, P.; Firestein, G.S.; Kavanaugh, A.; McInnes, I.B.; Solomon, D.H.; Strand, V.; et al. Rheumatoid arthritis. *Nat. Rev. Dis. Primers* **2018**, *4*, 18001. [CrossRef] [PubMed]

3. Turesson, C.; O'Fallon, W.M.; Crowson, C.S.; Gabriel, S.E.; Matteson, E.L. Extra-articular disease manifestations in rheumatoid arthritis: Incidence trends and risk factors over 46 years. *Ann. Rheum. Dis.* **2003**, *62*, 722–727. [CrossRef] [PubMed]
4. Deal, C. Bone loss in rheumatoid arthritis: Systemic, periarticular, and focal. *Curr. Rheumatol. Rep.* **2012**, *14*, 231–237. [CrossRef] [PubMed]
5. Bader, M. Tissue renin-angiotensin-aldosterone systems: Targets for pharmacological therapy. *Annu. Rev. Pharm. Toxicol.* **2010**, *50*, 439–465. [CrossRef] [PubMed]
6. Tamargo, J.; Caballero, R.; Delpón, E. The Renin–Angiotensin System and Bone. *Clin. Rev. Bone Miner. Metab.* **2015**, *13*, 125–148. [CrossRef]
7. Paul, M.; Poyan Mehr, A.; Kreutz, R. Physiology of local renin-angiotensin systems. *Physiol. Rev.* **2006**, *86*, 747–803. [CrossRef] [PubMed]
8. Kagami, S. Involvement of glomerular renin-angiotensin system (RAS) activation in the development and progression of glomerular injury. *Clin. Exp. Nephrol.* **2012**, *16*, 214–220. [CrossRef] [PubMed]
9. Zhao, J.; Yang, H.; Chen, B.; Zhang, R. The skeletal renin-angiotensin system: A potential therapeutic target for the treatment of osteoarticular diseases. *Int. Immunopharmacol.* **2019**, *72*, 258–263. [CrossRef] [PubMed]
10. Izu, Y.; Mizoguchi, F.; Kawamata, A.; Hayata, T.; Nakamoto, T.; Nakashima, K.; Inagami, T.; Ezura, Y.; Noda, M. Angiotensin II type 2 receptor blockade increases bone mass. *J. Biol. Chem.* **2009**, *284*, 4857–4864. [CrossRef] [PubMed]
11. Shimizu, H.; Nakagami, H.; Osako, M.K.; Hanayama, R.; Kunugiza, Y.; Kizawa, T.; Tomita, T.; Yoshikawa, H.; Ogihara, T.; Morishita, R. Angiotensin II accelerates osteoporosis by activating osteoclasts. *FASEB J.* **2008**, *22*, 2465–2475. [CrossRef] [PubMed]
12. Gu, S.S.; Zhang, Y.; Li, X.L.; Wu, S.Y.; Diao, T.Y.; Hai, R.; Deng, H.W. Involvement of the skeletal renin-angiotensin system in age-related osteoporosis of ageing mice. *Biosci. Biotechnol. Biochem.* **2012**, *76*, 1367–1371. [CrossRef] [PubMed]
13. Yongtao, Z.; Kunzheng, W.; Jingjing, Z.; Hu, S.; Jianqiang, K.; Ruiyu, L.; Chunsheng, W. Glucocorticoids activate the local renin-angiotensin system in bone: Possible mechanism for glucocorticoid-induced osteoporosis. *Endocrine* **2014**, *47*, 598–608. [CrossRef] [PubMed]
14. Price, A.; Lockhart, J.C.; Ferrell, W.R.; Gsell, W.; McLean, S.; Sturrock, R.D. Angiotensin II type 1 receptor as a novel therapeutic target in rheumatoid arthritis: In vivo analyses in rodent models of arthritis and ex vivo analyses in human inflammatory synovitis. *Arthritis Rheum.* **2007**, *56*, 441–447. [CrossRef] [PubMed]
15. Pattacini, L.; Casali, B.; Boiardi, L.; Pipitone, N.; Albertazzi, L.; Salvarani, C. Angiotensin II protects fibroblast-like synoviocytes from apoptosis via the AT1-NF-kappaB pathway. *Rheumatology* **2007**, *46*, 1252–1257. [CrossRef] [PubMed]
16. Kaneko, K.; Ito, M.; Fumoto, T.; Fukuhara, R.; Ishida, J.; Fukamizu, A.; Ikeda, K. Physiological function of the angiotensin AT1a receptor in bone remodeling. *J. Bone Min. Res.* **2011**, *26*, 2959–2966. [CrossRef] [PubMed]
17. Asaba, Y.; Ito, M.; Fumoto, T.; Watanabe, K.; Fukuhara, R.; Takeshita, S.; Nimura, Y.; Ishida, J.; Fukamizu, A.; Ikeda, K. Activation of renin-angiotensin system induces osteoporosis independently of hypertension. *J. Bone Min. Res.* **2009**, *24*, 241–250. [CrossRef] [PubMed]
18. Brewster, U.C.; Setaro, J.F.; Perazella, M.A. The renin-angiotensin-aldosterone system: Cardiorenal effects and implications for renal and cardiovascular disease states. *Am. J. Med. Sci.* **2003**, *326*, 15–24. [CrossRef] [PubMed]
19. Siragy, H.M.; Carey, R.M. Role of the intrarenal renin-angiotensin-aldosterone system in chronic kidney disease. *Am. J. Nephrol.* **2010**, *31*, 541–550. [CrossRef] [PubMed]
20. Schett, G.; Gravallese, E. Bone erosion in rheumatoid arthritis: Mechanisms, diagnosis and treatment. *Nat. Rev. Rheumatol.* **2012**, *8*, 656–664. [CrossRef] [PubMed]
21. Terenzi, R.; Manetti, M.; Rosa, I.; Romano, E.; Galluccio, F.; Guiducci, S.; Ibba-Manneschi, L.; Matucci-Cerinic, M. Angiotensin II type 2 receptor (AT2R) as a novel modulator of inflammation in rheumatoid arthritis synovium. *Sci. Rep.* **2017**, *7*, 13293. [CrossRef] [PubMed]
22. Sakuta, T.; Morita, Y.; Satoh, M.; Fox, D.A.; Kashihara, N. Involvement of the renin-angiotensin system in the development of vascular damage in a rat model of arthritis: Effect of angiotensin receptor blockers. *Arthritis Rheum.* **2010**, *62*, 1319–1328. [CrossRef] [PubMed]

23. Hayward, M.D.; Jones, B.K.; Saparov, A.; Hain, H.S.; Trillat, A.C.; Bunzel, M.M.; Corona, A.; Li-Wang, B.; Strenkowski, B.; Giordano, C.; et al. An extensive phenotypic characterization of the hTNFalpha transgenic mice. *BMC Physiol.* **2007**, *7*, 13. [CrossRef] [PubMed]
24. Ito, M.; Oliverio, M.I.; Mannon, P.J.; Best, C.F.; Maeda, N.; Smithies, O.; Coffman, T.M. Regulation of blood pressure by the type 1A angiotensin II receptor gene. *Proc. Natl. Acad. Sci. USA* **1995**, *92*, 3521–3525. [CrossRef] [PubMed]
25. Umebayashi, R.; Uchida, H.A.; Kakio, Y.; Subramanian, V.; Daugherty, A.; Wada, J. Cilostazol Attenuates Angiotensin II-Induced Abdominal Aortic Aneurysms but Not Atherosclerosis in Apolipoprotein E-Deficient Mice. *Arter. Thromb. Vasc. Biol.* **2018**, *38*, 903–912. [CrossRef] [PubMed]
26. Uchida, H.A.; Sugiyama, H.; Takiue, K.; Kikumoto, Y.; Inoue, T.; Makino, H. Development of angiotensin II-induced abdominal aortic aneurysms is independent of catalase in mice. *J. Cardiovasc. Pharm.* **2011**, *58*, 633–638. [CrossRef]
27. Mukai, T.; Gallant, R.; Ishida, S.; Yoshitaka, T.; Kittaka, M.; Nishida, K.; Fox, D.A.; Morita, Y.; Ueki, Y. SH3BP2 gain-of-function mutation exacerbates inflammation and bone loss in a murine collagen-induced arthritis model. *PLoS ONE* **2014**, *9*, e105518. [CrossRef] [PubMed]
28. Mukai, T.; Gallant, R.; Ishida, S.; Kittaka, M.; Yoshitaka, T.; Fox, D.A.; Morita, Y.; Nishida, K.; Rottapel, R.; Ueki, Y. Loss of SH3 domain-binding protein 2 function suppresses bone destruction in tumor necrosis factor-driven and collagen-induced arthritis in mice. *Arthritis. Rheumatol.* **2015**, *67*, 656–667. [CrossRef] [PubMed]
29. Mukai, T.; Ishida, S.; Ishikawa, R.; Yoshitaka, T.; Kittaka, M.; Gallant, R.; Lin, Y.L.; Rottapel, R.; Brotto, M.; Reichenberger, E.J.; et al. SH3BP2 cherubism mutation potentiates TNF-alpha-induced osteoclastogenesis via NFATc1 and TNF-alpha-mediated inflammatory bone loss. *J. Bone Min. Res.* **2014**, *29*, 2618–2635. [CrossRef] [PubMed]
30. Fujita, S.; Mukai, T.; Mito, T.; Kodama, S.; Nagasu, A.; Kittaka, M.; Sone, T.; Ueki, Y.; Morita, Y. Pharmacological inhibition of tankyrase induces bone loss in mice by increasing osteoclastogenesis. *Bone* **2018**, *106*, 156–166. [CrossRef]
31. Bouxsein, M.L.; Boyd, S.K.; Christiansen, B.A.; Guldberg, R.E.; Jepsen, K.J.; Muller, R. Guidelines for assessment of bone microstructure in rodents using micro-computed tomography. *J. Bone Min. Res.* **2010**, *25*, 1468–1486. [CrossRef] [PubMed]
32. Danks, L.; Komatsu, N.; Guerrini, M.M.; Sawa, S.; Armaka, M.; Kollias, G.; Nakashima, T.; Takayanagi, H. RANKL expressed on synovial fibroblasts is primarily responsible for bone erosions during joint inflammation. *Ann. Rheum. Dis.* **2016**, *75*, 1187–1195. [CrossRef] [PubMed]
33. Fujii, Y.; Inoue, H.; Arai, Y.; Shimomura, S.; Nakagawa, S.; Kishida, T.; Tsuchida, S.; Kamada, Y.; Kaihara, K.; Shirai, T.; et al. Treadmill Running in Established Phase Arthritis Inhibits Joint Destruction in Rat Rheumatoid Arthritis Models. *Int. J. Mol. Sci.* **2019**, *20*, 5100. [CrossRef] [PubMed]
34. Nagasu, A.; Mukai, T.; Iseki, M.; Kawahara, K.; Tsuji, S.; Nagasu, H.; Ueki, Y.; Ishihara, K.; Kashihara, N.; Morita, Y. Sh3bp2 Gain-Of-Function Mutation Ameliorates Lupus Phenotypes in B6.MRL-Fas(lpr) Mice. *Cells* **2019**, *8*, 402. [CrossRef] [PubMed]

International Journal of
Molecular Sciences

MDPI

Article

Global Gene Expression Analysis Identifies Age-Related Differences in Knee Joint Transcriptome during the Development of Post-Traumatic Osteoarthritis in Mice

Aimy Sebastian [1], Deepa K. Murugesh [1], Melanie E. Mendez [1,2], Nicholas R. Hum [1,2], Naiomy D. Rios-Arce [1], Jillian L. McCool [1,2], Blaine A. Christiansen [3] and Gabriela G. Loots [1,2,*]

1 Physical and Life Sciences Directorate, Lawrence Livermore National Laboratories, Livermore, CA 94550, USA; sebastian4@llnl.gov (A.S.); murugesh2@llnl.gov (D.K.M.); mendez20@llnl.gov (M.E.M.); hum3@llnl.gov (N.R.H.); riosarce1@llnl.gov (N.D.R.-A.); mccool1@llnl.gov (J.L.M.)
2 Molecular and Cell Biology, School of Natural Sciences, UC Merced, Merced, CA 95343, USA
3 Department of Orthopedic Surgery, UC Davis Medical Center, Sacramento, CA 95101, USA; bchristiansen@ucdavis.edu
* Correspondence: loots1@llnl.gov; Tel.: +1-925-423-0923

Received: 6 December 2019; Accepted: 29 December 2019; Published: 6 January 2020

Abstract: Aging and injury are two major risk factors for osteoarthritis (OA). Yet, very little is known about how aging and injury interact and contribute to OA pathogenesis. In the present study, we examined age- and injury-related molecular changes in mouse knee joints that could contribute to OA. Using RNA-seq, first we profiled the knee joint transcriptome of 10-week-old, 62-week-old, and 95-week-old mice and found that the expression of several inflammatory-response related genes increased as a result of aging, whereas the expression of several genes involved in cartilage metabolism decreased with age. To determine how aging impacts post-traumatic arthritis (PTOA) development, the right knee joints of 10-week-old and 62-week-old mice were injured using a non-invasive tibial compression injury model and injury-induced structural and molecular changes were assessed. At six-week post-injury, 62-week-old mice displayed significantly more cartilage degeneration and osteophyte formation compared with young mice. Although both age groups elicited similar transcriptional responses to injury, 62-week-old mice had higher activation of inflammatory cytokines than 10-week-old mice, whereas cartilage/bone metabolism genes had higher expression in 10-week-old mice, suggesting that the differential expression of these genes might contribute to the differences in PTOA severity observed between these age groups.

Keywords: osteoarthritis; aging; PTOA; gene expression; RNA-seq; cartilage degeneration; scRNA-seq; chondrocytes

---

1. Introduction

Osteoarthritis (OA) is a degenerative joint disease characterized by progressive cartilage loss, bone remodeling, synovial inflammation, and significant joint pain, often resulting in disability [1]. According to Center for Disease Control statistics, approximately 30 million people in the United States are estimated to have OA. Currently, there are no approved therapies available to prevent degeneration or rebuild articular cartilage destroyed by OA. Existing treatments mainly target the symptoms, and advanced OA often requires joint replacement [1]. A more in-depth understanding of the pathophysiology of the disease will likely lead to the development of novel therapeutic strategies for the prevention and/or treatment of OA.

Aging is a key risk factor for the development of OA. It is estimated that, by 2050, people over the age of 60 will account for more than 20% of the world's population. Of that, ~15–20% will have symptomatic OA, and one-third of these people will be severely disabled. In addition to age, joint injury is also a common risk factor for OA. OA that develops because of a joint injury is defined as post-traumatic OA (PTOA). Clinical statistics reveal that ~50% of people with injury to the anterior cruciate ligament (ACL) or the meniscus will develop PTOA within 1–2 decades of the injury [2]. It has also been suggested that age and joint injury interact and have a combined effect on the development and progression of OA following joint trauma. The average time from meniscal injury to the onset of radiographic signs of OA in patients older than 30 was five years; in sharp contrast, patients between 17 and 30 years of age were asymptomatic for up to 15 years [3]. Although several studies have investigated the role of age and injury in the development of OA, the mechanisms by which age and injury interact to contribute to OA pathogenesis are still not well understood [4–7].

Recently, using a noninvasive tibial compression (TC) injury model of PTOA, we investigated molecular and structural changes in the knee joints of young (10-16 weeks-old) mice following ACL injury [8–10]. These mice showed significant cartilage erosion, subchondral bone loss, and osteophyte formation as early as 4–6 weeks post-injury [8–10]. Gene expression analysis using RNA-seq revealed that a significant number of genes associated with inflammatory responses were elevated shortly after the injury (one-day post-injury) and several genes associated with cartilage and bone remodeling were elevated at 1–6 weeks post-injury [8,10].

In the present study, we compared OA-associated changes in the knee joints of mice ranging in age from 10 to 95 weeks old, to determine the contribution of age to OA pathogenesis. First, we identified age-related molecular changes in healthy (uninjured) knee joints by comparing gene expression in 10-week-old, 62-week-old, and 95-week-old mice. Then, using the TC injury model [11], we compared molecular and structural changes associated with PTOA development between 10- and 62-week-old mice, to better understand how age and joint injury interact to contribute to the development of PTOA. We found that the old mice displayed a more severe cartilage degeneration phenotype and increased osteophyte formation in response to injury compared with the younger mice. We also identified significant differences in injury-induced response genes between old and young mice, including an increased expression of inflammatory-response related genes and reduced expression of genes involved in cartilage and bone development in old mice, which could have contributed to the more severe PTOA phenotype observed in old mice.

2. Results

2.1. *Aging Up-Regulated Inflammatory Response-Related Genes and Down-Regulated Genes Associated with Cartilage Development and Homeostasis in Mouse Knee Joints*

To determine aging-related molecular changes in healthy (uninjured) knee joints, we profiled the knee joint transcriptome of 10-week-old, 62-week-old, and 95-week-old mice using RNA-seq. Compared with 10-week-old mice, 974 and 1732 genes were up-regulated and 1006 and 1386 genes were down-regulated in 62-week-old mice and 95-week-old mice, respectively (Figure 1A,B, Table S1). Six-hundred and four genes including 42 arthritis-associated genes (*Mmp3*, *Ccl3*, *Ccr5*, *Csf3*, *Cxcr6*, *Lyz1*, *Il33*, and *Tnfsf15*, among others), 110 genes associated with immune response (*Tlr7*, *Csf3*, *Cd3d*, *Cd4*, *Nlrp1b*, and *Cd8a*, among others) and 47 inflammatory response-related genes (*Ccl5*, *Ccr5*, *Cxcl1*, and *Cxcl5*, among others) were up-regulated in both 62-week-old and 95-week-old old mice compared with 10-week-old mice (Figure S1A, Figure 1C). Of these common up-regulated genes, 143 genes including several key regulators of immune/inflammatory responses such as *Il5ra*, *Il17re*, *Cxcr3*, *Cxcr6*, *Cxcl5*, *Cxcl9*, *Ccl3*, and *Ccl4* had a significantly higher expression in 95-week-old mice compared with 62-week-old mice, suggesting a progressive increase in the levels of inflammatory mediators in the joint with age (Figure 1C,E). Genes down-regulated in both 62-week-old and 95-week-old mice compared with 10-week-old mice included 39 genes associated with cartilage development (*Col2a1*, *Col9a1*, *Sox9*, *Acan*, and *Comp*, among others), 40 genes associated with bone development (*Col1a1*, *Alpl*, *Sparc*, *Bglap*, and *Runx2*, among others), 35 genes involved in osteoblast differentiation, and 22 genes involved in chondrocyte differentiation (Figure 1D, Figure S1B–D). Several key regulators of cartilage development and homeostasis including *Sox9*, *Col2a1*, and *Acan* had the lowest expression in 95-week-old mice, indicating a reduction in cartilage anabolic responses with age (Figure 1F).

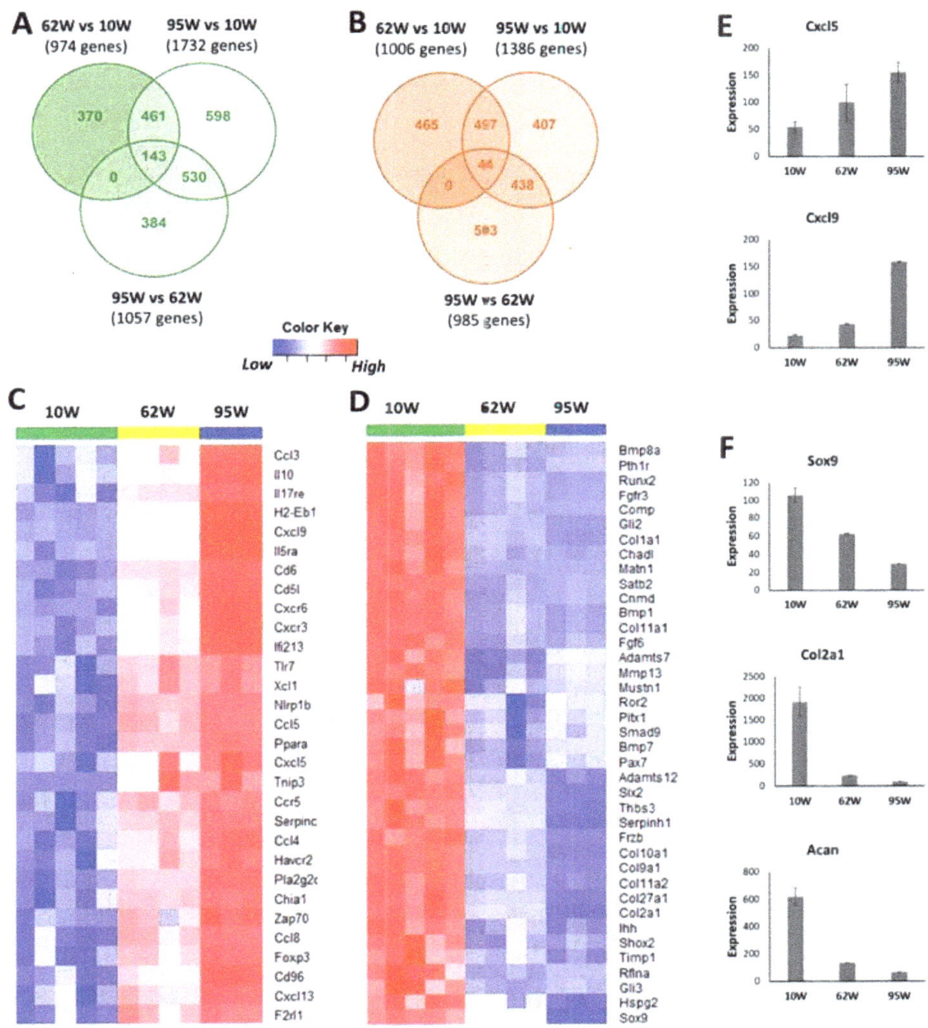

Figure 1. Age-related changes in the knee joint gene expression. Genes up- (**A**) and down-regulated (**B**) in 62-week-old (62W) mice and 95-week-old (95W) mice compared with 10-week-old (10W) mice and in 95-week-old mice compared with 62-week-old mice. (**C**) Inflammatory response-related genes up-regulated in both 62-week-old and 95-week-old compared with 10-week-old mice (top 30 genes). (**D**) Cartilage development-associated genes down-regulated in both 62-week-old and 95-week-old compared with 10-week-old mice. (**E**) Examples of inflammatory response genes showing progressive increase with age. (**F**) Key cartilage development-associated genes showing an age-related decrease in expression.

2.2. Injury-Induced Knee Joint Degeneration was Accelerated in Old Mice

To understand how aging impacts PTOA development after injury, we investigated structural changes in the knee joints of 62-week-old and 10-week-old mice six weeks after an ACL injury. Ten-week-old mice represent young adult humans whose cartilage is normally healthy, whereas 62-week-old mice represent a ~50–60 year-old human, an age group in which OA is prevalent. By six-week post-injury, both 10-week-old and 62-week-old mice exhibited severe cartilage degradation in the injured joints (Figure 2A,B). OA lesions were more severe in 62-week-old mice than in 10-week-old mice, where the majority of the femoral head was lacking the articular cartilage layer in the injured 62-week old mice (Figure 2A). Osteophyte formation was observed in both age groups by six-week post-injury, and 62-week-old mice had significantly more osteophytes than 10-week-old mice (Figure 2C). ACL injury also resulted in a significant reduction in subchondral bone volume in the femoral epiphysis in both age groups (Figure 2D). Older, 62-week-old mice displayed a significantly lower subchondral bone volume than 10-week-old mice before injury, and they also lost more subchondral bone (25% loss) than younger mice (18% loss) by six weeks after injury (Figure 2D).

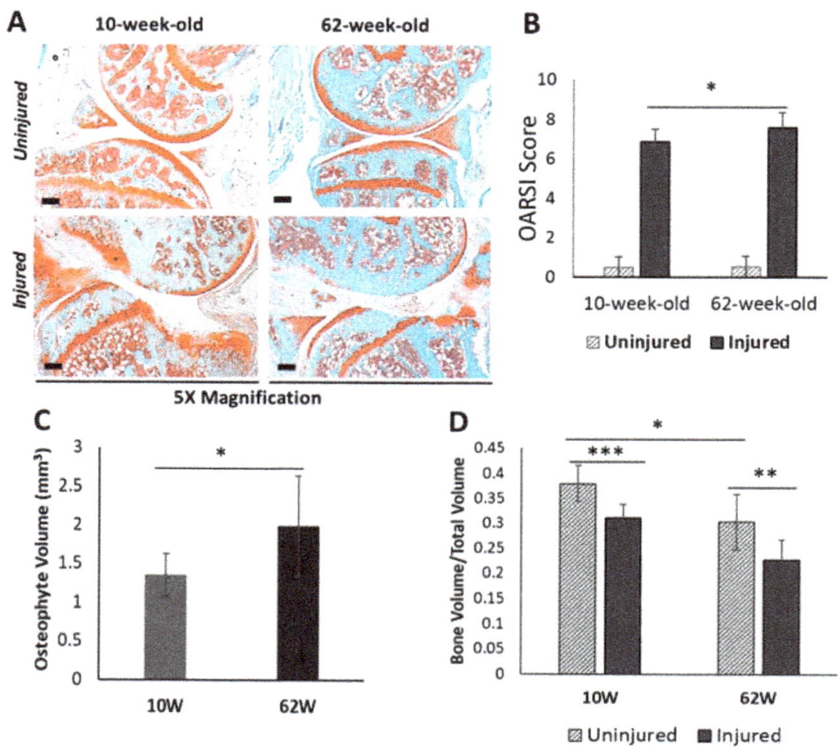

Figure 2. Characterization of post-traumatic osteoarthritis (PTOA)-associated structural changes in 10-week-old and 62-week-old mice. (**A**) Histological evaluation of uninjured contralateral joints and injured joints at six-week post-injury using Safranin-O and Fast Green staining which stains cartilage in red and surrounding tissue in green (5× magnification). Scale bars: 200 µm. (**B**) Osteoarthritis Research Society International (OARSI) scoring of histological sections of injured and uninjured contralateral joints at six-week post-injury. (**C**) Osteophyte volume at six-week post-injury. (**D**) Epiphyseal trabecular bone volume fraction (BV/TV) of the distal femur was quantified using µCT and analyzed between injured and uninjured contralateral joints at six-week post-injury. 10W: 10-week-old; 62W: 62-week-old. * $p < 0.05$, ** $p < 0.01$, *** $p < 0.001$.

2.3. Age-Related Differences in ACL Injury-Induced Gene Expression Changes in the Knee Joints

To determine how aging impacts PTOA development at the molecular level, we compared injury-induced gene expression changes in both 10-week-old and 62-week-old mice at six-week post-injury. RNA-seq analysis identified 699 and 255 genes differentially expressed in injured knee joints of 10-week-old mice and 62-week-old mice, respectively, compared with respective uninjured contralateral joints (Figure 3A, Table S2). Of these genes, 184 up-regulated genes were common to both age groups (Figure 3B). These genes included 41 genes involved in extracellular matrix organization (*Htra1*, *Fn1*, *Comp*, *Tnc*, *Dcn*, *Bgn*, *Sulf1*, *Loxl1*, *Loxl2*, *Has1*, *Lum*, *Plod2*, and *Collagens*, among others), 19 genes involved in collagen metabolic process (*Collagens*, *Mmp2*, and *Mmp3*, among others), 14 genes involved in cartilage development (*Col2a1*, *Col10a1*, *Comp*, *Ror2*, *Osr2*, *Pth1r*, *Thbs3*, *Sulf1*, and *Loxl2*, among others), and 24 genes involved in bone development and metabolism (*Cthrc1*, *Ibsp*, *Sparc*, *Pth1r*, and *Enpp1*, among others). Of these common up-regulated genes, 113 genes including several regulators of cartilage and bone development/metabolism such as *Chad*, *Col10a1*, *Col2a1*, *Comp*, *Pth1r*, *Ror2*, *Ibsp*, and *Sparc* had higher expression in injured joints of 10-week-old mice compared with injured joints of 62-week-old mice, suggesting a more active cartilage and bone remodeling in young mice after injury (Figure 3B,C, Table S2).

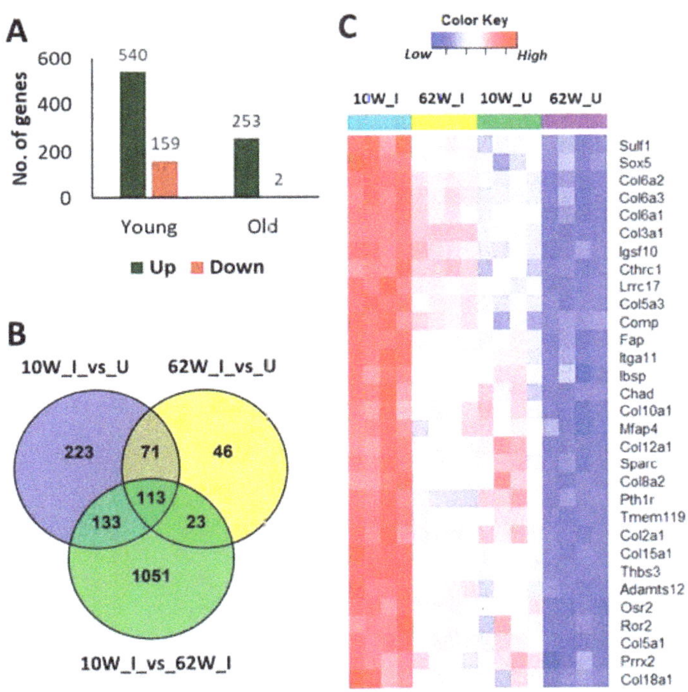

Figure 3. Age related differences in anterior cruciate ligament (ACL) injury-induced gene expression changes at six-week post-injury. (**A**) Number of genes differentially expressed in response to injury in 10-week-old and 62-week-old mice at six-week post-injury. (**B**) Overlap between genes up-regulated in 10-week-old and 62-week-old mice compared with respective uninjured controls and genes up-regulated in injured joints of 10-week-old compared with injured joints of 62-week-old mice. (**C**) Injury-induced regulators of cartilage and bone development/metabolism showing highest expression in injured joints of 10-week-old-mice. 10W_I: injured joints of 10-week-old; 10W_U: uninjured joints of 10-week-old; 62W_I: injured joints of 62-week-old; 62W_U: uninjured joints of 62-week-old.

We also identified 356 genes up-regulated only in 10-week-old injured joints, which included several regulators of skeletal system development (*Phex*, *Sulf2*, *Fbn1*, *Fbn2*, *Sfrp1*, *Tnfrsf11b*, *Hapln1*, *Igf1*, and *Rspo2*, among others), extracellular matrix organization (*Dmp1*, *Mmp12*, *Mmp19*, *Adamts2*, *Tnc*, and *Loxl1*, among others), inflammatory response (*Cxcl10*, *C3ar1*, *C4b*, *Ccr5*, *Ccl8*, and *Il33*, among others), and Wnt signaling (*Fzd1*, *Nfatc4*, *Wnt16*, *Sfrp1*, *Sfrp4*, *Nkd2*, *Prickle2*, *Rspo2*, *Rspo1*, and *Dkk3*, among others) (Figure 3B, Table S2). Sixty-nine genes were specifically up-regulated in 62-week-old mice compared with respective uninjured controls, which included several regulators of bone development and metabolism (*Postn*, *Bmp1*, *Sfrp2*, *Gja1*, *Ptn*, *Alpl*, *Sp7*, and *Mmp14*, among others) (Figure 3B, Table S2). However, 23 of these 69 genes including *Alpl*, *Sp7*, *Bmp1*, and *Mmp14* had higher expression in both injured and uninjured joints of 10-week-old mice compared with 62-week-old mice (Table S2). Two genes (*Kcna3* and *Gm30934*) were down-regulated in 62-week-old mice, whereas 159 genes were down-regulated in 10-weekold mice in response to injury, and none of these genes overlapped with genes down-regulated in 62-week-old mice (Table S2).

We have previously shown that, in young mice, inflammatory response genes were highly up-regulated immediately post-injury and a large number of genes associated with cartilage and bone remodeling were highly elevated at one-week and two weeks post-injury [8,10]. To identify the differences in injury-induced early molecular changes between the young and old, we profiled the knee joint transcriptome of 62-week-old mice at one-day, one-week, and two weeks post-injury. Our analysis identified 779, 1486, and 1299 genes differentially expressed in injured knee joints of old mice at one-day, one-week, and two-weeks post injury, respectively, compared with respective uninjured contralateral joints (Figure 4A, Table S2). In 10-week-old mice, 755, 811, and 596 genes were differentially expressed at one-day, one-week, and two weeks post injury, respectively (Figure 4B, Table S2). We also observed a huge overlap between genes up-regulated in both age groups at early post-injury timepoints (Table 1). This included 48 genes up-regulated in both age groups at all post-injury timepoints examined in this study (Table 2).

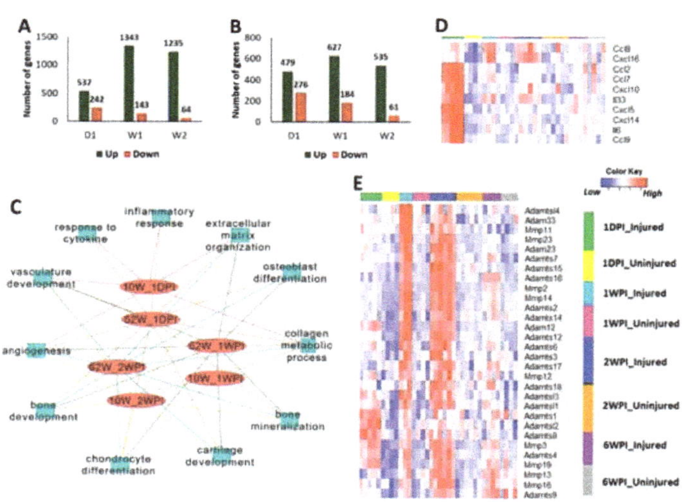

Figure 4. Injury-induced transcriptional changes at early post-injury timepoints. Number of genes up- and down-regulated in injured knee joints of 62-week-old (**A**) and 10-week-old (**B**) mice at one-day (1D), one-week (1W), and two weeks (2W) post-injury compared with uninjured contralateral joints. (**C**) Key biological processes associated with genes up-regulated in 62-week-old mice and 10-week-old mice at early timepoints. (**D**) Inflammatory cytokines up-regulated at one-day post-injury in 62-week-old mice. (**E**) Matrix degrading enzymes up-regulated in 62-week-old mice after injury. Majority of these had highest expression at 1–2 weeks post-injury. 10W: 10-week-old; 62W: 62-week-old; 1DPI: one-day post-injury; 1WPI: one-week post-injury; 2WPI: two weeks post-injury.

Table 1. Table showing up-regulated genes shared between 10-week-old and 62-week-old mice at various post-injury timepoints.

Time Post-Injury		62-Week-Old			
		1 Day (Total: 537)	1 Week (Total: 1343)	2 Weeks (Total: 1235)	6 Weeks (Total: 253)
10-week-old	1 Day (Total: 479)	246	288	256	78
	1 Week (Total: 627)	227	536	534	179
	2 Weeks (Total: 535)	196	465	462	177
	6 Weeks (Total: 540)	170	427	430	184

Injury-induced genes in both young and old mice showed enrichment for similar biological processes at early post-injury timepoints (Figure 4C). Similar to what we have previously shown for young mice [10], 62-week-old mice also displayed an up-regulation of inflammatory response related genes at one-day post-injury (Figure 4C,D, Table S2). These genes included several cytokines that also showed an increase in expression with age such as *Ccl8*, *Cxcl5*, and *Il33* (Table S1). As in the case of young mice [10], a large number of genes involved in extracellular matrix organization and cartilage/bone metabolism including core matrix proteins such as collagens, *Fn1*, *Dcn*, *Eln*, *Fbn1*, *Fbn2*, *Bgn*, *Acan*, *Cthrc1*, *Postn*, *Prelp*, *Prg4*, and *Vcan* and matrix degrading enzymes such as *Mmp2*, *Mmp3*, *Adamts2*, and *Adamts3* showed an increased expression in the injured joints of 62-week-old mice compared with uninjured controls (Figure 4E, Figure S2, Table S2). The majority of these genes had the highest expression at 1–2 weeks post-injury, indicating a more active tissue remodeling at this timepoint (Figure 4E, Figure S2). We also observed that a number of collagen processing enzymes such as *Lox*, *Loxl2*, *Loxl3*, and *Plod2* were activated by injury in both age groups (Figure S3A). Using single-cell RNAseq (scRNA-seq) data from adult mouse knee joint cartilage, we also determined that mature chondrocytes robustly express *Loxl2*, *Loxl3*, and *Plod2*, whereas *Lox* expression was more restricted to immature chondrocytes/mesenchymal progenitors (Figure S3B).

Table 2. Genes up-regulated in injured joints of both young and old mice at all timepoints examined. Fold change (log2 scale) values are shown in the table (false discovery rate (FDR) < 0.05 for all genes).

Age	Young				Old			
Gene	1 Day	1 Week	2 Weeks	6 Weeks	1 Day	1 Week	2 Weeks	6 Weeks
Adamts12	0.649	1.324	0.917	0.783	1.225	2.363	1.898	0.804
AW551984	1.397	1.863	1.662	1.048	1.479	2.865	2.787	1.106
Bmper	1.402	1.245	1.039	1.023	1.436	1.447	1.443	0.813
Col14a1	1.112	2.110	1.552	1.424	0.730	2.939	2.508	1.016
Col18a1	0.741	1.263	1.124	0.606	1.003	2.268	1.758	0.689
Col3a1	1.543	2.075	1.683	1.594	2.395	4.267	3.878	2.270
Col5a1	0.916	1.441	0.995	0.781	1.053	3.080	2.482	1.078
Col5a2	0.725	1.157	0.793	1.036	1.304	3.118	2.815	1.381
Col5a3	0.670	1.119	0.735	1.080	0.690	2.137	1.783	1.007
Col6a1	0.752	1.674	1.282	0.992	0.934	3.155	2.603	1.256
Col6a2	0.752	1.688	1.287	1.162	0.993	3.170	2.639	1.156
Col6a3	0.930	1.807	1.156	1.292	1.436	3.188	2.564	1.270
Col8a1	0.609	0.748	0.615	0.590	0.965	1.681	1.537	0.701
Crabp2	1.600	2.440	2.452	1.956	1.842	3.802	4.167	1.867
Cthrc1	1.686	2.050	1.281	1.488	1.765	4.493	3.955	1.914
Dab2	0.994	1.056	0.888	0.606	1.200	1.697	1.668	0.772
Dsel	0.692	1.267	0.736	0.919	0.686	1.764	1.700	1.005
Enpp1	0.685	1.408	0.789	1.393	0.860	1.914	2.009	1.265
Fcrls	1.990	1.288	1.208	0.895	2.233	2.501	2.223	1.005
Fndc1	0.825	1.977	1.474	1.413	0.668	2.795	2.227	1.023
Fstl1	1.196	1.500	1.217	0.895	1.278	2.371	2.128	0.745

Table 2. *Cont.*

Age	Young				Old			
Gene	1 Day	1 Week	2 Weeks	6 Weeks	1 Day	1 Week	2 Weeks	6 Weeks
Has1	1.367	1.921	1-.955	3.181	3.310	2.894	2.648	1.590
Hhipl1	1.551	1.644	1.067	1.431	1.357	1.896	1.780	1.386
Igsf10	0.990	1.772	1.072	1.405	0.750	2.965	2.662	1.479
Kcnj15	1.108	2.295	1.724	2.637	1.566	2.779	2.562	1.192
Lrrc17	2.079	1.925	1.112	0.871	1.316	2.565	2.359	0.912
Mfap5	1.189	1.732	1.322	1.094	1.214	2.235	2.038	0.893
Mmp3	1.648	1.988	2.032	1.094	3.513	2.440	3.143	2.060
Mrgprf	1.071	1.967	1.493	1.309	0.848	2.582	2.138	0.988
Nox4	1.343	1.028	1.303	1.185	1.240	1.604	1.489	1.066
P4ha3	2.305	2.528	1.917	1.187	2.206	4.191	3.840	1.621
Plce1	0.648	0.863	0.672	0.668	0.657	1.160	1.099	0.704
Prg4	0.733	1.228	1.273	1.817	1.618	1.526	1.471	1.620
Prrx2	1.492	1.385	1.176	0.838	1.773	3.217	2.546	1.032
Ptgfrn	0.726	1.164	0.802	0.754	1.131	2.010	1.697	0.775
Slc16a2	1.413	1.655	0.950	0.792	1.360	1.783	1.654	0.782
Slc1a4	0.984	1.629	1.206	1.143	1.566	2.347	1.991	1.319
Slc41a2	0.727	0.814	0.619	0.621	1.026	1.096	1.438	0.711
Srpx2	0.842	1.219	0.867	1.054	1.207	2.155	2.032	0.839
Sulf1	0.896	1.245	0.911	1.029	1.333	1.743	1.713	0.903
Thbs2	0.958	1.614	0.831	0.733	0.684	2.893	2.294	1.086
Thbs3	0.643	1.773	1.330	1.429	1.115	3.018	2.660	1.214
Thbs4	0.832	0.925	0.974	0.695	1.349	1.717	1.546	1.052
Timp1	2.037	1.193	1.059	1.132	4.129	2.886	2.697	1.377
Tmem45a	0.606	1.129	0.788	0.940	1.361	2.375	2.159	0.990
Tnfaip6	1.941	1.804	1.345	2.636	3.897	3.911	3.240	1.722
Tnn	1.117	1.722	1.019	1.056	1.098	4.072	3.469	1.830

Although injury activated a large number of genes involved in cartilage anabolism in both age groups, histological analysis (Figure 2) suggested that this was not sufficient to prevent joint degeneration. To further investigate this, we performed immunohistochemistry analysis of two injury-induced genes: chondroadherin (*Chad*), a leucine rich repeat extracellular matrix protein that is synthesized by chondrocytes and reported to promote their attachment [12]; and *Plod2*, an enzyme involved in collagen synthesis [13]. Consistent with gene expression data (Table S1), immunohistochemistry showed lower Chad and Plod2 protein expression in the articular cartilage of old mice compared with young mice, confirming a decrease in expression with age (Figure 5C,D). However, in contrast to an increase in the transcript levels observed after injury (Table S2), injured joints of both age groups had significantly lower Chad and Plod2 protein expression compared with respective uninjured controls, suggesting that the increase in gene expression in response to injury failed to translate into increased protein expression. Alternatively, other cells in the joint may have up-regulated the transcript levels of these genes, in which case the non-cartilage derived RNA would account for higher transcript levels in the injured joints.

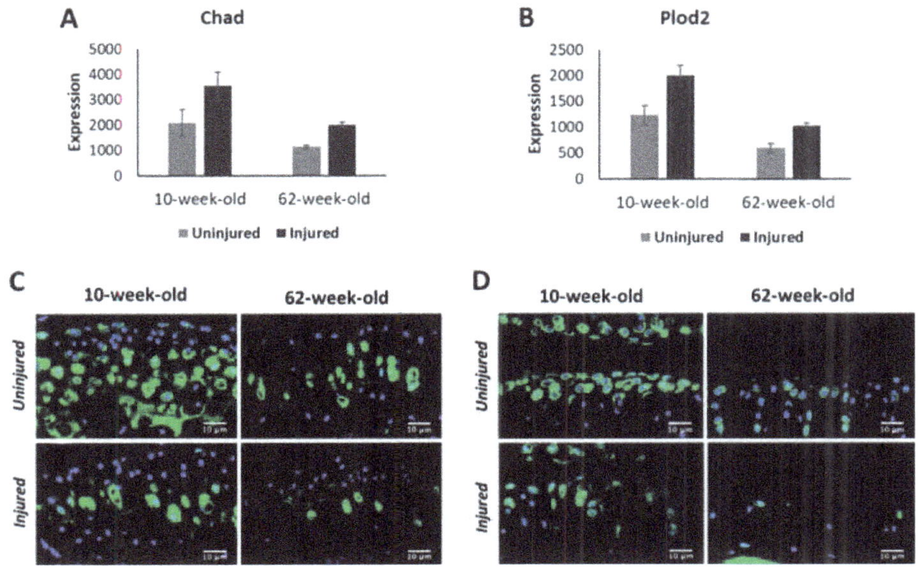

Figure 5. *Chad* (**A**) and *Plod2* (**B**) gene expression at six-week post injury in 10-week-old and 62-week-old mice. Chad (**C**) and Plod2 (**D**) protein expression in 10-week-old and 62-week-old mice Green: protein staining. Blue: DAPI staining marking the nucleus. (40× magnification).

The number of genes down-regulated in response to injury was much lower than the number of up-regulated genes in both age groups, at all timepoints examined (Figure 4A,B). At one-day post-injury, 68 genes were down-regulated in both 10-week-old and 62-week-old mice including several genes involved glucose catabolic process in such as *Pfkfb1*, *Pgam2*, and *Eno3* (Table S2). Thirty-seven genes including several regulators of muscle structure and function such as *Myh1*, *Myh2*, *Myl2*, *Myl3*, *Actn2*, and *Ankrd2* were down-regulated in both age groups at one-week post-injury (Table S2). Cytokine-like 1 (*Cytl1*) [14,15], a gene potentially involved in chondrogenesis and cartilage development, was down-regulated in 10-week-old mice at all post-injury timepoints and in 62-weeks old mice at one-day, one-week, and two weeks post-injury (Figure 6A), and this trend was consistent when protein levels were analyzed by immunohistochemistry (Figure 6B), suggesting that *Cytl1* correlates with PTOA severity. scRNA-seq analysis of adult mouse knee joint cartilage showed that *Cytl1* was robustly expressed by a specific chondrocyte subpopulation, which also expressed high levels of *Bmp2*, *Wif1*, and *Prg4*, genes that play a role in chondrocyte differentiation and maintenance [16–18] (Figure 6C–E), indicating a spatially restricted expression pattern for this gene in the cartilage and a potential role in the development and maintenance of the articular cartilage.

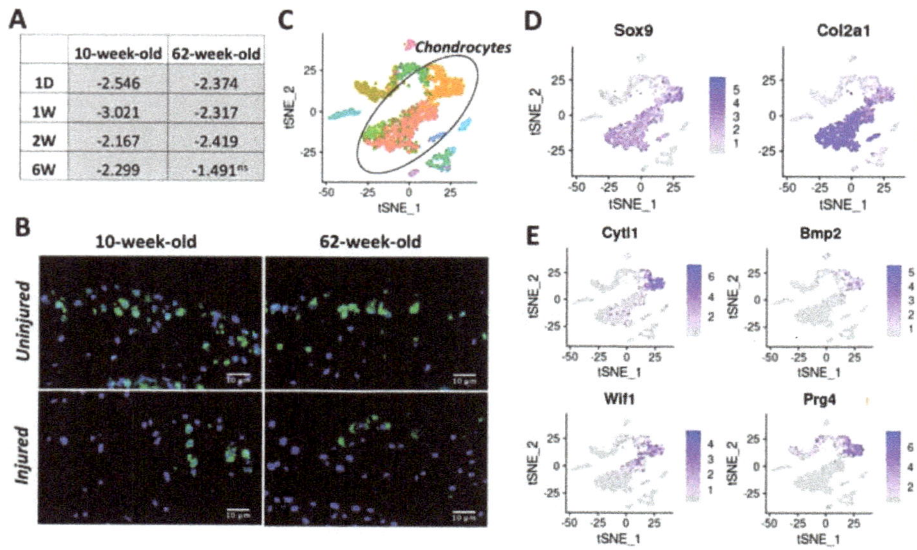

Figure 6. (**A**) Table showing *Cytl1* fold down-regulation in injured joints compared with uninjured controls at various post-injury timepoints, in both 10-week-old and 62-week-old mice. (**B**) Cytl1 protein expression at six-week post injury in 10-week-old and 62-week-old mice. Green: protein staining. Blue: DAPI staining marking the nucleus. (40× magnification) (**C**) tSNE plot of mouse cartilage cells identified using scRNA-seq. Each color represents a distinct cell type/subtype. Chondrocyte subtypes identified in mouse cartilage based on the expression of chondrocyte markers *Col2a1*, *Acan*, and *Sox9* are shown in black oval. (**D**) Expression of chondrocyte markers *Sox9* and *Col2a1* in scRNA-seq data. (**E**) *Cytl1* expression is restricted to a chondrocyte subtype that also express high levels of *Bmp2*, *Wif1*, and *Prg4* at high levels. Ns: not significant.

3. Discussion

Aging and injury are two key risk factors for OA. Several studies have investigated how aging and injury independently contribute to OA pathogenesis; however, very limited data are available on how aging and injury interact to influence OA progression [4]. In this study, we investigated the differences in molecular responses of young and old mice to knee joint injury using RNA-seq. Our study identified several age-related structural and molecular changes in mouse knee joint during PTOA development and progression.

Histological analysis showed that both 10-week-old and 62-week-old mice exhibited significant joint degeneration by six-week post-injury. Consistent with previous reports [4], older mice had more severe articular cartilage degeneration compared with young mice. Both age groups had deficits in epiphyseal trabecular bone in the injured joint and exhibited considerable osteophyte formation, which was more severe in older animals. Old mice also showed lower trabecular bone volume fraction (BV/TV) compared with the young mice, suggesting an age-dependent bone loss. Our previous study showed peak trabecular bone changes at approximately two weeks post injury, while mineralized osteophytes were not observable by μCT until about four weeks [19]. In this study, we only examined six-week post-injury joints using μCT and histology, and the joints were severely damaged in both age groups by six-week post-injury. Examining an earlier time point (e.g., 2–4 weeks post-injury) would potentially allow us to more clearly see differences in PTOA progression between old and young mice and determine whether aging accelerates PTOA.

At a molecular level, older mice had significantly higher expression of inflammatory signaling genes including *Ccl3*, *Ccl4*, *Ccl5*, *Ccl8*, *Cxcl5*, *Cxcl9*, *Cxcl13*, *Il6*, and *Il33* compared with young mice and the expression of many of these inflammatory cytokines increased with age, with 95-week-old mice showing the highest expression (Figure 1C). A study comparing gene expression in joint tissues from 12-week-old mice and 12-month-old mice has shown that the expressions of *Il6*, *Il33*, *Cxcl9*, *Cxcl13*, *Ccl8*, and *Ccl5*, were significantly up-regulated in the old mice compared with the young [4], which is consistent with our observation. We also found that knee joint injury further activated the expression of many of these genes in both young and old mice at one-day post-injury, and the majority of these genes reverted to the uninjured control level by 1–2 weeks post-injury in both age groups. It has been suggested that inflammation plays a key role in the pathogenesis of osteoarthritis; inflammatory mediators may promote cartilage degradation either directly or indirectly through the induction of proteolytic enzymes [20,21]. Low innate production of interleukin (IL)-6 has been shown to be associated with the absence of osteoarthritis in old age [22]. It has also been shown that STR/ort, a mouse strain with high susceptibility to OA, expresses high levels of inflammatory markers, whereas MRL/MpJ, a mouse strain resistant to PTOA, had low expression values for these genes [10,23,24]. These data together suggest that an increase in the levels of inflammatory mediators with age might have played a role in the enhanced joint degeneration observed in older mice.

Consistent with previous studies demonstrating an age-related decline in chondrocyte anabolic responses [4,25], we observed a significant reduction in the expression of genes involved in cartilage development and metabolism including *Sox9* [26], *Col2a1*, *Col9a1-a3* [27], *Acan*, *Comp*, *Perlecan (Hspg2)* [28], and *Hapln1* [29] with age (Table S1). *Emp7*, a key regulator cartilage homeostasis and cartilage repair [30], also showed reduced expression in old animals. Chondroadherin (Chad), a cartilage matrix protein thought to mediate chondrocyte adhesion, also displayed a down-regulation with age [12]. However, knee joint injury activated the expression of many of these cartilage anabolic genes in both 10-week-old and 62-week-old mice (Table S2). These observations are consistent with previous data showing up-regulation of these genes in human OA cartilage compared with normal cartilage [31]. We also found that injured joints of 10-week-old mice had higher expression of these genes compared with injured joints of 62-week-old mice, suggesting that young mice are more actively trying to repair the cartilage after injury (Figure 3C). However, immunohistochemical analysis of Chad showed a significant reduction in protein expression in the injured joints of both 10-week-old and 62-week-old mice at six-week post-injury. This suggests that increased expression of cartilage anabolic genes after injury was not sufficient to prevent cartilage degeneration.

Cartilage intermediate layer protein 2 (CILP-2) is a protein that is localized in the deeper intermediate zone of the articular cartilage extracellular matrix and was down-regulated in mouse OA cartilage [32]. Serum levels of CILP-2 appear to be associated with loss of cartilage thickness in certain individuals with increased risk of developing knee osteoarthritis [33]. We found that *Cilp2* showed an age-dependent decrease in expression (Table S1). Our data also showed down-regulation of *Cilp2* immediately post-injury in both 10-week-old and 62-week-old mice; however, it was up-regulated at later timepoints in both age groups (Table S2). Several genes involved in matrix degradation including MMPs (*Mmp2*, *-3*, *-12*, *-14*, *-19*), ADAMTS (*Adamts4*, *-6*, *-12*, *-15*, *-16*) and HtrA serine peptidase 1 and 3 were also up-regulated in both young and old mice after injury and may play a role in tissue remodeling after joint injury.

Expression of collagen crosslinking enzymes lysyl oxidases (*Lox*, *Loxl2*, and *loxl3*) also decreased with age (Figure S3C). Lysyl oxidases play a key role in physiological and pathological remodeling of extracellular matrix and it has been shown that systemic LOXL2 adenovirus or LOXL2 genetic overexpression in mice can protect against OA [34]. Procollagen-lysine,2-oxoglutarate 5-dioxygenase 2 (*Plod2*), another collagen processing enzyme, also had significantly lower expression in old mice compared with young. Mutations in *PLOD2* cause Bruck syndrome (BS), a rare congenital connective tissue disorder characterized by a combination of joint contractures with various skeletal anomalies [35]. It has been suggested that PLOD2 plays a role in synovial fibrosis, a major contributor to joint stiffness in OA [36]. scRNA-seq analysis of adult mouse knee joints cartilage indicated that chondrocytes robustly express this gene (Figure S3B), suggesting that Plod2 plays a role in maintaining cartilage homeostasis.

We observed a significant up-regulation of transcripts encoding these collagen processing enzymes after injury in both age groups at various post injury timepoints, possibly as a mechanism to prevent cartilage damage (Table S2). However, immunohistochemistry analysis of Plod2 showed a decrease in protein expression in injured joint at six-week post-injury, which was consistent with what we observed for cartilage matrix protein Chad (Figure 5C,D). We only examined the cartilage for protein expression, and other cells in the joint such as osteoblasts, fibroblasts, or immune cells may have contributed to the up-regulation of the transcript levels of these genes, in which case the non-chondrocyte derived RNA would account for higher transcript levels in the injured joints. Differences in the rates of RNA and protein metabolism could also have contributed to this inconsistency. Further studies are required to understand how protein metabolism is regulated after injury and how this plays a role in cartilage degeneration.

Very few genes were down-regulated in both age groups after injury. Cytokine-like 1 (CYTL1) is a cytokine that has been shown to promote chondrogenic differentiation of mesenchymal stem cells [14], and *Cytl1* knock-out mice were more sensitive to osteoarthritic (OA) cartilage destruction than wildtype mice [15]. Cytokine-like 1 (CYTL1) was down-regulated in both young and old mice after injury (Table S2). Cytl1 also showed a reduced expression in 62-week-old mice compared with 10-week-old mice. Furthermore, we found that in adult mice *Cytl1* expression is restricted to a subset of chondrocytes, which also express high levels of *Bmp2*, a key regulator of chondrogenic differentiation [16]; Wnt inhibitor *Wif1*; and lubricin (*Prg4*), a gene involved in boundary lubrication [37] (Figure 6C–E). Wif1 is expressed at cartilage-mesenchyme interfaces and neutralizes Wnt3a-mediated inhibition of chondrogenesis [17]. It has been shown that Prg4-expressing cells located at the embryonic joint surface serve as a progenitor population for all deeper layers of the mature articular cartilage [38]. It has also been shown that Prg4 plays an important anti-inflammatory role in regulating synoviocyte proliferation in OA and reduces basal and IL-1β-stimulated expression of matrix degrading enzymes [18]. Co-localization of Cytl1 with these genes indicate that Cytl1 plays a role in chondrocyte differentiation and maintenance. Consistent with our RNA-seq data, immunohistochemical analysis showed that Cytl1 expression is reduced after injury in both age groups (Figure 6A,B). Our data suggest that age- or injury-induced decrease of Cytl1 could negatively affect cartilage homeostasis and contribute to joint degeneration.

Our study shows clear age-related structural and transcriptional differences in the murine knee joints after injury. One major limitation of this study is the use of mouse models instead of human subjects. The murine models may not fully recapitulate the changes seen in the human joints as a result of age or injury. Several studies have used human biopsy samples to investigate OA pathogenesis, but there are limitations in terms of the types of studies that can be conducted using human subjects as it is difficult to obtain biopsy samples from healthy and diseased human knee joints at multiple timepoints. However, murine models allow us to overcome some of the limitations of human data, by allowing us to conduct longitudinal studies and gain insights into PTOA development and progression. Another limitation of our study is that injury-induced transcriptional changes were identified relative to uninjured contralateral joint, which may have caused us to underestimate injury-induced systemic changes that may affect both joints. Our previous studies have shown that the expression of several inflammatory cytokines was up-regulated in both injured and uninjured contralateral joints in response to injury, although the level of activation in the contralateral was significantly lower than injured joints. Using contralateral joints as controls may not accurately capture such injury-induced systemic changes. Also, transcriptome data were obtained from whole joints, which makes it difficult to tease out the cell type-specific gene expressions changes. To overcome this challenge, we have examined tissue specific expression of selected proteins using other techniques such as immunohistochemistry and scRNA-seq. Nevertheless, this study provides novel insights into genes and molecular pathways involved in the PTOA development in young and old. Our data suggest that increased inflammation and reduced cartilage anabolism as a result of aging may contribute to a severe PTOA phenotype in old individuals. Keeping inflammation under control after joint injury may be beneficial in preventing or at least slowing down cartilage damage. This study also identified several potential therapeutic targets for PTOA including collagen metabolism enzymes such as lysyl oxidases and Plod2 and proteins such as Cytl1. In summary, this study highlights several new genes and molecular pathways that play a role in PTOA pathogenesis in young and old mice, and the data presented herein could help facilitate future research, which could aid the development of novel therapeutic approaches for PTOA.

4. Materials and Methods

4.1. Tibial Compression Overload Injury

Right knee joints of 10-week-old and 62-week-old C57BL/6J mice (Jackson Laboratory, Bar Harbor, ME, USA; Stock No: 000664) received a single non-invasive tibial compression overload at 1 mm/s displacement rate until ACL rupture using an electromagnetic material testing system (ElectroForce 3200, TA Instruments, New Castle, DE, USA), as previously described [8,10,19]. Buprenorphine was administered immediately post-injury (0.01 mg/kg) for pain relief. All animal experimental procedures were completed in accordance with the Institutional Animal Care and Use Committee (IACUC) guidance at Lawrence Livermore National Laboratory and the University of California, Davis in AAALAC-accredited facilities under protocol 168 approved in February 2019.

4.2. Histological Assessment of Disease Severity

Injured and uninjured (contralateral) joints were collected at six-week post-injury and processed as previously described for histology [10]. Briefly, dissected joints were fixed in 4% paraformaldehyde, decalcified using 0.5 M EDTA, processed, and embedded intact into paraffin. The joints were sectioned in the sagittal plane and serial medial sections that included the femoral condyles, menisci, and tibial plateaus were cut at 4 µm; stained on glass slides using 0.1% Safranin-O (0.1%, Sigma, St. Louis, MO, USA; S8884) and 0.05% Fast Green (0.05%, Sigma, St. Louis, MO, USA; F7252) using standard procedures (IHC World, Woodstock, MD, USA); and imaged using a Leica DM5000 microscope. Blinded slides were evaluated by seven scientists (six with and one without expertise in OA) utilizing modified (sagittal) Osteoarthritis Research Society International (OARSI) scoring parameters because of the severity of the phenotype six weeks following TC injury. Modified scoring scores (0) for intact cartilage staining with strong red staining on the femoral condyle and tibia, (1) for minor fibrillation without cartilage loss, (2) for clefts below the superficial zone, (3) for cartilage thinning on the femoral condyle and tibia, (4) for lack of staining on the femoral condyle and tibia, (5) for staining present on 90% of the entire femoral condyle with tibial resorption, (6) for staining present on over 80% of the femoral condyle with tibial resorption, (7) for staining present on 75% of the femoral condyle with tibial resorption, (8) for staining present on over 50% of the femora condyle with tibial resorption, (9), for staining present in 25% of the femoral condyle with tibial resorption, and (10) for staining present in less than 10% of the femoral condyle with tibial resorption.

4.3. Micro-Computed Tomography (µCT)

Whole knee joints from both young and old mice ($n \geq 5$ per group) were scanned using µCT (SCANCO µCT 35, Brüttisellen, Switzerland) at six-week post injury as previously described [10], according to the rodent bone structure analysis guidelines (X-ray tube potential = 55 kVp, intensity = 114 µA, 10 µm isotropic nominal voxel size, integration time = 900 ms). Trabecular bone in the distal femoral epiphysis was analyzed by manually drawing contours on 2D transverse slides. The distal femoral epiphysis was designated as the region of trabecular bone enclosed by the growth plate and subchondral cortical bone plate. Epiphyseal trabecular bone volume fraction was determined by quantifying trabecular bone volume per total volume (BV/TV). Mineralized osteophyte volume in injured and contralateral joints was quantified by drawing contours around all heterotropic mineralized tissue attached to the distal femur and proximal tibia as well as the whole fabellae, menisci, and patella. Total mineralized osteophyte volume was then determined as the volumetric difference in mineralized tissue between injured and uninjured joints. Statistical analysis was performed using a paired *t*-test to compare injured and contralateral knees.

4.4. Immunohistochemistry (IHC)

Sagittal six-micrometer sections from injured and uninjured samples from both age groups of C57Bl/6J mice were used for IHC. Unitrieve was used as an antigen retrieval method for 30 min at 65 °C. Primary antibodies: CYTL1 (Proteintech, Rosemont, IL, USA; 15856-1-AP(1:75)), PLOD2 (Invitrogen, Carlsbad, CA, USA; PA5-69194(1:100)), and CHAD (Invitrogen, Carlsbad, CA, USA; PA5-53761(1:300)) were used and incubated overnight at room temperature in a dark, humid chamber. Negative control slides were incubated with secondary antibody-only. Stained slides were mounted with Prolong Gold with DAPI (Molecular Probes, Eugene, OR, USA). Slides were imaged using a Leica DM5000 microscope. ImagePro Plus V7.0 Software and a QIClick CCD camera (QImaging, Surrey, BC, Canada) were used for imaging and photo editing.

4.5. Bulk RNA Sequencing and Data Analysis

The knee joint RNA from 10-week-old, 62-week-old, and 95-week-old mice was isolated as described before [10]. Briefly, injured and contralateral joints (n = 3–6 per group) were dissected, chopped, and homogenized in Qiazol (79306, Qiagen, Valencia, CA, USA). Total RNA was purified using RNeasy Mini Kit (QIAGEN Inc., Germantown, MD, USA) according to the manufacturer's protocol and the RNA integrity was assessed using a bioanalyzer (Agilent Technologies, Santa Clara, CA, USA). Poly(A)+-enriched cDNA libraries were generated using the Illumina TruSeq RNA Library Prep kit v2 (Illumina Inc., Hayward, CA, USA). The sequencing was performed using an Illumina (Illumina Inc., Hayward, CA, USA) NextSeq 500 instrument to generate 75 bp single-end reads. The quality of sequencing data was checked using FastQC (version 0.11.5) software [http://www.bioinformatics.bbsrc.ac.uk/projects/fastqc]. Sequence reads were mapped to the mouse reference genome (mm10) using STAR (version 2.6) [39]. A matrix of raw counts per gene was generated using "featureCounts" from Rsubread package (version 1.30.5) [40]. RUVseq was used to determine factors of unwanted variation [41]. Differentially expressed genes were identified using edgeR, adjusting for factors of unwanted variation [42]. Genes with fold changes >1.5 and false discovery rate (FDR) adjusted p-value less than 0.05 were considered as significantly differentially expressed. Heatmaps were generated using heatmap.2 function in R package 'gplots'.

4.6. Single Cell RNA-Seq (scRN-Aseq) and Data Analysis

Ten-week-old C57Bl/6J mice were euthanized, and right and left hindlimbs were collected by removing the leg at the hip joint and storing on ice in Dulbecco's Modified Eagle Medium Nutrient Mixture F-12 (DMEM/F-12) (Thermo Fisher Scientific, Waltham, MA, USA). The articular cartilage of the knee joint was isolated from the femur and tibia by cutting 0.5–1 mm of tissue from the end of both long bones. Cartilage tissue was digested to a single cell suspension in 1 mL of 0.2% Collagenase 2 solution (Thermo Fisher Scientific, Waltham, MA, USA) while shaking at 37 °C for 2 h. Fractions were collected at 30 min intervals, filtered through a 70 μm Nylon cell strainer, and then resuspended in DMEM/F12 with 10% fetal bovine serum (FBS). Remaining undigested cartilage tissue was further incubated in 1 mL of fresh Collagenase 2 digestion media.

Following digestion, cell suspensions were pelleted via centrifugation for 10 min at 500 G, then resuspended in ACK lysis buffer (Thermo Fisher Scientific, Waltham, MA, USA), and incubated for 10 min on ice in order to remove red blood cells. Cell suspensions were next resuspended in 100 uL of PBS + 10% FBS. CD45+ and Ter119+ cell depletion was accomplished using CD45 and Ter119 MACSmicrobeads (Miltenti Biotec, Sunnyvale, CA, USA) and running cell samples on an LS MACScolumns (Miltenti Biotec, Sunnyvale, CA, USA) following the manufacturer's instructions. Final cell counts were performed using a hemocytometer and cells were resuspended in PBS + 0.04% nonacetylated BSA before introduction into a Chromium Controller (10x Genomics, Pleasanton, CA,

USA). Library preparation was performed using Chromium Single Cell 3′ GEM, Library & Gel Bead Kit v3 (10x Genomics, Pleasanton, CA, USA; Catalog no. 1000075) following the manufacturer's protocol and sequenced using Illumina NextSeq 500. Sequencing data were demultiplexed, quality controlled, and aligned to the mouse genome (mm10) using Cell Ranger (10x Genomics, Pleasanton, CA, USA). Data analysis was performed using Seurat (version 3.1.1) [43].

4.7. Functional Annotation

Gene ontology analysis was performed using ToppGene and ToppCluster [44] and enriched gene ontology terms and pathways (p-value < 0.01) were identified. Cytoscape (version 3.6.1) was used for ontology and pathway visualization [45].

Supplementary Materials: Supplementary materials can be found at http://www.mdpi.com/1422-0067/21/1/364/s1.

Author Contributions: Study design: A.S. and G.G.L.; Data acquisition: A.S., D.K.M., M.E.M., N.D.R.-A., N.R.H., J.L.M., and B.A.C. Data analysis and interpretation: A.S., B A.C., and G.G.L. A.S. and G.G.L wrote the manuscript. All authors have read and agreed to the published version of the manuscript.

Funding: A.S., D.K.M., N.R.H., and G.G.L. were supported by Lawrence Livermore National Laboratory LDRD grants 20-LW-002 and 16-ERD-007. G.G.L. and B.A.C. were supported by DOD PR180268/P1 and NIH R01 AR075013.

Acknowledgments: This work was performed under the auspices of the U.S. Department of Energy by Lawrence Livermore National Laboratory under Contract DE-AC52-07NA27344.

Conflicts of Interest: The authors declare no conflict of interest. The funders had no role in the design of the study; in the collection, analyses, or interpretation of data; in the writing of the manuscript, or in the decision to publish the results.

Abbreviations

ACL	Anterior cruciate ligament
OA	Osteoarthritis
PTOA	Post-traumatic osteoarthritis
scRNA-seq	Single-cell RNA sequencing
TC	Tibial compression
μCT	Microcomputed tomography

References

1. Matthews, G.L.; Hunter, D.J. Emerging drugs for osteoarthritis. *Expert Opin. Emerg. Drugs* **2011**, *16*, 479–491. [CrossRef]
2. Lohmander, L.S.; Englund, P.M.; Dahl, L.L.; Roos, E.M. The long-term consequence of anterior cruciate ligament and meniscus injuries: Osteoarthritis. *Am. J. Sports Med.* **2007**, *35*, 1756–1769. [CrossRef]
3. Roos, H.; Adalberth, T.; Dahlberg, L.; Lohmander, L.S. Osteoarthritis of the knee after injury to the anterior cruciate ligament or meniscus: The influence of time and age. *Osteoarthr. Cartil.* **1995**, *3*, 261–267. [CrossRef]
4. Loeser, R.F.; Olex, A.L.; McNulty, M.A.; Carlson, C.S.; Callahan, M.F.; Ferguson, C.M.; Chou, J.; Leng, X.; Fetrow, J.S. Microarray analysis reveals age-related differences in gene expression during the development of osteoarthritis in mice. *Arthritis Rheum.* **2012**, *64*, 705–717. [CrossRef]
5. Ramos, Y.F.; den Hollander, W.; Bovee, J.V.; Bomer, N.; van der Breggen, R.; Lakenberg, N.; Keurentjes, J.C.; Goeman, J.J.; Slagboom, P.E.; Nelissen, R.G.; et al. Genes involved in the osteoarthritis process identified through genome wide expression analysis in articular cartilage; the RAAK study. *PLoS ONE* **2014**, *9*, e103056. [CrossRef]
6. Gardiner, M.D.; Vincent, T.L.; Driscoll, C.; Burleigh, A.; Bou-Gharios, G.; Saklatvala, J.; Nagase, H.; Chanalaris, A. Transcriptional analysis of micro-dissected articular cartilage in post-traumatic murine osteoarthritis. *Osteoarthr. Cartil.* **2015**, *23*, 616–628. [CrossRef]
7. Blaker, C.L.; Clarke, E.C.; Little, C.B. Using mouse models to investigate the pathophysiology, treatment, and prevention of post-traumatic osteoarthritis. *J. Orthop Res.* **2017**, *35*, 424–439. [CrossRef]

8. Chang, J.C.; Sebastian, A.; Murugesh, D.K.; Hatsell, S.; Economides, A.N.; Christiansen, B.A.; Loots, G.G. Global molecular changes in a tibial compression induced ACL rupture model of post-traumatic osteoarthritis. *J. Orthop Res.* **2017**, *35*, 474–485. [CrossRef]
9. Chang, J.C.; Christiansen, B.A.; Murugesh, D.K.; Sebastian, A.; Hum, N.R.; Collette, N.M.; Hatsell, S.; Economides, A.N.; Blanchette, C.D.; Loots, G.G. SOST/Sclerostin Improves Posttraumatic Osteoarthritis and Inhibits MMP2/3 Expression After Injury. *J. Bone Min. Res.* **2018**, *33*, 1105–1113. [CrossRef]
10. Sebastian, A.; Chang, J.C.; Mendez, M.E.; Murugesh, D.K.; Hatsell, S.; Economides, A.N.; Christiansen, B.A.; Loots, G.G. Comparative Transcriptomics Identifies Novel Genes and Pathways Involved in Post-Traumatic Osteoarthritis Development and Progression. *Int. J. Mol. Sci.* **2018**, *19*, 2657. [CrossRef]
11. Christiansen, B.A.; Guilak, F.; Lockwood, K.A.; Olson, S.A.; Pitsillides, A.A.; Sandell, L.J.; Silva, M.J.; van der Meulen, M.C.; Haudenschild, D.R. Non-invasive mouse models of post-traumatic osteoarthritis. *Osteoarthr. Cartil.* **2015**, *23*, 1627–1638. [CrossRef] [PubMed]
12. Hessle, L.; Stordalen, G.A.; Wenglen, C.; Petzold, C.; Tanner, E.; Brorson, S.H.; Baekkevold, E.S.; Onnerfjord, P.; Reinholt, F.P.; Heinegard, D. The skeletal phenotype of chondroadherin deficient mice. *PLoS ONE* **2014**, *8*, e63080. [CrossRef] [PubMed]
13. Qi, Y.; Xu, R. Roles of PLODs in Collagen Synthesis and Cancer Progression. *Front. Cell Dev. Biol.* **2018**, *6*, 66. [CrossRef] [PubMed]
14. Kim, J.S.; Ryoo, Z.Y.; Chun, J.S. Cytokine-like 1 (Cytl1) regulates the chondrogenesis of mesenchymal cells. *J. Biol. Chem.* **2007**, *282*, 29359–29367. [CrossRef] [PubMed]
15. Jeon, J.; Oh, H.; Lee, G.; Ryu, J.H.; Rhee, J.; Kim, J.H.; Chung, K.H.; Song, W.K.; Chun, C.H.; Chun, J.S. Cytokine-like 1 knock-out mice (Cytl1-/-) show normal cartilage and bone development but exhibit augmented osteoarthritic cartilage destruction. *J. Biol. Chem.* **2011**, *286*, 27206–27213. [CrossRef] [PubMed]
16. Zhou, N.; Li, Q.; Lin, X.; Hu, N.; Liao, J.Y.; Lin, L.B.; Zhao, C.; Hu, Z.M.; Liang, X.; Xu, W.; et al. BMP2 induces chondrogenic differentiation, osteogenic differentiation and endochondral ossification in stem cells. *Cell Tissue Res.* **2016**, *366*, 101–111. [CrossRef] [PubMed]
17. Surmann-Schmitt, C.; Widmann, N.; Dietz, U.; Saeger, B.; Eitzinger, N.; Nakamura, Y.; Rattel, M.; Latham, R.; Hartmann, C.; von der Mark, H.; et al. Wif-1 is expressed at cartilage-mesenchyme interfaces and impedes Wnt3a-mediated inhibition of chondrogenesis. *J. Cell Sci.* **2009**, *122*, 3627–3637. [CrossRef]
18. Alquraini, A.; Jamal, M.; Zhang, L.; Schmidt, T.; Jay, G.D.; Elsaid, K.A. The autocrine role of proteoglycan-4 (PRG4) in modulating osteoarthritic synoviocyte proliferation and expression of matrix degrading enzymes. *Arthritis Res. Ther.* **2017**, *19*, 89. [CrossRef]
19. Christiansen, B.A.; Anderson, M.J.; Lee, C.A.; Williams, J.C.; Yik, J.H.; Haudenschild, D.R. Musculoskeletal changes following non-invasive knee injury using a novel mouse model of post-traumatic osteoarthritis. *Osteoarthr. Cartil.* **2012**, *20*, 773–782. [CrossRef]
20. Sokolove, J.; Lepus, C.M. Role of inflammation in the pathogenesis of osteoarthritis: Latest findings and interpretations. *Ther. Adv. Musculoskelet. Dis.* **2013**, *5*, 77–94. [CrossRef]
21. Greene, M.A.; Loeser, R.F. Aging-related inflammation in osteoarthritis. *Osteoarthr. Cartil.* **2015**, *23*, 1966–1971. [CrossRef]
22. Goekoop, R.J.; Kloppenburg, M.; Kroon, H.M.; Frolich, M.; Huizinga, T.W.; Westendorp, R.G.; Gussekloo, J. Low innate production of interleukin-1beta and interleukin-6 is associated with the absence of osteoarthritis in old age. *Osteoarthr. Cartil.* **2010**, *18*, 942–947. [CrossRef]
23. Kyostio-Moore, S.; Nambiar, B.; Hutto, E.; Ewing, P.J.; Piraino, S.; Berthelette, P.; Sookdeo, C.; Matthews, G.; Armentano, D. STR/ort mice, a model for spontaneous osteoarthritis, exhibit elevated levels of both local and systemic inflammatory markers. *Comp. Med.* **2011**, *61*, 346–355.
24. Lewis, J.S., Jr.; Furman, B.D.; Zeitler, E.; Huebner, J.L.; Kraus, V.B.; Guilak, F.; Olson, S.A. Genetic and cellular evidence of decreased inflammation associated with reduced incidence of posttraumatic arthritis in MRL/MpJ mice. *Arthritis Rheum.* **2013**, *65*, 660–670. [CrossRef]
25. Loeser, R.F. Aging and osteoarthritis: The role of chondrocyte senescence and aging changes in the cartilage matrix. *Osteoarthr. Cartil.* **2009**, *17*, 971–979. [CrossRef]
26. Bi, W.; Deng, J.M.; Zhang, Z.; Behringer, R.R.; de Crombrugghe, B. Sox9 is required for cartilage formation. *Nat. Genet.* **1999**, *22*, 85–89. [CrossRef]

27. Fassler, R.; Schnegelsberg, P.N.; Dausman, J.; Shinya, T.; Muragaki, Y.; McCarthy, M.T.; Olsen, B.R.; Jaenisch, R. Mice lacking alpha 1 (IX) collagen develop noninflammatory degenerative joint disease. *Proc. Natl. Acad. Sci. USA* **1994**, *91*, 5070–5074. [CrossRef]
28. Arikawa-Hirasawa, E.; Watanabe, H.; Takami, H.; Hassell, J.R.; Yamada, Y. Perlecan is essential for cartilage and cephalic development. *Nat. Genet.* **1999**, *23*, 354–358. [CrossRef]
29. Watanabe, H.; Yamada, Y. Mice lacking link protein develop dwarfism and craniofacial abnormalities. *Nat. Genet.* **1999**, *21*, 225–229. [CrossRef]
30. Chubinskaya, S.; Hurtig, M.; Rueger, D.C. OP-1/BMP-7 in cartilage repair. *Int. Orthop.* **2007**, *31*, 773–781. [CrossRef]
31. Aigner, T.; Fundel, K.; Saas, J.; Gebhard, P.M.; Haag, J.; Weiss, T.; Zien, A.; Obermayr, F.; Zimmer, R.; Bartnik, E. Large-scale gene expression profiling reveals major pathogenetic pathways of cartilage degeneration in osteoarthritis. *Arthritis Rheum.* **2006**, *54*, 3533–3544. [CrossRef]
32. Bernardo, B.C.; Belluoccio, D.; Rowley, L.; Little, C.B.; Hansen, U.; Bateman, J.F. Cartilage intermediate layer protein 2 (CILP-2) is expressed in articular and meniscal cartilage and down-regulated in experimental osteoarthritis. *J. Biol. Chem.* **2011**, *286*, 37758–37767. [CrossRef]
33. Boeth, H.; Raffalt, P.C.; MacMahon, A.; Poole, A.R.; Eckstein, F.; Wirth, W.; Buttgereit, F.; Onnerfjord, P.; Lorenzo, P.; Klint, C.; et al. Association between changes in molecular biomarkers of cartilage matrix turnover and changes in knee articular cartilage: A longitudinal pilot study. *J. Exp. Orthop.* **2019**, *6*, 19. [CrossRef]
34. Tashkandi, M.; Ali, F.; Alsaqer, S.; Alhousami, T.; Cano, A.; Martin, A.; Salvador, F.; Portillo, F.; Gerstenfeld, L.C.; Goldring, M.B.; et al. Lysyl Oxidase-Like 2 Protects against Progressive and Aging Related Knee Joint Osteoarthritis in Mice. *Int. J. Mol. Sci.* **2019**, *20*, 4798. [CrossRef]
35. Gistelinck, C.; Witten, P.E.; Huysseune, A.; Symoens, S.; Malfait, F.; Larionova, D.; Simoens, P.; Dierick, M.; Van Hoorebeke, L.; De Paepe, A.; et al. Loss of Type I Collagen Telopeptide Lysyl Hydroxylation Causes Musculoskeletal Abnormalities in a Zebrafish Model of Bruck Syndrome. *J. Bone Min. Res.* **2016**, *31*, 1930–1942. [CrossRef]
36. Remst, D.F.; Blom, A.B.; Vitters, E.L.; Bank, R.A.; van den Berg, W.B.; Blaney Davidson, E.N.; van der Kraan, P.M. Gene expression analysis of murine and human osteoarthritis synovium reveals elevation of transforming growth factor beta-responsive genes in osteoarthritis-related fibrosis. *Arthritis Rheum.* **2014**, *66*, 647–656. [CrossRef]
37. Coles, J.M.; Zhang, L.; Blum, J.J.; Warman, M.L.; Jay, G.D.; Guilak, F.; Zauscher, S. Loss of cartilage structure, stiffness, and frictional properties in mice lacking PRG4. *Arthritis Rheum.* **2010**, *62*, 1666–1674. [CrossRef]
38. Kozhemyakina, E.; Zhang, M.; Ionescu, A.; Ayturk, U.M.; Ono, N.; Kobayashi, A.; Kronenberg, H.; Warman, M.L.; Lassar, A.B. Identification of a Prg4-expressing articular cartilage progenitor cell population in mice. *Arthritis Rheum.* **2015**, *67*, 1261–1273. [CrossRef]
39. Dobin, A.; Davis, C.A.; Schlesinger, F.; Drenkow, J.; Zaleski, C.; Jha, S.; Batut, P.; Chaisson, M.; Gingeras, T.R. STAR: Ultrafast universal RNA-seq aligner. *Bioinformatics* **2013**, *29*, 15–21. [CrossRef]
40. Liao, Y.; Smyth, G.K.; Shi, W. featureCounts: An efficient general purpose program for assigning sequence reads to genomic features. *Bioinformatics* **2014**, *30*, 923–930. [CrossRef]
41. Risso, D.; Ngai, J.; Speed, T.P.; Dudoit, S. Normalization of RNA-seq data using factor analysis of control genes or samples. *Nat. Biotechnol.* **2014**, *32*, 896–902 [CrossRef] [PubMed]
42. Robinson, M.D.; McCarthy, D.J.; Smyth, G.K. edgeR: A Bioconductor package for differential expression analysis of digital gene expression data. *Bioinformatics* **2010**, *26*, 139–140. [CrossRef] [PubMed]
43. Butler, A.; Hoffman, P.; Smibert, P.; Papalexi, E.; Satija, R. Integrating single-cell transcriptomic data across different conditions, technologies, and species. *Nat. Biotechnol.* **2018**, *36*, 411–420. [CrossRef]
44. Chen, J.; Bardes, E.E.; Aronow, B.J.; Jegga, A.G. ToppGene Suite for gene list enrichment analysis and candidate gene prioritization. *Nucleic Acids Res.* **2009**, *37*, W305–W311. [CrossRef]
45. Shannon, P.; Markiel, A.; Ozier, O.; Baliga, N.S.; Wang, J.T.; Ramage, D.; Amin, N.; Schwikowski, B.; Ideker, T. Cytoscape: A software environment for integrated models of biomolecular interaction networks. *Genome Res.* **2003**, *13*, 2498–2504. [CrossRef]

International Journal of
Molecular Sciences

MDPI

Article

The Systemic Immune Response to Collagen-Induced Arthritis and the Impact of Bone Injury in Inflammatory Conditions

José H. Teixeira [1,2], Andreia M. Silva [1,2], Maria Inês Almeida [1], Mafalda Bessa-Gonçalves [1,2], Carla Cunha [1], Mário A. Barbosa [1,2] and Susana G. Santos [1,2,*]

1 i3S—Instituto de Investigação e Inovação em Saúde and INEB—Instituto Nacional de Engenharia Biomédica, University of Porto, 4200-135 Porto, Portugal; jhteixeira@ineb.up.pt (J.H.T.); andreiamacsilva@gmail.com (A.M.S.); ines.Almeida@ineb.up.pt (M.I.A.); mafalda.goncalves@i3s.up.pt (M.B.-G.); carla.cunha@ineb.up.pt (C.C.); mbarbosa@i3s.up.pt (M.A.B.)

2 Department of Molecular Biology, ICBAS—Instituto de Ciências Biomédicas Abel Salazar, University of Porto, 4050-313 Porto, Portugal

* Correspondence: susana.santos@ineb.up.pt; Tel.: +351-220-408-800

Received: 20 September 2019; Accepted: 29 October 2019; Published: 31 October 2019

Abstract: Rheumatoid arthritis (RA) is a systemic disease that affects the osteoarticular system, associated with bone fragility and increased risk of fractures. Herein, we aimed to characterize the systemic impact of the rat collagen-induced arthritis (CIA) model and explore its combination with femoral bone defect (FD). The impact of CIA on endogenous mesenchymal stem/stromal cells (MSC) was also investigated. CIA induction led to enlarged, more proliferative, spleen and draining lymph nodes, with altered proportion of lymphoid populations. Upon FD, CIA animals increased the systemic myeloid cell proportions, and their expression of co-stimulatory molecules CD40 and CD86. Screening plasma cytokine/chemokine levels showed increased tumor necrosis factor-α (TNF-α), Interleukin (IL)-17, IL-4, IL-5, and IL-12 in CIA, and IL-2 and IL-6 increased in CIA and CIA+FD, while Fractalkine and Leptin were decreased in both groups. CIA-derived MSC showed lower metabolic activity and proliferation, and significantly increased osteogenic and chondrogenic differentiation markers. Exposure of control-MSC to TNF-α partially mimicked the CIA-MSC phenotype in vitro. In conclusion, inflammatory conditions of CIA led to alterations in systemic immune cell proportions, circulating mediators, and in endogenous MSC. CIA animals respond to FD, and the combined model can be used to study the mechanisms of bone repair in inflammatory conditions.

Keywords: rheumatoid arthritis; collagen-induced arthritis; microenvironment; inflammation; mesenchymal stem/stromal cells; bone injury; repair/regeneration

1. Introduction

Rheumatoid arthritis (RA) is an autoimmune condition, characterized by symmetrical joint inflammation, that affects approximately 1% of the world's population [1]. RA is characterized mainly by synovium hyperplasia and a joint destruction process. In this scenario, immune cells and the inflammatory microenvironment that they create in affected joints are key components in the pathophysiology of RA. Moreover, it is well-described that during the inflammatory stages of the disease, extra-articular manifestations are common, which involve other tissues or organs [2].

RA patients are at risk of systemic complications and several co-morbidities, including osteoporosis and frequent vertebral and hip fragility fractures [3,4]. The incidence rate of overall fractures in RA patients is 33 per 1000 person-years [5], and the risk is increased with disease activity and associated with overexpression of pro-inflammatory cytokines that can disturb the bone remodeling process [4,6,7].

Over the last decades, animal models—especially the rodent models—have been crucial tools for understanding the biologic process of RA [8], and their use can aid in developing new therapeutic strategies for fracture healing in RA inflammatory conditions. Collagen induced-arthritis (CIA) animal models have been one of the most widely used models in RA research. Originally described by Trentham [9], CIA is a reproducible animal experimental model of RA [10,11]. In fact, the similarity to human RA regarding the disease clinical, histological, and immunological signals—including high articular levels of inflammatory cytokines—like tumor necrosis factor-α (TNF-α) [12,13], make it an invaluable model to study the pathologic process and to search new therapeutic strategies [14–16]. The response to rat CIA has been reported to involve macrophages, T and B lymphocytes, and mediators such as TNF-α, Interleukin (IL)-1β, IL-6, and IL-17 [17]. Nonetheless, the systemic response in this model has not been well characterized so far.

Importantly, current RA treatments do not promote joint repair, and several efforts are being made to develop new therapies, especially based in cell approaches using mesenchymal stem/stromal cells (MSC) [18,19]. MSC are multipotent progenitor cells with the potential to differentiate into mesenchymal lineage tissues (e.g., bone, cartilage, and adipose tissue), described to have immunomodulatory roles [20], being capable of recruiting different cell types and promoting tissue repair [21]. The transplantation of MSC has been reported to ameliorate or delay RA onset in CIA animals, partially mediated by inflammatory signaling suppression [22,23], and thereby reducing joint swelling and destruction [24,25]. Although the available evidence supports the use of MSC transplantation as a cell-based strategy in CIA animals, data on the biology of endogenous CIA animals-derived MSC in basal conditions is scarce. Moreover, the impact of the systemic inflammatory condition on biological properties of endogenous MSC has not been explored yet.

Herein, we propose CIA as a reliable model to study bone regeneration in inflammatory conditions, and additionally we investigate the effect of RA induction on the biological behavior of endogenous MSC as crucial cells involved in repair/regeneration.

Our results have shown that the combination of the two models is feasible and that CIA animals respond to the bone injury with a significant increase of systemic myeloid cells number and their co-stimulatory molecules (CD40 and CD86) expression, accompanied by increased levels of IL-13, IL-2, and IL-6 in plasma. The systemic inflammatory environment created by the arthritis induction leads to decreased metabolic activity and proliferation of CIA-derived MSC, and increased differentiation capacity determined by the expression of osteogenic (runt-related transcription factor 2 (RUNX2) and alkaline phosphatase (ALP)), and chondrogenic (aggrecan (ACAN)) markers in basal conditions.

2. Results

2.1. Collagen-induced arthritis (CIA) as a Model to Study Bone Injury in Inflammatory Conditions

First, we established if the CIA model in the rat would be suitable to study the response to bone injury under inflammatory conditions by inducing it in otherwise healthy female Wistar rats and performing a critical size bone defect at day 21 after CIA induction (Figure 1).

Arthritis induction was effective in all animals, with macroscopic evidences of erythema and swelling in hind paws, and significant increases in swelling after day 14 when compared to the non-immunized/control animals (Figure S1A,B). The arthritis index score increased along the monitoring time until hitting a plateau between day 17 and 21 (Figure S1C).

At day 21 after immunization, a group of CIA animals with evident signals of arthritis were subjected to a cylindrical femoral bone defect (FD), as illustrated in the x-ray of Figure 1A, and followed up to three days post-injury. The combination of CIA with FD (CIA+FD) did not compromise animal welfare beyond the impact of CIA itself, with CIA+FD animals recovering well from surgery and keeping to a similar body weight as the control and CIA groups (Figure 1B). Hind paw swelling of CIA+FD animals showed a slight decrease at day 3 post-injury, albeit not significant (Figure 1C).

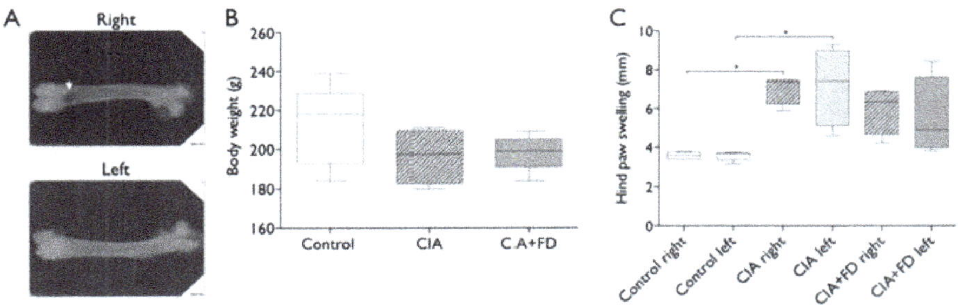

Figure 1. Combination of collagen-induced arthritis (CIA) model with femoral defect (FD). CIA was induced and allowed to develop for 21 days, before a cylindrical defect was performed in the femur of a half of the CIA animals to combine both animal models (CIA+FD) (**A**) X-ray of cylindrical defect performed on the right femur (white arrow indicates the defect site) of CIA animals at day 3 after surgery. (**B**) Body weight evaluation 3 days after bone defect. (**C**) Measurements of paw swelling in both paws (right and left) of control, CIA and CIA+FD, 3 days after bone injury. Box plots represent min-to-max distribution of $n = 4$ to 5 animals per group. * $p < 0.05$, determined by Kruskal–Wallis test and Dunn's multiple comparisons test.

2.2. The Impact of CIA and Bone Injury in Secondary Lymphoid Organs

Next, we wanted to ascertain if CIA and its combination with a bone defect correlated with acute systemic changes in secondary lymphoid organs. Spleen from CIA and CIA+FD groups were collected three days after bone injury and found to be enlarged when compared to control, with a significant increase in weight for CIA+FD animals (Figure 2A). Cell proliferation was assessed by Ki-67 staining, and was also increased in both CIA and CIA+FD groups, but a statistically significant increase was only observed for the CIA group (Figure 2B). Lymph nodes draining the hind paws were also collected and found to be enlarged in CIA and CIA+FD groups (Figure 2C). Cell proliferation in lymph nodes was quantified across the different animals and found significantly increased in CIA animals when compared to controls (Figure 2D). Overall, these results support that spleen and lymph nodes are responding to CIA induction with increased cell proliferation.

To further determine the impact of CIA and CIA+FD in systemic immune cell populations, we performed multicolor flow cytometry analysis of cells from blood, draining lymph nodes and spleen. The gating strategy is illustrated in Supplementary Figure S2. Results obtained are summarized in Figure 3 and show significant changes in the proportion of lymphoid and myeloid cells in blood, draining lymph nodes and spleen. Concerning the lymphoid lineage populations (Figure 3A), we observed a significant increase in the percentage of B lymphocytes in blood and lymph nodes from CIA animals relative to control animals, but no differences were observed in spleen. T cell percentage was significantly decreased in lymph nodes of CIA animals, while Natural Killer (NK) cells were increased ($p = 0.0571$) in the spleen of those animals. The proportions of $CD8^+$ and $CD4^+$ T cells were similar between all groups in blood and spleen, but significant differences were observed in CIA lymph nodes. Results showed an increased percentage of $CD8^+$ and decreased $CD4^+$ T cells in CIA animals when compared to control animals. Bone injury (CIA+FD) did not induce further significant changes in lymphoid cell proportion in CIA animals at three days post-injury, except for a significant increase in NK cells in blood at day 3 after bone defect.

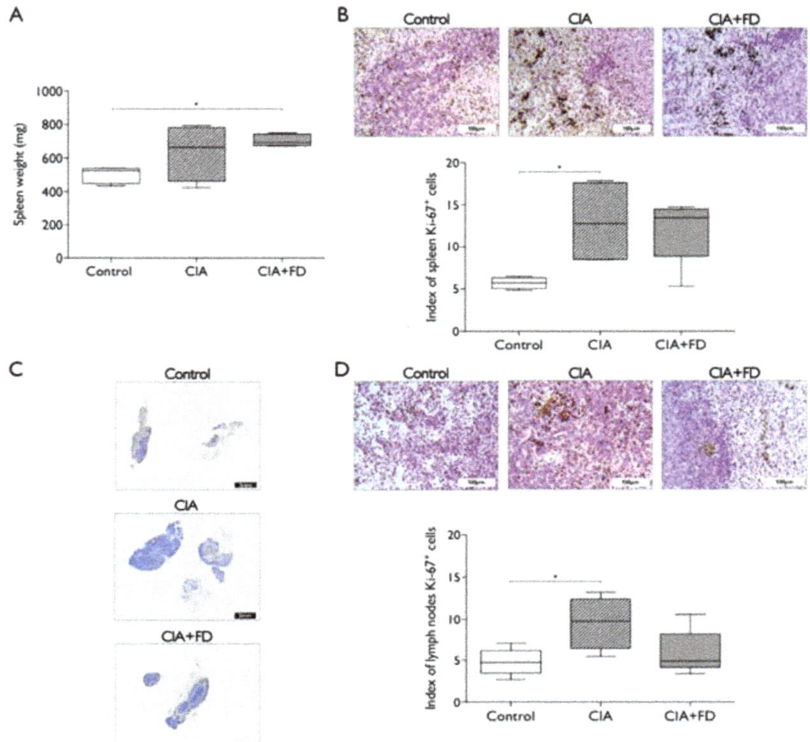

Figure 2. Arthritis induction and the combination with femoral defect promotes alterations in rat secondary lymphoid organs. (**A**) Spleen weight from control, CIA, and CIA+FD animals. (**B**) Representative spleen paraffin-section showing immunohistochemistry (IHQ) staining for the proliferation marker Ki-67, and quantitative staining evaluation across different sections of all animals. (**C**) Draining lymph nodes general view of histological analysis. (**D**) Higher magnification showing Ki-67 IHQ staining, and quantitative staining evaluation across different sections of all animals. Box plots represent min-to-max distribution of n = 4 to 5 animals per group. * $p < 0.05$ determined by Mann–Whitney test. Scale bar: 3 mm (black), 100 µm (white).

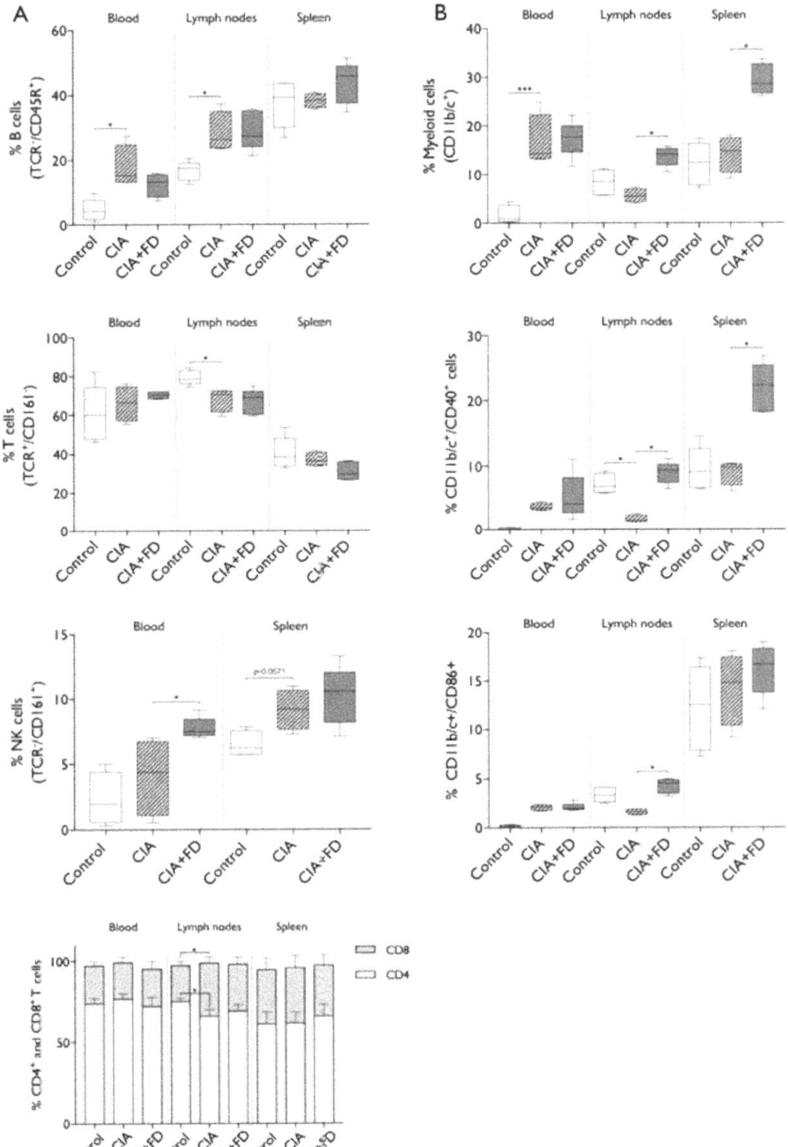

Figure 3. CIA and CIA+FD lead to alterations in systemic immune cell proportions. The percentages of lymphoid and myeloid populations at systemic level were analyzed in blood, draining lymph nodes and spleen of control, CIA, and CIA+FD animals, by multicolor flow cytometry. (**A**) Percentage of main lymphoid populations: B cells (TCR$^-$/CD45$^+$), T cells (TCR$^+$/CD161$^-$), NK cells (TCR$^-$/CD161$^+$), and CD4 (TCR$^+$/CD4$^+$) and CD8 (TCR$^+$/CD8$^+$) T cells. (**B**) Myeloid cells (CD11b/c$^+$), and their activation status as determined by co-expression of the co-stimulatory markers CD40 and CD86. Box plots represent min-to-max distribution of n = 4 to 5 animals per group. * $p < 0.05$, *** $p < 0.001$ determined by Kruskal–Wallis test and Dunn's multiple comparisons test.

Analyzing the myeloid cells (Figure 3B) revealed a significantly higher percentage of myeloid cells in blood of the CIA group, which did not change with bone injury. Conversely, in draining the lymph nodes and spleen, no increases were observed in the CIA group, but there were significant increases in percentages of myeloid cells 3 days after bone injury. To further explore these results, expression of co-stimulatory molecules CD40 and CD86 was analyzed to investigate myeloid cell activation. Cells in circulation from CIA animals present increased the percentage of cells expressing each molecule, albeit not significant, while lymph node cells showed a significant decrease of the percentage of myeloid cells expressing CD40, with CD86 following the same tendency. Importantly, 3 days after bone injury, myeloid cells showed increased expression of both co-stimulatory molecules CD40 and CD86, in lymph nodes, and for CD40 also in spleen, when compared to the CIA group. Overall, these evidences suggest a persistent systemic immune response in CIA animals that are nonetheless still able to respond to an acute injury, particularly increasing their myeloid cells proportion and activation.

2.3. *The Impact of CIA and Bone Defect in Circulating Inflammatory Mediators*

To further investigate the systemic inflammatory impact of CIA and the combination with bone injury, 27 chemokines and cytokines were quantified in plasma. From these, epidermal growth factor (EGF), growth-regulated oncogenes/keratinocyte chemoattractant (GRO/KC), Macrophage inflammatory protein-2 (MIP-2, CXCL2), and Granulocyte-macrophage colony-stimulating factor (GM-CSF) were out of the detection range for this assay. From the remaining 23 cytokines/chemokines detected, IL-13 was not detected in the control group, but was detected in the other two animal groups and thus was considered in the analysis. Results obtained are illustrated in Figure 4 and show that, relative to the control group, CIA animals had a significant upregulation of 8 molecules and a downregulation of 5. Among the significantly up-regulated mediators IL-13, IL-2, and IL-6 were also significantly up-regulated in the CIA+FD group, while TNF-α, IL-17 A, IL-4, IL-5, and IL-12 (p70) lost significance in the CIA+FD group. Nonetheless, the tendency for increase was maintained, and in the case of IL-5 it was close to statistical significance ($p = 0.0534$). Also, Monocyte chemoattractant protein-1/C-C motif chemokine ligand 2 (MCP-1/CCL2) and Eotaxin were close to statistical significance in CIA ($p = 0.0552$ and $p = 0.0620$, respectively), and MCP-1 was significantly up-regulated for the CIA+FD group. Regarding the downregulated mediators identified in CIA plasma, Vascular endothelial growth factor (VEGF), Fractalkine, IL-18, C-X-C motif chemokine 5 (CXCL5, LIX), and Leptin, only Fractalkine and Leptin levels were statistically significantly lower in the CIA+FD group, relative to control. The only molecule that showed a significant difference between the CIA and CIA+FD groups was the regulated on activation, normal T cell expressed and secreted (RANTES) chemokine, which was significantly downregulated in CIA when compared to CIA+FD, but neither group had a significant difference to the control group.

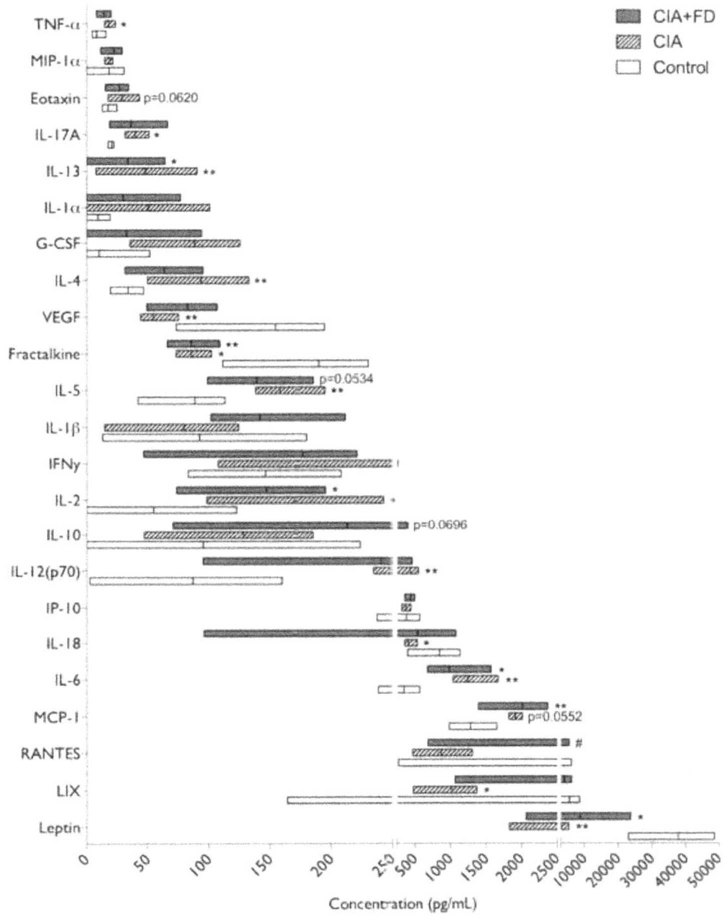

Figure 4. Changes in plasma cytokine and chemokine profile in CIA and CIA+FD. Quantitative results of the multiplex cytokine/chemokine array performed for all animals in each group. Box plots represent min-to-max distribution of $n = 4$ to 5 animals per group. * $p < 0.05$, ** $p < 0.01$ in relation to control group, and # $p < 0.05$ relatively to CIA group, determined by Kruskal–Wallis test and Dunn's multiple comparisons test.

2.4. CIA Induction Impacts Endogenous MSC Biologic Behavior

To evaluate the impact of chronic inflammation on endogenous MSC we next isolated and culture bone marrow-derived MSC (BM-MSC) from CIA and control animals. The number of bone marrow cells recovered was similar between the CIA and control animal groups, and after selective culture and expansion, cells obtained were highly positive for the classical stromal markers CD29 and CD90, and did not express the haematopoietic marker CD45 (Supplementary Figure S3). The bone marrow isolated cells showed the ability to differentiate into the chondrogenic, osteogenic, and adipogenic lineages (Supplementary Figure S4). All together, these data confirmed the successful isolation of MSC from bone marrow of both CIA and control animals.

BM-MSC were then used to evaluate the impact of the cells source microenvironment on their biological properties and behavior. CIA and control BM-MSC were metabolic active along 1, 3, and 7 days of culture, but CIA-MSC showed lower metabolic activity that did not increase along time, when compared to control cells (Figure 5A). In line with these results, the Ki-67 fluorescent immuno-staining analysis also showed a tendency for reduced proliferation of CIA-MSC (Figure 5B,C). To access if exposure to the inflammatory microenvironment could be conditioning, MSC proliferation control cells were cultured in the presence of TNF-α or IL-4. Interestingly, even low doses of TNF-α produced significant reductions in the percentage of proliferating cells, while IL-4 had no significant impact (Figure 5D).

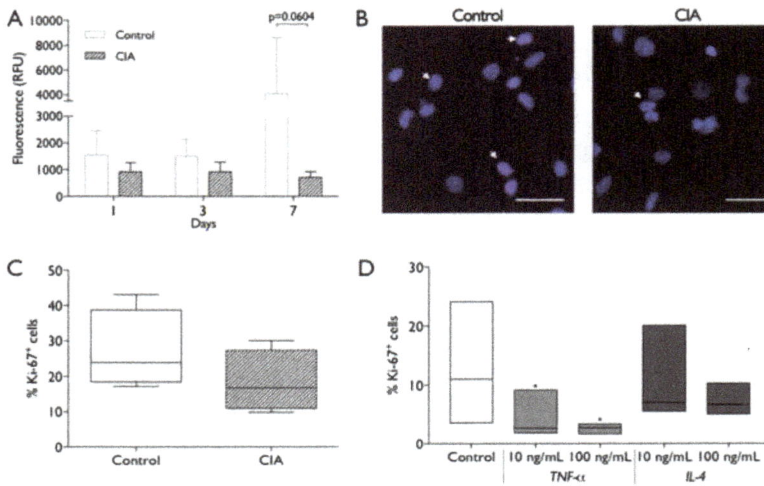

Figure 5. MSC metabolic activity and proliferation capacity. (**A**) Metabolic activity was measured at 1, 3 and 7 days of MSC culture by resazurin assay. RFU: relative fluorescence units. Statistical differences were evaluated by 2-way ANOVA followed by Turkey's multiple comparison test (**B**) Representative images of nuclei (Dapi, blue) and Ki-67 immunostaining (pink, white arrows) of control and CIA-derived MSC after 2 days in culture. Scale bar: 50 µm. (**C**). Percentage of Ki-67$^+$ control and CIA-derived MSC, across different experiments. Statistical differences were evaluated by Mann–Whitney test. (**D**) Percentage of Ki-67$^+$ control- derived MSC after 2 days in absence/presence of 10 ng/mL or 100 ng/mL of TNF-α or IL-4. Box plots represent min-to-max distribution of $n = 4$ to 5 animals per group. * $p < 0.05$ by Friedman test followed by Dunn's multiple comparisons test.

The endogenous differentiation ability of BM-MSC from CIA and control animals was evaluated at 3 and 7 days of culture, in the absence of chemical and molecular inductors. The results obtained showed that CIA animals-derived MSC had increased expression of osteogenic genes, with significantly higher ALP expression, relative to control cells, at 7 days, and a significant increase in RUNX2 expression from 3 to 7 days in CIA-MSC, which was not observed in control-MSC (Figure 6A). When analyzing chondrogenic differentiation capacity of CIA-MSC in basal conditions, results indicate a significantly higher expression of ACAN at 3 days compared to control cells, and that significantly decreased by day 7, while expression of SOX9 did not show significant differences between the cells of CIA and control animals, or along time (Figure 6B). Then we explored if exposure to cytokines could impact MSC differentiation in the absence of chemical induction. Results obtained show that exposure to TNF-α or IL-4 increased ALP gene expression with IL-4 exposure producing significant increases, even when compared to the positive control, using chemical inductors (Figure 6C). Interestingly, IL-4 exposure led to increased ACAN expression, to levels similar to those obtained with chondrogenic induction and for CIA- MSC, while TNF-α did not lead to the increases observed for MSC from CIA animals (Figure 6D).

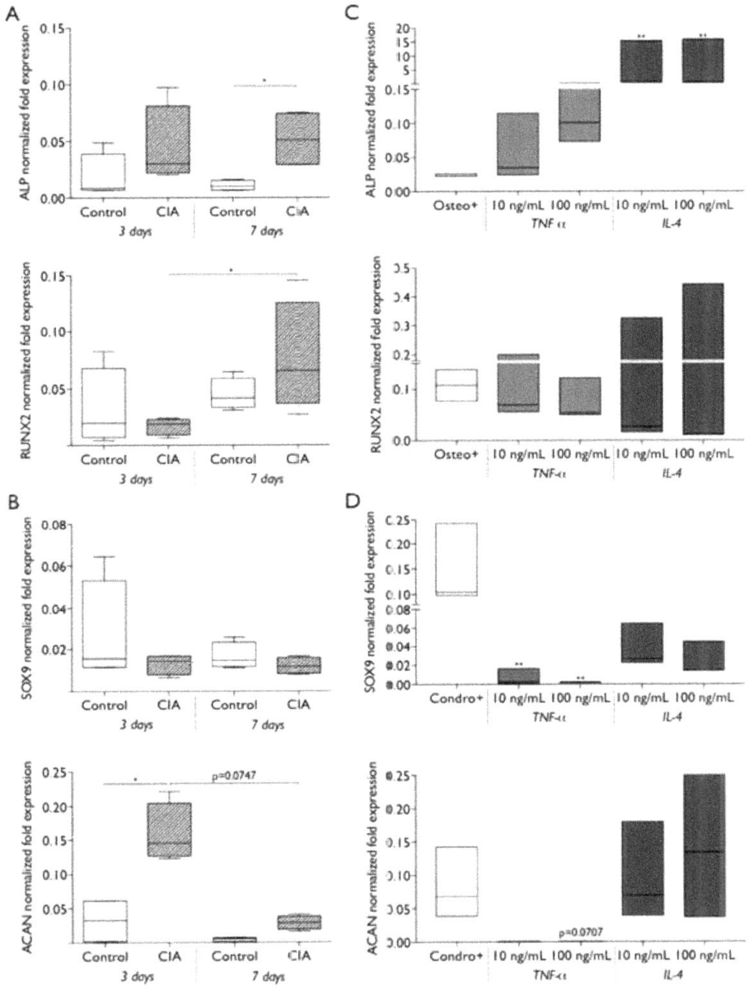

Figure 6. The capacity of MSC differentiation is affected by arthritis induction. The differentiation of control and CIA-MSC were evaluated in absence of chemical inductors, at 3 and 7 days of culture by reverse transcription-quantitative polymerase chain reaction (RT-qPCR) for (**A**) osteogenic marker genes ALP and RUNX2, and (**B**) chondrogenic differentiation genes SOX9 and ACAN. Box plots represent min-to-max distribution of $n = 2$ to 3 different animals per group, in 2 independent experiments. * $p < 0.05$ by Kruskal–Wallis test followed by Dunn's multiple comparisons test. The effect of 10 ng/mL or 100 ng/mL of TNF-α and IL-4 in the differentiation of control MSC, were evaluated in basal conditions at 3 days by RT-qPCR for (**C**) osteogenic and (**D**) chondrogenic markers. Cells cultured with osteogenic and chondrogenic inductors were used as positive controls for osteogenic (osteo+) and chondrogenic (chond+) differentiation. * $p < 0.05$, ** $p < 0.01$ determined by Friedman test followed by Dunn's multiple comparisons test.

Taken together, these results indicate that exposure to hallmark arthritis cytokines like TNF-α can partially mimic the CIA impact on MSC.

3. Discussion

In the current study, arthritis was induced in all animals and reached a plateau in its score by 17 to 21 days after CII-IFA (Collagen type II-Incomplete Freund's adjuvant) immunization. This is in line with previous reports on this model [26]. Histologically, our data shows hind paws swelling and inflammation in digital joints, visible by the infiltration of inflammatory cells and hyperplasia of the synovial membrane, which constitute hallmarks of human RA pathology [27] and have been previously reported in CIA animal model [11,28,29]. The CIA model was combined with a critical size femoral bone defect model in a load-bearing site without the need for fixation material [30] and without significant acute implications for animal welfare and paw swelling. Enlargement of secondary lymphoid organs was similar between CIA and CIA+FD at 3 days post-bone injury, albeit slightly decreased percentages of proliferating cells in CIA+FD were observed. This is in line with previous work in the CIA model, such as in the report by Ibraheem where the injection of different collagen types combined with adjuvant to induce arthritis in rats led to enlarged lymph nodes with histologic alterations [31] and the reports of splenomegaly in the most severe states of adjuvant-induced arthritis [11,32]. Also, a previous report induced a mid-shaft femur fracture with fracture fixation in the CIA rat model and showed delayed healing in CIA animals, but the authors do not analyze inflammation in their study [33]. In fact, the current study is, to the best of our knowledge, the first one addressing the interplay between inflammation and bone injury in these RA models.

To determine the systemic immune cell response to CIA induction and the combination with bone injury, we evaluated the main immune cell populations that are the key cell players involved in the development and maintenance of the inflammation in CIA model [10], in blood and secondary lymphoid organs. Our results show a significant increase in B cells in blood and draining lymph nodes of CIA animals and also increased myeloid cells in blood. This change in proportions may suggest that these cells migrate from the blood to the inflamed tissues. A previous report in the mouse CIA model described similar increases in the percentage of B cells, which they correlate with increased anti-collagen antibodies in serum [34]. Activated B cells have been reported to produce anti-collagen antibodies that bind to cartilage collagen and form an immune complex, generating a localized inflammatory response and attracting monocytes, granulocytes, and T cells to the joint [10,17].

Interestingly, CIA animals responded to the bone injury with significant increases in myeloid cells and their activation, particularly in secondary lymphoid organs. Myeloid cells are important regulators that contribute to the perpetuation of inflammation in RA [35]. Moreover, in a murine model of early RA, increased myeloid dendritic cells were reported in draining lymph nodes before the appearance of joint histological changes, indicating their role in the early stage of murine RA [36]. A significant decrease in T cell proportions was found in lymph nodes of CIA rats, accompanied by a decrease in CD4/CD8 ratios. These data may suggest that T cells are attracted to the joints, but this requires further confirmation. The immune response mediated by T cells is described as crucial for the development of mouse [10,17] and rat CIA, with athymic rats being resistant to CIA induction, but T cell transfer alone was reported to have induced only a mild response [10]. The role of NK cells in RA and CIA is not yet clear, with some evidence that they may contribute to [37,38] or protect against [39] inflammation. Here, we did not observe differences in the percentage of NK cells in peripheral blood as described in a previous study in CIA mice [34], but observed an increase in the CIA+FD group. The same work showed a decrease in splenic NK cells proportion at day 37, different from the increasing tendency that was observed in the current study at day 21 after CIA induction. Interestingly, the changes observed here in systemic immune cell proportions are different from those previously observed in the same model of bone injury, but in healthy animals at day 6 post-surgery [40]. This might be explained by the inflammatory conditions, but also by different times post-injury, as in the same model in healthy animals we observed an acute response at day 3, and resolution of that response at day 14 post-surgery [41].

In the current study, a broad quantitative analysis of plasma cytokines/chemokines comparing control, CIA, and CIA+FD animals was performed. We found increased levels of the hallmark cytokine

TNF-α in the plasma of CIA animals. High TNF-α levels in affected joints or in peripheral blood serum are strongly associated with RA disease severity [42,43]. This pro-inflammatory cytokine was described in different RA animal models [43,44], including the transgenic mouse expressing human TNF-α [45] and the CIA model [12,13]. TNF-α has also been reported as accelerating arthritis signals when injected into animals [43]. In response to TNF-α, RA synovial fibroblasts are described to produce MCP-1/CCL2, which was also found increased in the plasma of CIA animals in the current study, particularly after bone injury. MCP-1 is a potent chemokine that mediates monocyte ingress and activation in joints [46]. This was clearly demonstrated in vivo by the injection of a rabbit model with MCP-1/CCL2, resulting in a marked macrophage infiltration of the affected joints [47]. Macrophages have been previously described as a major source of MCP-1/CCL2 [48]. In our results, $CD68^+$ macrophages were also found in the inflamed synovium.

Levels of IL-17, IL-2, and IL-5 were also increased in CIA animals, and maintained the same tendency (albeit not always significant) in the CIA+FD group. These cytokines are related to the T cell function and response in vivo. Systemic IL-17 levels intensify RA and induce a chronic and erosive form of the disease [49]. A recent report in CIA model in Dark Agouti rats demonstrated that the Th-17 response in draining lymph nodes is greater in females than in males, correlating the Th-17/Treg (regulatory T cell) axis with sexual differences in CIA severity [50]. IL-2 is a positive regulator of T cell proliferation, and administration of IL-2 can mediate a pro-inflammatory effect on CIA mice, increasing the animals' arthritic scores [51]. A recent report shows that IL-2-Anti-IL-2 monoclonal antibody immune complexes can inhibit CIA by increasing Treg cell functions [52]. IL-5 is a cytokine with pleiotropic effects on target cells, including eosinophils and B cells, inducing cell proliferation, survival, and differentiation [53], its role in RA remains unknown, but a recent work found elevated serum levels of IL-5 in 59% of seropositive RA patients [54]. Also, it was reported that lymph node cells isolated from CIA-susceptible mice lines showed a higher number of IL-5 producing cells in culture than cells from resistant mice [55]. Fractalkine was found downregulated in CIA animals with and without bone injury, which is not in agreement with reports indicating amelioration of arthritis symptoms and joint destruction when Fractalkine is suppressed [56,57]. Also, Leptin was found significantly reduced in the plasma of CIA and CIA+FD animals, but its role in arthritis is still controversial. In the mouse CIA model, Leptin injection has been reported to worsen disease via Th-17 cells [58], but has also been reported as anti-inflammatory when collagen-antibody-induced arthritis is induced in mice overexpressing Leptin [59]. Also, its levels have been reported as increased in other models of RA and in patient's plasma, but reduced at the joint level, indicating its consumption [60]. RANTES (or CCL5) was the only molecule that showed a significant difference between the CIA and CIA+FD groups. A recent report on bioinformatic analysis of human RA gene expression data indicates that CCL5 might have a negative impact on the development of RA [61], while another recent report in mouse indicates that peritoneal levels of several CC chemokines, including CCL5, could be related with mouse strain susceptibility to experimental arthritis [62]. However, as in our study, neither group had a significant difference to control, and so the biological meaning of this result remains unclear.

Although the use of MSC as therapeutics for RA is being intensely studied, the effect of CIA induction and its inflammatory milieu on the biological behavior of endogenous bone marrow-derived MSC had not been explored so far. Growing evidence indicates that bone marrow is actively involved in the RA disease process. In RA patient samples, the interaction between synovial inflammatory tissue and bone marrow reportedly results from the disruption of cortical bone leading to bone marrow invasion [63]. Furthermore, previous work described in vivo a significant enlargement of vascularized bone canals that link the bone marrow and the synovium tissue, in joints with synovial hyperplasia [64]. Also, it has been suggested that bone marrow-derived immature mesenchymal cells may migrate through the joint space to replace synovial cells, similar to what happens with inflammatory cells [65,66]. In fact, even if bone marrow is not primarily affected, this interaction, together with the aberrant cytokine production, can potentially affect the biological behavior, namely the survival and proliferation of bone marrow cells [67].

The current work shows that culture-expanded MSC from CIA animals were morphologically and immunophenotypically similar to controls, expressing the characteristic mesenchymal markers (Figure S1C). Nevertheless, the metabolic activity and percentage of proliferative cells were lower in the CIA-MSC cultures. This had not been described in RA animal models thus far, but agrees with what was described in cells derived from RA patients [68,69]. RA-MSC display proliferation defects in culture without significant differences in the percentages of apoptotic cells [68,69], and high levels of the cell cycle inhibitor p21, which can mediate the defects in cell growth and replicative capacity [69]. Mice treated with anti-TNF-α at an early CIA stage showed a reduction in the number of MSC in the bone marrow and synovium [64]. Conversely, a previous report described that the proportion of $CD34^+$ bone marrow progenitor cells increase after the anti-TNF-α treatment in RA patients, with the number of bone marrow mononuclear cells in clonogenic assays being higher when compared to the pretreatment values [67]. In our study, a significant reduction in the percentage of proliferative MSC was observed in control cells exposed to TNF-α, an important pro-inflammatory cytokine found increased in the plasma of CIA animals. This reduction in healthy MSC proliferation in the presence of TNF-α could have consequences for MSC-based therapies for RA.

Our results show increased osteogenic gene expression of CIA-MSC in basal conditions when compared to control MSC. Contrasting data has been reported on the osteogenic and chondrogenic potential of MSC isolated from RA patients. Previous reports indicate that ALP expression was comparable between the cells from RA and healthy donors [68,69], and that RA MSC do not differ significantly from the normal cells on their chondrogenic differentiation [70]. MSC differentiation in the CIA animal model has been analyzed in response to the chemical/molecular stimulation protocols commonly used in vitro, but not in basal conditions, and further detailed analysis is still required. Previous work showed that control and CIA-derived mouse BM-MSC respond to osteogenic stimulation with similar increases in RUNX2 and ALP gene expression [71]. In our work the cells were isolated from the same site and from animals with the same age and sex. Thus, our results support that the alterations in proliferative and differentiation capacities are not site or age-dependent, but are likely associated with the disease condition of the animals. We also explored if CIA conditions could be mimicked by exposure to TNF-α and observed an increase, albeit not statistically significant in ALP gene expression. This agrees with previous reports showing that exposure to these concentrations of TNF-α impairs MSC proliferation/survival [72]. The same authors also found impaired MSC response to osteogenesis induction upon exposure to these concentrations of TNF-α, but the response of the cells in the absence of osteogenic induction was not analyzed. In the RA model of human TNF-α transgene, previous reports showed the deleterious effects of high levels of this cytokine on fracture repair [45], and in the CIA model fracture healing was also impaired [33]. Further studies are required to analyze if such impairments are related to changes in MSC proliferation and differentiation, and the role of chronic inflammation in bone repair [72].

In conclusion, arthritis induction creates a systemic inflammatory environment, with changes in immune cells and circulating cytokine/chemokine levels. Also, bone marrow-derived MSC isolated from CIA animals display impaired proliferation and increased differentiation in basal conditions. Further studies are needed to clarify the relation between exposure to inflammatory cytokines like TNF-α and MSC phenotype impairments, and their consequences for bone repair in RA. Furthermore, the current work supports the viability of using the CIA model to investigate the mechanisms of bone repair/regeneration in chronic inflammatory conditions, and the development of therapeutic strategies more appropriate to treat bone fractures in RA patients.

4. Materials and Methods

4.1. Bovine Collagen Type II Emulsion Preparation

Bovine collagen type II (CII, 2 mg/mL, Chondrex, Redmond, WA, USA) was added in a 1:1 proportion of incomplete Freund's adjuvant (IFA, Chondrex, Redmond WA, USA) and homogenized in an ice water bath, according to the manufacturer's instructions. Then, the emulsion was kept at 4 °C until injection, without this period exceeding 1 h.

4.2. Collagen-Induced Arthritis (CIA) Rat Model

Animal procedures were performed in accordance with the ethical animal welfare and experimentation, and approved by the Portuguese official authority regulating laboratory animal sciences (DGAV). Fifteen female Wistar rats (7–8 weeks old) were purchased from Charles River Laboratories (Barcelona, Spain) and housed in a clean environment. Animals were randomly divided into CIA (n = 10) and healthy control (n = 5) groups. On day 0, CIA rats were immunized with 200 µL of CII-IFA emulsion (200 µg collagen/rat) with a 25-gauge needle via subcutaneous injection at the base of the tail. Seven days after, a booster injection of CII-IFA emulsion was administrated to ensure a high incidence and severity of arthritis. Animals were maintained under general isoflurane anesthesia during these interventions, and all the arthritis-inducing procedures were performed according to the guidelines of Chondrex and based in previous reports [9,15]. At day thirteen after CIA induction, one animal from CIA group was lost due to a problem of gastric obstruction.

4.3. Monitoring of Clinical Arthritis Development

The animal health condition and physical activity was monitored daily according to the recent guidelines of refinement in RA research [32]. Three times per week the animals were weighed, paw swelling was measured with digital caliper at the metacarpus level, and x-ray was performed. Each rat paw was scored individually according to signs of joints (interphalangeal, metacarpophalangeal, carpal and tarsal) inflammation, adapting the Chondrex arthritis scoring system: (0) normal, (1) mild redness and swelling of the ankle or digits, (2) moderate redness and swelling of ankle or wrist, (3) severe redness of the entire paw, (4) maximally inflamed limb with the involvement of multiple joints. The arthritis index was determined by the sum of the score of each front and hind paw with the total maximum of 16.

4.4. CIA Rat Model Combined with Bone Injury Model

Twenty-one days after arthritis induction, a critical size femur defect was performed in 5 CIA rats, as previously described by our group [30]. Briefly, knees were shaved and disinfected, and then an incision was made in the skin and muscles surrounding the right femur were retracted. After lateral knee arthrotomy, a cylindrical defect (FD, 3 × 4 mm, diameter × depth) was created using a surgical drill (micromotor, K-control TLC 4965) in the anterolateral wall of the lateral condyle of the femur. Surgeries were performed under general anesthesia with volatile isoflurane. After surgery, analgesia was provided by subcutaneous administration of buprenorphine (0.05 mg/kg) twice a day. Three days after the bone injury, animals were euthanized for blood and organ collection.

4.5. Blood, Spleen and Lymph Nodes Collection and Processing

At day 24, animals were maintained under general anesthesia with volatile isoflurane and whole blood was collected by cardiac puncture into tubes containing anticoagulant citrate-phosphate-dextrose solution (Sigma-Aldrich Inc., St Louis, MO, USA). Blood was centrifuged, and plasma and buffy coats collected and processed as described previously [41]. Plasma was further centrifuged twice at 2500× g for 15 min and supernatant stored at −80 °C until further analysis. Collected buffy coats were diluted in phosphate buffered saline (PBS), overlaid on Lymphoprep (Axis-Shield Diagnostics, Dundee, Scotland) in a 1:1 ratio and centrifuged at 800× g for 30 min at RT to isolate peripheral blood mononuclear cells (PBMC).

Animals were dissected for the collection of spleen and draining lymph nodes (inguinal and popliteal nodes). Spleen was clean from adjacent tissue and weighted, and then a half portion of spleen and lymph nodes were preserved in formalin 10% for further histology processing, whereas the remaining parts were used to isolate single cells for flow cytometry analysis, as described previously [41].

Briefly, spleen was digested with 1 mg/mL Collagenase I (Sigma-Aldrich Inc., St Louis, MO, USA), both spleen and lymph nodes were gently crushed, and strained to obtain cell suspensions. Red blood cells in spleen cell suspension were then lysed by incubation with NH_4Cl 150 mM in Tris 10 mM. Obtained cells were washed with PBS.

4.6. Histology and Immunohistochemistry Analysis

Animal hind paws were collected, fixed in formalin 10% for 48h, and then decalcified in 10% EDTA solution, for 1 month. Tissue was embedded in paraffin and sections of 4 μm thickness were cut and stained with hematoxylin and eosin (H&E). Spleen and draining lymph nodes were fixed for 24 h, paraffin embedded and 3 μm thickness paraffin sections were cut for H&E staining and immunohistochemistry (IHQ).

Expression of proliferation marker Ki-67 and macrophage marker CD68 was assessed by IHQ. NovolinkTM Polymer Detection Kit (Leica Biosystems, Newcastle, UK) was used following the manufacturer's instructions. Antigen retrieval was performed by sections incubation in citrate buffer (98 °C, citrate buffer 10 mM, pH 6.0). After endogenous peroxidase neutralization, permeabilization with Triton X-100 0.3% was performed for Ki-67 immunostaining. Sections were incubated with Block protein solution and then in primary antibodies: anti-Ki-67 (1:50, clone SP6, ThermoFisher Scientific, Waltham, MA, USA) and anti-CD68 (1:100, clone ED1, Bio-Rad Laboratories, Irvine, CA, USA) for 45 min at RT. Positive staining was revealed after 30 min of incubation with NovoLinkTM Polymer and 5 min of incubation with peroxidase-substrate solution DAB. Finally, sections were counterstained with hematoxylin and slides mounted. Sections incubated without primary antibody were used as negative controls. Representative images of positive staining were taken using Olympus CX31 light microscope (20× objective). Nine images per slide were analyzed using Fiji software, and the number of nuclei Ki-67$^+$ and Ki-67$^-$ nuclei were counted. Proliferation index was calculated as the ratio of Ki-67$^+$ nuclei to the total number of nuclei counted.

4.7. Flow Cytometry Analysis

Cells from blood, spleen, and lymph nodes were incubated with 1 μL per sample of mouse anti-Rat CD32 (clone D34-485, 20 μg/mL, BD biosciences, San Jose, CA, USA) diluted in staining buffer (0.5% bovine serum albumin (BSA) and 0.01% sodium azide in PBS), to prevent unspecific bindings. Then, cells were immunostained for 30 min on ice for the presence of T cells, B cells, NK cells, and myeloid cells by the following surface antibodies: anti-TCR-PerCP (clone R73, 4 μg/mL), anti-CD4-APC (clone OX-35, 4 μg/mL), anti-CD8a-V450 (clone OX-8, 8 μg/mL), anti-CD45R-PE (clone His24, 8 μg/mL), anti-CD161a-FITC (clone10/78, 2 μg/mL), anti-CD11b/c-PE-Cy7 (clone OX-42, 1.6 μg/mL), anti-CD40-FITC (clone HM40-3, 40 μg/mL), anti-CD86-PE (clone 24F, 16 μg/mL) all from BD biosciences. Cells stained with the corresponding isotype antibodies were used as control. Cells were washed 4 times in PBS and fixed with paraformaldehyde 1%. Samples were analyzed on a FACSCanto flow cytometer (Becton Dickinson), with acquisition of 10.000 events in gate for each sample, and data analyzed with FlowJo software.

4.8. Plasma Cytokine Quantification

Plasma cytokines were quantified at Eve Technologies Corp. (Calgary, AB, Canada) using the Rat Cytokine Array/Chemokine Array 27-Plex Discovery Assay. Plasma samples, 30 μL, were diluted twice in PBS prior analysis, according to the manufacturer's indications. The sensitivity of the assay for the markers analyzed ranged from 0.1 to 15.7 pg/mL.

4.9. Isolation of MSC, Primary Culture and Phenotypic Characterization

Rat MSC were isolated form CIA and control femurs, as previously described [41]. Briefly, bone marrow was flushed with PBS and bone debris were removed by filtering the cell suspension through a 100 μm cell strainer. After red blood cells lysis, cells were counted and seeded in minimum essential medium alpha modification (α-MEM) supplemented with 10% MSC-qualified fetal bovine serum (ThermoFisher Scientific, Waltham, MA, USA MA, USA) and 1% penicillin G-streptomycin (P/S; Invitrogen, Carlsbad, CA, USA), at 10^6/100 mm plate. MSC were selected by adherence to plastic surface, expanded and cryopreserved for forward use. Isolated and cultured MSC identity was confirmed by multicolor flow cytometry based on classical cell surface markers $CD29^+$ (anti-CD29-APC, HMβ1-1, BioLegend, San Diego, CA, USA), $CD90^+$ (anti-CD90-PE, MRC OX-7, Immunotools, Friesoythe, Germany) and $CD45^-$ (anti-CD45-FITC, MRC OX-30, Immunotools, Friesoythe, Germany) staining, and by ability of cells to differentiate into the osteogenic, chondrogenic and adipogenic lineages. Cells from CIA and control animals were maintained in a humidified incubator, at 37 °C and 5% CO2, and used for experiments between passages 4 and 8.

4.10. MSC Metabolic Activity and Proliferation Assays

MSC were seeded in a 96-well plate at 2000 cells/well and allowed to reach 40% to 60% confluence. Then, metabolic activity and proliferation assays were performed. Metabolic activity was evaluated by resazurin assay, incubating cells with 10% Alamar blue (ThermoFisher Scientific, Waltham, MA, USA) in MSC culture conditions for 4 h. Fluorescence was measured (530 nm excitation and 590 nm emission) in a Synergy HT Multi-Mode Microplate Reader (BioTek Instruments, Winooski, VT, USA). This procedure was repeated at 1, 3 and 7 days of culture in five replicates. Samples without cells were used as negative controls.

To determine the MSC proliferation index, cells were fixed after 48 h in culture in absence/presence of TNF-α or IL-4 (Immunotools, Friesoythe, Germany) at 10 ng/mL and 100 ng/mL. After permeabilization step with Triton X-100 0.1% and block with 5% BSA, cells were labelled for Ki-67 (1:150; clone SP6, ThermoFisher Scientific, Waltham, MA, USA) followed by AlexaFluor647-conjugated secondary antibody, and nuclei stained with DAPI 1 μg/mL. Cells incubated with secondary antibody only were used as a negative control. Immunofluorescence images were acquired in the IN Cell Analyzer 2000 (GE Healthcare, Chicago, IL, USA) using a Nikon 20x/0.45 NA Plan Fluor objective, capturing 30 sequential and non-overlapping images of the center of each well. Images were analyzed by Fiji Software and proliferation index determined by counting number of cells with $Ki\text{-}67^+$ labelling inside the nuclei relative to the total number of nuclei counted.

4.11. MSC Differentiation Assay

For MSC characterization, cells were seeded in 6 well-plate at a density of 6000 cells/well and grow until reached 40–60% of confluence. Then, cells were incubated in basal or differentiation MSC media without/with osteogenic (α-MEM 10^{-7} M dexamethasone (Sigma-Aldrich Inc., St Louis, MO, USA), 10^{-2} M β-glycerophosphate and 5×10^{-5} M ascorbic acid) and adipogenic (10^{-4} M dexamethasone, 5×10^{-4} M IBMX, 10 μg/mL insulin, 10^{-4} M indomethacin) supplements for 21 and 28 days, respectively. Media was changed twice a week and at the end of the osteogenic or adipogenic differentiation, and cells were fixed and stained with Alizarin red or Oil red O, respectively.

For chondrogenic differentiation, a cell pellet of 2×10^5 cells was incubated in 15 mL falcon conical tubes in differentiation media (α-MEM supplemented with 4.5 g/L glucose, 2.5×10^{-4} M ascorbic acid, 40 μg/mL L-proline, 100 μg/mL sodium pyruvate, 100 μg/mL ITS, 10^{-7} M dexamethasone, and 10 ng/mL TGF-β3) for 28 days. Then, cell pellet was fixed with paraformaldehyde 4%, processed for histologic analysis, and stained by H&E and Toluidine blue stain.

For MSC gene expression, cells were cultured in basal conditions for 3 and 7 days, in absence/presence of TNF-α or IL-4 (10 ng/mL and 100 ng/mL). Cells stimulated with osteogenic and chondrogenic media as above were used as positive controls. Cells were collected for RNA isolation and expression of gene markers for osteogenic and chondrogenic differentiation was analyzed.

4.12. RNA Isolation and Reverse Transcription-Quantitative Polymerase Chain Reaction (RT-qPCR)

For gene expression analysis, MSC RNA was extracted using TRizol (Invitrogen, Carlsbad, CA, USA) reagent following manufacturer's instructions, quantified by NanoDrop ND-1000 (ThermoFisher Scientific, Waltham, MA, USA) and integrity assessed by agarose electrophoresis. RNA (900 ng of total RNA) was digested with TURBO DNA-free Kit (Life Technologies, Carlsbad, CA, USA), according to manufacturer's protocol, and complementary DNA (cDNA) was synthesized with random hexamers (Life Technologies, Carlsbad, CA, USA) and dNTPs using SuperScript III Reverse Transcriptase (Life Technologies, Carlsbad, CA, USA). RT-qPCR was performed in an iQ5 Real-Time PCR Detection System (Bio-Rad Laboratories, Irvine, CA, USA) using cDNA, gene specific primers for osteogenic and chondrogenic differentiation markers (Table 1), and iQ SYBR Green Supermix (Bio-Rad Laboratories, Irvine, CA, USA). Relative gene expression was calculated using the $2^{-\Delta CT}$ method and normalized with the GAPDH reference gene, considering threshold cycles <35.

Table 1. Sequences of primers used for gene expression analysis by RT-qPCR.

Gene	Primer Sequence
ALP	Forward 5′-GACAAGAAGCCCTTCACAGC-3′ Reverse 5′-CTGGGCCTGGTAGTTGTTGT-3′
RUNX2	Forward 5′-CCGATGGGACCGTGGTT-3′ Reverse 5′-CAGCAGAGGCATTTCGTAGCT-3′
SOX9	Forward 5′-CTGAAGGGCTACGACTGGAC-3′ Reverse 5′-TACTGGTCTGCCAGCTTCCT-3′
ACAN	Forward 5′-CTTGGGCAGAAGAAAGATCG-3′ Reverse 5′-GTGCTTGTAGGTGTTGGGGT-3′
GAPDH	Forward 5′-TGCCACTCAGAAGACTGTGG-3′ Reverse 5′-TTCAGCTCTGGGATGACCTT-3′

4.13. Statistical Analysis

Data analysis were performed using GraphPad Prism v7.0 software. Normality distribution of data was tested by D'Agostino and Pearson normality test. For weight, paw swelling measurements and arthritis score, 2-way ANOVA followed by Tukey's multiple comparisons was used. For non-parametric data, when two groups were compared, Mann–Whitney test was performed. To compare multiple unpaired groups, Kruskal–Wallis test was used, followed by uncorrected Dunn's multiple comparison test. To compare multiple paired groups, Friedman test followed by uncorrected Dunn's multiple comparisons was performed. Statistical significance was considered whenever * $p < 0.05$; ** $p < 0.01$; *** $p < 0.001$; **** $p < 0.0001$.

Supplementary Materials: Supplementary materials can be found at http://www.mdpi.com/1422-0067/20/21/5436/s1.

Author Contributions: J.H.T., M.A.B. and S.G.S. planned all the experiments. J.H.T., A.M.S., M.I.A., M.B.-G., C.C. and S.G.S. performed animal experiments and sample collection. J.H.T., A.M.S., S.G.S. executed experiments, acquired and analyzed the data. J.H.T. and S.G.S. wrote the main manuscript text. J.H.T., A.M.S., M.I.A., M.B.-G., C.C., M.A.B. and S.G.S. discussed and approved the manuscript.

Funding: This research was funded by the project NORTE-01-0145-FEDER-000012, supported by Norte Portugal Regional Operational Programme (NORTE 2020), under the PORTUGAL 2020 Partnership Agreement, through the European Regional Development Fund (ERDF), and AO Foundation-Switzerland (project S-15-83S). J.H.T, A.M.S, M.B.G, M.I.A and C.C were supported by FCT-Fundação para a Ciência e a Tecnologia, through the fellowships SFRH/BD/112832/2015, SFRH/BD/85968/2012, PD/BD/135489/2018, DL 57/2016/CP1360/CT0008 and DL 57/2016/CP1360/CT0004, respectively.

Acknowledgments: Authors thank to Sofia Lamas for the guidance on the animal welfare and support with animal experiments (Animal facility, i3S); Catarina Meireles for the help on flow cytometry analysis (Translational Cytometry Unit, i3S) and Cláudia Ribeiro-Machado for the support with the histological procedures and analysis.

Conflicts of Interest: The authors declare no conflict of interest. The funders had no role in the design of the study; in the collection, analyses, or interpretation of data; in the writing of the manuscript, or in the decision to publish the results.

Abbreviations

CIA	Collagen-induced arthritis
MSC	Mesenchymal stem/stromal cells
TNF-α	Tumor necrosis factor-alpha
IL	Interleukin
RA	Rheumatoid Arthritis
FD	Femoral defect
CIA+FD	Collagen-induced arthritis with femoral defect
RT-qPCR	Reverse transcription-quantitative polymerase chain reaction
CII-IFA	Collagen type II-Incomplete Freund's adjuvant

References

1. Van der Woude, D.; van der Helm-van Mil, A.H.M. Update on the epidemiology, risk factors, and disease outcomes of rheumatoid arthritis. *Best Pract. Res. Clin. Rheumatol.* **2018**, *32*, 174–187. [CrossRef] [PubMed]
2. Cojocaru, M.; Cojocaru, I.M.; Silosi, I.; Vrabie, C.D.; Tanasescu, R. Extra-articular manifestations in rheumatoid arthritis. *Maedica (Buchar)* **2010**, *5*, 286–291. [PubMed]
3. Barreira, S.C.; Fonseca, J.E. The impact of conventional and biological disease modifying antirheumatic drugs on bone biology. Rheumatoid arthritis as a case study. *Clin. Rev. Allergy Immunol.* **2016**, *51*, 100–109. [CrossRef] [PubMed]
4. Heinlen, L.; Humphrey, M.B. Skeletal complications of rheumatoid arthritis. *Osteoporos. Int.* **2017**, *28*, 2801–2812. [CrossRef] [PubMed]
5. Jin, S.; Hsieh, E.; Peng, L.; Yu, C.; Wang, Y.; Wu, C.; Wang, Q.; Li, M.; Zeng, X. Incidence of fractures among patients with rheumatoid arthritis: A systematic review and meta-analysis. *Osteoporos. Int.* **2018**, *29*, 1263–1275. [CrossRef] [PubMed]
6. Ghazi, M.; Kolta, S.; Briot, K.; Fechtenbaum, J.; Paternotte, S.; Roux, C. Prevalence of vertebral fractures in patients with rheumatoid arthritis: Revisiting the role of glucocorticoids. *Osteoporos. Int.* **2012**, *23*, 581–587. [CrossRef] [PubMed]
7. Claes, L.; Recknagel, S.; Ignatius, A. Fracture healing under healthy and inflammatory conditions. *Nat. Rev. Rheumatol.* **2012**, *8*, 133–143. [CrossRef]
8. Kannan, K.; Ortmann, R.A.; Kimpel, D. Animal models of rheumatoid arthritis and their relevance to human disease. *Pathophysiology* **2005**, *12*, 167–181. [CrossRef]
9. Trentham, D.E.; Townes, A.S.; Kang, A.H. Autoimmunity to type ii collagen an experimental model of arthritis. *J. Exp. Med.* **1977**, *146*, 857–868. [CrossRef]
10. Bevaart, L.; Vervoordeldonk, M.J.; Tak, P.P. Evaluation of therapeutic targets in animal models of arthritis: How does it relate to rheumatoid arthritis? *Arthritis Rheum.* **2010**, *62*, 2192–2205. [CrossRef]
11. Bendele, A. Animal models of rheumatoid arthritis. *J. Musculoskelet Neuronal Interact* **2001**, *1*, 377–385. [PubMed]
12. Mussener, A.; Litton, M.J.; Lindroos, E.; Klareskog, L. Cytokine production in synovial tissue of mice with collagen-induced arthritis (cia). *Clin. Exp. Immunol.* **1997**, *107*, 485–493. [CrossRef] [PubMed]
13. Marinova-Mutafchieva, L.; Williams, R.O.; Mason, L.J.; Mauri, C.; Feldmann, M.; Maini, R.N. Dynamics of proinflammatory cytokine expression in the joints of mice with collagen-induced arthritis (cia). *Clin. Exp. Immunol.* **1997**, *107*, 507–512. [CrossRef] [PubMed]
14. Wang, T.; Qiao, H.; Zhai, Z.; Zhang, J.; Tu, J.; Zheng, X.; Qian, N.; Zhou, H.; Lu, E.; Tang, T. Plumbagin ameliorates collagen-induced arthritis by regulating treg/th17 cell imbalances and suppressing osteoclastogenesis. *Front. Immunol.* **2018**, *9*, 3102. [CrossRef]
15. Rosloniec, E.F.; Cremer, M.; Kang, A.; Myers, L.K Collagen-induced arthritis. *Curr. Protoc. Immunol.* **2001**, *20*, 15.5.1–15.5.24.

16. Endale, M.; Lee, W.M.; Kwak, Y.S.; Kim, N.M.; Kim, B.K.; Kim, S.H.; Cho, J.; Kim, S.; Park, S.C.; Yun, B.S.; et al. Torilin ameliorates type ii collagen-induced arthritis in mouse model of rheumatoid arthritis. *Int. Immunopharmacol.* **2013**, *16*, 232–242. [CrossRef]

17. Luross, J.A.; Williams, N.A. The genetic and immunopathological processes underlying collagen-induced arthritis. *Immunology* **2001**, *103*, 407–416. [CrossRef]
18. Alvaro-Gracia, J.M.; Jover, J.A.; Garcia-Vicuna, R.; Carreno, L.; Alonso, A.; Marsal, S.; Blanco, F.; Martinez-Taboada, V.M.; Taylor, P.; Martin-Martin, C.; et al. Intravenous administration of expanded allogeneic adipose-derived mesenchymal stem cells in refractory rheumatoid arthritis (cx611): Results of a multicentre, dose escalation, randomised, single-blind, placebo-controlled phase ib/iia clinical trial. *Ann. Rheum. Dis.* **2017**, *76*, 196–202. [CrossRef]
19. Park, E.H.; Lim, H.S.; Lee, S.; Roh, K.; Seo, K.W.; Kang, K.S.; Shin, K. Intravenous infusion of umbilical cord blood-derived mesenchymal stem cells in rheumatoid arthritis: A phase ia clinical trial. *Stem Cells Transl. Med.* **2018**, *7*, 636–642. [CrossRef]
20. Gao, F.; Chiu, S.M.; Motan, D.A.; Zhang, Z.; Chen, L.; Ji, H.L.; Tse, H.F.; Fu, Q.L.; Lian, Q. Mesenchymal stem cells and immunomodulation: Current status and future prospects. *Cell Death Dis.* **2016**, *7*, e2062. [CrossRef]
21. Ansboro, S.; Roelofs, A.J.; De Bari, C. Mesenchymal stem cells for the management of rheumatoid arthritis: Immune modulation, repair or both? *Curr. Opin. Rheumatol.* **2017**, *29*, 201–207. [CrossRef] [PubMed]
22. Chen, M.; Su, W.; Lin, X.; Guo, Z.; Wang, J.; Zhang, Q.; Brand, D.; Ryffel, B.; Huang, J.; Liu, Z.; et al. Adoptive transfer of human gingiva-derived mesenchymal stem cells ameliorates collagen-induced arthritis via suppression of th1 and th17 cells and enhancement of regulatory t cell differentiation. *Arthritis Rheum.* **2013**, *65*, 1181–1193. [CrossRef] [PubMed]
23. Yan, X.; Cen, Y.; Wang, Q. Mesenchymal stem cells alleviate experimental rheumatoid arthritis through microrna-regulated ikappab expression. *Sci. Rep.* **2016**, *6*, 28915. [CrossRef] [PubMed]
24. Augello, A.; Tasso, R.; Negrini, S.M.; Cancedda, R.; Pennesi, G. Cell therapy using allogeneic bone marrow mesenchymal stem cells prevents tissue damage in collagen-induced arthritis. *Arthritis Rheum.* **2007**, *56*, 1175–1186. [CrossRef]
25. Liu, R.; Li, X.; Zhang, Z.; Zhou, M.; Sun, Y.; Su, D.; Feng, X.; Gao, X.; Shi, S.; Chen, W.; et al. Allogeneic mesenchymal stem cells inhibited t follicular helper cell generation in rheumatoid arthritis. *Sci. Rep.* **2015**, *5*, 12777. [CrossRef]
26. Palmblad, K.; Erlandsson-Harris, H.; Tracey, K.J.; Andersson, U. Dynamics of early synovial cytokine expression in rodent collagen-induced arthritis: A therapeutic study using a macrophage-deactivating compound. *Am. J. Pathol.* **2001**, *158*, 491–500. [CrossRef]
27. Komatsu, N.; Takayanagi, H. Inflammation and bone destruction in arthritis: Synergistic activity of immune and mesenchymal cells in joints. *Front. Immunol.* **2012**, *3*, 77. [CrossRef]
28. Asquith, D.L.; Miller, A.M.; McInnes, I.B.; Liew, F.Y. Animal models of rheumatoid arthritis. *Eur. J. Immunol.* **2009**, *39*, 2040–2044. [CrossRef]
29. Trentham, D.E.; Dynesius, R.A.; David, J.R. Passive transfer by cells of type ii collagen-induced arthritis in rats. *J. Clin. Investig.* **1978**, *62*, 359–366. [CrossRef]
30. Santos, S.G.; Lamghari, M.; Almeida, C.R.; Oliveira, M.I.; Neves, N.; Ribeiro, A.C.; Barbosa, J.N.; Barros, R.; Maciel, J.; Martins, M.C.; et al. Adsorbed fibrinogen leads to improved bone regeneration and correlates with differences in the systemic immune response. *Acta Biomater.* **2013**, *9*, 7209–7217. [CrossRef]
31. Ibraheem, A.S.; El-Sayed, M.F.; Ahmed, R.A. Lymph node histopathological studies in a combined adjuvant–collagen induced arthritis model in albino rat rattus rattus. *J. Basic Appl. Zool.* **2013**, *66*, 195–205. [CrossRef]
32. Hawkins, P.; Armstrong, R.; Boden, T.; Garside, P.; Knight, K.; Lilley, E.; Seed, M.; Wilkinson, M.; Williams, R.O. Applying refinement to the use of mice and rats in rheumatoid arthritis research. *Inflammopharmacology* **2015**, *23*, 131–150. [CrossRef] [PubMed]
33. Hu, Y.; Zhang, T.; Huang, H.; Cheng, W.; Lai, Y.; Bai, X.; Chen, J.; Yue, Y.; Zheng, Z.; Guo, C.; et al. Fracture healing in a collagen-induced arthritis rat model: Radiology and histology evidence. *J. Orthop. Res.* **2018**, *36*, 2876–2885. [CrossRef] [PubMed]
34. Richter, J.; Capkova, K.; Hribalova, V.; Vannucci, L.; Danyi, I.; Maly, M.; Fiserova, A. Collagen-induced arthritis: Severity and immune response attenuation using multivalent n-acetyl glucosamine. *Clin. Exp. Immunol.* **2014**, *177*, 121–133. [CrossRef]
35. Alivernini, S.; Tolusso, B.; Ferraccioli, G.; Gremese, E.; Kurowska-Stolarska, M.; McInnes, I.B. Driving chronicity in rheumatoid arthritis: Perpetuating role of myeloid cells. *Clin. Exp. Immunol.* **2018**, *193*, 13–23. [CrossRef]

36. Benson, R.A.; Patakas, A.; Conigliaro, P.; Rush, C.M.; Garside, P.; McInnes, I.B.; Brewer, J.M. Identifying the cells breaching self-tolerance in autoimmunity. *J. Immunol.* **2010**, *184*, 6378–6385. [CrossRef]
37. Dalbeth, N.; Callan, M.F. A subset of natural killer cells is greatly expanded within inflamed joints. *Arthritis Rheum.* **2002**, *46*, 1763–1772. [CrossRef]
38. De Matos, C.T.; Berg, L.; Michaelsson, J.; Fellander-Tsai, L.; Karre, K.; Soderstrom, K. Activating and inhibitory receptors on synovial fluid natural killer cells of arthritis patients: Role of cd94/nkg2a in control of cytokine secretion. *Immunology* **2007**, *122*, 291–301. [CrossRef]
39. Lo, C.K.; Lam, Q.L.; Sun, L.; Wang, S.; Ko, K.H.; Xu, H.; Wu, C.Y.; Zheng, B.J.; Lu, L. Natural killer cell degeneration exacerbates experimental arthritis in mice via enhanced interleukin-17 production. *Arthritis Rheum.* **2008**, *58*, 2700–2711. [CrossRef]
40. Vasconcelos, D.M.; Goncalves, R.M.; Almeida, C.R.; Pereira, I.O.; Oliveira, M.I.; Neves, N.; Silva, A.M.; Ribeiro, A.C.; Cunha, C.; Almeida, A.R.; et al. Fibrinogen scaffolds with immunomodulatory properties promote in vivo bone regeneration. *Biomaterials* **2016**, *111*, 163–178. [CrossRef]
41. Silva, A.M.; Almeida, M.I.; Teixeira, J.H.; Ivan, C.; Oliveira, J.; Vasconcelos, D.; Neves, N.; Ribeiro-Machado, C.; Cunha, C.; Barbosa, M.A.; et al. Profiling the circulating mirnome reveals a temporal regulation of the bone injury response. *Theranostics* **2018**, *8*, 3902–3917. [CrossRef] [PubMed]
42. Choy, E. Understanding the dynamics: Pathways involved in the pathogenesis of rheumatoid arthritis. *Rheumatology (Oxford)* **2012**, *51* (Suppl. 5), v3–v11. [CrossRef]
43. Szekanecz, Z.; Halloran, M.M.; Volin, M.V.; Woods, J.M.; Strieter, R.M.; Haines, G.K., 3rd; Kunkel, S.L.; Burdick, M.D.; Koch, A.E. Temporal expression of inflammatory cytokines and chemokines in rat adjuvant-induced arthritis. *Arthritis Rheum.* **2000**, *43*, 1266–1277. [CrossRef]
44. Fuseler, J.W.; Conner, E.M.; Davis, J.M.; Wolf, R.E.; Grisham, M.B. Cytokine and nitric oxide production in the acute phase of bacterial cell wall-induced arthritis. *Inflammation* **1997**, *21*, 113–131. [CrossRef] [PubMed]
45. Timmen, M.; Hidding, H.; Wieskotter, B.; Baum, W.; Pap, T.; Raschke, M.J.; Schett, G.; Zwerina, J.; Stange, R. Influence of antitnf-alpha antibody treatment on fracture healing under chronic inflammation. *BMC Musculoskelet Disord* **2014**, *15*, 184. [CrossRef] [PubMed]
46. Szekanecz, Z.; Vegvari, A.; Szabo, Z.; Koch, A.E. Chemokines and chemokine receptors in arthritis. *Front. Biosci (Schol Ed.)* **2010**, *2*, 153–167. [CrossRef] [PubMed]
47. Akahoshi, T.; Wada, C.; Endo, H.; Hirota, K.; Hosaka, S.; Takagishi, K.; Kondo, H.; Kashiwazaki, S.; Matsushima, K. Expression of monocyte chemotactic and activating factor in rheumatoid arthritis. Regulation of its production in synovial cells by interleukin-1 and tumor necrosis factor. *Arthritis Rheum.* **1993**, *36*, 762–771. [CrossRef]
48. Kinne, R.W.; Brauer, R.; Stuhlmuller, B.; Palombo-Kinne, E.; Burmester, G.R. Macrophages in rheumatoid arthritis. *Arthritis Res.* **2000**, *2*, 189–202. [CrossRef]
49. Sarkar, S.; Cooney, L.A.; White, P.; Dunlop, D.B.; Endres, J.; Jorns, J.M.; Wasco, M.J.; Fox, D.A. Regulation of pathogenic il-17 responses in collagen-induced arthritis: Roles of endogenous interferon-gamma and il-4. *Arthritis Res. Ther.* **2009**, *11*, R158. [CrossRef]
50. Dimitrijevic, M.; Arsenovic-Ranin, N.; Kosec, D.; Bufan, B.; Nacka-Aleksic, M.; Pilipovic, I.; Leposavic, G. Sexual dimorphism in th17/treg axis in lymph nodes draining inflamed joints in rats with collagen-induced arthritis. *Brain Behav. Immun.* **2019**, *76*, 198–214. [CrossRef]
51. Thornton, S.; Boivin, G.P.; Kim, K.N.; Finkelman, F.D.; Hirsch, R. Heterogeneous effects of il-2 on collagen-induced arthritis. *J. Immunol.* **2000**, *165*, 1557–1563. [CrossRef] [PubMed]
52. Yokoyama, Y.; Iwasaki, T.; Kitano, S.; Satake, A.; Nomura, S.; Furukawa, T.; Matsui, K.; Sano, H. Il-2-anti-il-2 monoclonal antibody immune complexes inhibit collagen-induced arthritis by augmenting regulatory t cell functions. *J. Immunol.* **2018**, *201*, 1899–1906. [CrossRef] [PubMed]
53. Kouro, T.; Takatsu, K. Il-5- and eosinophil-mediated inflammation: From discovery to therapy. *Int. Immunol.* **2009**, *21*, 1303–1309. [CrossRef] [PubMed]
54. Chalan, P.; Bijzet, J.; van den Berg, A.; Kluiver, J.; Kroesen, B.J.; Boots, A.M.; Brouwer, E. Analysis of serum immune markers in seropositive and seronegative rheumatoid arthritis and in high-risk seropositive arthralgia patients. *Sci. Rep.* **2016**, *6*, 26021. [CrossRef]

55. De Franco, M.; Gille-Perramant, M.F.; Mevel, J.C.; Couderc, J. T helper subset involvement in two high antibody responder lines of mice (biozzi mice): Hi (susceptible) and hii (resistant) to collagen-induced arthritis. *Eur. J. Immunol.* **1995**, *25*, 132–136. [CrossRef]
56. Hoshino-Negishi, K.; Ohkuro, M.; Nakatani, T.; Kubo, Y.; Nishimura, M.; Ida, Y.; Kakuta, J.; Hamaguchi, A.; Kumai, M.; Kamisako, T.; et al. Role of anti-fractalkine antibody in suppression of joint destruction by inhibiting migration of osteoclast precursors to the synovium in experimental arthritis. *Arthritis Rheumatol.* **2019**, *71*, 222–231. [CrossRef]
57. Nanki, T.; Urasaki, Y.; Imai, T.; Nishimura, M.; Muramoto, K.; Kubota, T.; Miyasaka, N. Inhibition of fractalkine ameliorates murine collagen-induced arthritis. *J. Immunol.* **2004**, *173*, 7010–7016. [CrossRef]
58. Deng, J.; Liu, Y.; Yang, M.; Wang, S.; Zhang, M.; Wang, X.; Ko, K.H.; Hua, Z.; Sun, L.; Cao, X.; et al. Leptin exacerbates collagen-induced arthritis via enhancement of th17 cell response. *Arthritis Rheum.* **2012**, *64*, 3564–3573. [CrossRef]
59. Okano, T.; Koike, T.; Tada, M.; Sugioka, Y.; Mamoto, K.; Inui, K.; Okihana, H.; Ebihara, K.; Nakao, K.; Nakamura, H. Hyperleptinemia suppresses aggravation of arthritis of collagen-antibody-induced arthritis in mice. *J. Orthop. Sci.* **2015**, *20*, 1106–1113. [CrossRef]
60. Tian, G.; Liang, J.N.; Wang, Z.Y.; Zhou, D. Emerging role of leptin in rheumatoid arthritis. *Clin. Exp. Immunol.* **2014**, *177*, 557–570. [CrossRef]
61. Huang, Y.; Zheng, S.; Wang, R.; Tang, C.; Zhu, J.; Li, J. Ccl5 and related genes might be the potential diagnostic biomarkers for the therapeutic strategies of rheumatoid arthritis. *Clin. Rheumatol.* **2019**, *38*, 2629–2635. [CrossRef] [PubMed]
62. Rossato, C.; Albuquerque, L.L.; Katz, I.S.S.; Borrego, A.; Cabrera, W.H.K.; Spadafora-Ferreira, M.; Ribeiro, O.G.; Starobinas, N.; Ibanez, O.M.; De Franco, M.; et al. Early peritoneal cc chemokine production correlates with divergent inflammatory phenotypes and susceptibility to experimental arthritis in mice. *J. Immunol. Res.* **2019**, *2019*, 2641098. [CrossRef] [PubMed]
63. Jimenez-Boj, E.; Redlich, K.; Turk, B.; Hanslik-Schnabel, B.; Wanivenhaus, A.; Chott, A.; Smolen, J.S.; Schett, G. Interaction between synovial inflammatory tissue and bone marrow in rheumatoid arthritis. *J. Immunol.* **2005**, *175*, 2579–2588. [CrossRef] [PubMed]
64. Marinova-Mutafchieva, L.; Williams, R.C.; Funa, K.; Maini, R.N.; Zvaifler, N.J. Inflammation is preceded by tumor necrosis factor-dependent infiltration of mesenchymal cells in experimental arthritis. *Arthritis Rheum.* **2002**, *46*, 507–513. [CrossRef]
65. Santiago-Schwarz, F.; Sullivan, C.; Rappa, D.; Carsons, S.E. Distinct alterations in lineage committed progenitor cells exist in the peripheral blood of patients with rheumatoid arthritis and primary sjogren's syndrome. *J. Rheumatol.* **1996**, *23*, 439–446.
66. Tomita, T.; Takeuchi, E.; Toyosaki-Maeda, T.; Oku, H.; Kaneko, M.; Takano, H.; Sugamoto, K.; Ohzono, K.; Suzuki, R.; Ochi, T. Establishment of nurse-like stromal cells from bone marrow of patients with rheumatoid arthritis: Indication of characteristic bone marrow microenvironment in patients with rheumatoid arthritis. *Rheumatology (Oxford)* **1999**, *38*, 854–863. [CrossRef]
67. Papadaki, H.A.; Kritikos, H.D.; Gemetzi, C.; Koutala, H.; Marsh, J.C.; Boumpas, D.T.; Eliopoulos, G.D. Bone marrow progenitor cell reserve and function and stromal cell function are defective in rheumatoid arthritis: Evidence for a tumor necrosis factor alpha-mediated effect. *Blood* **2002**, *99*, 1610–1619. [CrossRef]
68. Kastrinaki, M.C.; Sidiropoulos, P.; Roche, S.; Ringe, J.; Lehmann, S.; Kritikos, H.; Vlahava, V.M.; Delorme, B.; Eliopoulos, G.D.; Jorgensen, C.; et al. Functional, molecular and proteomic characterisation of bone marrow mesenchymal stem cells in rheumatoid arthritis. *Ann. Rheum. Dis.* **2008**, *67*, 741–749. [CrossRef]
69. Sun, Y.; Deng, W.; Geng, L.; Zhang, L.; Liu, R.; Chen, W.; Yao, G.; Zhang, H.; Feng, X.; Gao, X.; et al. Mesenchymal stem cells from patients with rheumatoid arthritis display impaired function in inhibiting th17 cells. *J. Immunol. Res.* **2015**, *2015*, 284215. [CrossRef]
70. Dudics, V.; Kunstar, A.; Kovacs, J.; Lakatos, T.; Geher, P.; Gomor, B.; Monostori, E.; Uher, F. Chondrogenic potential of mesenchymal stem cells from patients with rheumatoid arthritis and osteoarthritis: Measurements in a microculture system. *Cells Tissues Organs* **2009**, *189*, 307–316. [CrossRef]

71. Tong, Y.; Niu, M.; Du, Y.; Mei, W.; Cao, W.; Dou, Y.; Yu, H.; Du, X.; Yuan, H.; Zhao, W. Aryl hydrocarbon receptor suppresses the osteogenesis of mesenchymal stem cells in collagen-induced arthritic mice through the inhibition of beta-catenin. *Exp. Cell Res.* **2017**, *350*, 349–357. [CrossRef] [PubMed]
72. Huang, H.; Zhao, N.; Xu, X.; Xu, Y.; Li, S.; Zhang, J.; Yang, P. Dose-specific effects of tumor necrosis factor alpha on osteogenic differentiation of mesenchymal stem cells. *Cell Prolif.* **2011**, *44*, 420–427. [CrossRef] [PubMed]

International Journal of *Molecular Sciences*

MDPI

Article

Treadmill Running in Established Phase Arthritis Inhibits Joint Destruction in Rat Rheumatoid Arthritis Models

Yuta Fujii [1], Hiroaki Inoue [1], Yuji Arai [2,*], Seiji Shimomura [1], Shuji Nakagawa [2], Tsunao Kishida [3], Shinji Tsuchida [1], Yoichiro Kamada [1], Kenta Kaihara [1], Toshiharu Shirai [1], Ryu Terauchi [1], Shogo Toyama [1], Kazuya Ikoma [1], Osam Mazda [3] and Yasuo Mikami [4]

1 Department of Orthopaedics, Graduate School of Medical Science, Kyoto Prefectural University of Medicine, Kawaramachi-Hirokoji, Kamigyo-ku, Kyoto 602-8566, Japan; y-fujii@koto.kpu-m.ac.jp (Y.F.); hinoue@koto.kpu-m.ac.jp (H.I.); s-shimo@koto.kpu-m.ac.jp (S.S.); tuchi-kf@koto.kpu-m.ac.jp (S.T.); kamada-y@koto.kpu-m.ac.jp (Y.K.); kaihara5@koto.kpu-m.ac.jp (K.K.); shirai.t77@gmail.com (T.S.); ryutel@mbox.kyoto-inet.or.jp (R.T.); shogot@koto.kpu-m.ac.jp (S.T.); kazuya@koto.kpu-m.ac.jp (K.I.)

2 Department of Sports and Para-Sports Medicine, Graduate School of Medical Science, Kyoto Prefectural University of Medicine, Kawaramachi-Hirokoji, Kamigyo-ku, Kyoto 602-8566, Japan; shushi@koto.kpu-m.ac.jp

3 Department of Immunology, Graduate School of Medical Science, Kyoto Prefectural University of Medicine, Kawaramachi-Hirokoji, Kamigyo-ku, Kyoto 602-8566, Japan; tsunao@koto.kpu-m.ac.jp (T.K.); mazda@koto.kpu-m.ac.jp (O.M.)

4 Department of Rehabilitation Medicine, Graduate School of Medical Science, Kyoto Prefectural University of Medicine, Kawaramachi-Hirokoji, Kamigyo-ku, Kyoto 602-8566, Japan; mikami@koto.kpu-m.ac.jp

* Correspondence: y123arai@koto.kpu-m.ac.jp; Tel.: +81-75-251-5139; Fax.: +81-75-251-5433

Received: 13 September 2019; Accepted: 13 October 2019; Published: 15 October 2019

Abstract: Exercise therapy inhibits joint destruction by suppressing pro-inflammatory cytokines. The efficacy of pharmacotherapy for rheumatoid arthritis differs depending on the phase of the disease, but that of exercise therapy for each phase is unknown. We assessed the differences in the efficacy of treadmill running on rheumatoid arthritis at various phases, using rat rheumatoid arthritis models. Rats with collagen-induced arthritis were used as rheumatoid arthritis models, and the phase after immunization was divided as pre-arthritis and established phases. Histologically, the groups with forced treadmill running in the established phase had significantly inhibited joint destruction compared with the other groups. The group with forced treadmill running in only the established phase had significantly better bone morphometry and reduced expression of connexin 43 and tumor necrosis factor α in the synovial membranes compared with the no treadmill group. Furthermore, few cells were positive for cathepsin K immunostaining in the groups with forced treadmill running in the established phase. Our results suggest that the efficacy of exercise therapy may differ depending on rheumatoid arthritis disease activity. Active exercise during phases of decreased disease activity may effectively inhibit arthritis and joint destruction.

Keywords: rheumatoid arthritis; exercise therapy; autoimmune disorder; treadmill running; exercise; articular cartilage; collagen-induced arthritis; pro-inflammatory cytokine; connexin 43; osteoporosis

1. Introduction

Rheumatoid arthritis (RA) is an autoimmune disorder that particularly affects the synovial membranes. Affected synovial membranes produce an excess of pro-inflammatory cytokines and chemokines, such as tumor necrosis factor (TNF)-α, interleukin (IL)-6, IL-1b, and stromal cell-derived factor 1, which destroy the joints and cause pain and a restricted range of motion [1–3]. Other than the joints, RA also affects major internal organs, including the heart, lungs, liver, and brain [4]. The progress of these arthritic and systemic symptoms reduces patients' activities of daily living (ADL), and because it causes a variety of disabilities, RA is a disease of public health importance, and it must be managed as such.

In RA treatment, priority is given to pharmacotherapy. In recent years, a paradigm shift has occurred in RA pharmacotherapy due to the arrival of biological disease-modifying anti-rheumatic drugs (bDMARDs), and it has become possible to minimize joint destruction [5–7]. However, bDMARDs have the disadvantages of adverse drug reactions and high costs, and they can only be used in limited cases [8,9]. Exploring other modalities of treatment of RA is therefore becoming increasingly important. One of such methods is exercise therapy. Exercise therapy is a safe and economical treatment that is widely used for the treatment of several systemic diseases; not only joint diseases. Exercise therapy was conducted based on the experience of individual doctors or therapists. In recent years, its mechanisms are becoming clearer, and evidence is accumulating. Among the various available exercise options, exercise therapy using treadmills works to protect articular cartilage and subchondral bone [10]. In osteoarthritis (OA), it inhibits the formation of bone spurs and bone destruction [11], and it thereby reduces joint symptoms. Treadmill exercise has also been reported to improve cardio-pulmonary function and ADL for patients with heart or lung disease [12,13]. Exercise therapy for RA is strongly recommended by a Cochrane review [14], and it has been reported to improve bodily functions and ADL, clinical indicators of joint symptoms, muscle strength, and cardio-pulmonary function [15,16]. In recent years, treadmill running in rat RA models was reported to inhibit the production of connexin 43 (Cx43) and TNF-α in the synovial membranes, as well as prevent the degeneration of articular cartilage and subchondral bone [17]. It was also revealed that exercise therapy inhibits joint destruction through bio-molecular mechanisms by suppressing pro-inflammatory cytokines.

The natural course of RA is divided into an induction phase following immunological sensitization, a pre-arthritis phase during which autoantibodies are produced, and an established phase during which arthritis occurs and progresses [18]. The effectiveness of treatment may vary with the phase of disease. Dekkers et al. used animal models to study the differences in efficacy of pharmacotherapy for each phase, and they established that pharmacotherapy is more effective in the established phase than in the pre-arthritis phase [19]. It was found that compared with the pre-arthritis phase, in which cytokine production increases sharply, it is easier to get efficacy from anti-TNF-α antibodies in the established phase, during which cytokine quantities are stable. Thus, phase-related differences in cytokine production influence the efficacy of pharmacotherapy [20]. However, phase-related differences in the efficacy of exercise therapy are unknown. Since exercise therapy also demonstrates efficacy in suppressing cytokines, we posed the hypothesis that it would be more effective to suppress arthritis and joint destruction with treadmill running during the established phase than in the pre-arthritis phase.

Based on the above context, the objective of this study was to assess the differences in efficacy of treadmill running during each phase of RA, using rat RA models.

2. Results

2.1. Kinetic Change in Body Weight and Paw Volume

Body weight in each group (no intervention (control) group, pre-arthritis intervention short (PAS) group, pre-arthritis intervention long (PAL) group, and therapeutic intervention (T) group) gradually increased from day 0 to day 12, decreased from day 12 to day 20, and increased again starting on day 21. Paw volume in each group increased from day 14, reaching its maximum between day 20 and day 23, and gradually decreasing thereafter. No significant differences in either body weight or paw volume were observed among groups from day 0 to day 42 (Figure 1A–C).

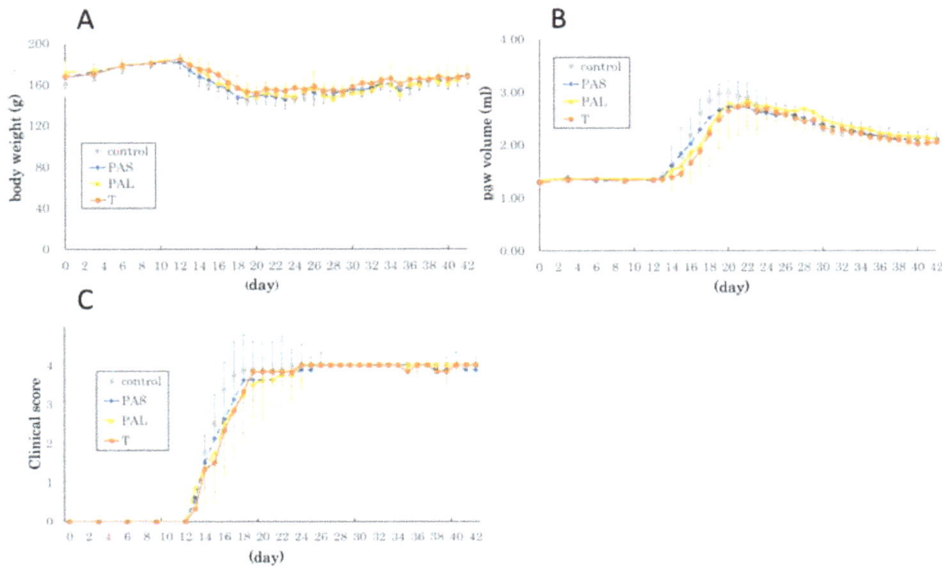

Figure 1. Kinetic change in (**A**) body weight, (**B**) paw volume, and (**C**) clinical score after immunization. The parameters were measured once every three days until day 12 and every day thereafter. There were no significant differences among the four groups (no intervention group, control; pre-arthritis intervention short group, PAS; pre-arthritis intervention long group, PAL; therapeutic intervention group, T) on all days.

2.2. *Effect of Treadmill Running on Articular Cartilage*

To assess the histological effects of treadmill running on joints and their cartilage, we stained the articular cartilage from the rat paws with hematoxylin and eosin (H&E), and safranin O on day 42 (Figure 2A–D). In the control group and the PAS group, we observed intra-articular infiltration by inflammatory cells and pannus formation in hyperplastic synovial membranes. Joint structure destruction was also more severe in these groups than in the T group and the PAL group. Furthermore, safranin O staining in the control and PAS groups was less than in the T and PAL groups. The histological scores were significantly lower in the T and PAL groups than in the control and PAS groups. There was no difference in histological score between the PAS and control groups (Figure 2E,F).

2.3. *Influence of Treadmill Running on the Production of TNF-α and Cx43 in the Synovium*

Following past reports, we conducted immunostaining for TNF-α and Cx43 [17]. TNF-α expression was aggravated throughout the synovial membranes, but the level of staining was significantly lower for the T group than for the control group (Figure 3A,C). For Cx43, the level of staining was significantly lower for the T group than for the control and PAS groups (Figure 3B,D).

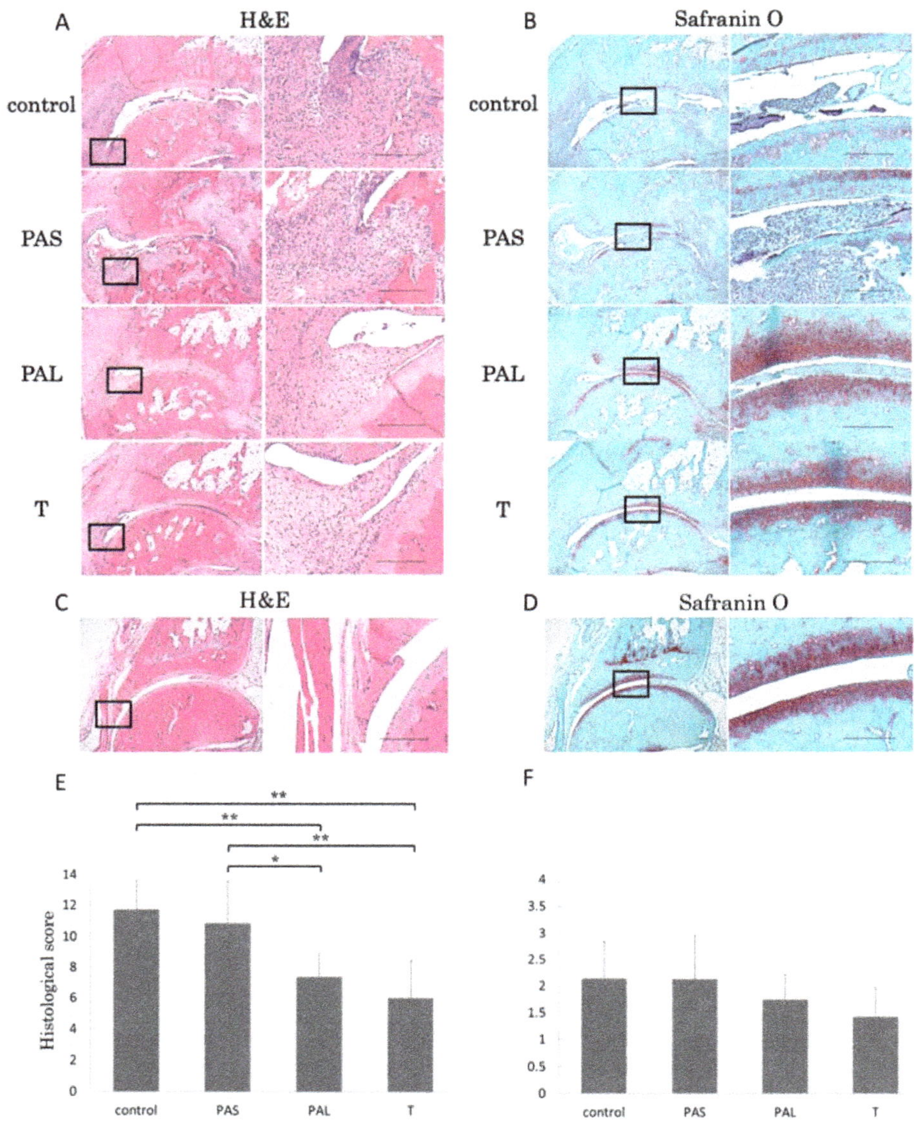

Figure 2. Representative micrographs of (**A**) hematoxylin and eosin, and (**B**) safranin O-stained sagittal sections. Representative micrographs of (**C**) hematoxylin and eosin, and (**D**) safranin O-stained sagittal sections in a normal rat without treadmill running. (**E**) The histological scores (mean ± standard deviation) and (**F**) only the cartilage evaluation scored based on the histological score (mean ± standard deviation) are shown. The PAL and T groups had suppressed destruction of the ankle joint more than the control and PAS groups. ** $p < 0.01$, * $p < 0.05$. Scale bar = 200 μm. The black spot represents the position in the high-magnification figure.

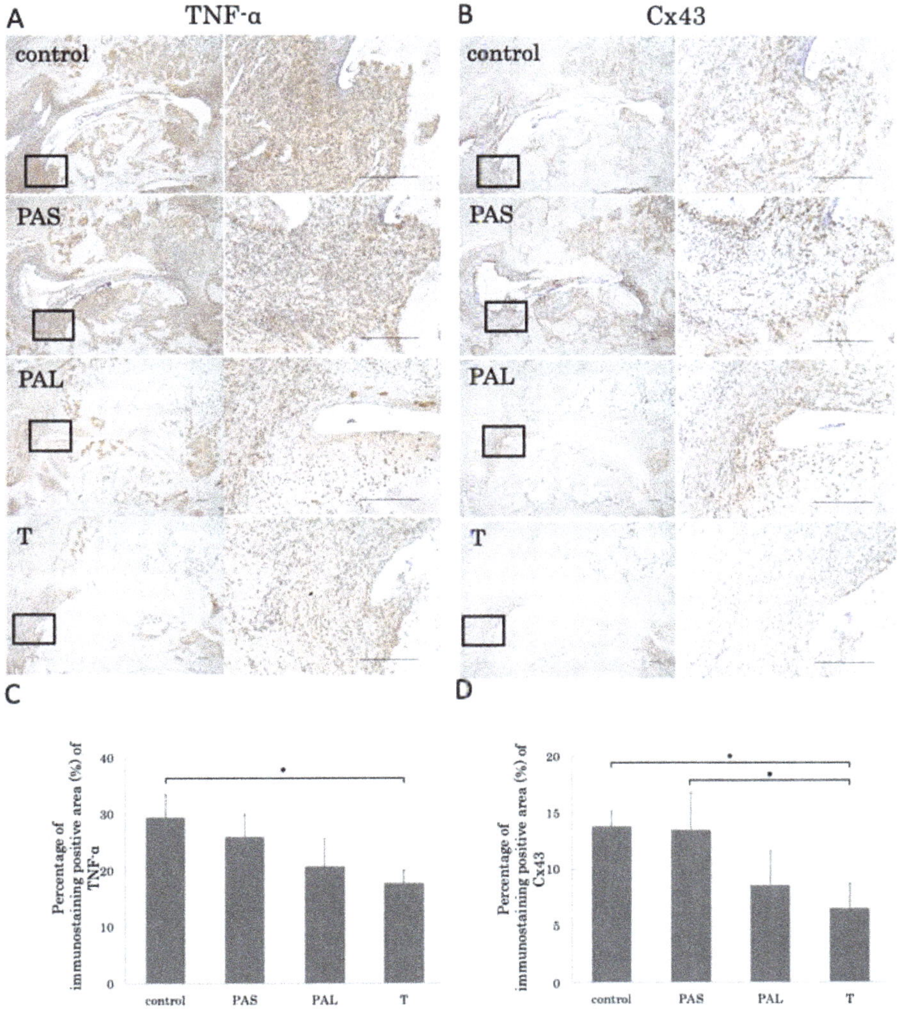

Figure 3. Representative micrographs of immunohistochemical staining for (**A**) TNF-α and (**B**) Cx43 are shown. All images were evaluated semi-quantitatively using ImageJ for (**C**) TNF-α and (**D**) Cx43. T group had significantly suppressed TNF-α and Cx43 expression. * $p < 0.05$. Scale bar = 200 μm. The black spot represents the position in the high-magnification figure.

2.4. Prevention of Bone Loss by Treadmill Running

We used micro-computed tomography (μ-CT) to assess periarticular skeletal composition changes (Figure 4). The T group had higher bone volume fraction (BV/TV), trabecular thickness (Tb.Th), and bone mineral content per tissue volume (BMC/TV) than the control group (Figure 4A,B,D). Furthermore, marrow star volume (MSV) values were significantly lower for the T group than for the control group (Figure 4C).

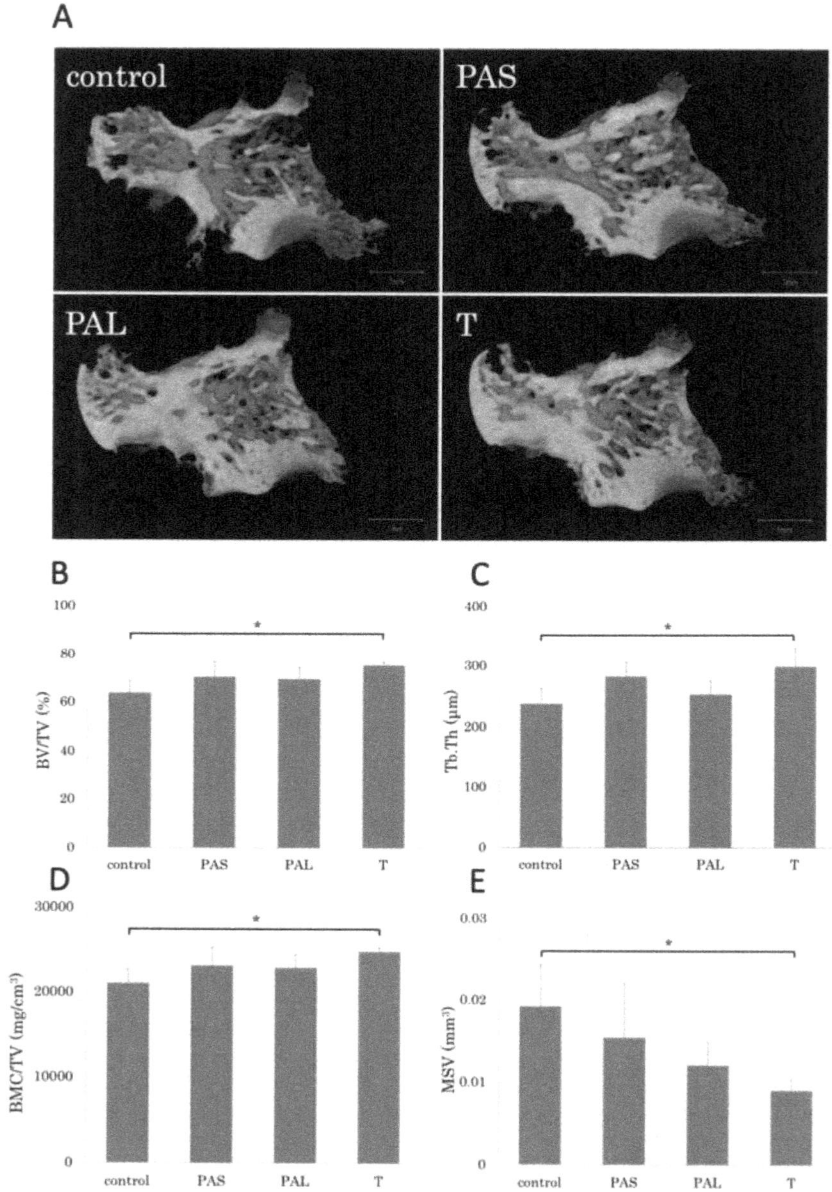

Figure 4. Representative three-dimensional reconstruction of (**A**) the sagittal sections of the talus architecture. Trabecular bone parameters such as (**B**) bone volume fraction (BV/TV), (**C**) trabecular thickness (Tb.Th), (**D**) bone mineral content per tissue volume (BMC/TV), and (**E**) marrow star volume (MSV) of the whole talus are shown. T group had improved bone loss. $n = 4$ in each group. * $p < 0.05$.

2.5. *Effects of Treadmill Running on Bone Erosion*

We used μ-CT to assess the effects of treadmill running on bone erosion (Figure 5). The eroded bone surface per repaired bone surface (Es/Rps) value for T group was significantly lower than that of the control group (Figure 5B,C). To assess its effects on bone metabolism, we conducted immunostaining with cathepsin K, one of the osteoclast marker that serves as an indicator of the degree of bone resorption [21,22]. Many cathepsin K-positive cells were observed in the pannus areas of the control and PAS groups. Fewer cathepsin K-positive cells were in the T and PAL groups than in the control and PAS groups (Figure 5A).

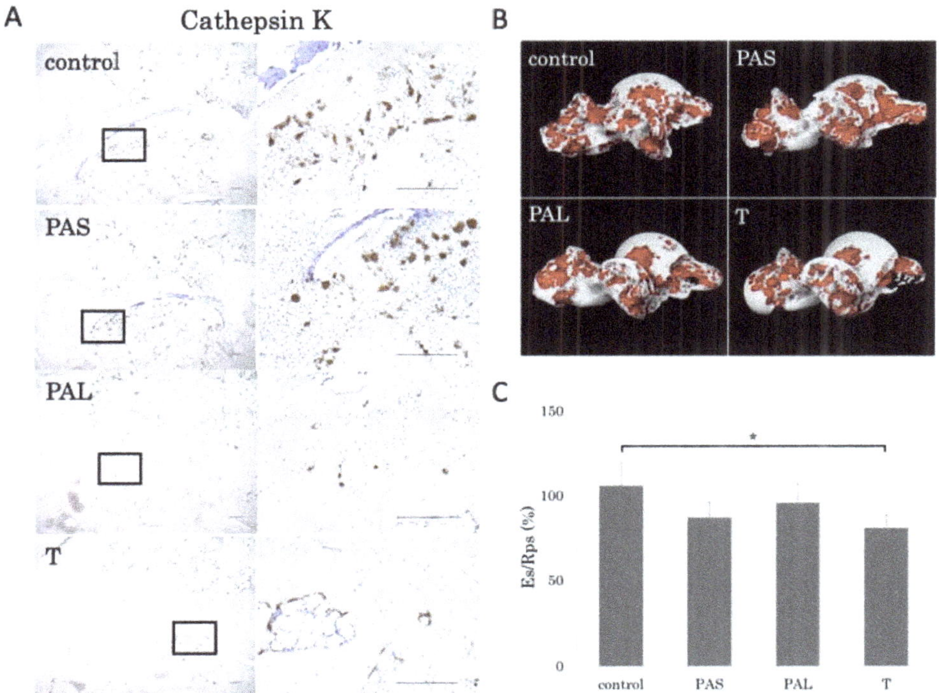

Figure 5. (**A**) Representative micrographs of cathepsin K immunohistochemical staining. Cathepsin K positive cells were fewer in the PAL and T groups. (**B**) Representative 3D reconstruction of bone erosion area in the whole talus architecture. Red area is bone erosion area. (**C**) The eroded bone surface (Es) and repaired bone surface (Rps) was calculated using 3D-μ-CT, and Es/Rps values are shown for the four groups. Es/Rps was significantly lower in the **T** group compared to the control group. * $p < 0.05$. Scale bar = 200 μm. The black spot represents the position in the high-magnification figure.

3. Discussion

In this study, we conducted comparative analyses on four groups of rat RA models to assess the differences in the efficacy of treadmill running treatment in each phase of RA. We studied a control group that was raised freely after immunological sensitization, a PAS group that did treadmill running only during the pre-arthritis phase, a PAL group that did treadmill running from the pre-arthritis phase to the established phase, and a T group that did treadmill running only during the established phase. The results revealed that there were no differences in body weight among the groups, and that even if 12 m/min treadmill running was conducted in any phase, there were no effects on the general condition of the rats. Furthermore, there were no differences among the groups in terms of paw volume, but histologically, joint destruction was significantly suppressed in the PAL and T groups when compared with the control and PAS groups.

Based on these results, we concluded that treadmill running more effectively suppresses joint destruction during the established phase of RA than during the pre-arthritis phase.

We also analyzed the role of Cx43 as a key gene in synovial membrane inflammation in RA. Studies have shown that, in collagen-induced arthritis (CIA) rats, Cx43 induces joint destruction through pro-inflammatory cytokines such as TNF-α and IL-6, and that joint destruction is suppressed not only if Cx43 expression is suppressed in small interfering ribonucleic acid, but also by suppressing Cx43 expression through treadmill running as well [17,23,24]. Cx43 expression changes with mechanical stress such as stretching stimuli and shearing forces in cardiomyocytes and osteocytes [25,26]; therefore, it may also change due to the addition of mechanical stress to the synovial membranes by treadmill running. In this study, TNF-α expression in the synovial membranes of the T group was significantly lower than that of the control group, but there were no differences in TNF-α expression between the control and PAS groups. As with TNF-α, Cx43 expression in the synovial membranes of the T group was significantly lower than in the control and PAS groups.

Taking these results and the structural results into consideration together, we are of the opinion that treadmill running during the pre-arthritis phase is unable to suppress the sudden spike in Cx43 and TNF-α expression that has been described to occur in this phase, and does not completely suppress arthritis or joint destruction. However, treadmill running during the established phase can suppress the expression of these substances in their steady state, and thus suppress arthritis and joint destruction.

In this study, our analysis of the efficacy of treadmill running in suppressing bone destruction during each phase of RA found that with respect to bone morphometry, BV/TV, Tb.Th, and BMC/TV increased in the T group relative to the control group. MSV tended to be lower for the three groups that did treadmill running than for the control group, and it was especially low in the T group. These results made it clear that treadmill running was most effective in suppressing bone destruction in the established phase of RA. Furthermore, talus surface absorption area (Es/Rps)—which is an indicator of bone destruction—was suppressed in the T group. The T and PAL also groups had fewer cathepsin K immunostaining positive cells than the control and PAS groups.

Osteoclasts that differentiate from bone marrow-derived monocyte-macrophage progenitors play an important role in bone destruction in RA, and suppressing their differentiation is essential for suppressing bone destruction. Differentiation from progenitor cells into osteoclasts is facilitated by TNF-α [27], and because TNF-α is suppressed by mechanical stress [28], we conclude that in this study, bone destruction was suppressed through treadmill running during the established phase, in which mechanical stress exerted on the synovial membranes suppressed TNF-α expression, and the stress itself directly suppressed osteoclast differentiation. Furthermore, the receptor activator of the nuclear factor-kappa B ligand (RANKL) is also the key cytokine that induces osteoclast formation. In RA, osteoclasts are responsible for bone erosion, and they undergo differentiation and activation by RANKL, which is secreted by synovial fibroblasts, T cells, and B cells. Sato et al. reported that the inflammatory cytokines enhance RANKL expression in osteoclastogenesis-supporting cells and activate osteoclast precursor cells by synergizing with RANKL signaling [29]. Therefore, the decrease in the inflammatory cytokines, such as TNF-α, due to treadmill running may partly suppress osteoclast differentiation via RANKL.

The results of this study revealed the potential for efficacy of exercise therapy to differ depending on RA disease activity. We suggest that in phases with high disease activity, that is when arthritis is exacerbated, it may be possible to more effectively suppress arthritis and joint destruction by using pharmacotherapy in a central role, and at the same time using active exercise therapy during phases in which disease activity declines and inflammatory cytokine production is in a steady state.

There were several limitations to this study. First, we did not conduct a detailed study on the mechanisms through which treadmill running suppresses Cx43 and TNF-α. Second, when considering clinical applications, pharmacotherapy is necessary, but we did not study the efficacy of combined pharmacotherapy and exercise therapy. Third, we only investigated immunostaining with cathepsin K as an osteoclast marker without using tartrate-resistant acid phosphatase staining and measuring the serum C-telopeptide of type I collagen level.

4. Materials and Methods

This study was conducted in accordance with the animal research guidelines of the Kyoto Prefectural University of Medicine, Kyoto, Japan (code no. M29-22, 1 April 2017).

4.1. CIA Model

Rat CIA models have many points of similarity with human RA and are widely used for RA studies in vivo. To create such models for this study, type II collagen (CII; Collagen Research Center, Tokyo, Japan) and Freund's incomplete adjuvant (FIA; Sigma-Aldrich, Saint Louis, MO, USA) were blended and emulsified on ice in a 1:1 ratio. Then, to create rat CIA models, 200 μL of the CII/FIA solution was intracutaneously injected into 32 8-week-old male Dark Agouti (DA) rats (Shimizu Laboratory Suppliers, Kyoto, Japan) at the base of the tail [30]. The rats weighed between 140 and 190 g.

4.2. Treadmill Running Protocol

Based on the study by Dekkers et al. [19], we divided all the induced rats into the following groups: the control group ($n = 8$), which was freely raised at random; and the pre-arthritis intervention short (PAS) ($n = 8$), pre-arthritis intervention long (PAL) ($n = 8$), and therapeutic intervention (T) ($n = 8$) groups, which were made to run on a treadmill (TMS8D; MEQUEST, Toyama, Japan) from day 14 to 28, day 14 to 42, and day 28 to 42, respectively. The running conditions for the PAS, PAL, and T groups were set for efficacy of suppression of joint destruction in rat OA models and rat RA models from a previous study: 5 times/week, speed of 12 m/min, 30 min/day [17,31]. Rats with CIA may have reduced activity due to inflammation and pain. To ensure uniform activity, we applied slightly electric stimulation to encourage the rat from behind if it stopped on the treadmill machine. In this study, all rats ran without electric stimulation, so they all had the same performance. The running protocols for each group are shown in Figure 6. The rats were raised in 12-h light:dark cycles and allowed free access to food and water. All the rats were sacrificed on day 42.

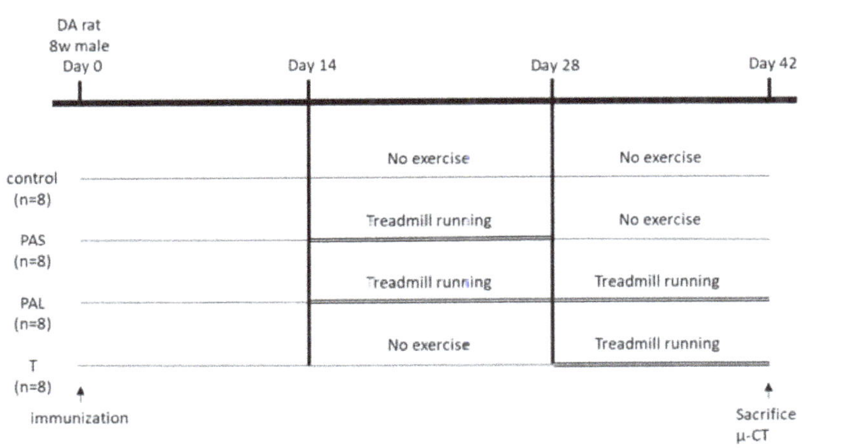

Figure 6. Experimental protocols. Eight-week-old male Dark Agouti rats were randomly divided into four groups: control, PAS, PAL, and T groups. PAS ($n = 8$), run from day 14 to 28; PAL ($n = 8$), run from day 14 to 42; and T ($n = 8$), run from day 28 to 42.

4.3. Body Weight, Paw Volume, and Clinical Score

Body weight, paw volume, and clinical score were measured on days 0, 3, 6, 9, and 12, and daily from then (Figure 2). Paw volume was measured with a water replacement plethysmometer (Unicom

Japan, Tokyo, Japan). The clinical score was defined as follows: score 0, normal paw; score 1, inflammation and swelling of one toe; score 2, inflammation and swelling of > 1 toe with inflammation and swelling of the entire paw or mild swelling of the entire paw; score 3, inflammation and swelling of the entire paw; score 4, severe inflammation and swelling of the entire paw or ankylosed paw [32]. Specimens with maximum paw volume < 2.5 mL were excluded because immunization of those rats is insufficient. Thus, two rats were excluded, one in the control group and another in the T group.

4.4. Histochemical Analyses and Semi-Quantitative Analyses

After the end of the treadmill running protocol, the right ankle joints of the rats were removed and set in 4% paraformaldehyde (Wako, Osaka, Japan). They were then decalcified with 20% ethylenediaminetetraacetic acid and embedded in paraffin. The center of each ankle joint was sliced in 6-μm thick sagittal slices, and stained with H&E and safranin O. Arthritic changes, such as infiltration of inflammatory cells, synovial proliferation, destruction of articular cartilage, and bone erosion, were then evaluated histologically, and we measured the histological score as described by Weinberger et al. [33]. In brief, the infiltration of mononuclear cells (0–3 points) and histiocytes (0–3 points) into the synovium, cartilage destruction (0–3 points), and bone erosion (0–5 points) were measured.

4.5. Immunohistochemical Analyses

For immunohistochemistry of TNF-α, Cx43, and cathepsin K, paraffin-embedded joint tissue sections were de-paraffinized in xylene, rehydrated with graded alcohol, and immersed in 0.4 mg/mL of phosphate buffered saline (PBS). Antigen activation was conducted in 8-min intervals with proteinase K, and endogenous peroxidase activity block was conducted at 5-min intervals with 3% H_2O_2. Rabbit polyclonal anti-TNF-α antibodies (ab6671, Abcam, Cambridge, UK) at a concentration of 1:150, and anti-Cx43 antibodies (#3512, Cell Signaling Technology, Danvers, MA, USA) at a concentration of 1:50 were incubated overnight at 4 °C. Rabbit polyclonal anti-cathepsin K (111239-1-AP, Proteintech, Chicago, IL, USA) at a concentration of 1:2000 was incubated for 50 min at room temperature. The sections were incubated in Histofine Simple Stain Rat MAX-PO for 30 min at room temperature, after extensive washing with PBS. Immunostaining was detected by 3,3′-diaminobenzidine (DAB) staining. Counter staining was done with Mayer's hematoxylin. We confirmed that there is no nonspecific staining. TNF-α and Cx43 staining areas of the synovial membrane interstitial cells were calculated using ImageJ® with modifying a method reported by Mane et al. [34]. In detail, three fields of view with a magnification of 400× were taken randomly. The images were deconvoluted and showed only DAB immunoreaction. A standard threshold was maintained without any adjustment. The percentage of the immunostained-positive area was averaged. Validation of ImageJ® analysis was performed by two expert orthopedists. Quantification of all the images was blinded.

4.6. Micro-Computed Tomography Analysis

The left ankle joints of the rats were fixed in 70% ethanol and scanned with a μ-CT system (TOSCANER-32300μFD, Toshiba, Tokyo, Japan). The reconstructed data sets were examined with three-dimensional data analysis software (TRI/3-D-BON, Ratoc System Engineering Co., Tokyo, Japan; $n = 4$ for each group) [35]. The regions of interest were defined in the whole talus bones. To analyze the talus, the following trabecular bone parameters in the whole talus were evaluated: bone volume fraction, Tb.Th, and bone mineral content per tissue volume (BMC/TV). We also assessed indirect parameters, including MSV, which is the mean volume of all the parts of an object that can be unobscured in all the directions from a point inside the object [36]. The degree of bone erosion and bone formation were also analyzed using 3D-μ-CT. Eroded bone surface per repaired bone surface (Es/Rps) on whole talus was determined with the software automatically according to the software program. We set the concave surface search range up to 0.5 mm, and the absorption surface extraction radius of curvature was 240 μm or less.

4.7. Statistical Analysis

All data were presented as the mean and standard deviation and analyzed with Statistical Package for Social Sciences (SPSS) 26.0 for Windows (SPSS Inc., Chicago, IL, USA). The data were analyzed by analysis of variance, and post hoc testing was performed with the Tukey–Kramer test. In all analyses, $p < 0.05$ was defined as statistically significant.

5. Conclusions

This study was the first to report on the varying effects of treadmill running, at different phases of RA, on the synovial membranes, articular cartilages, and bones of rat RA models. For RA patients as well, it may be possible for therapeutic exercise in the appropriate phases to increase bio-molecular suppression of arthritis through the suppression of inflammatory cytokine expression, and to consequently suppress joint destruction.

Author Contributions: Conceptualization, Y.F., S.S., H.I., and S.N.; Methodology, T.K.; Software, Y.F.; Validation, S.T. (Shinji Tsuchida), R.T., T.S., and K.I.; Formal analysis, Y.F. and S.T. (Shogo Toyama); Investigation, Y.F., S.S., Y.K., and K.K.; Resources, Y.A.; Data curation, Y. F., H.I., and Y.A.; Writing–original draft preparation, Y.F.; Writing–review and editing, all authors; Visualization, Y.F.; Supervision, T.K. and O.M.; Project administration, Y.A. and Y.M.; Funding acquisition, Y.F., S.T. (Shogo Toyama), S.N., and Y.A.

Funding: This work was supported by JSPS KAKENHI (grant numbers 17H02136, 18K10752, and 19K19914) and Grant of Japan Sports Medicine Foundation, 2018.

Acknowledgments: We would like to thank Editage (www.editage.com) for English language editing.

Conflicts of Interest: The authors declare no conflict of interest.

Abbreviations

μ-CT	micro-computed tomography
ADL	activities of daily living
bDMARDs	biological disease-modifying anti-rheumatic drugs
BMC/TV	bone mineral content per tissue volume
BV/TV	bone volume fraction
CIA	collagen-induced arthritis
Cx43	connexin 43
Es/Rps	eroded bone surface per repaired bone surface
H&E	hematoxylin and eosin
IL	interleukin
MSV	marrow star volume
OA	osteoarthritis
PAL	pre-arthritis intervention long
PAS	pre-arthritis intervention short
RA	rheumatoid arthritis
SPSS	Statistical Package for Social Sciences
T	therapeutic intervention
Tb.Th	trabecular thickness
TNF	tumor necrosis factor

References

1. Nanki, T.; Hayashida, K.; El-Gabalawy, H.S.; Suson, S.; Shi, K.; Girschick, H.J.; Yavuz, S.; Lipsky, P.E. Stromal cell-derived factor-1-CXC chemokine receptor 4 interactions play a central role in CD4+ T cell accumulation in rheumatoid arthritis synovium. *J. Immunol.* **2000**, *165*, 6590–6598. [CrossRef] [PubMed]
2. Aletaha, D.; Neogi, T.; Silman, A.J.; Funovits, J.; Felson, D.T.; Bingham, C.O.; Birnbaum, N.S.; Burmester, G.R.; Bykerk, V.P.; Cohen, M.D.; et al. Rheumatoid arthritis classification criteria: An American College of Rheumatology/European League Against Rheumatism collaborative initiative. *Arthritis Rheum.* **2010**, *62*, 2569–2581. [CrossRef] [PubMed]

3. Mcknnes, I.B.; Schett, G. The pathogenesis of rheumatoid arthritis. *N. Engl. J. Med.* **2011**, *365*, 2205–2219. [CrossRef] [PubMed]
4. Alam, J.; Jantan, I.; Bukhari, S.N.A. Rheumatoid arthritis: Recent advances on its etiology, role of cytokines and pharmacotherapy. *Biomed. Pharm.* **2017**, *92*, 615–633. [CrossRef]
5. Maini, R.; St Clair, E.W.; Breedveld, F.; Furst, D.; Kalden, J.; Weisman, M.; Smolen, J.; Emery, P.; Harriman, G.; Feldmann, M.; et al. Infliximab (chimeric anti-tumour necrosis factor α monoclonal antibody) versus placebo in rheumatoid arthritis patients receiving concomitant methotrexate: A randomised phase III trial. *Lancet* **1999**, *354*, 1932–1939. [CrossRef]
6. Lipsky, P.E.; Van der Heijde, D.M.; St Clair, E.W.; Furst, D.E.; Breedveid, F.C.; Kalden, J.R.; Smolen, J.R.; Weisman, M.; Emery, P.; Feldmann, M.; et al. Infliximab and methotrexate in the treatment of rheumatoid arthritis. Anti-tumor necrosis factor trial in rheumatoid arthritis with concomitant therapy study group. *N. Engl. J. Med.* **2000**, *343*, 1594–1602. [CrossRef]
7. Smolen, J.S.; Weinblatt, M.E.; Sheng, S.; Zhuang, Y.; Hsu, B. Sirukumab. A human anti-interleukin-6 monoclonal antibody: A randomised, 2-part (proof-of-concept and dose-finding), phase II study in patients with active rheumatoid arthritis despite methotrexate therapy. *Ann. Rheum. Dis.* **2014**, *73*, 1616–1625. [CrossRef]
8. Genovese, M.C.; McKay, J.D.; Nasonov, E.L.; Mysler, E.F.; da Silva, N.A.; Alecock, E.; Woodworth, T.; Gomez-Reino, J.J. Interleukin-6 receptor inhibition with tocilizumab reduces disease activity in rheumatoid arthritis with inadequate response to disease-modifying antirheumatic drugs: The tocilizumab in combination with traditional disease-modifying antirheumatic drug therapy study. *Arthritis Rheum.* **2008**, *58*, 2968–2980.
9. Singh, J.A.; Wells, G.A.; Christensen, R.; Tanjong Ghogomu, E.; Maxwell, L.; Macdonald, J.K.; Filippini, G.; Skoetz, N.; Francis, D.; Lopes, L.C.; et al. Adverse effects of biologics: A network meta-analysis and Cochrane overview. *Cochrane Database Syst. Rev.* **2011**, CD008794. [CrossRef]
10. Zhang, W.; Nuki, G.; Moskowitz, R.W.; Abramson, S.; Altman, R.D.; Arden, N.K.; Bierma-Zeinstra, S.; Brandt, K.D.; Croft, P.; Doherty, M.; et al. OARSI recommendations for the management of hip and knee osteoarthritis, Part III: Changes in evidence following systematic cumulative update of research published through January 2009. *Osteoarthr. Cartil.* **2010**, *18*, 476–499. [CrossRef]
11. Iijima, H.; Aoyama, T.; Ito, A.; Yamaguchi, S.; Nagai, M.; Tajino, J.; Zhang, X.; Kuroki, H. Effects of short-term gentle treadmill walking on subchondral bone in a rat model of instability-induced osteoarthritis. *Osteoarthr. Cartil.* **2015**, *23*, 1563–1574. [CrossRef] [PubMed]
12. Ingle, L. Theoretical rationale and practical recommendations for cardiopulmonary exercise testing in patients with chronic heart failure. *Heart Fail. Rev.* **2007**, *12*, 12–22. [CrossRef] [PubMed]
13. Salcedo, P.A.; Lindheimer, J.B.; Klein-Adams, J.C.; Sotolongo, A.M.; Falvo, M.J. Effects of exercise training on pulmonary function in adults with chronic lung disease: A meta-analysis of randomized controlled trials. *Arch. Phys. Med. Rehabil.* **2018**, *99*, 2561–2569. [CrossRef] [PubMed]
14. Hurkmans, E.; van der Giesen, F.J.; Vliet Vlieland, T.P.; Schoones, J.; Van den Ende, E.C. Dynamic exercise programs (aerobic capacity and/or muscle strength training) in patients with rheumatoid arthritis. *Vet. Res. Commun.* **2009**. [CrossRef] [PubMed]
15. Van den Ende, C.H.; Hazes, J.M.; le Cessie, S.; Mulder, W.J.; Belfor, D.G.; Breedveld, F.C.; Dijkmans, B.A. Comparison of high and low intensity training in well controlled rheumatoid arthritis. Results of a randomised clinical trial. *Ann. Rheum. Dis.* **1996**, *55*, 798–805. [CrossRef] [PubMed]
16. Baillet, A.; Vaillant, M.; Guinot, M.; Juvin, R.; Gaudin, P. Efficacy of resistance exercises in rheumatoid arthritis: Meta-analysis of randomized controlled trials. *Rheumatology.* **2012**, *51*, 519–527. [CrossRef]
17. Shimomura, S.; Inoue, H.; Arai, Y.; Nakagawa, S.; Fujii, Y.; Kishida, T.; Ichimaru, S.; Tsuchida, S.; Shirai, T.; Ikoma, K.; et al. Treadmill running ameliorates destruction of articular cartilage and subchondral bone, not only synovitis, in a rheumatoid arthritis rat model. *Int. J. Mol. Sci.* **2018**, *19*, 1653. [CrossRef]
18. Batsalova, T.; Lindh, I.; Backlund, J.; Dzhambazov, B.; Holmdahl, R. Comparative analysis of collagen type II-specific immune responses during development of collagen-induced arthritis in two B10 mouse strains. *Arthritis Res. Ther.* **2012**, *14*, R237. [CrossRef]
19. Dekkers, J.S.; Schoones, J.W.; Huizinga, T.W.; Toes, R.E.; van der Helm-van Mil, A.H. Possibilities for preventive treatment in rheumatoid arthritis? Lessons from experimental animal models of arthritis: A systematic literature review and meta-analysis. *Ann. Rheum. Dis.* **2017**, *76*, 458–467. [CrossRef]

20. Bokarewa, M.; Tarkowski, A. Local infusion of infliximab for the treatment of acute joint inflammation. *Ann. Rheum. Dis.* **2003**, *62*, 783–784. [CrossRef]
21. Drake, M.T.; Clarke, B.L.; Ourler, M.J.; Khosla, S. Cathepsin K inhibitors for osteoporosis: Biology, potential clinical utility, and lessons learned. *Endcr. Rev.* **2017**, *38*, 325–350. [CrossRef] [PubMed]
22. Wilson, S.R.; Peters, C.; Saftig, P.; Bromme, D. Cathepsin K activity-dependent regulation of osteoclast actin ring formation and bone resorption. *J. Biol. Chem.* **2009**, *284*, 2584–2592. [CrossRef] [PubMed]
23. Tsuchida, S.; Arai, Y.; Kishida, T.; Takahashi, K.A.; Honjo, K.; Terauchi, R.; Inoue, H.; Oda, R.; Mazda, O.; Kubo, T. Silencing the expression of connexin 43 decreases inflammation and joint destruction in experimental arthritis. *J. Orthop. Res.* **2013**, *31*, 525–530. [CrossRef] [PubMed]
24. Matsuki, T.; Arai, Y.; Tsuchida, S.; Terauchi, R.; Oda, R.; Fujiwara, H.; Mazda, O.; Kubo, T. Expression of connexin 43 in synovial tissue of patients with rheumatoid arthritis. *Arch. Rheumatol.* **2016**, *31*, 55–63. [CrossRef]
25. Manuel, A.R.; Sirisha, B.; Rekha, K.; Paul, D.L.; Jean, X J. Mitogen-activated protein kinase (MAPK) activated by prostaglandin E2 phosphorylates connexin 43 and closes osteocytic hemichannels in response to continuous flow shear stress. *J. Biol. Chem.* **2015**, *47*, 28321–28328.
26. Bivi, N.; Pacheco-Costa, R.; Brun, L.R.; Murphy, T.R.; Farlow, N.R.; Robling, A.G.; Bellido, T.; Plotkin, L.I. Absence of Cx43 selectively from osteocytes enhances responsiveness to mechanical force in mice. *J. Orthop. Res.* **2013**, *31*, 1075–1081. [CrossRef]
27. Yokota, K.; Sato, K.; Miyazaki, T.; Kitaura, H.; Kayama, H.; Miyoshi, F.; Araki, Y.; Akiyama, Y.; Takeda, K.; Mimura, T. Combination of tumor necrosis factor and interleukin-6 induces mouse osteoclast-like cells with bone resorption activity both in vitro and in vivo. *Arthritis Rheum.* **2014**, *66*, 121–129. [CrossRef]
28. Suzuki, N.; Yoshimura, Y.; Deyama, Y.; Suzuki, K.; Kitagawa, Y. Mechanical stress directly suppresses osteoclast differentiation in RAW264.7 cells. *Int. J. Mol. Med.* **2008**, *21*, 291–296. [CrossRef]
29. Sato, K.; Suematsu, A.; Okamoto, K.; Yamaguchi, A.; Morishita, Y.; Kadono, Y.; Tanaka, S.; Kodama, T.; Akira, S.; Iwakura, Y.; et al. Th17 functions as an osteoclastogenic helper T cell subset that links T cell activation and bone destruction. *J. Exp. Med.* **2006**, *203*, 2673–2682. [CrossRef]
30. Bakharevski, O.; Stein-Oakley, A.N.; Thomson, N.M.; Ryan, P.F. Collagen induced arthritis in rats. Contrasting effect of subcutaneous versus intradermal inoculation of type II collagen. *J. Rheumatol.* **1998**, *25*, 1945–1952.
31. Nam, J.; Perera, P.; Liu, J.; Wu, L.C.; Rath, B.; Butterfield, T.A.; Agarwal, S. Transcriptome-wide gene regulation by gentle treadmill walking during the progression of monoiodoacetate-induced arthritis. *Arthritis Rheum.* **2011**, *63*, 1613–1625. [CrossRef] [PubMed]
32. Jin, H.; Ma, N.; Li, X.; Kang, M.; Guo, M.; Song, L. Application of GC/MS-based metabonomic profiling in studying the therapeutic effects of *Aconitum carmichaeli* with *Ampelopsis japonica* extract on collagen-induced arthritis in rats. *Molecules* **2019**, *24*, 1934. [CrossRef] [PubMed]
33. Weinberger, A.; Halpern, M.; Zahalka, M.A.; Quintana, F.; Traub, L.; Moroz, C. Placental immunomodulator ferritin, a novel immunoregulator, suppresses experimental arthritis. *Arthritis Rheum.* **2003**, *48*, 846–853. [CrossRef] [PubMed]
34. Mane, D.R.; Kale, A.K.; Belaldavar, C. Validation of immunoexpression of tenascin-C in oral precancerous and cancerous tissues using ImageJ analysis with novel immunohistochemistry profiler plugin: An immunohistochemical quantitative analysis. *J. Oral Maxillofac. Pathol.* **2017**, *21*, 211–217. [CrossRef]
35. Munemoto, M.; Kido, A.; Sakamoto, Y.; Inoue, K.; Yokoi, K.; Shinohara, Y.; Tanaka, Y. Analysis of trabecular bone microstructure in osteoporotic femoral heads in human patients: In vivo study using multidetector row computed tomography. *BMC Musculoskelet Disord.* **2016**, *17*, 13. [CrossRef]
36. Vesterby, A.; Gundersen, H.J.; Melsen, F. Star volume of marrow space and trabeculae of the first lumber vertebra: Sampling efficiency and biological variation. *Bone* **1989**, *10*, 7–13. [CrossRef]

International Journal of *Molecular Sciences*

MDPI

Review

The Role of Collagen Triple Helix Repeat-Containing 1 Protein (CTHRC1) in Rheumatoid Arthritis

Askhat Myngbay [1], Limara Manarbek [2], Steve Ludbrook [3] and Jeannette Kunz [2,*]

1. PhD Program in Science Engineering and Technology, Nazarbayev University, Nur-Sultan 010000, Kazakhstan; askhat.myngbay@nu.edu.kz
2. Department of Biology, School of Sciences and Humanities, Nazarbayev University, Nur-Sultan 010000, Kazakhstan; lmanarbek@nu.edu.kz
3. GlaxoSmithKline Research & Development, Stevenage SG1 2NY, UK; Steve.B.Ludbrook@gsk.com

* Correspondence: jeannette.kunz@nu.edu.kz; Tel.: +7-702-411-0463

Abstract: Rheumatoid arthritis (RA) is a chronic autoimmune disease causing inflammation of joints, cartilage destruction and bone erosion. Biomarkers and new drug targets are actively sought and progressed to improve available options for patient treatment. The Collagen Triple Helix Repeat Containing 1 protein (CTHRC1) may have an important role as a biomarker for rheumatoid arthritis, as CTHRC1 protein concentration is significantly elevated in the peripheral blood of rheumatoid arthritis patients compared to osteoarthritis (OA) patients and healthy individuals. CTHRC1 is a secreted glycoprotein that promotes cell migration and has been implicated in arterial tissue-repair processes. Furthermore, high *CTHRC1* expression is observed in many types of cancer and is associated with cancer metastasis to the bone and poor patient prognosis. However, the function of CTHRC1 in RA is still largely undefined. The aim of this review is to summarize recent findings on the role of CTHRC1 as a potential biomarker and pathogenic driver of RA progression. We will discuss emerging evidence linking CTHRC1 to the pathogenic behavior of fibroblast-like synoviocytes and to cartilage and bone erosion through modulation of the balance between bone resorption and repair.

Keywords: collagen triple helix repeat containing 1; CTHRC1; rheumatoid arthritis; biomarker; bone erosion; cartilage destruction; fibroblast-like synoviocytes; Wnt signaling

Citation: Myngbay, A.; Manarbek, L.; Ludbrook, S.; Kunz, J. The Role of Collagen Triple Helix Repeat-Containing 1 Protein (CTHRC1) in Rheumatoid Arthritis. *Int. J. Mol. Sci.* **2021**, *22*, 2426. https://doi.org/10.3390/ijms22052426

Received: 28 December 2020
Accepted: 14 January 2021
Published: 28 February 2021

1. Introduction

Rheumatoid arthritis (RA) is a chronic systemic autoimmune disease, which affects around 1% of the population according to the World Health Organization [1]. RA is characterized by cartilage degradation and bone erosion within both small and larger joints including hand, wrist, knee and feet, leading to disability in a proportion of patients [2]. Although several genetic and environmental factors have been linked to an increased risk for RA, the definitive pathogenesis remains obscure, making the development of effective treatment strategies challenging. Some breakthroughs, including the introduction of anti-tumor necrosis factor alpha (anti-TNF-α), in the treatment of RA, which occurred in the mid-1990s, showed efficacy towards inflammation and joint destruction and led to an improvement of clinical outcomes of RA [3]. However, cytokine antagonists against TNF-α, Interleukin-6 (IL-6) and Interleukin-1 (IL-1) lacked efficacy in a significant fraction of patients, and the persistence of efficacy remains a tremendous problem even in responsive patients [3]. Likewise, the therapeutic effects of B cell depletion and T cell co-stimulation blockers were not observed in all patients [4,5]. Indeed, accumulating evidence suggests that differences in genetic background and exposure to environmental stimuli among patients require treatment strategies to be more personalized as particular patients' response can be TNF-α-dominant, T cell-dominant, and B cell-dominant [4,5].

While significant efforts have been undertaken to identify biomarkers to diagnose RA, there is still a lack of diagnostic and prognostic biomarkers for better patient stratification.

ACPA (anti-citrullinated protein antibody) and RF (rheumatoid factor) are two widely accepted autoantibodies used in clinical practice as biologic markers of RA [6]. Nonetheless, neither of these two markers has sufficient specificity or sensitivity for effective diagnosis of all RA patients, and neither autoantibody allows classification of patient subpopulations or patient outcome [6]. Recently, CTHRC1 has emerged as a new biomarker that may contribute to improved RA diagnosis and assessment of disease activity [7,8]. CTHRC1 protein levels are increased in the plasma of RA patients but were either absent or detected only at very low levels in healthy individuals or patients suffering from other forms of arthritis, such as OA or reactive arthritis (ReA) [7]. These findings suggest that CTHRC1 may enhance differential diagnosis of RA when used in a wider panel of markers. In addition, emerging evidence suggests that CTHRC1 is directly involved in the disease course. Accordingly, CTHRC1 is expressed in subsets of activated fibroblast-like (FLS) cells of the synovium associated with RA pathophysiology [9]. Furthermore, CTHRC1 acts as a critical modulator of bone resorption and formation by regulating osteoclast–osteoblast crosstalk [10,11], thus raising the possibility that CTHRC1 levels may reflect a more direct role—pathological or protective—in cartilage and bone erosion in RA. In this review, we will discuss the role and diagnostic potential of CTHRC1 in RA and provide an overview of the signaling processes modulated by CTHRC1.

2. CTHRC1 Domain Structure

CTHRC1 is a secreted 28 kDa glycoprotein that is highly conserved from chordates to vertebrates [12]. The human protein contains an N-terminal hydrophobic signal peptide of 30 amino acids in length that directs CTHRC1 for secretion, a short collagen triple helix repeat (CTHR) domain consisting of 12 repeats of the Gly-X-Y motif located between amino acids 57 and 93 [12], and a highly conserved C-terminal domain with structural homology to the globular C1q domain of collagens VIII and X domain (Figure 1) [13]. The CTHR domain may promote CTHRC1 dimer or trimer formation and mediate interaction with a variety of ligands [12,13]. The domain structure of CTHRC1 is similar to that of adiponectin, which belongs to the C1q/tumor necrosis factor (TNF)-related protein superfamily [14]. Thus, secreted CTHRC1 may share structural characteristics with this protein superfamily and similarly assemble into trimers and multimers composed of CTHRC1 trimers. CTHRC1 is also a cysteine-rich protein: 10 conserved cysteine residues are distributed between residues 55 to 243 (9 of which are located within the C1q domain; Figure 1) and account for 4.7% of amino acid residues present in the mature protein [12]. The single putative N-glycosylation site at amino acid 186 (Figure 1) has been reported to stabilize the protein and may promote the tethering of secreted CTHRC1 to the plasma membrane [15]. Several shorter alternatively spliced transcripts have been described [12], one of which lacks the N-terminal hydrophobic signal peptide and may not be secreted. However, only the longest transcript has so far been functionally characterized in more detail.

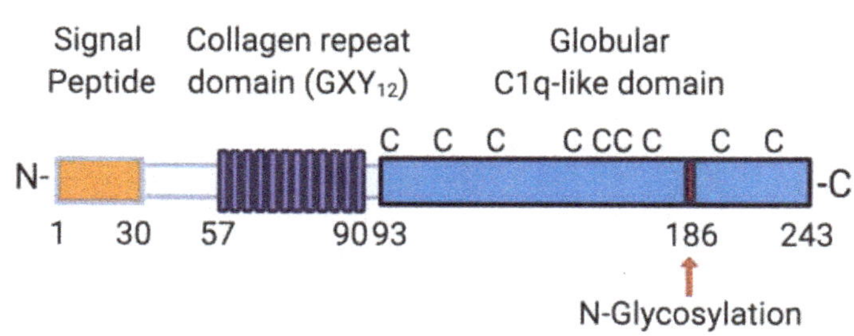

Figure 1. Domain structure of human CTHRC1. The longest CTHRC1 variant encodes a 243 amino acid protein with a 30 amino acid cleavable signal sequence, followed by a short collagen repeat domain consisting of 12 GXY repeats (where G stands for glycine, X for any amino acid and Y for tyrosine). CTHRC1 also contains a globular cysteine-rich (C indicates the positions of individual

cysteine residues) domain with structural similarity to C1q. CTHRC1 is glycosylated, and a single potential glycosylation site is indicated with a red arrow. Aminoterminal (N-) and carboxyterminal (-C) ends of the protein are indicated. Numbers specify amino acid positions within the human protein. Created with BioRender.com.

3. Identification and Physiological Function of CTHRC1

CTHRC1 was first identified by Pyagay et al., who reported the transiently upregulated expression of *CTHRC1* in rat arteries on adventitial and intimal smooth muscle following injury [12]. Increased levels of CTHRC1 protein were also observed in the matrix of calcifying human atherosclerotic plaques [12]. Notably, CTHRC1 was not detectable in normal arteries, indicating that the protein plays a specific role in the wound-healing response and promotes vascular remodeling during arterial injury [12,16]. Mechanistically, increased CTHRC1 levels are associated with a significant decrease in collagen type I and type III mRNA and protein levels, leading to a reduction of collagen deposition, and enhanced migration [12]. Consistent with such a role, CTHRC1 expression has been correlated with conditions and processes associated with deregulated wound and tissue repair, including, among others, liver and lung fibrosis and myocardial infarction [17–24], liver injury caused by Hepatitis B infection [20,25,26], tumor angiogenesis and metastasis [27,28].

4. Expression of *CTHRC1*

Under non-pathological conditions, *CTHRC1* expression is detected mainly during embryonic development in the visceral endoderm, the notochord and neural tube and is also significantly associated with developing cartilage and bone, especially in calcified tissues [29]. In the adult body, expression of *CTHRC1* is much more restricted and observed mainly in the bone matrix and periosteum, in the myocardium and in renal arteries [29]. In general, *CTHRC1* expression is detected and increased specifically in stromal cell types, including myofibroblasts and smooth muscle cells [29,30]. In addition, *CTHRC1* is expressed in human pituitary glands and was proposed to act as a circulatory hormone [31]. Overall, the restricted expression in the adult body likely accounts for the low levels of CTHRC1 protein normally detected in circulation.

5. Signaling Roles of CTHRC1

The pathways modulated by CTHRC1 reflect its role in tissue remodeling after injury, regulation of ossification and other physiological processes, most significantly cancer development and progression to metastasis. Extensive evidence links CTHRC1 to two major signaling pathways: The transforming growth factor β (TGF-β) pathway and canonical/noncanonical Wnt signaling pathways.

5.1. Role of CTHRC1 in the TGF-β Pathway

The TGF-β superfamily of signaling pathways regulates diverse developmental and homeostatic processes and alterations in these pathways are associated with a variety of human pathologies, including developmental disorders, vascular and immune diseases, fibrosis, and cancer [32–34]. The relationship between CTHRC1 with members of the TGF-β superfamily is highlighted by their overlap in expression patterns in specific cell types and tissues [10,16] and the finding that the promoter region of CTHRC1 has a consensus binding site for SMAD transcription factors, which are downstream components of TGF-β/BMP4 pathways [35]. Consistent with this, CTHRC1 expression was shown to be induced by TGF-β and TGF-β superfamily members, including Bone morphogenetic protein 2 and 4 (BMP2/4) and activin [10,16,36].

The link between TGF-β and CTHRC1 was first reported in injured arteries and has since also been reported in other cell types [11,17,19,21,22,29]. TGF-β is a central growth factor involved in vascular development in the embryo and the wound healing response in adult tissues [12,16,36]. During vascular development and upon injury, TGF-β mediates several negative regulatory effects during vessel repair by upregulating collagen synthesis via activation of SMAD2/3 complexes, leading to increased collagen deposition and smooth muscle cell proliferation [16]. Activation of the TGF-β signaling pathway also induces expression of *CTHRC1* [36]. Interestingly, CTHRC1 has been shown to act as an inhibitor of TGF-β, impacting neointimal formation and proliferation and migration of smooth muscle cells after vascular injury [10,16,36]. Accordingly, sustained activation of *CTHRC1* expression confers an antagonistic effect on TGF-β signaling with CTHRC1, leading to reduced SMAD2/3 phosphorylation in vascular cells (Figure 2) [36]. Elevated levels of CTHRC1 thereby promote vessel repair by inhibiting the expression of the TGF-β target genes collagen type I and III, which, in turn, reduces collagen deposition and enhances cell migration during vascular remodeling [12,16,36]. This regulatory feedback loop (summarized in Figure 2) may allow for tight control of CTHRC1 activity to balance the effects of TGF-β during the wound repair process.

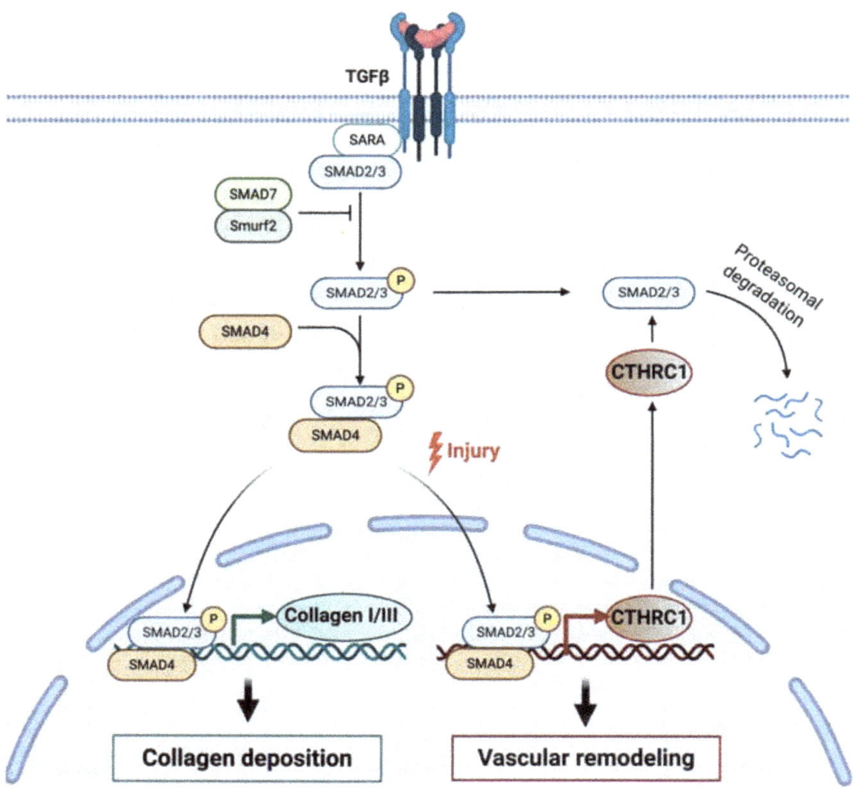

Figure 2. Model for CTHRC1 modulating collagen deposition and vascular repair following injury through the TGF-β signaling pathway. TGF-β is known to stimulate collagen deposition in various cell types by activating receptor-associated SMAD proteins (SMAD2 and SMAD3). Activated SMAD2 and SMAD3 oligomerize with SMAD4. The complex then translocates into the nucleus, where it regulates the expression of TGF-β-responsive genes, including genes encoding collagen I and III, and CTHRC1. Elevated levels of CTHRC1 eventually lead to attenuation of TGF-β signaling by inhibiting SMAD2/3 phosphorylation [36], possibly leading to SMAD2/3 degradation [21]. Created with BioRender.com.

5.2. CTHRC1 Is a Component of Canonical and Non-Canonical Wnt Signaling Pathways

CTHRC1 activity has also been linked to Wnt signaling. Canonical Wnt signaling is implicated in embryonic development, cancer, and stem cell differentiation [37,38]. Activation of the canonical Wnt signaling pathway leads to the stabilization and nuclear translocation of the transcriptional activator β-catenin into the cell nucleus, where β-catenin promotes the transcription of Wnt-associated genes [37]. Besides the canonical branch, there are several non-canonical branches of the pathway, which do not lead to the cytoplasmic stabilization of β-catenin. One of these pathways is the planar cell polarity (PCP) pathway, which regulates cell motility and adhesion via Dishevelled, RhoA, and actin cytoskeletal reorganization [37]. Canonical and noncanonical Wnt signaling pathways are also considered to be major modulators of RA pathogenesis [39].

Prevailing evidence suggests that canonical and non-canonical Wnt pathways converge at the level of CTHRC1. N-glycosylation by the Dolichyl-Phosphate N-Acetylglucosaminephosphotransferase 1 (DPAGT1) was reported to stabilize CTHRC1 protein stability and promote the secretion and pro-migratory function of CTHRC1 [40]. DPAGT1 expression is induced by activation of Wnt/β-catenin signaling [41], thus providing a link between Wnt/β-catenin and CTHRC1 (Figure 3) [40]. CTHRC1 may also positively promote the transcriptional activity of either β-catenin or the β-catenin/TCF complex [40], although it remains to be delineated exactly how CTHRC1 regulates Wnt/β-catenin signaling. Notably, in vitro studies showed upregulated expression of β-catenin in RA-FLS, leading to their chronic activation, indicating that Wnt signaling is induced in RA-FLS [42].

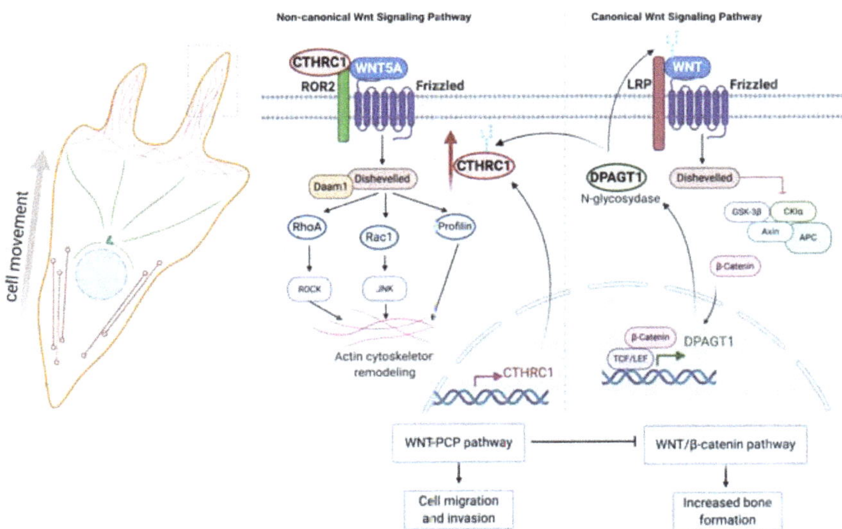

Figure 3. Role and regulation of CTHRC1 in canonical and noncanonical Wnt signaling. Expression of the N-glycosidase *DPAGT1* is induced in response to activation of canonical Wnt/β-catenin signaling. DPAGT1 mediates the N-glycosylation of Wnt ligands and of CTHRC1, thereby enhancing protein stability and secretion of CTHRC1. CTHRC1, in turn, attenuates signaling by the canonical Wnt/β-catenin pathway and induces cytoskeletal reorganization and cell movement via activation of noncanonical Wnt/PCP signaling. Secreted CTHRC1 activates the Wnt/PCP pathway by acting as a co-receptor and promoting the formation of the WNT5A/FZD/ROR2 complex. Created with BioRender.com.

Various studies have shown that CTHRC1 can activate the Wnt/PCP signaling pathway by acting as a coreceptor for formation of WNT/FZD/ROR2 complexes [15]. Consistent with such a role, CTHRC1 has been reported to interact with several PCP core components, including multiple FZD (Frizzled) receptors (FZD3, FZD5 and FZD6), WNT5A and the non-canonical co-receptor ROR2 (Receptor Tyrosine Kinase Like Orphan Receptor 2), but not with LRP6 (Low-density lipoprotein receptor-related protein 6) and the PCP component VANGL2 (VANGL planar cell polarity protein 2) [15]. CTHRC1 promotes the binding of WNT5A to ROR2, leading to enhanced WNT5A-ROR2 complex formation and stimulation of RhoA and Rac1 small GTPase activation, indicating that CTHRC1 can modulate both cascades of the Wnt/PCP pathway (Figure 2) [15]. Furthermore, Wnt/PCP and CTHRC1 may be part of an autocrine feedback mechanism, because CTHRC1 gene expression has been reported to be induced upon activation of FZD6/WNT/PCP (Figure 2) [43].

A recent study further identified the vertebrate-specific transmembrane protein Wnt-activated inhibitory factor 1 (WAIF1, also known as trophoblast glycoprotein, TPBG; 5T4 oncofetal trophoblast glycoprotein) as a receptor for secreted CTHRC1. Wnt-Activated Inhibitory Factor 1 (WAIF1)/5T4 has been shown to inhibit Wnt/β-catenin signaling and to concomitantly activate noncanonical Wnt pathways [44]. Taken together, these data suggest that CTHRC1 expression and function are positively regulated by the canonical Wnt signaling pathway. CTHRC1, in turn, acts as a switch between canonical and noncanonical Wnt pathways, leading to the inhibition of the canonical branch and activation of the noncanonical WNT/PCP branch of the pathway (Figure 3).

6. CTHRC1 Is Associated with RA Development and Disease Severity

CTHRC1 was first linked to RA pathogenesis through the genetic association of *Cthrc1* gene polymorphisms with attenuation of proteoglycan-induced (PGIA) and collagen antibody-induced murine arthritis (CAIA) [45–48]. *Cthrc1* is located within the proteoglycan induced arthritis 8 (*Pgia8*) locus of mouse chromosome 15, which controls PGIA severity in a sex-specific manner [45–48]. In *Pgia8*-congenic male mice, expression of all genes located within the entire locus was suppressed by 30–50%, and this was linked to resistance to arthritis development [46]. However, of the over 200 genes located within this locus, *Cthrc1* expression exhibited the strongest correlation with arthritis severity and levels of the pro-inflammatory cytokines IL-6 and IL-1β [46].

Notably, while *Cthrc1* was the most significantly down-regulated gene in the locus, it also exhibited marked co-expression with several other genes located within the *Pgia8* locus: the Wnt signaling components R-spondyn (*Rspo2*) and Syndecan 2 (*Sdc2*), ADAM metallopeptidase with thrombospondin type 1 motif 12 (*Adamts12*), as well as Complement C1q and tumor necrosis factor related protein 3 (*C1qtnf3*) [46]. All these genes were significantly repressed in male mice and linked to inflammation. Co-expression of *Cthrc1* with *Rspo2* and *Sdc2* supports the notion that CTHRC1 and the Wnt signaling pathways are linked in RA. *Adamts12* is genetically associated with several inflammatory conditions, including asthma, Crohn's disease, and RA [49,50]. In RA, ADAMTS12 is one of the enzymes triggering cartilage destruction by degrading cartilage oligomeric matrix protein (COMP) [46,51]. C1QTNF3 (also named CTRP3 for "C1q/TNF-related protein-3") is an adipokine with broad immunomodulatory and metabolic functions [52]. *C1qtnf3/Ctrp3* is highly expressed in several mouse models of arthritis and attenuates systemic inflammation and arthritis severity, suggestive of a protective role [53,54].

Importantly, the syntenic region to the *Pgia8* locus of mouse chromosome 15 in the human genome is also associated with RA development, serum rheumatoid factor and efficacy of anti-TNF-α treatment of RA patients [55–58]. The linkage of CTHRC1 with arthritis development and disease severity in mice therefore raised the question of whether the corresponding human locus may be similarly linked to RA development in patients. Consistent with such a notion, we recently showed that CTHRC1 protein is significantly and specifically elevated in the plasma of RA patients [7]. Importantly, CTHRC1 plasma levels were low or undetectable in healthy controls, as well as in OA and ReA patients [7]. In addition, CTHRC1 levels were positively associated with RA disease markers, such as RF, anti-citrullinated protein antibodies (ACPA) and C-reactive protein (CRP). CTHRC1 also correlated significantly with RA disease activity based on the combined index of the 28-joint disease activity score (DAS28), the combined score DAS28-CRP, and with a panel of pro-inflammatory cytokines, including interleukin 1 beta (IL-1β), interleukin 6 (IL-6), interleukin 8 (IL-8) and interferon gamma (IFNγ) [7]. A recent study independently confirmed that CTHRC1 is a specific marker for the diagnosis of RA, particularly when used in combination with other markers, such as anti-mutated citrullinated vimentin antibodies (anti-MCV) [8]. Together, these findings corroborate observations in murine models of arthritis and indicate that CTHRC1 may have potential use as a biomarker for enhanced differential RA diagnosis. Moreover, CTHRC1 was also identified as a novel serum biomarker associated with disease activity in systemic lupus erythematosus (SLE, [59]). Interestingly, CTHRC1 protein serum levels were highest in a subgroup of SLE patients with arthritis [59]. Thus, CTHRC1 may serve as a marker for the development of arthritis in SLE.

7. Invasive Synoviocytes Are Key Drivers of Joint Destruction in RA

Synovial hyperplasia is a hallmark of RA pathogenesis and characterized by the formation of pannus. The arthritic pannus is a multicellular vascularized tissue composed of cells of both mesenchymal and hematopoietic origin [34,35]. In response to synovial inflammation, pannus tissue invades cartilage and bone, resulting in major damage of the intimal lining and sub lining layers of the synovial tissue and, eventually, results in joint destruction. Fibroblast-like synoviocytes (FLS) in the synovial intimal lining are key drivers of bone erosion in RA; these cells become hyperproliferative and acquire an aggressive migratory and invasive phenotype [60–64]. These cells are also a source of numerous pro-inflammatory cytokines, growth factors and cartilage- and bone-degrading proteases. (Figure 4A,B) [60–64]. RA-FLS are also known to co-operate with macrophage-like progenitor cells, leading to local formation of osteoclasts, which invade the subchondral bone using acid attack and acidic proteinases (Figure 4A). Pro-inflammatory cytokines like TNF-α and IL-1β further protect FLS from Fas-mediated cell death (Figure 4A), thus preventing the elimination of RA-FLS from the inflamed synovium [64,65]. RA-FLSs thereby establish an autocrine feedback network that perpetuates synovial hyperplasia, contributes to the inflammatory microenvironment and promotes pannus invasion through increased synoviocyte motility and invasion [64].

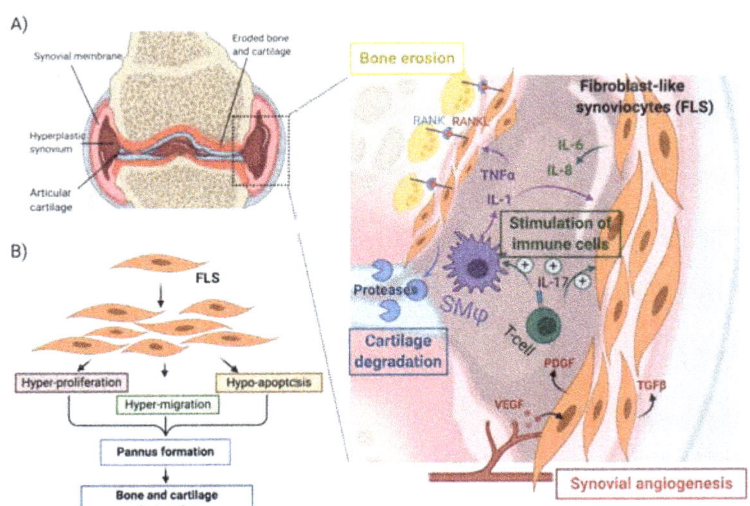

Figure 4. Role of synoviocytes in pannus formation and bone erosion in rheumatoid arthritis (**A**) and (**B**) activation of fibroblast-like synoviocytes by cytokines (TNF-α and IL-1β) secreted by synovial macrophages. (SMф) leads to the acquisition of a hyper-proliferative, hyper-migratory and hypo-apoptotic phenotype that contributes to the formation of a hyperplastic synovium and ultimately leads to bone and cartilage erosion Activated synoviocytes in the pannus play a central role in the recruitment and stimulation of immune cells, the vascularization of the pannus through activation of angiogenesis, and the promotion of cartilage and bone erosion. Created with BioRender.com.

8. RA-FLS Are One Source of CTHRC1

Significantly, the immunohistochemical analysis of CAIA mouse synovium showed that CTHRC1 protein levels were highly elevated in pannus compared to normal synovial tissue and concentrated in FLSs located at the invasive leading edge of pannus [66–68]. Consistent with these murine studies, CTHRC1 was recently reported to be highly expressed in two synovium fibroblast subtypes isolated from tissues of RA patients. One FLS subtype, characterized by the presence of CD34 and cadherin 11 (CDH11) and the absence of THY1/CD90, was implicated in monocyte recruitment in the RA synovium through secretion of IL-6, CXCL12 (C-X-C Motif Chemokine Ligand 12) and CCL2 (C-C Motif Chemokine Ligand 2) [9,69]. A second fibroblast subtype ($CD34^-$ $THY1/CD90^+$ $CDH11^+$) was significantly expanded in RA versus OA and exhibited the highest association with RA pathology [9,69]. Both *CTHRC1*-expressing FLS subtypes—the $CD34^-THY1^+$ and $CD34^+$ subsets—also showed induced expression of several other genes related to migration and invasion, including *TWIST1*, *POSTN*, *LOXL2*, *PDGFRB* and *MMP14* [9,69]. Accordingly, both FLS subtypes exhibited enhanced migration and invasion in vitro. Thus, CTHRC1 may promote pathological changes in the synovium by modulating the migration and invasion of different FLS populations and, potentially, by contributing to the recruitment of immune cells to the inflamed synovium.

Nevertheless, at present, we can only speculate about the function of CTHRC1 in RA-FLS subpopulations and the mechanisms governing CTHRC1 expression in these cells. CTHRC1 might act as part of either Wnt or TGF-β signaling pathways. Canonical and noncanonical branches of the Wnt signaling pathway are considered to play major roles in RA pathogenesis, in part, by modulating the activation of FLS and by promoting the production of pro-inflammatory cytokines and chemokines [39]. Accordingly, upregulated expression of β-catenin and of non-canonical Wnt/PCP pathway members is observed in the RA synovium [70–72]. This is associated with chronic activation of RA-FLS and a pro-inflammatory microenvironment that promotes the local recruitment of immune cells [70–72]. Kim et al. demonstrated that WNT5A is a key inducer of cytokine production during inflammation [73]. *WNT5A* expression was observed in RA-FLS but not in normal tissue [74], and overexpression of *WNT5A* in RA-FLS led to enhanced production of pro-inflammatory cytokines and chemokines [72,73]. Conversely, blockade of non-canonical WNT5A/FZD5 signaling leads to downregulation of IL-6, IL-15 and RANKL, which inhibited RA-FLS activation [39,75]. These data indicate that WNT5A-mediated signaling induces the secretion of cytokines and chemokines that promote the recruitment of leukocytes into the synovium. The WNT5A/ROR2 complex also plays a crucial role in bone-marrow-derived mesenchymal stem cell differentiation into osteoblasts, suggesting that activation of non-canonical Wnt signaling in the arthritic synovium also affects bone homeostasis by modulating osteoblastogenesis [73]. Given that CTHRC1 is known to stabilize the Wnt/Frizzled complex [40], CTHRC1 could promote Wnt/PCP signaling in the synovium, thus potentially modulating inflammatory cell migration and cell differentiation, as well as bone remodeling.

While the importance of canonical and noncanonical Wnt signaling pathways in the arthritic synovium is well established, the role of TGF-β in the synovium and in RA disease pathogenesis is not well defined. TGF-β is known to modulate pathogenic and inflammatory responses in the RA synovium and to regulate osteoblast differentiation [76]. TGF-β1 may also promote synovial lining hyperplasia synergistically with TNF-α and IL-1β through the regulation of RA-FLS proliferation, invasion and migration (Figure 4) [77]. Future work will be important to characterize the functional roles of the unique fibroblast subsets of FLS marked by *CTHRC1* expression and to elucidate the specific mode of action and regulation of CTHRC1 in these FLSs.

9. CTHRC1 Plays a Central Role in Bone Remodeling

Bone erosion is a central aspect of RA and is associated with disease severity [78]. Bone lesions both within and around the affected joints often appear early in the disease and can be accompanied by widespread osteoporosis in some patients without effective treatment. These lesions are the result of deregulated bone homeostasis due to enhanced osteoclast differentiation associated with bone resorption and the inhibition of osteoblast-mediated bone formation [78]. Osteoclasts are multinucleated cells that differentiate from monocyte/macrophage precursors under osteoblast/osteocyte control [78]. Osteoblasts regulate osteoclast differentiation and function via colony stimulating factor-1 (CSF-1) and RANKL (Receptor activator of nuclear factor κB/Receptor activator of nuclear factor kappa-B ligand, Figure 5) [78]. RANKL, which binds to the receptor RANK expressed on the surface of osteoclast precursors [79], is also secreted by osteocytes (Figure 5). In addition, osteoclast differentiation through RANK-RANKL interactions can be initiated by RA-FLSs, which also express RANKL on their surface [80].

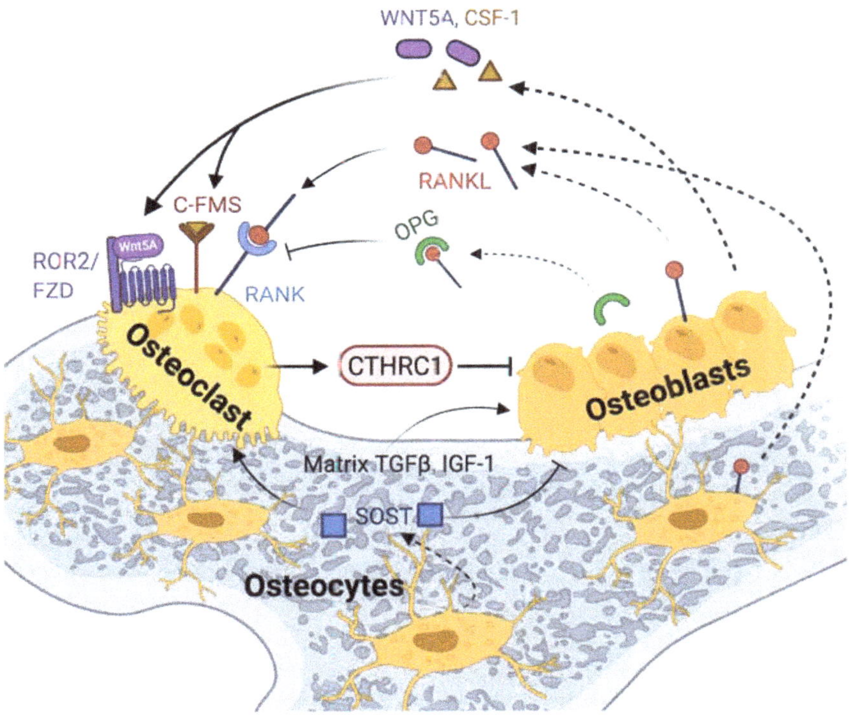

Figure 5. A model of CTHRC1 action in osteoclast–osteoblast crosstalk is shown, highlighting the effects of some of the key players involved. Membrane-bound and soluble RANKL produced by cells of the osteoblast lineage and by immune cells induces osteoclastogenesis upon binding to the receptor RANK on osteoclast precursors. RANKL action is opposed by the decoy receptor OPG secreted by osteoblasts or osteocytes. The inflammatory bone environment in RA results in increased production of RANKL by immune cells, osteoblastic cells and synovial fibroblasts. This exacerbates osteoclast differentiation and bone erosion. WNT5A binds to ROR2 receptors and activates non-canonical signaling, thereby promoting osteoclast differentiation and bone resorption. Likewise, signals generated by the binding of stromal-cell-produced colony-stimulating factor 1 (CSF-1) to the C-FMS receptor promote osteoclast differentiation and osteoclastogenesis. TGF-β and other factors, including IGF-1 released from the bone matrix during bone resorption, stimulate osteoblastogenesis [81]. CTHRC1 expression and secretion by osteoclasts points to an autoregulatory mechanism promoting osteoblastogenesis for enhanced bone formation [10,11,82,83], potentially by activating noncanonical Wnt signaling through the co-receptor WAIF1/5T4 [15,83]. An alternative model proposed by Jin et al. implicates osteoblast- and osteocyte-secreted CTHRC1 in the negative regulation of osteoclast differentiation through inhibition of RANKL-RANK signaling [84]. Created with BioRender.com.

Osteoblasts and osteocytes also balance osteoblast and osteoclast differentiation through secretion of additional factors. Osteoblasts secrete osteoprotegerin (OPG), a soluble receptor for RANKL, which inhibits osteoclastogenesis by blocking the RANKL-RANK interaction, and WNT5A, which contributes to the regulation of osteoclastogenesis through activation of noncanonical Wnt signaling (Figure 5) [85]. Studies showed that RANKL/RANK-deficient mice develop osteopetrosis, whereas OPG-deficient mice develop osteoporosis of trabecular and cortical bone [48–51]. Osteocytes also produce sclerostin (SOST), a secreted protein that attenuates osteoblast differentiation and promotes osteoclastogenesis by inhibiting the Wnt/β-catenin pathway [86]. While osteoclast-mediated bone resorption and osteoblast-mediated bone formation are normally tightly coupled to maintain bone homeostasis, the inflammatory bone environment in RA results in increased production of RANKL by immune cells, osteoblastic cells and synovial fibroblasts [78,87]. This shifts the balance towards pathological osteoclastogenesis and bone resorption.

Importantly, CTHRC1 has emerged as a critical coupling factor that links bone resorption to bone formation by controlling osteoblast-osteoclast cross-talk [10,11,82,83]. The essential regulatory role of CTHRC1 in bone homeostasis has been clearly demonstrated in vivo in mouse studies. Accordingly, loss of CTHRC1 function in mice was shown to result in decreased bone mass and decreased bone formation due to impaired coupling processes [10,11,84]. Conversely, overexpression of *Cthrc1* increased bone mass through stimulation of bone formation in transgenic animals [10,11,84].

However, the cellular source of secreted CTHRC1 and its precise role in bone biology are currently somewhat controversial, and any role of CTHRC1 in bone erosion in RA patients remains to be defined. While CTHRC1 may modulate osteoclastogenesis in the synovium via its expression in specific RA-FLS subsets [9,69], CTHRC1 clearly also plays an independent role in the regulation of bone formation/resorption. Several studies reported that CTHRC1 is secreted from osteoclasts and stimulates osteoblast differentiation (Figure 5 and Table 1) [10,11,82,83]. This effect may in part be mediated through WAIF1/5T4, a regulator of Wnt/β-catenin signaling expressed on stromal cells [15,83]. WAIF1/5T4 has been proposed to act as a receptor for osteoclast-derived CTHRC1, leading to the formation of a ternary complex by CTHRC1, WAIF1 and ROR2 on the osteoblast surface, which then mediates osteoblast-osteoclast crosstalk for bone remodeling [15,83]. Consistent with the notion that CTHRC1 is produced by osteoclasts to influence bone formation, the cell-type-specific ablation of *Cthrc1* expression in murine osteoblasts had no significant effect on bone mass, whereas osteoclast-specific deletion of *Cthrc1* led to bone loss [11]. Based on these data, Takeshita and coworkers concluded that CTHRC1 is secreted by osteoclasts and plays a major role in bone formation [11].

Table 1. Potential cellular sources of CTHRC1 and effects within the joint.

Cell Type	Potential Effect on Cells	Reference
Rheumatoid arthritis fibroblast-like synoviocytes (RA-FLS)	Proliferation, migration, initiation of cartilage destruction	[66]
Osteoclasts	Inhibition of osteoblast differentiation and osteoblast driven bone formation; activates WAIF1/PKCδ/ERK pathway necessary for RANKL expression leading to reduced bone resorption and formation	[10,11,82,83] [83]
Osteoblasts	Inhibition of monocyte-osteoclast differentiation and osteoclast-driven bone resorption in trabecular bone, inhibition of NFκB-dependent signaling; CTHRC1 may additionally suppress RANKL expression	[84]
Osteocytes	Inhibition of monocyte-osteoclast differentiation and osteoclast driven bone resorption in trabecular bone, inhibition of NFκB-dependent signaling; CTHRC1 may additionally suppress RANKL expression	[84]

In contrast to the aforementioned studies, Jin et al. reported that murine CTHRC1 is produced by osteocytes and osteoblasts, but not osteoclasts. Accordingly, *Cthrc1* was highly expressed by osteoblasts lining the trabecular and cortical bone surface and by some osteocytes but was absent from multinucleated osteoclasts [84]. Loss of *Cthrc1* expression in *Cthrc1* null mice was associated with a significant decrease in trabecular bone mass due to upregulated bone resorption, whereas cortical bone formation was only minimally affected [84]. Notably, bone-marrow-derived monocytes isolated from *Cthrc1* null mice showed normal osteoclast differentiation in vitro [84]. However, osteoclastogenesis could be blocked by the addition of recombinant CTHRC1 to these cells, indicating that CTHRC1 acts exogenously. Overall, these results led the authors to conclude that osteoblast- and osteocyte-derived CTHRC1 plays a critical role in negatively regulating osteoclast differentiation (Table 1, [84]). CTHRC1 may block osteoclastogenesis through suppression of RANKL expression and by inhibiting RANKL-induced NFκB activation (Table 1, [84]).

Overall, the molecular and cellular basis for the discrepancy between data reported from different laboratories remains to be defined. Contributing factors may be the use of different Cre-lox recombination approaches to generate cell-specific gene inactivation of *Cthrc1* in mice and the distinct detection methods used to visualize CTHRC1 protein. Alternatively, CTHRC1 may affect bone homeostasis through a combination of mechanisms and pathways depending on the tissue context and the presence or absence of inflammatory conditions. Additional studies in cellular and in vivo systems will be required to resolve the discrepancy between the data reported by different investigators and to clarify the precise physiological activity CTHRC1 in bone homeostasis. Regardless of this discrepancy, the role of CTHRC1 in bone remodeling has been firmly established in animal models and this may also have implications for the development of cartilage and bone erosion in RA patients.

Significantly, recent studies in mice focused on a potential role of CTHRC1 in joint destruction. Jin et al. assessed the role of murine CTHRC1 in arthritis development by studying the effect of *Cthrc1* ablation on collagen antibody-induced arthritis [84]. Interestingly, *Cthrc1* null mice exhibited exacerbated arthritis with extensive inflammatory cell infiltration and pannus formation and significant bone erosion. Thus, CTHRC1 appears to confer potent anti-inflammatory effects in the synovium and may play an important and broader role in the regulation of the immune response in this mouse model of arthritis. It remains to be seen whether these effects also translate to RA patients and whether elevated levels of CTHRC1 confer anti-inflammatory effects and act to reduce arthritic joint destruction.

10. Sex Disparity and CTHRC1

Rheumatoid arthritis occurs more frequently in women (about 75%), and symptoms are more pronounced in this population [88]. In particular, the influence of sex hormones on the immune response is well established [89], and estrogens are one of the causes of female predominance in RA and highly linked to disease severity and effects on bone remodeling [90]. In this regard, it is interesting to note that the murine *pgia8* locus conferred sex-specific attenuation of arthritis only in male, but not female mice [46]. Furthermore, the expression of *Cthrc1*, metalloproteinase *Adamts12*, *Rspo2* and *Sdc2* genes was not only highly associated with disease severity but was also linked to the sex-specific effects conferred by the *pgia8* locus on arthritis resistance [46]. The attenuation of *Cthrc1* expression in male mice was linked to the *pgia8* locus because CTHRC1 mRNA levels were equal in wild-type male and female mice [46]. The molecular basis for these sex-specific effects is not known. However, recent studies reported by Jin et al. show that CTHRC1 also has a diverse effect on bone formation in male and female mice. Bone histomorphometry, micro-computed tomography analysis and functional readouts of bone strength showed bone formation impairment of trabecular and cortical bone in male *Cthrc1* null mice with a significant reduction in bone mass, whereas female *Cthrc1* null mice exhibited impairment only in trabecular bone [84]. Taken together, these results indicate that in mice the sex-specific disparities in RA are linked to transcriptional regulation of *Cthrc1* and genes involved in cartilage degradation (*Adamts12*) and canonical and noncanonical Wnt signalling (*Rspo2*, *Sdc2*). Likewise, CTHRC1 confers sex-specific effects to bone formation in mice. Whether *CTHRC1* expression or function is also linked to the sex-bias phenotype of RA in human patients remains to be shown.

11. Conclusions

In this review, we described recent advances examining the role of CTHRC1 in RA pathogenesis. Available data suggest that CTHRC1 represents a promising new diagnostic and, potentially, also prognostic biomarker of RA. Additional studies will be necessary to reveal the precise function of CTHRC1 in RA pathogenesis in patients, such as the role of CTHRC1 in the RA synovium and the development of bone erosion. Additional studies will also be required to further address the mechanisms controlling CTHRC1 expression and function. In particular, the possibility that CTHRC1 signaling has different functional effects in specific cell types, where it may modulate TGF-β and/or Wnt signals depending on cellular context. Nevertheless, the similarities in CTHRC1 expression and function in rodent models of arthritis and RA patients are intriguing and provide a basis for future studies exploring the therapeutic and diagnostic potential of CTHRC1.

Author Contributions: A.M.: conceptualization, writing—original draft preparation; L.M.: writing—figure conceptualization and preparation, editing; S.L.: writing—original draft preparation; J.K.: conceptualization; writing—original draft preparation, editing and revision, funding acquisition. All authors have read and agreed to the published version of the manuscript.

Funding: This work was funded by a Nazarbayev University research award (Project ID 16135673, award number 064.01.01 SST 2016022 awarded to J.K.).

Conflicts of Interest: The authors declare no conflict of interest.

Abbreviations

ACPA	Anti-citrullinated protein antibody
ADAMTs12	A disintegrin and metallopeptidase with thrombospondin type 1 motif 12
Ang2	angiopoietin 2
BMP2/4	Bone morphogenetic protein 2/4
CAIA	Collagen Antibody-Induced Arthritis
CCL2	C-C Motif Chemokine Ligand 2
CD34, CD90	Cluster of differentiation 34/90
CDH11	cadherin 11
COMP	cartilage oligomeric matrix protein
C1qtnf3	Complement C1q tumor necrosis factor-related protein 3
CRP	C-reactive protein
CSF-1	Colony stimulating factor 1
CTHRC1	Collagen triple helix repeat-containing 1 protein
CXCL12	C-X-C Motif Chemokine Ligand 12
Daam2	Dishevelled associated activator of morphogenesis
DPAGT 1	Dolichyl-Phosphate N-Acetylglucosaminephosphotransferase 1
Dvl	Dishevelled
FZD	Frizzled
GSK3β	Glycogen synthase kinase 3beta
IL-1/6/8/11/15	Interleukin 1/6/8/11/15
INF-γ	Interferon gamma
LRP	Lipoprotein receptor-related protein
OA	Osteoarthritis
OPG	Osteoprotegerin
PCP Pathway	Planar cell polarity pathway
Pgia8	Proteoglycan induced arthritis 8

RA	Rheumatoid arthritis
RA-FLS	Rheumatoid arthritis fibroblast like synoviocyte
RANKL	Receptor Activator of Nuclear Factor-Kappa B ligand
RF	Rheumatoid factor
ROR2	Receptor tyrosine kinase-like orphan receptor 2
RSPO2	R-spondin 2
Sdc2	Syndecan 2
SLE	Systemic lupus erythematosus
SMAD 2/3/4	The abbreviation refers to the homologies to the *Caenorhabditis elegans* "small" worm phenotype and Drosophila MAD ("Mothers Against Decapentaplegic") family of genes
SOST	Sclerostin
TPBG	trophoblast glycoprotein
TCF	T cell factor
TGF-β	Transforming growth factor beta
TNF-α	Tumor necrosis factor alpha
THY1	Thy-1 Cell Surface Antigen
VANGL2	VANGL planar cell polarity protein 2
WAIF1	Wnt-activated inhibitory factor 1
Wnt	Wingless and Int-1

References

1. Gibofsky, A. Epidemiology, pathophysiology, and diagnosis of rheumatoid arthritis: A Synopsis. *Am. J. Manag. Care* **2014**, *20*, S128–S135.
2. Smolen, J.S.; Aletaha, D.; Barton, A.; Burmester, G.R.; Emery, P.; Firestein, G.S.; Kavanaugh, A.; McInnes, I.B.; Solomon, D.H.; Strand, V.; et al. Rheumatoid arthritis. *Nat. Rev. Dis Primers* **2018**, *4*, 18001. [CrossRef]
3. Feldmann, M. Development of anti-TNF therapy for rheumatoid arthritis. *Nat. Rev. Immunol.* **2002**, *2*, 364–371. [CrossRef]
4. Rein, P.; Mueller, R.B. Treatment with Biologicals in Rheumatoid Arthritis: An Overview. *Rheumatol. Ther.* **2017**, *4*, 247–261. [CrossRef]
5. Brzustewicz, E.; Bryl, E. The role of cytokines in the pathogenesis of rheumatoid arthritis–Practical and potential application of cytokines as biomarkers and targets of personalized therapy. *Cytokine* **2015**, *76*, 527–536. [CrossRef]
6. Van Delft, M.A.M.; Huizinga, T.W.J. An overview of autoantibodies in rheumatoid arthritis. *J. Autoimmun.* **2020**, *110*, 102392. [CrossRef]
7. Myngbay, A.; Bexeitov, Y.; Adilbayeva, A.; Assylbekov, Z.; Yevstratenko, B.P.; Aitzhanova, R.M.; Matkarimov, B.; Adarichev, V.A.; Kunz, J. CTHRC1: A New Candidate Biomarker for Improved Rheumatoid Arthritis Diagnosis. *Front. Immunol.* **2019**, *10* 1353. [CrossRef]
8. Hu, T.; Liu, Y.; Tan, L.; Huang, J.; Yu, J.; Wu, Y.; Pei, Z.; Zhang, X.; Li, J.; Song, L.; et al. Value of serum collagen triple helix repeat containing-1(CTHRC1) and 14-3-3eta protein compared to anti-CCP antibodies and anti-MCV antibodies in the diagnosis of rheumatoid arthritis. *Br. J. Biomed. Sci.* **2020**, 1–5. [CrossRef]
9. Mizoguchi, F.; Slowikowski, K.; Wei, K.; Marshall, J.L.; Rao, D.A.; Chang, S.K.; Nguyen, H.N.; Noss, E.H.; Turner, J.D.; Earp, B.E.; et al. Functionally distinct disease-associated fibroblast subsets in rheumatoid arthritis. *Nat. Commun.* **2018**, *9*, 789. [CrossRef]
10. Kimura, H.; Kwan, K.M.; Zhang, Z.; Deng, J.M.; Darnay, B.G ; Behringer, R.R.; Nakamura, T.; de Crombrugghe, B.; Akiyama, H Cthrc1 is a positive regulator of osteoblastic bone formation. *PLoS ONE* **2008**, *3*, e3174. [CrossRef]
11. Takeshita, S.; Fumoto, T.; Matsuoka, K.; Park, K.A.; Aburatani, H.; Kato, S.; Ito, M.; Ikeda, K. Osteoclast-secreted CTHRC1 in the coupling of bone resorption to formation. *J. Clin. Investig.* **2013**, *123*, 3914–3924. [CrossRef]
12. Pyagay, P.; Heroult, M.; Wang, Q.; Lehnert, W.; Belden, J.; Liaw, L.; Friesel, R.E.; Lindner, V. Collagen triple helix repeat containing 1, a novel secreted protein in injured and diseased arteries, inhibits collagen expression and promotes cell migration. *Circ. Res.* **2005**, *96*, 261–268. [CrossRef]
13. Leclere, L.; Nir, T.S.; Bazarsky, M.; Braitbard, M.; Schneidman-Duhovny, D.; Gat, U. Dynamic Evolution of the Cthrc1 Genes, a Newly Defined Collagen-Like Family. *Genome Biol. Evol.* **2020**, *12*, 3957–3970. [CrossRef]
14. Kishore, U.; Gaboriaud, C.; Waters, P.; Shrive, A.K.; Greenhough, T.J.; Reid, K.B.; Sim, R.B.; Arlaud, G.J. C1q and tumor necrosis factor superfamily: Modularity and versatility. *Trends Immunol.* **2004**, *25*, 551–561. [CrossRef]
15. Yamamoto, S.; Nishimura, O.; Misaki, K.; Nishita, M.; Minami, Y.; Yonemura, S.; Tarui, H.; Sasaki, H. Cthrc1 selectively activates the planar cell polarity pathway of Wnt signaling by stabilizing the Wnt-receptor complex. *Dev. Cell* **2008**, *15*, 23–36. [CrossRef]
16. LeClair, R.; Lindner, V. The role of collagen triple helix repeat containing 1 in injured arteries, collagen expression, and transforming growth factor beta signaling. *Trends Cardiovasc. Med.* **2007**, *17*, 202–205. [CrossRef]

17. Jin, J.; Togo, S.; Kadoya, K.; Tulafu, M.; Namba, Y.; Iwai, M.; Watanabe, J.; Nagahama, K.; Okabe, T.; Hidayat, M.; et al. Pirfenidone attenuates lung fibrotic fibroblast responses to transforming growth factor-beta1. *Respir. Res.* **2019**, *20*, 119. [CrossRef]
18. Bauer, Y.; Tedrow, J.; de Bernard, S.; Birker-Robaczewska, M.; Gibson, K.F.; Guardela, B.J.; Hess, P.; Klenk, A.; Lindell, K.O.; Poirey, S.; et al. A novel genomic signature with translational significance for human idiopathic pulmonary fibrosis. *Am. J. Respir. Cell Mol. Biol.* **2015**, *52*, 217–231. [CrossRef]
19. Li, J.; Wang, Y.; Ma, M.; Jiang, S.; Zhang, X.; Zhang, Y.; Yang, X.; Xu, C.; Tian, G.; Li, Q.; et al. Autocrine CTHRC1 activates hepatic stellate cells and promotes liver fibrosis by activating TGF-beta signaling. *EBioMedicine* **2019**, *40*, 43–55. [CrossRef]
20. Li, Y.K.; Li, Y.M.; Li, Y.; Wei, Y.R.; Zhang, J.; Li, B.; You, Z.R.; Chen, Y.; Huang, B.Y.; Miao, Q.; et al. CTHRC1 expression in primary biliary cholangitis. *J. Dig. Dis.* **2019**, *20*, 371–376. [CrossRef]
21. Bian, Z.; Miao, Q.; Zhong, W.; Zhang, H.; Wang, Q.; Peng, Y.; Chen, X.; Guo, C.; Shen, L.; Yang, F.; et al. Treatment of cholestatic fibrosis by altering gene expression of Cthrc1: Implications for autoimmune and non-autoimmune liver disease. *J. Autoimmun.* **2015**, *63*, 76–87. [CrossRef]
22. Binks, A.P.; Beyer, M.; Miller, R.; LeClair, R.J. Cthrc1 lowers pulmonary collagen associated with bleomycin-induced fibrosis and protects lung function. *Physiol. Rep.* **2017**, *5*, 1–9. [CrossRef]
23. Tsukui, T.; Sun, K.H.; Wetter, J.B.; Wilson-Kanamori, J.R.; Hazelwood, L.A.; Henderson, N.C.; Adams, T.S.; Schupp, J.C.; Poli, S.D.; Rosas, I.O.; et al. Collagen-producing lung cell atlas identifies multiple subsets with distinct localization and relevance to fibrosis. *Nat. Commun.* **2020**, *11*, 1920. [CrossRef]
24. Ruiz-Villalba, A.; Romero, J.P.; Hernandez, S.C.; Vilas-Zornoza, A.; Fortelny, N.; Castro-Labrador, L.; San Martin-Uriz, P.; Lorenzo-Vivas, E.; Garcia-Olloqui, P.; Palacio, M.; et al. Single-Cell RNA Sequencing Analysis Reveals a Crucial Role for CTHRC1 (Collagen Triple Helix Repeat Containing 1) Cardiac Fibroblasts After Myocardial Infarction. *Circulation* **2020**, *142*, 1831–1847. [CrossRef]
25. Bai, L.; Zhang, W.; Tan, L.; Yang, H.; Ge, M.; Zhu, C.; Zhang, R.; Cao, Y.; Chen, J.; Luo, Z.; et al. Hepatitis B virus hijacks CTHRC1 to evade host immunity and maintain replication. *J. Mol. Cell Biol.* **2015**, *7*, 543–556. [CrossRef]
26. Zhang, R.; Cao, Y.; Bai, L.; Zhu, C.; Li, R.; He, H.; Liu, Y.; Wu, K.; Liu, F.; Wu, J. The collagen triple helix repeat containing 1 facilitates hepatitis B virus-associated hepatocellular carcinoma progression by regulating multiple cellular factors and signal cascades. *Mol. Carcinog.* **2015**, *54*, 1554–1566. [CrossRef]
27. Wu, Q.; Yang, Q.; Sun, H. Role of collagen triple helix repeat containing-1 in tumor and inflammatory diseases. *J. Cancer Res. Ther.* **2017**, *13*, 621–624. [CrossRef]
28. Jiang, N.; Cui, Y.; Liu, J.; Zhu, X.; Wu, H.; Yang, Z.; Ke, Z. Multidimensional Roles of Collagen Triple Helix Repeat Containing 1 (CTHRC1) in Malignant Cancers. *J. Cancer* **2016**, *7*, 2213–2220. [CrossRef]
29. Durmus, T.; LeClair, R.J.; Park, K.S.; Terzic, A.; Yoon, J.K.; Lindner, V. Expression analysis of the novel gene collagen triple helix repeat containing-1 (Cthrc1). *Gene Expr. Patterns* **2006**, *6*, 935–940. [CrossRef]
30. Leclair, R.J.; Wang, Q.; Benson, M.A.; Prudovsky, I.; Lindner, V. Intracellular localization of Cthrc1 characterizes differentiated smooth muscle. *Arterioscler. Thromb. Vasc. Biol.* **2008**, *28*, 1332–1338. [CrossRef]
31. Duarte, C.W.; Stohn, J.P.; Wang, Q.; Emery, I.F.; Prueser, A.; Lindner, V. Elevated plasma levels of the pituitary hormone Cthrc1 in individuals with red hair but not in patients with solid tumors. *PLoS ONE* **2014**, *9*, e100449. [CrossRef] [PubMed]
32. Derynck, R.; Budi, E.H. Specificity, versatility, and control of TGF-beta family signaling. *Sci. Signal.* **2019**, *12*, eaav5183. [CrossRef] [PubMed]
33. Tzavlaki, K.; Moustakas, A. TGF-beta Signaling. *Biomolecules* **2020**, *10*, 487. [CrossRef] [PubMed]
34. Vander Ark, A.; Cao, J.; Li, X. TGF-beta receptors: In and beyond TGF-beta signaling. *Cell Signal.* **2018**, *52*, 112–120. [CrossRef]
35. Wang, P.; Wang, Y.C.; Chen, X.Y.; Shen, Z.Y.; Cao, H.; Zhang, Y.J.; Yu, J.; Zhu, J.D.; Lu, Y.Y.; Fang, J.Y. CTHRC1 is upregulated by promoter demethylation and transforming growth factor-beta1 and may be associated with metastasis in human gastric cancer. *Cancer Sci.* **2012**, *103*, 1327–1333. [CrossRef]
36. LeClair, R.J.; Durmus, T.; Wang, Q.; Pyagay, P.; Terzic, A.; Lindner, V. Cthrc1 is a novel inhibitor of transforming growth factor-beta signaling and neointimal lesion formation. *Circ. Res.* **2007**, *100*, 826–833. [CrossRef]
37. Kikuchi, K.; Kubo, M.; Sato, S.; Fujimoto, M.; Tamaki, K. Serum tissue inhibitor of metalloproteinases in patients with systemic sclerosis. *J. Am. Acad. Dermatol.* **1995**, *33*, 973–978. [CrossRef]
38. Clevers, H.; Nusse, R. Wnt/beta-catenin signaling and disease. *Cell* **2012**, *149*, 1192–1205. [CrossRef]
39. Miao, C.G.; Yang, Y.Y.; He, X.; Li, X.F.; Huang, C.; Huang, Y.; Zhang, L.; Lv, X.W.; Jin, Y.; Li, J. Wnt signaling pathway in rheumatoid arthritis, with special emphasis on the different roles in synovial inflammation and bone remodeling. *Cell Signal.* **2013**, *25*, 2069–2078. [CrossRef]
40. Liu, G.; Sengupta, P.K.; Jamal, B.; Yang, H.Y.; Bouchie, M.P.; Lindner, V.; Varelas, X.; Kukuruzinska, M.A. N-glycosylation induces the CTHRC1 protein and drives oral cancer cell migration. *J. Biol. Chem.* **2013**, *288*, 20217–20227. [CrossRef]
41. Sengupta, P.K.; Bouchie, M.P.; Kukuruzinska, M.A. N-glycosylation gene DPAGT1 is a target of the Wnt/beta-catenin signaling pathway. *J. Biol. Chem.* **2010**, *285*, 31164–31173. [CrossRef] [PubMed]
42. Xiao, C.Y.; Pan, Y.F.; Guo, X.H.; Wu, Y.Q.; Gu, J.R.; Cai, D.Z. Expression of beta-catenin in rheumatoid arthritis fibroblast-like synoviocytes. *Scand. J. Rheumatol.* **2011**, *40*, 26–33. [CrossRef] [PubMed]
43. Dong, B.; Vold, S.; Olvera-Jaramillo, C.; Chang, H. Functional redundancy of frizzled 3 and frizzled 6 in planar cell polarity control of mouse hair follicles. *Development* **2018**, *145*, dev168468. [CrossRef] [PubMed]

44. Kagermeier-Schenk, B.; Wehner, D.; Ozhan-Kizil, G.; Yamamoto, H.; Li, J.; Kirchner, K.; Hoffmann, C.; Stern, P.; Kikuchi, A.; Schambony, A.; et al. Waif1/5T4 inhibits Wnt/beta-catenin signaling and activates noncanonical Wnt pathways by modifying LRP6 subcellular localization. *Dev. Cell* **2011**, *21*, 1129–1143. [CrossRef]
45. Adarichev, V.A.; Nesterovitch, A.B.; Bardos, T.; Biesczat, D.; Chandrasekaran, R.; Vermes, C.; Mikecz, K.; Finnegan, A.; Glant, T.T. Sex effect on clinical and immunologic quantitative trait loci in a murine model of rheumatoid arthritis. *Arthritis Rheum.* **2003**, *48*, 1708–1720. [CrossRef]
46. Kudryavtseva, E.; Forde, T.S.; Pucker, A.D.; Adarichev, V.A. Wnt signaling genes of murine chromosome 15 are involved in sex-affected pathways of inflammatory arthritis. *Arthritis Rheum.* **2012**, *64*, 1057–1068. [CrossRef]
47. Adarichev, V.A.; Vegvari, A.; Szabo, Z.; Kis-Toth, K.; Mikecz, K.; Glant, T.T. Congenic strains displaying similar clinical phenotype of arthritis represent different immunologic models of inflammation. *Genes Immun.* **2008**, *9*, 591–601. [CrossRef]
48. Glant, T.T.; Szanto, S.; Vegvari, A.; Szabo, Z.; Kis-Toth, K.; Mikecz, K.; Adarichev, V.A. Two loci on chromosome 15 control experimentally induced arthritis through the differential regulation of IL-6 and lymphocyte proliferation. *J. Immunol.* **2008**, *181*, 1307–1314. [CrossRef]
49. Libioulle, C.; Louis, E.; Hansoul, S.; Sandor, C.; Farnir, F.; Franchimont, D.; Vermeire, S.; Dewit, O.; de Vos, M.; Dixon, A.; et al. Novel Crohn disease locus identified by genome-wide association maps to a gene desert on 5p13.1 and modulates expression of PTGER4. *PLoS Genet.* **2007**, *3*, e58. [CrossRef]
50. Kurz, T.; Hoffjan, S.; Hayes, M.G.; Schneider, D.; Nicolae, R.; Heinzmann, A.; Jerkic, S.P.; Parry, R.; Cox, N.J.; Deichmann, K.A.; et al. Fine mapping and positional candidate studies on chromosome 5p13 identify multiple asthma susceptibility loci. *J. Allergy Clin. Immunol.* **2006**, *118*, 396–402. [CrossRef]
51. Liu, C.J.; Kong, W.; Xu, K.; Luan, Y.; Ilalov, K.; Sehgal, B.; Yu, S.; Howell, R.D.; Di Cesare, P.E. ADAMTS-12 associates with and degrades cartilage oligomeric matrix protein. *J. Biol. Chem.* **2006**, *281*, 15800–15808. [CrossRef] [PubMed]
52. Li, Y.; Wright, G.L.; Peterson, J.M. C1q/TNF-Related Protein 3 (CTRP3) Function and Regulation. *Compr. Physiol.* **2017**, *7*, 863–878. [CrossRef] [PubMed]
53. Kim, J.Y.; Min, J.Y.; Baek, J.M.; Ahn, S.J.; Jun, H.Y.; Yoon, K.H.; Choi, M.K.; Lee, M.S.; Oh, J. CTRP3 acts as a negative regulator of osteoclastogenesis through AMPK-c-Fos-NFATc1 signaling in vitro and RANKL-induced calvarial bone destruction in vivo. *Bone* **2015**, *79*, 242–251. [CrossRef] [PubMed]
54. Murayama, M.A.; Kakuta, S.; Maruhashi, T.; Shimizu, K.; Seno, A.; Kubo, S.; Sato, N.; Saijo, S.; Hattori, M.; Iwakura, Y. CTRP3 plays an important role in the development of collagen-induced arthritis in mice. *Biochem. Biophys. Res. Commun.* **2014**, *443*, 42–48. [CrossRef]
55. Wei, Z.; Li, M. Genome-wide linkage and association analysis of rheumatoid arthritis in a Canadian population. *BMC Proc.* **2007**, *1* (Suppl. 1), S19. [CrossRef]
56. Jawaheer, D.; Seldin, M.F.; Amos, C.I.; Chen, W.V.; Shigeta, R.; Etzel, C.; Damle, A.; Xiao, X.; Chen, D.; Lum, R.F.; et al. Screening the genome for rheumatoid arthritis susceptibility genes: A replication study and combined analysis of 512 multicase families. *Arthritis Rheum.* **2003**, *48*, 906–916. [CrossRef]
57. Mukhopadhyay, N.; Halder, I.; Bhattacharjee, S.; Weeks, D.E. Two-dimensional linkage analyses of rheumatoid arthritis. *BMC Proc.* **2007**, *1* (Suppl. 1), S68. [CrossRef]
58. Plant, D.; Bowes, J.; Potter, C.; Hyrich, K.L.; Morgan, A.W.; Wilson, A.G.; Isaacs, J.D.; Wellcome Trust Case Control Consortium; British Society for Rheumatology Biologics Register; Barton, A. Genome-wide association study of genetic predictors of anti-tumor necrosis factor treatment efficacy in rheumatoid arthritis identifies associations with polymorphisms at seven loci. *Arthritis Rheum.* **2011**, *63*, 645–653. [CrossRef]
59. Wu, Q.; Yang, Q.; Sun, H. Collagen triple helix repeat containing-1: A novel biomarker associated with disease activity in Systemic lupus erythematosus. *Lupus* **2018**, *27*, 2076–2085. [CrossRef]
60. Zvaifler, N.J.; Firestein, G.S. Pannus and pannocytes. Alternative models of joint destruction in rheumatoid arthritis. *Arthritis Rheum.* **1994**, *37*, 783–789. [CrossRef]
61. Gravallese, E.M. Bone destruction in arthritis. *Ann. Rheum. Dis.* **2002**, *61* (Suppl. 2), ii84–ii86. [CrossRef] [PubMed]
62. Schett, G. Synovitis–an inflammation of joints destroying the bone. *Swiss Med. Wkly.* **2012**, *142*, w13692. [CrossRef] [PubMed]
63. Goldring, S.R.; Gravallese, E.M. Pathogenesis of bone lesions in rheumatoid arthritis. *Curr. Rheumatol. Rep.* **2002**, *4*, 226–231. [CrossRef] [PubMed]
64. Bartok, B.; Firestein, G.S. Fibroblast-like synoviocytes: Key effector cells in rheumatoid arthritis. *Immunol. Rev.* **2010**, *233*, 233–255. [CrossRef] [PubMed]
65. Ohshima, S.; Mima, T.; Sasai, M.; Nishioka, K.; Shimizu, M.; Murata, N.; Yoshikawa, H.; Nakanishi, K.; Suemura, M.; McCloskey, R.V.; et al. Tumour necrosis factor alpha (TNF-alpha) interferes with Fas-mediated apoptotic cell death on rheumatoid arthritis (RA) synovial cells: A possible mechanism of rheumatoid synovial hyperplasia and a clinical benefit of anti-TNF-alpha therapy for RA. *Cytokine* **2000**, *12*, 281–288. [CrossRef] [PubMed]
66. Shekhani, M.T.; Forde, T.S.; Adilbayeva, A.; Ramez, M.; Myngbay, A.; Bexeitov, Y.; Lindner, V.; Adarichev, V.A. Collagen triple helix repeat containing 1 is a new promigratory marker of arthritic pannus. *Arthritis Res. Ther.* **2016**, *18*, 171. [CrossRef] [PubMed]
67. Lindqvist, E.; Jonsson, K.; Saxne, T.; Eberhardt, K. Course of radiographic damage over 10 years in a cohort with early rheumatoid arthritis. *Ann. Rheum. Dis.* **2003**, *62*, 611–616. [CrossRef] [PubMed]

68. Machold, K.P.; Stamm, T.A.; Nell, V.P.; Pflugbeil, S.; Aletaha, D.; Steiner, G.; Uffmann, M.; Smolen, J.S. Very recent onset rheumatoid arthritis: Clinical and serological patient characteristics associated with radiographic progression over the first years of disease. *Rheumatology* **2007**, *46*, 342–349. [CrossRef]
69. Abuwarwar, M.H.; Knoblich, K.; Fletcher, A.L. A pathogenic hierarchy for synovial fibroblasts in rheumatoid arthritis. *Ann. Transl. Med.* **2018**, *6*, S75. [CrossRef]
70. Cheon, H.; Boyle, D.L.; Firestein, G.S. Wnt1 inducible signaling pathway protein-3 regulation and microsatellite structure in arthritis. *J. Rheumatol.* **2004**, *31*, 2106–2114.
71. Nakamura, Y.; Nawata, M.; Wakitani, S. Expression profiles and functional analyses of Wnt-related genes in human joint disorders. *Am. J. Pathol.* **2005**, *167*, 97–105. [CrossRef]
72. Sen, M.; Lauterbach, K.; El-Gabalawy, H.; Firestein, G.S.; Corr, M.; Carson, D.A. Expression and function of wingless and frizzled homologs in rheumatoid arthritis. *Proc. Natl. Acad. Sci. USA* **2000**, *97*, 2791–2796. [CrossRef] [PubMed]
73. Kim, J.; Kim, D.W.; Ha, Y.; Ihm, M.H.; Kim, H.; Song, K.; Lee, I. Wnt5a induces endothelial inflammation via beta-catenin-independent signaling. *J. Immunol.* **2010**, *185*, 1274–1282. [CrossRef] [PubMed]
74. Rauner, M.; Stein, N.; Winzer, M.; Goettsch, C.; Zwerina, J.; Schett, G.; Distler, J.H.; Albers, J.; Schulze, J.; Schinke, T.; et al. WNT5A is induced by inflammatory mediators in bone marrow stromal cells and regulates cytokine and chemokine production. *J. Bone Miner. Res.* **2012**, *27*, 575–585. [CrossRef] [PubMed]
75. Sen, M.; Chamorro, M.; Reifert, J.; Corr, M.; Carson, D.A. Blockade of Wnt-5A/frizzled 5 signaling inhibits rheumatoid synoviocyte activation. *Arthritis Rheum.* **2001**, *44*, 772–781. [CrossRef]
76. Larson, C.; Oronsky, B.; Carter, C.A.; Oronsky, A.; Knox, S.J.; Sher, D.; Reid, T.R. TGF-beta: A master immune regulator. *Expert Opin. Ther. Targets* **2020**, *24*, 427–438. [CrossRef]
77. Cheon, H.; Yu, S.J.; Yoo, D.H.; Chae, I.J.; Song, G.G.; Sohn, J. Increased expression of pro-inflammatory cytokines and metalloproteinase-1 by TGF-beta1 in synovial fibroblasts from rheumatoid arthritis and normal individuals. *Clin. Exp. Immunol.* **2002**, *127*, 547–552. [CrossRef]
78. Schett, G.; Gravallese, E. Bone erosion in rheumatoid arthritis: Mechanisms, diagnosis and treatment. *Nat. Rev. Rheumatol.* **2012**, *8*, 656–664. [CrossRef]
79. Kong, Y.Y.; Yoshida, H.; Sarosi, I.; Tan, H.L.; Timms, E.; Capparelli, C.; Morony, S.; Oliveira-dos-Santos, A.J.; Van, G.; Itie, A.; et al. OPGL is a key regulator of osteoclastogenesis, lymphocyte development and lymph-node organogenesis. *Nature* **1999**, *397*, 315–323. [CrossRef]
80. Geusens, P. The role of RANK ligand/osteoprotegerin in rheumatoid arthritis. *Ther. Adv. Musculoskelet. Dis.* **2012**, *4*, 225–233. [CrossRef]
81. Jann, J.; Gascon, S.; Roux, S.; Faucheux, N. Influence of the TGF-beta Superfamily on Osteoclasts/Osteoblasts Balance in Physiological and Pathological Bone Conditions. *Int. J. Mol. Sci.* **2020**, *21*, 7597. [CrossRef] [PubMed]
82. Wang, C.; Gu, W.; Sun, B.; Zhang, Y.; Ji, Y.; Xu, X.; Wen, Y. CTHRC1 promotes osteogenic differentiation of periodontal ligament stem cells by regulating TAZ. *J. Mol. Histol.* **2017**, *48*, 311–319. [CrossRef] [PubMed]
83. Matsuoka, K.; Kohara, Y.; Naoe, Y.; Watanabe, A.; Ito, M.; Ikeda, K.; Takeshita, S. WAIF1 Is a Cell-Surface CTHRC1 Binding Protein Coupling Bone Resorption and Formation. *J. Bone Miner. Res.* **2018**. [CrossRef] [PubMed]
84. Jin, Y.R.; Stohn, J.P.; Wang, Q.; Nagano, K.; Baron, R.; Bouxsein, M.L.; Rosen, C.J.; Adarichev, V.A.; Lindner, V. Inhibition of osteoclast differentiation and collagen antibody-induced arthritis by CTHRC1. *Bone* **2017**, *97*, 153–167. [CrossRef] [PubMed]
85. Tanaka, Y.; Ohira, T. Mechanisms and therapeutic targets for bone damage in rheumatoid arthritis, in particular the RANK-RANKL system. *Curr. Opin. Pharmacol.* **2018**, *40*, 110–119. [CrossRef] [PubMed]
86. Delgado-Calle, J.; Sato, A.Y.; Bellido, T. Role and mechanism of action of sclerostin in bone. *Bone* **2017**, *96*, 29–37. [CrossRef]
87. Goldring, S.R.; Purdue, P.E.; Crotti, T.N.; Shen, Z.; Flannery, M.R.; Binder, N.B.; Ross, F.P.; McHugh, K.P. Bone remodelling in inflammatory arthritis. *Ann. Rheum. Dis.* **2013**, *72* (Suppl. 2), ii52–ii55. [CrossRef]
88. Alpizar-Rodriguez, D.; Pluchino, N.; Canny, G.; Gabay, C.; Finckh, A. The role of female hormonal factors in the development of rheumatoid arthritis. *Rheumatology* **2017**, *56*, 1254–1263. [CrossRef]
89. Taneja, V. Sex Hormones Determine Immune Response. *Front. Immunol.* **2018**, *9*, 1931. [CrossRef]
90. Islander, U.; Jochems, C.; Lagerquist, M.K.; Forsblad-d'Elia, H.; Carlsten, H. Estrogens in rheumatoid arthritis; the immune system and bone. *Mol. Cell. Endocrinol.* **2011**, *335*, 14–29. [CrossRef]

International Journal of *Molecular Sciences*

MDPI

Review

Clinical Aspects of Janus Kinase (JAK) Inhibitors in the Cardiovascular System in Patients with Rheumatoid Arthritis

Przemysław J. Kotyla [1,*], Md Asiful Islam [2,*] and Małgorzata Engelmann [3]

1 Department of Internal Medicine, Rheumatology and Clinical Immunology, Faculty in Katowice, Medical University of Silesia, 40-635 Katowice, Poland

2 Department of Haematology, School of Medical Sciences, Universiti Sains Malaysia, Kubang Kerian 16150, Kelantan, Malaysia

3 Department of Physiotherapy in Internal Medicine, Academy of Physical Education in Katowice, 40-065 Katowice, Poland; m.engelmann@awf.katowice.pl

* Correspondence: pkotyla@sum.edu.pl (P.J.K.); asiful@usm.my or ayoncx70@yahoo.com (M.A.I.)

Received: 14 September 2020; Accepted: 3 October 2020; Published: 7 October 2020

Abstract: Janus kinase (JAK) inhibitors, a novel class of targeted synthetic disease-modifying antirheumatic drugs (DMARDs), have shown their safety and efficacy in rheumatoid arthritis (RA) and are being intensively tested in other autoimmune and inflammatory disorders. Targeting several cytokines with a single small compound leads to blocking the physiological response of hundreds of genes, thereby providing the background to stabilize the immune response. Unfortunately, blocking many cytokines with a single drug may also bring some negative consequences. In this review, we focused on the activity of JAK inhibitors in the cardiovascular system of patients with RA. Special emphasis was put on the modification of heart performance, progression of atherosclerosis, lipid profile disturbance, and risk of thromboembolic complications. We also discussed potential pathophysiological mechanisms that may be responsible for such JAK inhibitor-associated side effects.

Keywords: rheumatoid arthritis; JAK/STAT; Janus kinase inhibitors; cardiovascular system; heart failure; thromboembolic; lipid profile disturbances; cytokines

---

1. Introduction

Rheumatoid arthritis (RA) is the most common form of inflammatory polyarthropathies, affecting approximately 1% of the population worldwide. When the disease is not treated or treated insufficiently, it ultimately leads to permanent joint destruction, and subsequent disability [1]. In addition, as a member of systemic connective tissue diseases, RA is linked to an increased risk of internal organ involvements and systemic complications with premature atherosclerosis being the most important one. In the last two decades, significant therapeutic progress has been made and new therapeutic strategies implemented, resulting in better disease control and leading to a sustained remission or at least low disease activity. The new approach to RA treatment is based on the early introduction of synthetic disease-modifying antirheumatic drugs (DMARDs), mainly methotrexate (MTX), and is aimed to achieve remission or low disease activity. Unfortunately, only part of the patients responds well to such a treatment.

At the end of the last century, the therapeutic regimens for treating RA widened and new therapeutic strategies were implemented to the treatment repertoire. The new group of therapeutic molecules called biological DMARDs (bDMARDs) or simply biologics were introduced to the common clinical practice. The mode of action of biologics is based on blocking the inflammatory cytokines, depleting the population of antibody producing B-cells, and interfering in the co-stimulation of immunocompetent cells. This new approach revolutionized the treatment of RA. However, a substantial portion of patients still do not respond to such treatment. The limitation of these therapeutic strategies is the fact that biologics, which are high molecular weight compounds, are highly immunogenic and often produce adverse drug reactions such as tuberculosis, heart failure, neuropathies, and others [2–4]. Also of note is the fact that they are given parenterally, are expensive in manufacturing, and difficult to handle.

The progress made in immunology over the last 20 years contributed to the better understanding of the mechanisms of autoimmune diseases that translated directly to the development of new therapeutic approaches.

Among them, the Janus kinases/signal transducers and activators of transcription (JAK/STAT) pathway attracts high interest, and offers blockade of several cytokines with one small synthetic compound [5–8]. In line with the discovery of the JAK/STAT pathway, several synthetic compounds which are able to block this pathway have been developed [9]. This group of new synthetic DMARDs is called JAK inhibitors and indeed offer the blockade of many cytokines with one small compound (Table 1). Treatment with JAK inhibitors proven to be efficacious and relatively safe, and is recognized as equal and even superior to the conventional biologics [10]. This approach however may not be entirely free of risk of developing side effects. Blockade of several cytokines and interferons (IFNs) may bring many pathophysiological consequences as JAK/STAT pathway is deeply involved in several largely unknown regulatory networks and reduction of cytokine synthesis may contribute to the reduction of inflammatory process on one side in addition of dysregulating immune, cardiovascular, and nervous systems. As the example may serve tumor necrosis factor (TNF)-α inhibition that is responsible for worsening of the heart function in patients with congestive heart failure, lipid profile disturbances as the result of interleukin (IL)-6 inhibition, or increased risk of thromboembolism in the course of JAK inhibitor administration.

In this review, we tried to discuss the pathophysiological mechanism that may explain adverse drug reactions in the cardiovascular system during treatment with JAK inhibitors. Special emphasis was put on the role of cytokines blocked during the treatment with JAK inhibitors and their pathophysiological impacts on the functioning of the cardiovascular system.

Table 1. Currently available classes of disease-modifying antirheumatic drugs (DMARDs).

Typical Drug Representatives	Mode of Action	Side Effects
	csDMARDs	
Methotrexate	At lower doses (as used in rheumatology) methotrexate inhibits the 5-aminoimidazole-4-carboxamide ribonucleotide transformylase. As a result, it increases extracellular pool of adenosine leading to an overall immunomodulatory activity	Oral ulcers, alopecia, nausea, hepatic and hematologic toxicities, and pneumonitis
	tsDMARDs	
JAK inhibitors ▪ Tofacitinib ▪ Baricitinib ▪ Upadacitinib	Inhibition of JAK molecule and subsequently JAK stat pathway resulting in reducing expression of cytokine related genes	Lipid profile disturbances, higher risk of infections, and thromboembolic complications
	bDMARDs	
TNF-α inhibitors ▪ Infliximab ▪ Etanercept ▪ Golimumab ▪ Adalimumab ▪ Certolizumab pegol	Inhibit (ameliorate) TNF activity upon targeted cells resulting in blockade of inflammatory response driven by this cytokine.	Infections, latent tuberculosis reactivation, neuropathy development (anectodical data), contraindicated in patients with over or latent heart failure, and risk of malignancy

Table 1. Cont.

Typical Drug Representatives	Mode of Action	Side Effects
IL-6 inhibitors		
▪ Tocilizumab	Inhibit IL-6 activity upon targeted cells.	Infections and lipid profile disturbances
B-cell depletion		
▪ Rituximab	Antibody against B-cell (anti CD-20). Depletion of whole lines of B-cells expressing CD-20 molecule	Infections, infusion-related reactions, hepatitis B infection reactivation, cytokine released syndrome, and progressive multifocal leukoencephalopathy
Inhibitors of co-stimulation		
▪ Abatacept ▪ CTLA-4 (CD-152) molecule fused to an immunoglobulin G1 Fc part	CTLA-4 regulates T-cell priming, differentiation, and migration. CTLA-4 ensures homeostasis of regulatory T cells and mediates their immunosuppressive capacity.	serious allergic reactions including anaphylaxis and angioedema, latent tuberculosis reactivation, and higher risk for cancer (i.e., skin cancer)

DMARDs: disease-modifying antirheumatic drugs; csDMARDs: conventional synthetic DMARDs; tsDMARDs: targeted synthetic DMARDs; bDMARDs: biological DMARDs; TNF: tumor necrosis factor; IL: interleukin; CD: cluster of differentiation; CTLA: cytotoxic T-lymphocyte-associated protein.

2. JAK-STAT Pathway

JAKs are enzymes belonging to the tyrosine kinase family enzymes and their main function is to phosphorylate tyrosine residues to activate downstream signaling proteins and evoke physiological functions. When activated, they transfer extracellular signals provided by growth factors, cytokines, and chemokines that translate directly to the change of DNA transcription with the subsequent translation of several proteins. At the moment, four JAKs have been identified in mammalians (JAK1, JAK2, JAK3, and TYK2) which are specifically attached to receptors [11]. Activation of one specific JAK by the ligand-receptor can be recognized by the various receptor-ligand complexes as the one specific JAK and could be activated by several cytokines. *JAK1*, *JAK2*, and *TYK2* are expressed by many cells, contrary to this; hematopoietic, myeloid, and lymphoid cells express JAK3 [12]. The activation of JAK is a multi-step process. After a ligand is ligated to the receptor, the receptor's subunits dimerize and form an active receptor which is able to activate receptor-associated JAK [13]. Active phosphorylated JAK then phosphorylates tyrosine residues in the cytoplasmic part of the receptor enabling creation of docking sites for STAT. STATs are DNA-binding proteins which, when phosphorylated (activated), dimerize and translocate to the nucleus, followed by regulation of gene expression. It makes STATs the second key player in the transmission of signal. Currently, seven STAT proteins have been identified. The JAK/STAT system is responsible to transmit signals of more than 50 ligands and is recognized as one of the central communication systems of the immune response [14]. Active STATs then translocate to the nucleus where they interact with DNA regulatory elements, changing the expression of related genes [15,16].

JAK and more precisely JAK/STAT system is responsible for transmitting the signals provided by the wide spectrum of cytokines, which are ligands for class I and class II receptors. These receptors are protein complexes expressed on the surface of cells. They are built as one to four receptor chains. The typical structure of the receptor is formed from extracellular cytokine R homology domain (CHD) and a sequence acting as cytokine binding site. Slight structural differences in the CHD cytokine receptors enable to distinguish class I or class II family receptors [17]. Class I receptor family interacts with four cytokine families - gamma chains (γc), beta chains (βc), cytokines that utilize gp130 protein, and ILs that interact with a receptor's common subunit p40. Presence of γc in the receptor enables to interact with IL-2, IL-4, IL-7, IL-9, IL-15, and IL-21 [18], since βc is responsible for transducing the signals provided by granulocyte-macrophage colony-stimulating factor (GM-CSF), IL-3, and IL-5. Several cytokines utilize gp130 protein as a component of their receptor. This cytokine subfamily consists of IL-6, IL-11, IL-27, and IL-31. This receptor complex is also used by ciliary neurotrophic growth factor, oncostatin M, cardiotrophin1 and cardiotrophin-like cytokine factor 1 [19–21]. Recently, two other cytokines namely IL-35 and IL-39 have been added to gp130 family due to the fact that they use gp130 as a signal transmitting unit in the receptor complex [22,23]. The last cytokine family that utilize class I receptor consists of IL-12 and IL-23 receptors for heterodimeric cytokines that share the common subunit p40 [24,25]. Several hormone-like cytokines as growth hormone, leptin, erythropoietin, and thrombopoietin also transmit signals via the class I receptor. Plethora of cytokines, chemokines, and growth factors makes class I receptors the real crossroad of immune response, metabolism growth, tissue development, and indicates how important modulation of this pathway is. βc-the family of class II cytokines comprise a large group of signaling molecules. The most important members of this class are type I, II, and III IFNs (IFN-α, IFN-β, IFN- γ, IL-28, and IL-29) and cytokines belonging to IL-10-related family (IL-10, IL-19, IL-20, IL-22, IL-24, and IL-26) [17].

The transmission of signals from receptors requires two molecules of JAKs. JAK1 transmits signals provided by IL-6, IL-10, IL-11, IL-19, IL-20, and IL-22, and IFN-α, IFN-β, and IFN-γ, since JAK2 activation is responsible for the signaling of hormone-like cytokines-erythropoietin, thrombopoietin, growth hormone, GM-CSF, IL-3, and IL-5. [26]. JAK3 is exceptional member of JAK family which transmits signals as heterodimer of JAK1 and JAK3 molecules and is primarily expressed on hematopoietic cells. Attached to γ-chain transmits signals from IL-2, IL-4, IL-7, IL-9, IL-15, and IL-21 [26]. The last member of JAK family TYK2 facilitates signaling for IL-12, IL-23, and type I IFNs [27]. TYK2 creates heterodimers with either JAK1 or JAK2 [27]. Signaling the various cytokines by specific pairs of JAKs at least potentially creates a chance to target (inhibit) narrow branch of cytokines. However, one should remember that, contrary to biologic-targeted therapy, when one drug blocks only one cytokine, JAK inhibitor blocks many cytokines which utilize the same type of receptor.

3. The Role of JAK/STAT Pathway in Immunity and Autoimmunity

The results from many studies performed in the last two decades confirmed the involvement of the JAK/STAT pathway in several diseases associated with inflammation, cancer, immunity, and immune deficiency. This is not surprising as JAK mutations have been identified in immune deficiency syndromes including severe combined immune deficiency (SCID), in hematologic malignancies (leukemias and lymphomas) [28], and also in autoimmunity (hyper IgE-Job's syndrome) [29]. Some of the mutations in the JAK/STAT pathway directly increase the risk of developing well characterized autoimmune disorders like inflammatory bowel disease, psoriasis, ankylosing spondylitis, Behçet's disease [30–32], RA, Sjögren syndrome, or systemic lupus erythematosus (SLE) [33,34]. These findings underline the role of cytokine mediated regulation that affects such important pathophysiological processes as IFN-mediated immunity [35,36], T- and NK-cell-based immune response, regulation of function of lymphocytes, hematopoiesis, and nerve development. Recently, the role of IFNs in the development of several autoimmune disorders has been confirmed. In line with it, the term IFN signature has been coined indicating the special role of IFNs in the devolved of autoimmunity, specifically a prominent increase in the expression of type I IFN-regulated genes. This is especially a fact as far as SLE, inflammatory myopathies, and systemic sclerosis are concerned [37–41].

SLE is an autoimmune disease with a complex immunopathogenesis where B-cells have been implicated in humoral abnormalities and a prominent type I IFN signature is found in blood of majority of the SLE patients [42]. As the JAK/STAT cascade was identified to be responsible for the signal transduction from the activated IFN receptor to the nucleus, any disturbance in activity of this pathway may lead to the disease development. Indeed, the study on human lupus nephritis (LN) by Arakawa et al. [43] observed increased glomerular staining of STAT3 in renal biopsies of LN patients. Moreover, in patients with different types of glomerulonephritides, STAT3 activation highly correlated with glomerular and tubulointerstitial cell proliferation, interstitial fibrosis, and the level of renal injury. Obviously, the role of cytokines in the development of autoimmune diseases is not limited to IFNs. All known and perhaps not already known cytokines and chemokines create unique networks of self-interactions, activation, and regulatory loops. Any disturbance in this precise universe results directly to the development of autoimmunity, malignancy, allergy, or immunodeficiency. In addition, the second main player in autoimmunity, namely B-cells, are at least partially dependent upon cytokine stimulation utilizing the JAK/STAT system for signal transmission [44].

In the last four decades, the importance of cytokines in autoimmune diseases, as an executive arm of autoimmunity has been established. As the JAK/STAT pathway is one of the three most important signaling pathways in the cell, targeting of JAKs appears to be a rational strategy to stop the development of the diseases at a very early stage. In line with it, a great number of JAK inhibitors in various stages of preclinical development are being tested in clinical trials, and some of them have already been approved for the treatment.

4. JAK Inhibitors and Rheumatoid Arthritis

RA is a chronic inflammatory polyarthropathy characterized by the symmetrical involvement of peripheral joints, internal organ involvements, and systemic symptoms [1]. The etiology of the disease is not precisely understood but at the current level of knowledge and our understanding based on the disease mechanism, the pathogenesis is believed to be the mosaics of environmental, genetic, and lifestyle-related factors. All these factors when working together contribute to the aberrant immunological response and create the autoimmune reactions. Targeting many pro-inflammatory cytokines with a single small molecule created a unique opportunity to block several signaling pathways involved in the development of autoimmune diseases including RA. The obvious background to target JAK was to reduce the level of IL-6, one of the pivotal cytokines in RA. The other cytokines, although not directly involved into the pathogenesis of RA, create permissive background for inflammatory response contributing to the development of cellular response [45], including the Th1, Th2, and Th17 cells, which are directly involved in the development of autoimmune and inflammatory disorders [46]. Understanding the role of JAK in the pathogenesis of various autoimmune disorders led to the synthesis of several JAK inhibitors. Followed the approval of the first JAK inhibitor, tofacitinib, in the treatment of RA in 2012 and in 2017 in the USA and Europe, respectively, baricitinib and upadacitinib were subsequently approved for RA in DMARD failure patients.

Based on the selectivity of a given JAK molecule, JAK inhibitors are commonly subcategorized as first and next generation. First generation of JAK inhibitors (i.e., tofacitinib, baricitinib, and peficitinib, all approved for RA in Japan) block two or more JAK molecules resulting in inhibition of several cytokines. Consequently, inhibiting a JAK molecule may block more than one pathway, which may in part explain both the drug efficacy and some of the adverse effects observed with JAK inhibitor treatment [47]. In contrast, next generation of JAK inhibitors (i.e., upadacitinib and filgotinib, which are not approved for RA yet) is characterized by high selectivity, and thus administration of inhibitors blocks only one specific JAK molecule and selectively inhibits signal from one or limited number of cytokines. This provide the precise mechanism enabling to target one cytokine with one drug.

The current strategy for the treatment of RA is based on early starting classic synthetic DMARDs (csDMARDs), mainly methotrexate (which is still recognized as an anchor drug in the treatment regimen), administered alone or in combination with glucocorticosteroids. In case of MTX failure or intolerance, other csDMARDs (i.e., sulfasalazine or leflunomide) are available. The other group of therapeutic agents including bDMARDs or targeted synthetic DMARDs (tsDMARDs) with JAK inhibitors being the most important representative.

Blocking several cytokines with a single small molecule was a successful approach. In many clinical trials, JAK inhibitors were proven to be equal to bDMARDs [10,48,49]. Two studies designed as non-inferiority trials have shown statistical superiority of baricitinib or upadacitinib compared with adalimumab (all in combination with MTX) [50,51]. However, a third study using tofacitinib+MTX did not show such efficacy [52]. Therefore, the European League Against Rheumatism (EULAR) task force decided that clinical significance is too low to prefer tsDMARDs over bDMARDs. In line with this conclusion, current EULAR recommendation indicates adding bDMARD or a tsDMARD to the treatment regimen when the treatment target is not achieved with the first csDMARD strategy and poor prognostic factors are observed. Moreover, EULAR task force revised the preference of bDMARDs over tsDMARDs (proposed in earlier recommendation) because of new evidence regarding the successful long-term efficacy and safety of JAK inhibitors [53–55]. Currently, four JAK inhibitors are approved for the treatment of RA, namely tofacitinib, baricitinib, upadacitinib, and peficitinib (approved for RA in Japan), but many other compounds are currently tested in RA and other autoimmune diseases [56].

5. Safety Issues of JAK Inhibitors

Blocking several cytokines with one small molecule may potentially bring many pathophysiological consequences. It is especially true when we consider how blocking the different pathways translates to change the activity of various, sometime critical body systems. Firstly, targeting JAK3 attached to γ-cytokines leads to impairment of signaling via IL-2, IL-4, IL-7, IL-9, IL-15, and IL-21 (Figure 1). This is of the special importance as those cytokines are responsible for proper T-cell development and immunoglobulin synthesis. JAK3 blockade resembles severe immunodeficiency syndrome, with a switch off mutation in γ-chain resulting in X-linked SCID [57]. Therefore, infection, especially viral infections attracted the main attention of researches. Targeting JAK and blocking transmission of several cytokines may also lead to some safety issues in the cardiovascular system.

5.1. Heart Failure

JAK/STAT pathway transmits not only inflammatory signals, but also is deeply involved in the proper functioning of many systems of the body including the cardiovascular system. In neonatal rat, cardiocytes angiotensin II induces JAK2 phosphorylation and this process is critically depended on reactive oxygen species generation via membrane-bound NADP-oxidase. This may offer an important link between high glucose levels and glucose-dependent angiotensin II-mediated phosphorylation of JAK2. Of note is the fact that cardiac hypertrophy in non-failing heart is dependent on JAK2 phosphorylation [58]. This may potentially offer therapeutic approach in patients with RA, where insulin resistance and latent diabetes contribute to cardiac hypertrophy and heart failure. On the other hand, it was shown in a mice model that gp130 receptor and gp130 cytokines may offer survival pathway in transition to the heart failure (Figure 1) [59]. Thus, switching off this pathway via JAK inhibition ameliorates compensatory effect upon heart at risk for even failure. The pivotal role of cytokine that utilized gp130 receptor, namely IL-6 is still the matter of controversy. Contrary to TNF, which is known to contribute to heart insufficiency, the role of IL-6 is widely unknown. Quite recently, Hengdong et al. in their meta-analysis showed increased level of IL-6 was independently associated with higher risk of major adverse cardiovascular events (MACE), cardiovascular and all-causes of mortality in patients with acute coronary syndromes [60]. Although at this moment, it is not clear if IL-6 is the only valuable biomarker of heart failure or it is only pathophysiologically involved in heart failure. More information was obtained from the study of Liangjie et al. who assayed IL-6 and IL-17 in patients who underwent cardiac catherization. In this study, IL-6 and IL-17 levels were correlated with the levels of fibrotic parameters indicating the role of both cytokines in the development of heart insufficiency [61]. Recently, some indirect data suggested that targeting IL-1 with subsequent reduction of IL-6 exerted a significant effect on the primary cardiovascular end point [62]. IL-6 is the central inflammatory cytokine, and together with its downstream inflammatory biomarker CRP is linked to high cardiovascular risk [63].

Despite numerous experimental and clinical studies, the role of IL-6 on the development of heart failure has not yet been fully elucidated. It is believed that high concentration of IL-6 can lead at least partially to the development of heart failure [64] and may serve as an indicator of worse prognosis in patients with cardiovascular diseases [65]. Targeting JAK with subsequent blockade of gp130 mediated pathway may potentially facilitate to stabilize the heart function. At this moment, it is unclear whether this improvement is due to the direct reduction of IL-6 or this process is mediated via limitation of an inflammatory state. Blocking the JAK/STAT pathway may also bring many negative consequences. It is well known that activation of the JAK2/STAT3 pathway protects the myocardium against ischemia/reperfusion injury and inhibits apoptosis of the coronary artery endothelial cells [66], thus provide mechanism that are far beyond only cytokine signaling [67]. Contrary to this, in another study, inhibition of JAK2/STAT partially attenuated the pro-apoptotic effect of IL-23 (a member of

IL-12 family) upon cardiomyocytes [68]. Therefore, it is suggested that, in these circumstances, IL-23 promotes the activation of JAK2/STAT pathway and enhances the expression of IL-17, the cytokine deeply involved in myocardial ischemia/reperfusion injury (Figure 1) [69]. It is an identical fact when the other member from this cytokine family, IL-12, is concerned.

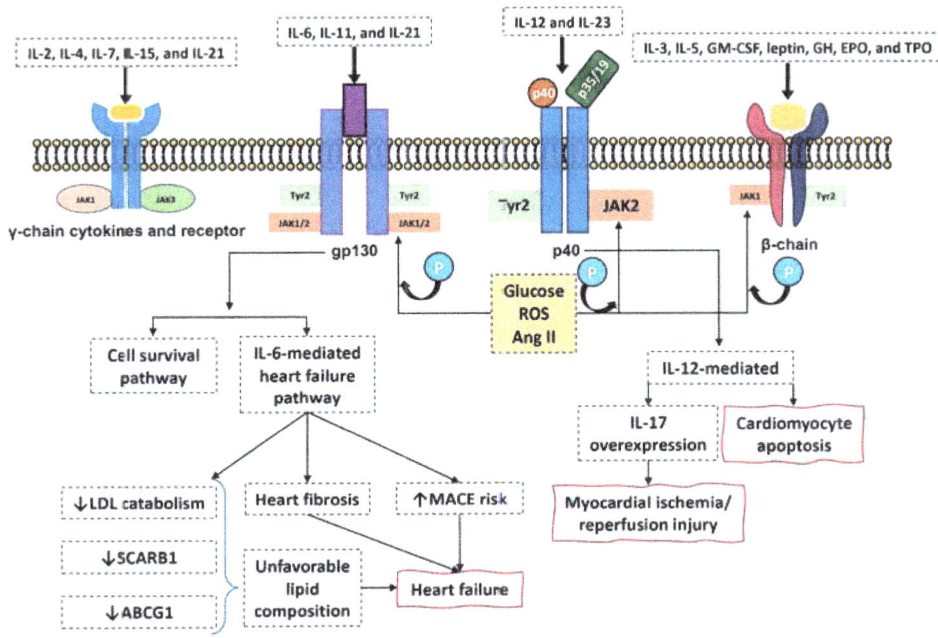

Figure 1. Several cytokine families utilize type I receptors. Receptors with gp130 component transmits signals from IL-6, IL-11, and IL-27 with subsequent activation of JAK1-JAK2 and TYK2 molecules. Cytokines activate (mainly IL-6) heart survival pathway resulting in stabilization of the heart function in ischemia/reperfusion conditions. The same pathway contributes however in deterioration of heart function and increases the risk of major adverse cardiovascular events (MACE), leading to heart fibrosis with subsequent development of heart failure. Cytokines IL-12 and IL-23 that interact with p40 receptor component transmit signals via activation of JAK2 and TYK2 molecules resulting in cardiomyocytes apoptosis. Moreover IL-12 facilitates IL-17 overexpression leading to myocardial/reperfusion injury. Blocking JAK/STAT pathway with JAK inhibitors may therefore result in blocking the heart failure survival pathway but also may reduce MACE incidence and fibrosis of the heart. Blocking of JAK/STAT pathway (mainly IL-6 mediated arm) is also responsible for unfavorable lipids profile changes mediated by reduced LDL catabolism, but this effect may be ameliorated by reduced expression of scavenger receptor class B and ATP-binding cassette G-1. Leading to improvement of lipid composition. Several pathological conditions upregulate JAK/STAT pathway activity (hyperglycemia, reactive oxygen species formation, and angiotensin II) facilitating transmission signals from proinflammatory cytokines.

Previous studies reported that plasma IL-12 concentrations were significantly increased in many types of atherosclerosis and atherosclerotic cardiovascular disease. At this moment, it is however unclear whether inhibition of signaling pathways via JAK/STAT system may attenuate the harmful effect of IL-12 upon the heart, which is not a surprising finding. The inhibition of JAK results in the reduced expression of many cytokines belonging to the various families. Moreover, even in the same cytokine family, some of them exert pro-inflammatory response since the other cytokines are recognized as anti-inflammatory ones. IL12 and IL-23 demonstrate strong pro-inflammatory properties. However, the other member of this family, IL-35, exerts anti-inflammatory potentials. Therefore, the direct effect of the inhibition of the JAK/STAT pathway is dependent on what cytokines are predominantly blocked when inhibition of the JAK/STAT pathway occurs (Figure 2).

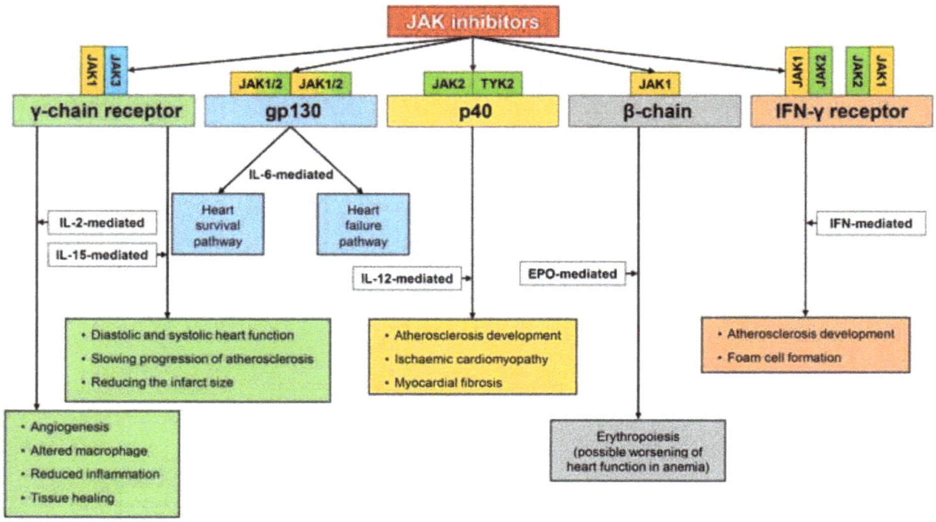

Figure 2. JAK inhibitors targeting JAKs of type I and II receptors. Based on cytokine profile inhibition of JAK/STAT pathway, diverse biological consequences are observed. Inhibition of JAK attached to γ-chain receptor resulting either in beneficial (blocking IL-15, high concentration mediated IL-2 transmission) or detrimental (inhibition of beneficial activity of low IL-2-impaired tissue healing and repair). Inhibition of JAK fused with gp130 receptor reduces IL-6 level. Based on the pathophysiological circumstances, reduced level of IL-6 may contribute to the reduction of heart survival pathway activity or favorably modify heart failure pathway. As far as IL-12 operating via p40 receptor subunit is concerned, inhibition of JAK results in reduction of IL-12-mediated signaling and exerts favorable effects on the cardiovascular system halting progression of atherosclerosis, reducing risk of developing ischemic cardiomyopathy, and myocardial fibrosis. Inhibition of JAK/STAT system transmitting signal from interferon receptor results in reduction of activity of IFN-dependent genes that translates directly to the reduction of foam cell formation and halting progression of atherosclerosis. Finally, some negative consequences may arise as the result of erythropoietin blockade with subsequent anemia development (indirectly contributing to worsening of heart function).

More data were provided from clinical studies where cardiovascular risk was assessed. Those studies demonstrated a low-incidence rate of MACE in RA patients, suggesting a good cardiovascular profile of JAK inhibitors [70]. Recently, these findings were substantiated by the first meta-analysis exploring the relationship between JAK inhibitor treatments and cardiovascular risks. According to the data from this study, short-term treatment with JAK inhibitor does not increase the risk of cardiovascular events when compared to placebo. Furthermore, with the exception of baricitinib, tofacitinib in both 5 and 10 mg doses and upadacitinib (15 mg and 30 mg doses) appeared to be equally safe [71]. Same conclusions were observed from analysis of clinical trials with tofacitinib [72]. The post-hoc analysis comprised in total eight trails - six phase III and long-term extension, respectively. The authors focused on MACE defined as any myocardial infarction, cerebrovascular event (i.e., stroke), or cardiovascular death (defined as death caused by coronary, cerebrovascular, or cardiac events) incidence in a large cohort of 4076 patients representing a total of 12,932 patient-years of tofacitinib exposure. In the study, MACE incidences were linked with older age, longer disease duration, higher mean body mass index, diabetes mellitus, hypertension, and lipid profile changes (higher total low-density lipoprotein (LDL), lower high-density lipoprotein (HDL) cholesterol, triglycerides, and higher total cholesterol to LDL ratio). Contrary to the previous studies linking disease activity with increased risk of poor cardiovascular outcome, in this study, disease activity parameters and inflammatory measured as baseline disease activity and inflammation measures were not significantly associated with MACE [72].

5.2. Lipid Profile

RA is linked with increased risk of cardiovascular events. In general population, the role-playing risk factors for atherosclerosis and poor cardiovascular outcome are obesity, sedentary lifestyle, smoking, and lipid profile disturbances. However, a significantly higher risk of developing cardiovascular events in RA patients cannot be explained by the presence of traditional risk factors alone. For many years, RA and other inflammatory conditions are recognized as the independent risk factors. In line with this, hampering the disease activity may add extra beneficial effect on the cardiovascular system.

Patients with RA often show lipid paradox, having lower total cholesterol and its subfractions as compared to unaffected population [73,74]. The most common explanation of this phenomena is suppression of cholesterol synthesis by inflammatory processes. Indeed, there is a strong link between C-reactive protein (a biomarker of inflammation) and circulating lipid levels [74]. Furthermore, treatment of RA may also impact lipid profile and some DMARDs exert the potentials to increase serum LDL and HDL cholesterol levels [75]. These phenomena cannot be explained only by the reduction of inflammation, since impact of various DMARDs on the lipid profile is variable, in spite of similar reductions in disease activity and systemic inflammatory parameters [76,77]. Followed observation on cholesterol increase in tocilizumab-treated RA patients, the interest on impact of various biologic and non-biologic DMARDs increased significantly. tocilizumab, an IL-6 receptor inhibitor, increases circulating LDL levels [77], but no increased risk of major cardiovascular events was observed [78,79]. It is established that tocilizumab reduces the LDL hypercatabolic state and diminishes the expression of LDL receptor on hepatocytes via a proprotein convertase subtilisin/kexin type-9-mediated mechanism [80,81]. Quite recently, Greco et al. showed that treatment with tocilizumab improves the activity of scavenger receptor class B member 1 and ATP binding cassette-G1 (ABCG1) which directly leads to favorable modifications of lipoprotein composition and functions in contributing to the reduced cardiovascular risk in tocilizumab-treated patients [82]. Therefore, contrary to the general population, changes in LDL composition are not translated to increased cardiovascular risk in patients with RA.

5.2.1. JAK Inhibitors and Lipid Profile

In the rabbit model, treatment with tofacitinib decreased systemic and synovial inflammation and increased circulating lipid levels have been observed. In this study, it failed to modify synovial macrophage density, however it reduced the lipid content within synovial macrophages. The study also confirmed the role IFN-γ in formation of foam cells, representing the key element for development of atherosclerosis. Inhibition of JAK/STAT pathway by tofacitinib contributed to lipid release via enhanced expression of cellular liver X receptor α and ATP-binding cassette transporter (ABCA1) synthesis [83]. Similarities in mechanisms of action in those two studies may suggest the role of IL-6 as a mediator of changes in lipid metabolism. The final effect may therefore be achieved by either IL-6 or JAK blockade (transmitting signals form IL-6-dependent receptor). Indeed, in an ex-vivo experiment, it was shown that tofacitinib decreased the expression of the IL-6 gene, having instead a variable effect on that of IL-8, TNF-α, and IL-10 genes [84]. Specifically, with ablation of JAK1 tofacitinib reduced signaling via IFN thus reducing TNF-α synthesis within macrophages. In a study with Chinese RA patients, the serum levels of TNF-α, IL-17, IL-6, and IFN-γ significantly decreased after the treatment with tofacitinib, parallel to an increase of IL-35, with subsequent T-reg lymphocyte response [85].

The role of IFN-γ in the modification of blood lipoproteins and promoting atherosclerosis development is postulated for many years. At the current level of knowledge, IFN signaling via JAK/STAT pathway regulates more than 2300 genes [85]. Signaling via IFN brings many pathophysiological consequences. Being a key element in immune response, IFN is also engaged in lipid metabolism and atherosclerosis development (Figure 3).

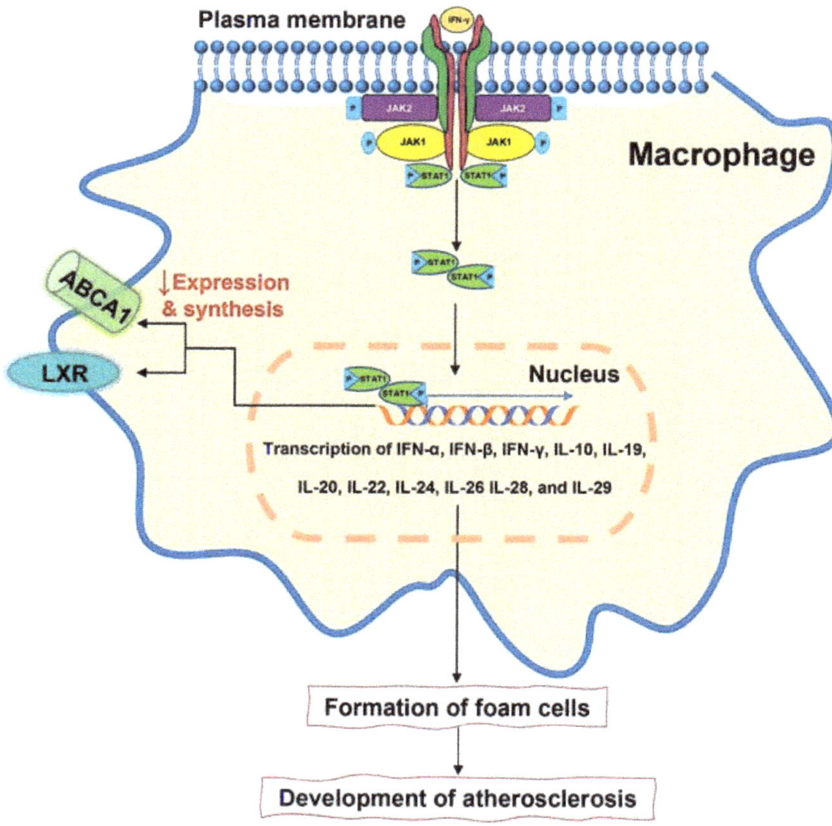

Figure 3. Interferons after ligating to type II receptors activate JAK/STAT pathway resulting in foam cells formation leading directly to atherosclerosis development. That same pathway that transmits signals from interferons contributes to reduced expression of the liver X receptor and decrease synthesis of ATP-binding cassette transporter leading to pro-atherosclerotic lipid composition.

Specifically, it can induce oxidative stress, promote foam cell accumulation, stimulate smooth muscle cell proliferation and migration into the arterial intima, enhance platelet-derived growth factor expression, and destabilize plaque [87]. This makes the IFN and STAT/JAK pathway the potential target to treat atherosclerosis. A few animal studies confirmed therapeutic potentials of IFN blockade resulting in inhibition of atherosclerotic plaque progression, stabilization of lipid- and macrophage-rich advanced plaques in ApoE knockout mice, and reduction of atherosclerosis in the graft vessels and the aorta in mice heart transplantation models [88–90]. Unfortunately, the inhibition of IFN blockade in atherosclerosis has not been tested in humans yet and studies on IFN inhibition in other indications (Crohn diseases and SLE) have been terminated prematurely due to lack of efficacy [87]. Another interesting study compared RA patients and healthy volunteers focusing on kinetics of cholesterol metabolism following a six-week tofacitinib treatment. In the study, the authors observed a reduction of the cholesterol ester fractional catabolic rate with subsequent increasing of HDL cholesterol and LDL cholesterol levels [91].

To summarize, blocking the JAK/STAT pathway may offer some potential to stop/reduce atherosclerosis development. The increment in lipid level did not translate to increased risk for atherosclerosis and is believed to be due to the transposition between several lipid compartments but not due to increased lipid synthesis. Moreover, as we already learned from the study with baricitinib, hypercholesterolemia, which occurred in less than 10% of the patients, was a dose-dependent event. Cholesterol level tends to increase during the first 12 weeks of the treatment, followed by stabilization of total cholesterol, LDL, and HDL serum levels when the treatment was continued [92].

5.2.2. Thromboembolic Events

Data from many clinical trials on JAK inhibitors suggesting increased risk of thromboembolic events in patients treated with JAK inhibitors. This risk is especially high in patients who already have risk factors for venous thromboembolic event (VTE), including history of cardiovascular disease, increased body mass, hypercoagulable states, neoplasm, and history of prior VTE, as well as patients receiving estrogens, patients undergoing major surgery, or patients with movement disabilities. The pathophysiological background of unprovoked thromboembolism, referring to both deep venous thrombosis and pulmonary embolism, is largely unknown, but it is believed to be linked with comorbidities, lifestyle, and risk factors. Recently, however, data on gene expression profiles provided a new insight into the pathogenesis of VTE. Among many mechanisms potentially involved into the progression of the diseases, leukocyte transendothelial migration and JAK-STAT signaling pathway and their related genes were found to be related with recurrent VTE [87]. Moreover, the regulatory network of recurrent VTE displayed that most of differentially expressed genes including intercellular adhesion molecule 1 and protein-tyrosine kinase 2-beta were regulated by STAT3. This may bring many clinical consequences as down regulated JAK/STAT related genes are directly linked to recurrent VTE, so the open question is whether continuation of JAK inhibitor after the first episode of VTE brings the hazard of recurrent VTE [87]. Contrary to this finding, Lu et al. suggested the role of the JAK2-STAT3 pathway in the regulatory network of platelet activation. According to the results from the study, collagen-induced platelet activation was mediated through the activation of JAK2-JNK/PKC-STAT3 signaling. So, the inhibition of this pathway may exert anti-platelet activity [88]. The opposite conclusions come from the study of Ayer et al., who investigated the role of mutation of JAK2 in the development of thrombosis in chronic myeloproliferative diseases, finding no relationship between thromboembolic events and JAK2 mutation [89]. Recently, the role of tissue factor (TF) and its regulatory mechanism attracted attention of many researchers. TFs may be regulated in several ways including this provided by heparanase. Heparanase (heparanase-1) is a mammalian enzyme (endo-β-D-glucuronidase) that degrades side chains of heparan sulfate [90]. Heparanase gene expression is regulated via many pro-inflammatory pathways (cytokines, reactive oxygen species, early growth response 1 transcription factor, and estrogens) and play a role as in the pathogenesis of several inflammatory disorders, such as inflammatory lung injury, cancer development, and chronic colitis [93]. Data from the literature suggests also the role of heparanase in the development of inflammatory arthritis including RA [93]. In line with it, dramatic hyperactivity of heparanase and angiogenesis gene expression in synovium of RA patients were found [94]. Data form patients with thalassemia showed very high activity of heparanase which in turn may activate the coagulation system, leading to thrombotic events. This is partially mediated by a high erythropoietin level which activates the JAK2 pathway. Therefore, the modulation of the JAK2 signaling pathway may help to reduce risk of thrombotic events mediated by heparinase [95]. The other beneficial effect that JAK inhibitors may exert on the coagulation pathway, reducing the risk of thromboembolic events, is the reduction of fibrinogen synthesis in hepatocytes. In this special instance, the effect is indirect and is related to total reduction of inflammatory response via inhibition of IL-6 signaling [96].

The potential mechanisms that lead to an increased risk of thromboembolic event in patients with RA treated with JAK inhibitors remain the subject of controversy. Blocking the JAK/STAT pathway may bring both harmful and beneficial effects depending on the pathophysiological environment.

Therefore, it may be suggested that not JAK inhibition alone, but comorbidities and risk factors presented in RA patients working together may in some predisposing patients increase the risk of thromboembolic complications.

6. Conclusions

The potent toll to halt inflammatory response has been given to rheumatologists and immunologists. So far, JAK inhibitors showed a high level of efficacy and satisfactorily level of safety. As with all novel compounds many questions arise regarding the safety profile and potential influence of these drugs on the functioning of vitally important internal organs, including the cardiovascular system. With the small synthetic compounds, we may block many cytokines belonging to several families, which exert both pro- and anti-inflammatory potentials. Parallel to this, we may change the expression of hundreds of related genes, creating a new environment for our patients. At the current level of knowledge, the direct influence of JAK inhibitors on the cardiovascular system is neutral or slightly beneficial. As we still accumulate knowledge on this impact, currently available data regarding this influence are not yet conclusive and more studies in this field are required. At this moment, it is still unclear which mechanisms may drive thromboembolic risk and this is the main concern regarding the administration of JAK inhibitors in patients with RA.

Author Contributions: Conceived and designed: P.J.K. and M.A.I.; wrote the original draft: P.J.K.; edited, critically reviewed, and revised the manuscript: M.A.I. and M.E.; drew figures: M.A.I. All authors have read and agreed to the published version of the manuscript.

Funding: This paper was funded by Medical University of Silesia, Katowice Poland.

Conflicts of Interest: The authors declare no conflict of interest.

Abbreviations

RA	Rheumatoid arthritis
DMARDs	Disease-modifying antirheumatic drugs
MTX	Methotrexate
JAK	Janus kinases
STAT	Signal transducers and activators of transcription
IFN	Interferon
TNF	Tumor necrosis factor
IL	Interleukin
SOCS	Suppressor of cytokine signaling
GM-CSF	Granulocyte-macrophage colony-stimulating factor
MACE	Major adverse cardiovascular events
LDL	Low-density lipoproteins
HDL	High-density lipoprotein
ABCA1	ATP-binding cassette transporter
VTE	Venous thromboembolic event
TF	Tissue factor

References

1. Smolen, J.S.; Aletaha, D.; McInnes, I.B. Rheumatoid arthritis. *Lancet* **2016**, *388*, 2023–2038. [CrossRef]
2. Kotyla, P.J.; Sliwinska-Kotyla, B.; Kucharz, E.J. Treatment with infliximab may contribute to the development of peripheral neuropathy among the patients with rheumatoid arthritis. *Clin. Rheumatol.* **2007**, *26*, 1595–1596. [CrossRef] [PubMed]
3. Kotyla, P.J. Bimodal function of anti-tnf treatment: Shall we be concerned about anti-tnf treatment in patients with rheumatoid arthritis and heart failure? *Int. J. Mol. Sci.* **2018**, *19*, 1739. [CrossRef] [PubMed]
4. Sartori, N.S.; de Andrade, N.P.B.; da Silva Chakr, R.M. Incidence of tuberculosis in patients receiving anti-tnf therapy for rheumatic diseases: A systematic review. *Clin. Rheumatol.* **2020**, *39*, 1439–1447. [CrossRef]

5. Angelini, J.; Talotta, R.; Roncato, R.; Fornasier, G.; Barbiero, G.; Dal Cin, L.; Brancati, S.; Scaglione, F. Jak-inhibitors for the treatment of rheumatoid arthritis: A focus on the present and an outlook on the future. *Biomolecules* **2020**, *10*, 1002. [CrossRef]
6. Jamilloux, Y.; El Jammal, T.; Vuitton, L.; Gerfaud-Valentin, M.; Kerever, S.; Sève, P. Jak inhibitors for the treatment of autoimmune and inflammatory diseases. *Autoimmun. Rev.* **2019**, *18*, 102390. [CrossRef]
7. Singh, S.; Singh, S. Jak-stat inhibitors: Immersing therapeutic approach for management of rheumatoid arthritis. *Int. Immunopharmacol.* **2020**, *86*, 106731. [CrossRef]
8. Xu, P.; Shen, P.; Yu, B.; Xu, X.; Ge, R.; Cheng, X.; Chen, Q.; Bian, J.; Li, Z.; Wang, J. Janus kinases (jaks): The efficient therapeutic targets for autoimmune diseases and myeloproliferative disorders. *Eur. J. Med. Chem.* **2020**, *192*, 112155. [CrossRef]
9. El Jammal, T.; Gerfaud-Valentin, M.; Sève, P.; Jamilloux, Y. Inhibition of jak/stat signaling in rheumatologic disorders: The expanding spectrum. *Jt. Bone Spine* **2020**, *87*, 119–129. [CrossRef]
10. Kotyla, P.J. Are janus kinase inhibitors superior over classic biologic agents in ra patients? *Biomed. Res. Int.* **2018**, *2018*, 7492904. [CrossRef]
11. Ghoreschi, K.; Laurence, A.; O'Shea, J.J. Janus kinases in immune cell signaling. *Immunol. Rev.* **2009**, *228*, 273–287. [CrossRef] [PubMed]
12. Kawamura, M.; McVicar, D.W.; Johnston, J.A.; Blake, T.B.; Chen, Y.-Q.; Lal, B.K.; Lloyd, A.R.; Kelvin, D.J.; Staples, J.E.; Ortaldo, J.R. Molecular cloning of l-jak, a janus family protein-tyrosine kinase expressed in natural killer cells and activated leukocytes. *Proc. Natl. Acad. Sci. USA* **1994**, *91*, 6374–6378. [CrossRef] [PubMed]
13. O'Shea, J.J.; Murray, P.J. Cytokine signaling modules in inflammatory responses. *Immunity* **2008**, *28*, 477–487. [CrossRef] [PubMed]
14. Villarino, A.V.; Kanno, Y.; O'Shea, J.J. Mechanisms and consequences of jak–stat signaling in the immune system. *Nat. Immunol.* **2017**, *18*, 374–384. [CrossRef] [PubMed]
15. Wang, Y.; Levy, D.E. Comparative evolutionary genomics of the stat family of transcription factors. *JAK-STAT* **2012**, *1*, 23–33. [CrossRef]
16. Zouein, F.A.; Duhé, R.J.; Booz, G.W. Jaks go nuclear: Emerging role of nuclear jak1 and jak2 in gene expression and cell growth. *Growth Factors* **2011**, *29*, 245–252. [CrossRef]
17. Schwartz, D.M.; Bonelli, M.; Gadina, M.; O'shea, J.J. Type i/ii cytokines, jaks, and new strategies for treating autoimmune diseases. *Nat. Rev. Rheumatol.* **2016**, *12*, 25. [CrossRef]
18. Waickman, A.T.; Park, J.-Y.; Park, J.-H. The common γ-chain cytokine receptor: Tricks-and-treats for t cells. *Cell. Mol. Life Sci.* **2016**, *73*, 253–269. [CrossRef]
19. Nicola, N.A.; Babon, J.J. Leukemia inhibitory factor (lif). *Cytokine Growth Factor Rev.* **2015**, *26*, 533–544. [CrossRef]
20. Boulanger, M.J.; Bankovich, A.J.; Kortemme, T.; Baker, D.; Garcia, K.C. Convergent mechanisms for recognition of divergent cytokines by the shared signaling receptor gp130. *Mol. Cell* **2003**, *12*, 577–589. [CrossRef]
21. Murakami, M.; Kamimura, D.; Hirano, T. Pleiotropy and specificity: Insights from the interleukin 6 family of cytokines. *Immunity* **2019**, *50*, 812–831. [CrossRef] [PubMed]
22. Collison, L.W.; Delgoffe, G.M.; Guy, C.S.; Vignali, K.M.; Chaturvedi, V.; Fairweather, D.; Satoskar, A.R.; Garcia, K.C.; Hunter, C.A.; Drake, C.G. The composition and signaling of the il-35 receptor are unconventional. *Nat. Immunol.* **2012**, *13*, 290. [CrossRef] [PubMed]
23. Wang, T.; Huang, W.; Costa, M.M.; Martin, S.A.; Secombes, C.J. Two copies of the genes encoding the subunits of putative interleukin (il)-4/il-13 receptors, il-4ralpha, il-13ralpha1 and il-13ralpha2, have been identified in rainbow trout (oncorhynchus mykiss) and have complex patterns of expression and modulation. *Immunogenetics* **2011**, *63*, 235–253. [CrossRef] [PubMed]
24. O'Shea, J.J.; Schwartz, D.M.; Villarino, A.V.; Gadina, M.; McInnes, I.B.; Laurence, A. The jak-stat pathway: Impact on human disease and therapeutic intervention. *Annu. Rev. Med.* **2015**, *66*, 311–328. [CrossRef]
25. Esch, A.; Masiarz, A.; Mossner, S.; Moll, J.M.; Grötzinger, J.; Schröder, J.; Scheller, J.; Floss, D.M. Deciphering site 3 interactions of interleukin 12 and interleukin 23 with their cognate murine and human receptors. *J. Biol. Chem.* **2020**, *295*, 10478–10492. [CrossRef]
26. Reddy, V.; Cohen, S. Jak inhibitors: What is new? *Curr. Rheumatol. Rep.* **2020**, *22*, 50. [CrossRef]

27. Tokumasa, N.; Suto, A.; Kagami, S.-i.; Furuta, S.; Hirose, K.; Watanabe, N.; Saito, Y.; Shimoda, K.; Iwamoto, I.; Nakajima, H. Expression of tyk2 in dendritic cells is required for il-12, il-23, and ifn-γ production and the induction of th1 cell differentiation. *Blood J. Am. Soc. Hematol.* **2007**, *110*, 553–560. [CrossRef]
28. O'Shea, J.J.; Holland, S.M.; Staudt, L.M. Jaks and stats in immunity, immunodeficiency, and cancer. *N. Engl. J. Med.* **2013**, *368*, 161–170. [CrossRef]
29. Holland, S.M.; DeLeo, F.R.; Elloumi, H.Z.; Hsu, A.P.; Uzel, G.; Brodsky, N.; Freeman, A.F.; Demidowich, A.; Davis, J.; Turner, M.L. Stat3 mutations in the hyper-ige syndrome. *N. Engl. J. Med.* **2007**, *357*, 1608–1619. [CrossRef]
30. Cho, J.H.; Gregersen, P.K. Genomics and the multifactorial nature of human autoimmune disease. *N. Engl. J. Med.* **2011**, *365*, 1612–1623. [CrossRef]
31. Remmers, E.F.; Cosan, F.; Kirino, Y.; Ombrello, M.J.; Abaci, N.; Satorius, C.; Le, J.M.; Yang, B.; Korman, B.D.; Cakiris, A. Genome-wide association study identifies variants in the mhc class i, il10, and il23r-il12rb2 regions associated with behcet's disease. *Nat. Genet.* **2010**, *42*, 698–702. [CrossRef] [PubMed]
32. Duerr, R.H.; Taylor, K.D.; Brant, S.R.; Rioux, J.D.; Silverberg, M.S.; Daly, M.J.; Steinhart, A.H.; Abraham, C.; Regueiro, M.; Griffiths, A. A genome-wide association study identifies il23r as an inflammatory bowel disease gene. *Science (N.Y.)* **2006**, *314*, 1461–1463. [CrossRef] [PubMed]
33. Remmers, E.F.; Plenge, R.M.; Lee, A.T.; Graham, R.R.; Hom, G.; Behrens, T.W.; De Bakker, P.I.; Le, J.M.; Lee, H.-S.; Batliwalla, F. Stat4 and the risk of rheumatoid arthritis and systemic lupus erythematosus. *N. Engl. J. Med.* **2007**, *357*, 977–986. [CrossRef] [PubMed]
34. Alunno, A.; Padjen, I.; Fanouriakis, A.; Boumpas, D.T. Pathogenic and therapeutic relevance of jak/stat signaling in systemic lupus erythematosus: Integration of distinct inflammatory pathways and the prospect of their inhibition with an oral agent. *Cells* **2019**, *8*, 898. [CrossRef] [PubMed]
35. Dupuis, S.; Jouanguy, E.; Al-Hajjar, S.; Fieschi, C.; Al-Mohsen, I.Z.; Al-Jumaah, S.; Yang, K.; Chapgier, A.; Eidenschenk, C.; Eid, P. Impaired response to interferon-α/β and lethal viral disease in human stat1 deficiency. *Nat. Genet.* **2003**, *33*, 388–391. [CrossRef]
36. Chapgier, A.; Kong, X.-F.; Boisson-Dupuis, S.; Jouanguy, E.; Averbuch, D.; Feinberg, J.; Zhang, S.-Y.; Bustamante, J.; Vogt, G.; Lejeune, J. A partial form of recessive stat1 deficiency in humans. *J. Clin. Investig.* **2009**, *119*, 1502–1514. [CrossRef]
37. Baechler, E.C.; Batliwalla, F.M.; Karypis, G.; Gaffney, P.M.; Ortmann, W.A.; Espe, K.J.; Shark, K.B.; Grande, W.J.; Hughes, K.M.; Kapur, V.; et al. Interferon-inducible gene expression signature in peripheral blood cells of patients with severe lupus. *Proc. Natl. Acad. Sci. USA* **2003**, *100*, 2610–2615. [CrossRef]
38. Barrat, F.J.; Crow, M.K.; Ivashkiv, L.B. Interferon target-gene expression and epigenomic signatures in health and disease. *Nat. Immunol.* **2019**, *20*, 1574–1583. [CrossRef]
39. Gallay, L.; Mouchiroud, G.; Chazaud, B. Interferon-signature in idiopathic inflammatory myopathies. *Curr. Opin. Rheumatol.* **2019**, *31*, 634–642. [CrossRef]
40. Marketos, N.; Cinoku, I.; Rapti, A.; Mavragani, C.P. Type i interferon signature in sjögren's syndrome: Pathophysiological and clinical implications. *Clin. Exp. Rheumatol.* **2019**, *37* (Suppl. 118), 185–191.
41. Rönnblom, L.; Eloranta, M.L. The interferon signature in autoimmune diseases. *Curr. Opin. Rheumatol.* **2013**, *25*, 248–253. [CrossRef] [PubMed]
42. Jiang, J.; Zhao, M.; Chang, C.; Wu, H.; Lu, Q. Type i interferons in the pathogenesis and treatment of autoimmune diseases. *Clin. Rev. Allergy Immunol.* **2020**, *59*, 248–272. [CrossRef] [PubMed]
43. Arakawa, T.; Masaki, T.; Hirai, T.; Doi, S.; Kuratsune, M.; Arihiro, K.; Kohno, N.; Yorioka, N. Activation of signal transducer and activator of transcription 3 correlates with cell proliferation and renal injury in human glomerulonephritis. *Nephrol. Dial. Transplant.* **2008**, *23*, 3418–3426. [CrossRef] [PubMed]
44. Justiz Vaillant, A.A.; Qurie, A. Interleukin. In *Statpearls*; StatPearls Publishing LLC.: Treasure Island, FL, USA, 2020.
45. Rochman, Y.; Spolski, R.; Leonard, W.J. New insights into the regulation of t cells by γ c family cytokines. *Nat. Rev. Immunol.* **2009**, *9*, 480–490. [CrossRef] [PubMed]
46. Kimura, A.; Kishimoto, T. Il-6: Regulator of treg/th17 balance. *Eur. J. Immunol.* **2010**, *40*, 1830–1835. [CrossRef]
47. Fragoulis, G.E.; McInnes, I.B.; Siebert, S. Jak-inhibitors. New players in the field of immune-mediated diseases, beyond rheumatoid arthritis. *Rheumatology (Oxford)* **2019**, *58*, i43–i54. [CrossRef]

48. Emery, P.; Pope, J.E.; Kruger, K.; Lippe, R.; DeMasi, R.; Lula, S.; Kola, B. Efficacy of monotherapy with biologics and jak inhibitors for the treatment of rheumatoid arthritis: A systematic review. *Adv. Ther.* **2018**, *35*, 1535–1563. [CrossRef]
49. Kerschbaumer, A.; Sepriano, A.; Smolen, J.S.; van der Heijde, D.; Dougados, M.; van Vollenhoven, R.; McInnes, I.B.; Bijlsma, J.W.J.; Burmester, G.R.; de Wit, M.; et al. Efficacy of pharmacological treatment in rheumatoid arthritis: A systematic literature research informing the 2019 update of the eular recommendations for management of rheumatoid arthritis. *Ann. Rheum. Dis.* **2020**, *79*, 744–759. [CrossRef]
50. Taylor, P.C.; Keystone, E.C.; van der Heijde, D.; Weinblatt, M.E.; del Carmen Morales, L.; Reyes Gonzaga, J.; Yakushin, S.; Ishii, T.; Emoto, K.; Beattie, S. Baricitinib versus placebo or adalimumab in rheumatoid arthritis. *N. Engl. J. Med.* **2017**, *376*, 652–662. [CrossRef]
51. Fleischmann, R.; Pangan, A.L.; Song, I.H.; Mysler, E.; Bessette, L.; Peterfy, C.; Durez, P.; Ostor, A.J.; Li, Y.; Zhou, Y. Upadacitinib versus placebo or adalimumab in patients with rheumatoid arthritis and an inadequate response to methotrexate: Results of a phase iii, double-blind, randomized controlled trial. *Arthritis Rheumatol.* **2019**, *71*, 1788–1800. [CrossRef]
52. Fleischmann, R.; Mysler, E.; Hall, S.; Kivitz, A.J.; Moots, R.J.; Luo, Z.; DeMasi, R.; Soma, K.; Zhang, R.; Takiya, L. Efficacy and safety of tofacitinib monotherapy, tofacitinib with methotrexate, and adalimumab with methotrexate in patients with rheumatoid arthritis (oral strategy): A phase 3b/4, double-blind, head-to-head, randomised controlled trial. *Lancet* **2017**, *390*, 457–468. [CrossRef]
53. Wollenhaupt, J.; Lee, E.-B.; Curtis, J.R.; Silverfield, J.; Terry, K.; Soma, K.; Mojcik, C.; DeMasi, R.; Strengholt, S.; Kwok, K. Safety and efficacy of tofacitinib for up to 9.5 years in the treatment of rheumatoid arthritis: Final results of a global, open-label, long-term extension study. *Arthritis Res. Ther.* **2019**, *21*, 89. [CrossRef] [PubMed]
54. Keystone, E.C.; Genovese, M.C.; Schlichting, D.E.; de la Torre, I.; Beattie, S.D.; Rooney, T.P.; Taylor, P.C. Safety and efficacy of baricitinib through 128 weeks in an open-label, longterm extension study in patients with rheumatoid arthritis. *J. Rheumatol.* **2018**, *45*, 14–21. [CrossRef] [PubMed]
55. Taylor, P.C.; Weinblatt, M.E.; Burmester, G.R.; Rooney, T.P.; Witt, S.; Walls, C.D.; Issa, M.; Salinas, C.A.; Saifan, C.; Zhang, X. Cardiovascular safety during treatment with baricitinib in rheumatoid arthritis. *Arthritis Rheumatol.* **2019**, *71*, 1042–1055. [CrossRef] [PubMed]
56. El Jammal, T.; Sève, P.; Gerfaud-Valentin, M.; Jamilloux, Y. State of the art: Approved and emerging jak inhibitors for rheumatoid arthritis. *Expert Opin. Pharmacother.* **2020**, 1–14. [CrossRef]
57. Spolski, R.; Gromer, D.; Leonard, W.J. The γ c family of cytokines: Fine-tuning signals from il-2 and il-21 in the regulation of the immune response. *F1000Research* **2017**, *6*, 1872. [CrossRef]
58. Fukuzawa, J.; Booz, G.W.; Hunt, R.A.; Shimizu, N.; Karoor, V.; Baker, K.M.; Dostal, D.E. Cardiotrophin-1 increases angiotensinogen mrna in rat cardiac myocytes through stat3: An autocrine loop for hypertrophy. *Hypertension* **2000**, *35*, 1191–1196. [CrossRef]
59. Hirota, H.; Chen, J.; Betz, U.A.; Rajewsky, K.; Gu, Y.; Ross, J., Jr.; Müller, W.; Chien, K.R. Loss of a gp130 cardiac muscle cell survival pathway is a critical event in the onset of heart failure during biomechanical stress. *Cell* **1999**, *97*, 189–198. [CrossRef]
60. Li, H.; Cen, K.; Sun, W.; Feng, B. Predictive value of blood interleukin-6 level in patients with acute coronary syndrome: A meta-analysis. *Immunol. Investig.* **2020**, 1–13. [CrossRef]
61. Xu, L.; Yan, J.; Zhang, F.; Zhou, C.; Fan, T.; Chen, X.; Cui, X.; Zhou, H.; Liang, Y. Use of inflammatory biomarkers and real-time cardiac catheterisation to evaluate the left ventricular diastolic function in patients with diastolic heart failure. *Heart Lung Circ.* **2020**. [CrossRef]
62. Ridker, P.M.; Libby, P.; MacFadyen, J.G.; Thuren, T.; Ballantyne, C.; Fonseca, F.; Koenig, W.; Shimokawa, H.; Everett, B.M.; Glynn, R.J. Modulation of the interleukin-6 signalling pathway and incidence rates of atherosclerotic events and all-cause mortality: Analyses from the canakinumab anti-inflammatory thrombosis outcomes study (cantos). *Eur. Heart J.* **2018**, *39*, 3499–3507. [CrossRef] [PubMed]
63. Ridker, P.M.; MacFadyen, J.G.; Glynn, R.J.; Bradwin, G.; Hasan, A.A.; Rifai, N. Comparison of interleukin-6, c-reactive protein, and low-density lipoprotein cholesterol as biomarkers of residual risk in contemporary practice: Secondary analyses from the cardiovascular inflammation reduction trial. *Eur. Heart J.* **2020**. [CrossRef]
64. Kanda, T.; Takahashi, T. Interleukin-6 and cardiovascular diseases. *Jpn. Heart J.* **2004**, *45*, 183–193. [CrossRef] [PubMed]

65. Gabriel, A.S.; Martinsson, A.; Wretlind, B.; Ahnve, S. Il-6 levels in acute and post myocardial infarction: Their relation to crp levels, infarction size, left ventricular systolic function, and heart failure. *Eur. J. Intern. Med.* **2004**, *15*, 523–528. [CrossRef] [PubMed]
66. Wang, K.; Li, B.; Xie, Y.; Xia, N.; Li, M.; Gao, G. Statin rosuvastatin inhibits apoptosis of human coronary artery endothelial cells through upregulation of the jak2/stat3 signaling pathway. *Mol. Med. Rep.* **2020**, *22*, 2052–2062. [CrossRef] [PubMed]
67. Wu, J.; Yu, J.; Xie, P.; Maimaitili, Y.; Wang, J.; Yang, L.; Ma, H.; Zhang, X.; Yang, Y.; Zheng, H. Sevoflurane postconditioning protects the myocardium against ischemia/reperfusion injury via activation of the jak2–stat3 pathway. *PeerJ* **2017**, *5*, e3196. [CrossRef] [PubMed]
68. Liao, Y.; Hu, X.; Guo, X.; Zhang, B.; Xu, W.; Jiang, H. Promoting effects of il-23 on myocardial ischemia and reperfusion are associated with increased expression of il-17a and upregulation of the jak2-stat3 signaling pathway. *Mol. Med. Rep.* **2017**, *16*, 9309–9316. [CrossRef]
69. Liao, Y.H.; Xia, N.; Zhou, S.F.; Tang, T.T.; Yan, X.X.; Lv, B.J.; Nie, S.F.; Wang, J.; Iwakura, Y.; Xiao, H.; et al. Interleukin-17a contributes to myocardial ischemia/reperfusion injury by regulating cardiomyocyte apoptosis and neutrophil infiltration. *J. Am. Coll. Cardiol.* **2012**, *59*, 420–429. [CrossRef]
70. Charles-Schoeman, C.; Wicker, P.; Gonzalez-Gay, M.A.; Boy, M.; Zuckerman, A.; Soma, K.; Geier, J.; Kwok, K.; Riese, R. Cardiovascular safety findings in patients with rheumatoid arthritis treated with tofacitinib, an oral janus kinase inhibitor. *Semin. Arthritis Rheum.* **2016**, *46*, 261–271. [CrossRef]
71. Xie, W.; Huang, Y.; Xiao, S.; Sun, X.; Fan, Y.; Zhang, Z. Impact of janus kinase inhibitors on risk of cardiovascular events in patients with rheumatoid arthritis: Systematic review and meta-analysis of randomised controlled trials. *Ann. Rheum. Dis.* **2019**, *78*, 1048–1054. [CrossRef]
72. Charles-Schoeman, C.; DeMasi, R.; Valdez, H.; Soma, K.; Hwang, L.J.; Boy, M.G.; Biswas, P.; McInnes, I.B. Risk factors for major adverse cardiovascular events in phase iii and long-term extension studies of tofacitinib in patients with rheumatoid arthritis. *Arthritis Rheumatol.* **2019**, *71*, 1450–1459. [CrossRef] [PubMed]
73. Choy, E.; Sattar, N. Interpreting lipid levels in the context of high-grade inflammatory states with a focus on rheumatoid arthritis: A challenge to conventional cardiovascular risk actions. *Ann. Rheum. Dis.* **2009**, *68*, 460–469. [CrossRef] [PubMed]
74. Johnsson, H.; Panarelli, M.; Cameron, A.; Sattar, N. Analysis and modelling of cholesterol and high-density lipoprotein cholesterol changes across the range of c-reactive protein levels in clinical practice as an aid to better understanding of inflammation–lipid interactions. *Ann. Rheum. Dis.* **2014**, *73*, 1495–1499. [CrossRef] [PubMed]
75. Robertson, J.; Peters, M.J.; McInnes, I.B.; Sattar, N. Changes in lipid levels with inflammation and therapy in ra: A maturing paradigm. *Nat. Rev. Rheumatol.* **2013**, *9*, 513. [CrossRef]
76. Souto, A.; Salgado, E.; Maneiro, J.R.; Mera, A.; Carmona, L.; Gómez-Reino, J.J. Lipid profile changes in patients with chronic inflammatory arthritis treated with biologic agents and tofacitinib in randomized clinical trials: A systematic review and meta-analysis. *Arthritis Rheumatol.* **2015**, *67*, 117–127. [CrossRef]
77. Smolen, J.S.; Beaulieu, A.; Rubbert-Roth, A.; Ramos-Remus, C.; Rovensky, J.; Alecock, E.; Woodworth, T.; Alten, R. Effect of interleukin-6 receptor inhibition with tocilizumab in patients with rheumatoid arthritis (option study): A double-blind, placebo-controlled, randomised trial. *Lancet* **2008**, *371*, 987–997. [CrossRef]
78. Singh, S.; Fumery, M.; Singh, A.G.; Singh, N.; Prokop, L.J.; Dulai, P.S.; Sandborn, W.J.; Curtis, J.R. Comparative risk of cardiovascular events with biologic and synthetic disease-modifying antirheumatic drugs in patients with rheumatoid arthritis: A systematic review and meta-analysis. *Arthritis Care Res.* **2020**, *72*, 561–576. [CrossRef]
79. Castagné, B.; Viprey, M.; Martin, J.; Schott, A.-M.; Cucherat, M.; Soubrier, M. Cardiovascular safety of tocilizumab: A systematic review and network meta-analysis. *PLoS ONE* **2019**, *14*, e0220178. [CrossRef]
80. Ferraz-Amaro, I.; Hernández-Hernández, M.V.; Tejera-Segura, B.; Delgado-Frías, E.; Macía-Díaz, M.; Machado, J.D.; Diaz-González, F. Effect of il-6 receptor blockade on proprotein convertase subtilisin/kexin type-9 and cholesterol efflux capacity in rheumatoid arthritis patients. *Horm. Metab. Res.* **2019**, *51*, 200–209. [CrossRef]
81. Strang, A.C.; Bisoendial, R.J.; Kootte, R.S.; Schulte, D.M.; Dallinga-Thie, G.M.; Levels, J.H.; Kok, M.; Vos, K.; Tas, S.W.; Tietge, U.J. Pro-atherogenic lipid changes and decreased hepatic ldl receptor expression by tocilizumab in rheumatoid arthritis. *Atherosclerosis* **2013**, *229*, 174–181. [CrossRef]

82. Greco, D.; Gualtierotti, R.; Agosti, P.; Adorni, M.P.; Ingegnoli, F.; Rota, M.; Bernini, F.; Meroni, P.L.; Ronda, N. Anti-atherogenic modification of serum lipoprotein function in patients with rheumatoid arthritis after tocilizumab treatment, a pilot study. *J. Clin. Med.* **2020**, *9*, 2157. [CrossRef] [PubMed]
83. Pérez-Baos, S.; Barrasa, J.I.; Gratal, P.; Larrañaga-Vera, A.; Prieto-Potin, I.; Herrero-Beaumont, G.; Largo, R. Tofacitinib restores the inhibition of reverse cholesterol transport induced by inflammation: Understanding the lipid paradox associated with rheumatoid arthritis. *Br. J. Pharmacol.* **2017**, *174*, 3018–3031. [CrossRef]
84. Hodge, J.A.; Kawabata, T.T.; Krishnaswami, S.; Clark, J.D.; Telliez, J.-B.; Dowty, M.E.; Menon, S.; Lamba, M.; Zwillich, S. The mechanism of action of tofacitinib-an oral janus kinase inhibitor for the treatment of rheumatoid arthritis. *Clin. Exp. Rheumatol.* **2016**, *34*, 318–328. [PubMed]
85. Li, Y.; Yuan, L.; Yang, J.; Lei, Y.; Zhang, H.; Xia, L.; Shen, H.; Lu, J. Changes in serum cytokines may predict therapeutic efficacy of tofacitinib in rheumatoid arthritis. *Mediat. Inflamm.* **2019**, *2019*. [CrossRef] [PubMed]
86. Rusinova, I.; Forster, S.; Yu, S.; Kannan, A.; Masse, M.; Cumming, H.; Chapman, R.; Hertzog, P.J. Interferome v2. 0: An updated database of annotated interferon-regulated genes. *Nucleic Acids Res.* **2012**, *41*, D1040–D1046. [CrossRef] [PubMed]
87. Xu, D.; Xu, R.; He, L.; Xu, T.; Zhang, Z.; Han, D.; Du, J. Comparison of pathogenic mechanisms underlying single and recurrent venous thromboembolism based on gene expression profiling. *Ann. Vasc. Surg.* **2016**, *36*, 252–259. [CrossRef] [PubMed]
88. Lu, W.J.; Lin, K.C.; Huang, S.Y.; Thomas, P.A.; Wu, Y.H.; Wu, H.C.; Lin, K.H.; Sheu, J.R. Role of a janus kinase 2-dependent signaling pathway in platelet activation. *Thromb. Res.* **2014**, *133*, 1088–1096. [CrossRef] [PubMed]
89. Ayer, M.; Menken, İ.; Yamak, M.; Ayer, F.A.; Kırkızlar, O.; Burak Aktuğlu, M. The impact of mean platelet volume (mpv) and jak-2 mutation on thrombosis in chronic myeloproliferative diseases. *Indian J. Hematol. Blood Transfus. Off. J. Indian Soc. Hematol. Blood Transfus.* **2017**, *33*, 181–187. [CrossRef]
90. Nadir, Y. Heparanase in the coagulation system. *Adv. Exp. Med. Biol.* **2020**, *1221*, 771–784.
91. Charles-Schoeman, C.; Fleischmann, R.; Davignon, J.; Schwartz, H.; Turner, S.M.; Beysen, C.; Milad, M.; Hellerstein, M.K.; Luo, Z.; Kaplan, I.V.; et al. Potential mechanisms leading to the abnormal lipid profile in patients with rheumatoid arthritis versus healthy volunteers and reversal by tofacitinib. *Arthritis Rheumatol. (Hoboken N.J.)* **2015**, *67*, 616–625. [CrossRef]
92. Smolen, J.S.; Genovese, M.C.; Takeuchi, T.; Hyslop, D.L.; Macias, W.L.; Rooney, T.; Chen, L.; Dickson, C.L.; Riddle Camp, J.; Cardillo, T.E.; et al. Safety profile of baricitinib in patients with active rheumatoid arthritis with over 2 years median time in treatment. *J. Rheumatol.* **2019**, *46*, 7–18. [CrossRef] [PubMed]
93. Goldberg, R.; Meirovitz, A.; Hirshoren, N.; Bulvik, B.; Binder, A.; Rubinstein, A.M.; Elkin, M. Versatile role of heparanase in inflammation. *Matrix Biol. J. Int. Soc. Matrix Biol.* **2013**, *32*, 234–240. [CrossRef] [PubMed]
94. Li, R.W.; Freeman, C.; Yu, D.; Hindmarsh, E.J.; Tymms, K.E.; Parish, C.R.; Smith, P.N. Dramatic regulation of heparanase activity and angiogenesis gene expression in synovium from patients with rheumatoid arthritis. *Arthritis Rheum. Off. J. Am. Coll. Rheumatol.* **2008**, *58*, 1590–1600. [CrossRef] [PubMed]
95. Ghoti, H.; Ackerman, S.; Rivella, S.; Casu, C.; Nadir, Y. Heparanase level and procoagulant activity are increased in thalassemia and attenuated by jak-2 inhibition. *Am. J. Pathol.* **2020**. [CrossRef]
96. Febvre-James, M.; Lecureur, V.; Fardel, O. Potent repression of c-reactive protein (crp) expression by the jak1/2 inhibitor ruxolitinib in inflammatory human hepatocytes. *Inflamm. Res.* **2020**, *69*, 51–62. [CrossRef]

International Journal of
Molecular Sciences

MDPI

Review

Molecular and Cellular Mechanisms of Arthritis in Children and Adults: New Perspectives on Applied Photobiomodulation

Laura Marinela Ailioaie [1,2] and Gerhard Litscher [3,*]

1 Department of Medical Physics, Alexandru Ioan Cuza University, 11 Carol I Boulevard, 700506 Iaşi, Romania; lauraailioaie@yahoo.com
2 Ultramedical & Laser Clinic, 83 Arcu Street, 700135 Iaşi, Romania
3 Research Unit of Biomedical Engineering in Anesthesia and Intensive Care Medicine, Research Unit for Complementary and Integrative Laser Medicine, and Traditional Chinese Medicine (TCM) Research Center Graz, Medical University of Graz, Auenbruggerplatz 39, 8036 Graz, Austria
* Correspondence: gerhard.litscher@medunigraz.at; Tel.: +43-316-385-83907

Received: 5 August 2020; Accepted: 2 September 2020; Published: 8 September 2020

Abstract: Juvenile idiopathic arthritis and adult rheumatoid arthritis are two major groups with chronic joint pain and inflammation, extra-articular manifestations, and high risk of comorbidities, which can cause physical and ocular disability, as well as create great socio-economic pressure worldwide. The pathogenesis of arthritis manifested in childhood and adulthood is multifactorial, unclear, and overly complex, in which immunity plays an important role. Although there are more and more biological agents with different mechanisms of action for the treatment of arthritis, the results are not as expected, because there are partial responses or non-responsive patients to these compounds, high therapeutic costs, side effects, and so on; therefore, we must turn our attention to other therapeutic modalities. Updating knowledge on molecular and cellular mechanisms in the comparative pathogenesis of chronic arthritis in both children and adults is necessary in the early and correct approach to treatment. Photobiomodulation (PBM) represents a good option, offering cost-effective advantages over drug therapy, with a quicker, more positive response to treatment and no side effects. The successful management of PBM in arthritis is based on the clinician's ability to evaluate correctly the inflammatory status of the patient, to seek the optimal solution, to choose the best technology with the best physical parameters, and to select the mode of action to target very precisely the immune system and the molecular signaling pathways at the molecular level with the exact amount of quantum light energy in order to obtain the desired immune modulation and the remission of the disease. Light is a very powerful tool in medicine because it can simultaneously target many cascades of immune system activation in comparison with drugs, so PBM can perform very delicate tasks inside our cells to modulate cellular dysfunctions, helping to initiate self-organization phenomena and finally, healing the disease. Interdisciplinary teams should work diligently to meet these needs by also using single-cell imaging devices for multispectral laser photobiomodulation on immune cells.

Keywords: adults; juvenile; cytokines; immune; laser blood irradiation; low-level laser; systemic

1. Introduction

Chronic arthritis is the most usual cause for joint pain, physical disability, and ocular invalidity worldwide. Juvenile idiopathic arthritis (JIA) and rheumatoid arthritis (RA) of the adult are two major groups with chronic joint inflammation, extra-articular manifestations, and high risk for comorbidities [1–5].

While in adults there are over 150 forms of chronic arthritis, in children, there are several dozen subtypes of the disease, but only juvenile polyarthritis with positive rheumatoid factor and the subtype of systemic arthritis also known as Still disease, which is more consistent with an autoinflammatory condition, have similar manifestations to adults [6].

Patients with systemic JIA require close keep under surveillance by a multidisciplinary team due to possible serious complications: macrophage activation syndrome, pericarditis, pulmonary hypertension, interstitial lung disease, infections, etc., which may be associated with increased mortality [7].

In the pathology of children, the oligoarticular manifestation is an entity that we do not find in the forms of rheumatic disease in adults and is characterized by often severe eye damage, localized growth disorders with elongation of a limb, and secondary posture disorders.

JIA is the type of chronic rheumatic disease that affects the child's daily activities due to pain, joint swelling, morning stiffness, and locomotor and possibly ocular infirmities, which causes short-term and long-term disabilities, until adulthood and sometimes throughout life [8].

Treatment available for patients with chronic arthritis aims to reduce pain, maintain joint function, improve well-being, and prevent disability and associated comorbidities.

Pharmacological therapy usually includes non-steroidal anti-inflammatory drugs, intra-articular or systemic steroids, to which will be added disease-modifying anti-rheumatic drugs (DMARDs) and biological agents administered on time in the "window of opportunity" to prevent irreversible complications [2].

Early use of intra-articular steroid therapy, methotrexate, and biological agents introduced in recent decades have improved the prognosis of children with arthritis, but those with polyarticular form can have serious problems with active disease as adults. Most children with the JIA oligoarticular subtype may enter remission, but a small number progress to a persistent polyarticular form as adults.

Concerns have been raised about the use of biological agents that may increase the risk of cancer in patients with chronic arthritis.

Based on the severity of the disease, which evolves progressively, the patient with chronic arthritis can become an important burden for the family, but especially for the society, through the enormous costs of direct health care, social assistance, loss in education, productivity, and jobs.

The first goal of this review was to update knowledge on molecular and cellular mechanisms through a parallelism between special forms of chronic arthritis present in both children and adults, for an introspection into the pathogenesis of these diseases, in an attempt to reveal to researchers and clinicians the latest discoveries regarding new molecules and signaling pathways.

The second objective of this review was to raise awareness and send a signal to rheumatologists on the need to change the treatment paradigms for arthritis through innovative therapies to stop the perpetuation of the disease from childhood to adulthood, the side effects, the inefficiency in some cases, and the high current costs, in order to overcome this human and economic burden.

The third purpose was to promote light or laser therapies (photobiomodulation) as an important complementary and alternative method, which has become increasingly known around the world in recent decades for reducing pain and sometimes even eliminating the cause of the pain itself, for inducing early remission before common destructive changes in joints begin, in all arthritis forms.

Last aim but not least is to signal that photobiomodulation (PBM) and the single-cell live tracking technology of immune cell activities are ready to precisely target the signaling pathways and to find the answers to the complex interaction of the laser with the immune system, for "undoing" arthritis!

Seeking and developing new treatments to interact smoothly with the immune system both in children and adults to handle immune-mediated diseases that are becoming more and more complex is urgently needed.

JIA, formerly known as juvenile rheumatoid arthritis in the Anglo-Saxon literature, and chronic juvenile arthritis for French speakers, is a chronic immune-mediated inflammatory disease of unknown etiology and a complex genetic component that is defined according to the criteria of the International

League of Associations for Rheumatology (ILAR) as inflammatory arthritis in one or more joints, which begins before the age of 16, persists for at least six weeks, and all other conditions that cause similar symptoms have been excluded [1,4].

A better understanding of the pathogenesis and the latest diagnostic tools are challenges for rheumatologists to update the classification. Based on ILAR criteria, there are seven main subgroups of JIA defined by clinical and laboratory data: systemic arthritis, rheumatoid factor (RF) polyarthritis—positive or negative, oligoarthritis (persistent or extensive), enthesitis-related arthritis (ERA), psoriatic arthritis (PsA), and a seventh category, undifferentiated arthritis, which includes those patients who do not fit any of the above forms of criteria [4,9].

1.1. RF-Positive Polyarticular JIA

RF-positive polyarticular juvenile idiopathic arthritis is defined by the existence of at least 5 inflamed joints over a period of 6 weeks, in the presence of RF found twice, at an interval of at least 3 months in the first 6 months after the onset of the disease. This category is considered clinically and biologically similar to adult RA by progressive destructive polyarticular manifestations in the knee, elbow, and foot.

In this case, arthritis in children is symmetrical and predominantly peripheral; it affects particularly small joints of the fingers and toes, but it may also affect the large joints of the knees, hips, ankles, and fist.

Other manifestations may include lower-level fever than in systemic form, rheumatoid nodules (tumors under the skin, most common in the elbow), anemia, and thrombocytosis.

Factors that determine disability include early age at onset, female gender, the presence of rheumatoid factor, and the presence of anti-cyclic citrullinated peptide antibodies (anti-CCP) [2,10].

As a peculiarity, it should be mentioned in children that it affects the temporomandibular joints and the upper cervical region (neck area).

Temporomandibular arthritis can limit mouth opening and discomfort in chewing. Arthritis of the neck area can cause instability or fusion of the cervical vertebrae, with a high potential for neurological injury of the spine to minor trauma.

Long-term studies show that the prognosis is severe in 50% of cases [11].

Most common complications are osteoporosis, vertebral collapse, dwarfism, pubertal delay, intercurrent viral, or bacterial infections in immunosuppressed children by disease or secondary to medication [12,13].

1.2. RF-Negative Polyarthritis

Rheumatoid factor negative polyarticular juvenile idiopathic arthritis is defined by inflammatory damage of 5 or more joints, in the first 6 months after onset, in the absence of RF [14].

According to some authors, this type of juvenile arthritis accounts for up to 30% of polyarticular forms of childhood, and in some cases, it has a rapidly disabling progression [15,16].

This category of polyarthritis is much more severe than oligoarthritis and is often associated with extra-articular manifestations that include salivary gland disease (Sjögren's Syndrome), lymphadenopathy within Felty's Syndrome, or juvenile vasculitis.

About 20% of this category of arthritis starts early, affects the female gender, to whom can be detected positive antinuclear antibodies (ANA), and in these cases, there is a high risk for iridocyclitis. The long-term functional prognosis of the disease is more severe than in the oligoarthritis subtypes, but it is better than in the RF-positive polyarticular JIA [2].

1.3. Systemic JIA

Systemic juvenile idiopathic arthritis (sJIA) is a subtype of the disease that occurs in childhood secondary to an immune disorder, which associates arthritis and systemic inflammatory symptoms [17].

sJIA is defined as arthritis accompanied or preceded by daily fever, with a minimum duration of 2 weeks, associated with the following extra-articular symptoms: erythematous rash, lymph node hypertrophy, hepato- and/or splenomegaly, and serositis [18].

The diagnosis is sustained by the prolonged fever for at least two weeks and is accompanied by two major criteria, or by one major criterion and two minor criteria. The major criteria are given by erythematous rash and arthritis. The minor criteria could be the following: generalized adenomegaly and/or hepatomegaly and/or splenomegaly; serositis; arthralgia lasting 2 weeks or more (in the absence of arthritis); and leukocytosis ($\geq$ 15,000 /µL) and increased numbers of neutrophils.

sJIA is similar to Still's disease in adults and for the correct diagnosis, the presence of fever is required alongside at least one major criterion; arthritis would no longer be necessary because, as in adults, it may be initially missing [19].

1.4. Enthesitis-Related Arthritis (ERA)

The enthesitis-related arthritis (ERA) has also been referred to by ILAR as an undifferentiated spondyloarthropathy, because the symptoms are mostly found in adulthood, but with a higher percentage of non-differentiated forms in children. In the current definition, an imagistic criterion was introduced by radiographic images or magnetic resonance images [20,21].

The diagnosis is supported by peripheral arthritis and enthesitis, or arthritis, or enthesitis, which are associated with $\geq$ 3 months of inflammatory back pain and sacroiliitis on X-ray or MRI images. Arthritis or enthesitis must persist for at least 6 weeks, to which are added the following symptoms: sensitivity of the sacroiliac joint; back pain, the presence of HLA-B27 antigen; previous acute uveitis (symptomatic); and a history of spondylarthritis in a first-degree relative [19,22,23].

Over the last decade, more and more evidence has been gathered suggesting that some of these categories appear to be quite homogeneous and are present both in children and adults; others are heterogeneous and cannot be better defined [24].

1.5. Psoriatic JIA

Psoriatic juvenile arthritis (psJIA) accounts for up to 10% of all JIA subtypes; it is a type of arthritis that affects both sexes and manifests itself in association with psoriatic skin lesions [25].

Psoriatic arthritis is defined within the ILAR classification as a persistent arthritis of more than 6 weeks and either the presence of a psoriatic rash or, in the absence of rash, at least 2 of the following minor criteria: first degree relative with psoriasis, nail pitting, onycholysis, dactylitis; the forms with positive RF and those associated with systemic manifestations are excluded. The peculiarity of psoriatic rheumatism is represented by the presence of ANA in more than 50% of cases and by its association with uveitis [4,25].

1.6. Oligoarticular JIA

Oligoarticular juvenile idiopathic arthritis, formerly referred to as pauciarthritis or juvenile rheumatoid arthritis with pauciarticular onset, is defined by the inflammatory involvement of one or less of five joints [2].

It is the most common subgroup in juvenile arthritis, accounting for about 50% of all cases. The oligoarticular JIA comprises two categories: the persistent form in which the number of inflamed joints remains the same throughout the disease, and the extensive form in which the number of active joints is five or cumulatively more, after the first 6 months onset [2,16].

A particular case is that of oligoarthritis as a more homogeneous entity observed only in childhood, with early onset and an association of positive antinuclear antibodies (ANA) [26], young age, and female gender, complicated with iridocyclitis [19,27–29].

1.7. Undifferentiated Arthritis

Undifferentiated JIA is a subtype of juvenile arthritis that does not exactly meet the criteria for the categories mentioned above, or it simultaneously meets several criteria for different subtypes of the disease [2].

The Paediatric Rheumatology INternational Trials Organisation (PRINTO) has a current project with the proposal to revise current JIA classification criteria after ILAR, using clinical evidence and common laboratory data available worldwide to classify those forms of chronic arthritis that are commonly encountered in children and that are the counterpart of childhood diseases observed in adults [19].

2. Molecular and Cellular Mechanisms of Systemic Arthritis

The pathogenesis of systemic arthritis manifested in childhood and adulthood is multifactorial, unclear, and very complex, in which the innate immunity plays an important role by activating neutrophils and macrophages, as well as the adaptive immunity, by increasing the percentage of pro-inflammatory cytokines: interleukin (IL)-1β, IL-6, IL-18, and interferon gamma (IFN)–γ [30–34].

sJIA accounts for about 10% of all forms of juvenile arthritis and is a chronic disease that results in significant morbidity and mortality in children [22,35].

The most significant manifestation of systemic arthritis is its association with macrophage activation syndrome, a secondary disorder of excessive, uncontrolled activation and non-malignant proliferation of T lymphocytes and macrophages, with a state of hypercitokinemia, on which the clinical–biological signs depend [36–38].

The underlying cause of the occurrence of chronic rheumatism in the JIA subtypes, including sJIA, is largely unknown. A current concept would be that triggering manifestations in sJIA would be due to an infectious aggression with an inappropriate immune response due to a genetic or acquired immune defect [33].

More and more studies have shown that in the pathogenesis of sJIA, the innate immune system is more involved, compared to the adaptive one [31,39,40].

Biological studies for sJIA describe a polymorphism of disease-promoting elements encoded by tumor necrosis factor alpha (TNFα), IL-6, IL-10, macrophage migration inhibitory factor (MIF), and IL-1 family (in particular, IL1A, IL1RN, IL1R2) [41–44].

More and more clinical and biological as well as translational research draw attention to the particularly important role of IL-1β, IL-6, and IL-18 in the complexity of disease manifestation and the limited role of TNF-α, as well as the relative absence of induced chemokines by interferon gamma (IFN-γ), IFN-γ-inducible protein 10 (IP-10, CXCL10), MIG, and I-TAC [31,40,45].

The IL-1 superfamily contains 11 cytokines, from which IL-1α and IL-1β have the most powerful pro-inflammatory effect. They have a natural antagonist IL-1Ra (IL-1 receptor antagonist), which is an endogenous inhibitor of IL-1 and works as a competitive inhibitor of IL-1 binding to IL-1R1. It is produced by inflamed synovial macrophages and initiates inflammatory responses [46].

IL-1 has a biphasic role in implicating innate immune mechanisms, but also in adaptive ones in triggering sJIA. At the onset of the disease, the disruption of immunity induced by IL-1 induces clinical manifestations of fever, rash, and early synovitis. Then, IL-1 intervenes in the mechanisms of adaptive regulation by activating and promoting the differentiation of T lymphocytes in Th17 cells with a pro-inflammatory role and by inhibiting the activity of T-regulatory cells [47].

Certain evidence of IL-1 involvement in the pathogenesis of sJIA is given by the successful treatment with IL-1 inhibitors, such as the biological agent anakinra, a soluble IL-1 receptor antagonist (IL-1Ra) that is similar to IL-1Ra, which has increased levels during the active disease observed also in polyarticular JIA. At the same time, with particularly good clinical results for anti-IL-1 therapy, the normalization of genes expressed by peripheral blood mononuclear cells (PBMCs) was observed [48–50].

Since the response to the IL-1β antagonist therapy of the anakinra product is limited by the large number of IL-1β receptors expressed on several different cell types and the rapid excretion of IL-1RA by healthy kidneys, two drugs (rilonacept and canakinumab) have appeared much more efficient [51].

However, not all patients with sJIA respond well to anti-IL-1 therapy. Clinical–biological research has shown that age at onset of disease, duration, number of active joints, polymorphonuclear, and serum ferritin levels can predict anti-IL-1 response. Elevated ferritin in patients' serum can be a valuable biological signal and parameter, which will guide us to explore macrophage activation syndrome (MAS), which can be effectively treated with anti-IL-1 agents. So far, the laboratory data have not revealed the presence of antibodies, and there is evidence that sJIA is actually a form of autoinflammatory disease, and not autoimmune [52].

The importance of IL-6 in the pathogenesis of sJIA has been demonstrated by correlating the serum and synovial concentration with the severe joint manifestations and the maximum level of fever [53].

Pro-inflammatory cytokines, such as IL-1, IL-6, and TNF-α, by stimulating similar receptors, induce IL-6 production in lymphocytes, macrophages, and synovial cells [54].

IL-6 has various functions in the pathogenesis of sJIA in children and rheumatoid arthritis in adults, in the sense that it induces an acute phase response as well as activates immune reactions and hematopoiesis.

The released IL-6 will induce the production of acute phase proteins (C-reactive protein and fibrinogen), which are known as biological markers of inflammation and the differentiation of naive T cells into Th17 cells [54,55].

The imbalance between Th17/Treg, where Th17 is activated significantly more than Treg, has a disastrous effect on RA development [56].

As IL-10 is a cytokine that would play a key anti-inflammatory role in the prevention of immune cascades from immune-mediated inflammatory diseases, conflicting results are reported in the literature regarding the poor involvement of this cytokine and the occurrence of manifestations in sJIA [43,44,57].

In a study published by Imbrechts et al., experimental evidence was provided on a mouse model that there would be a relationship between IL-10 insufficient production and its consequence in the innate cellular immune response from sJIA pathogenesis [58].

Both sJIA and macrophage activation syndrome are triggered by a cascade discharge of some cytokines such as interleukin 1β, IL-6 and IL-18.

To date, the exact role of interferon-gamma (IFN-γ), a cytokine with pro- and anti-inflammatory properties is being intensively investigated along with the role of NK cells providing IFN-γ [59].

Put K. found in its published PhD thesis on mice models that "the inflammatory environment in sJIA affects NK cells, causing an inflammatory transcriptional profile in these cells"; although there are very high plasma levels of IL-18, they do not influence NK cells, which causes IFN-y production to be low. Therefore, NK and IFN-y cells should be considered as limiting factors in sJIA pathogenesis [60].

Despite all previous knowledge that IL-18 is commonly recognized as the major inducer of IFN-y synthesis in NK cells, the paper published by Put K. et al. in patients with active systemic JIA shows that despite high plasma levels of IL-18, IFN-y levels remained low. In contrast, gene expression profiling was altered by the increased expression of innate genes, including TLR4 (Toll-Like Receptor 4) and S100A9 (S100 calcium-binding protein A9), and the decreased expression of immunity-regulating genes, such as IL-10RA (interleukin 10 receptor, alpha) and GZMK (granzyme K), as compared to cells from healthy controls. From these studies, it is believed that subtle defects in the pathways associated with NK cells, such as granzyme K expression and IFN-γ production determined by IL-18, may contribute to the immune aggregation of this disease [61].

Macrophages Activation Syndrome

Macrophage activation syndrome (MAS) or hemophagocytic syndrome is a complication of Still disease in children and adults, which can be life-threatening and is considered a subset of hemophagocytic lymphohistiocytosis (HLH) [62,63].

Macrophage activation syndrome generally has an unknown incidence because some forms are expressed by mild subclinical signs, but 10% of patients with sJIA could have a serious, potentially lethal complication [64].

From the biological point of view, MAS is expressed by a defect of the cytolytic pathways with an uncontrolled proliferation of cytotoxic cells and a hypersecretion of pro-inflammatory cytokines—that is, an increase in hematophagocytic T lymphocytes and macrophages that induce a cytokine storm with severe multiorgan injury [65,66].

In MAS, NK dysfunctions, mutations of the UNC13D, PRF1, STXBP2, and RAB27 genes, TLR-9 receptor dysfunction of IFN-γ, and activation pathways of IL-10 and IL-18 were observed [67–69].

Clinical symptoms include fever (96% of cases, often persistent), hepatomegaly (70%), splenomegaly (58%), and lymphadenopathy (51%). In 35% of cases, the neurological manifestations could be convulsions, drowsiness, irritability, confusion, headache, and coma. There may also be cardiac involvement even with pericarditis, pulmonary pleural effusion, hematuria, proteinuria, and signs of renal failure. Hemorrhagic manifestations range from purple rash, ecchymoses, gingival or gastrointestinal bleeding, and disseminated intravascular coagulation. MAS laboratory data include decreased ESR, WBC, platelet count and serum fibrinogen; as well as high and extremely high levels of ferritin, D-dimers, liver enzymes, lactate dehydrogenase, triglycerides, with the prolongation of prothrombin time (PT) and partial thromboplastin time (aPTT) [70–72].

Today, there are guidelines with diagnostic criteria for HLH, MAS associated with sJIA, or MAS associated with systemic lupus erythematosus. Selecting the right diagnostic criteria is essential for successful therapy [62].

3. Comparative Pathogenesis of Rheumatoid Arthritis in Adults and Children

The pathogenesis of RA and JIA is not yet very well known, although there is strong evidence that it involves the components of the immune system, especially T and B lymphocytes, as well as the antibodies and cytokines resulting from this immune conflict [7,73].

As is well known, the immune system has two main branches: the innate components and the adaptive immunity. The cells and receptors of the innate immune system play an extremely important role in rapidly recognizing the foreign infectious agent and initiating a defense response, which is known as pro-inflammatory [74].

In triggering an inflammatory action, innate immune cells—neutrophils, macrophages, monocytes, natural killer cells, dendritic cells (DC) and so on, playing the role of stopping the inflammatory process (infectious)—will inform, initiate, and direct the phenomena of the proliferation and differentiation of adaptive immune cells [74].

In response to the inflammatory aggression of B cells, the β- and γδ-selected T cells from the branch of innate immunity will be stimulated to proliferate and differentiate into cells specific to the functions appropriate to the immunological challenge, and they will eventually die and leave subsets of cells with memory. In rheumatoid arthritis, the activation of a naive T cell departing from the thymus to the lymphoid organs involves coordinated interactions between a number of molecules on the surface of this cell and an antigen-presenting cell (APC), that is, that carries an antigenic peptide derived from the infectious agent noncovalently linked to a major histocompatibility complex (MHC) class I or class II molecule.

When the APC cell is activated, various costimulatory ligands are expressed, allowing the activation, proliferation, and differentiation of T cells [74,75].

The T cells will express a series of inhibitory receptors for a fine regulation of the response appropriate to the inflammatory environment where they were being stimulated. Inhibitory receptors can act in two directions: to limit the costimulatory signaling, as well as to temporarily bind the costimulatory molecule [74].

At the synovial level, as result of inflammation, the differentiation of naive T cells in Th17 cells will occur. It was believed that this immune pathology would be mediated by Th1 cells (the first objectified), but today, the research has evolved, and it has been discovered that, in fact, Th17 cells are considered responsible for the pathogenesis in rheumatoid arthritis [76,77].

Current studies demonstrate that synovial fibroblasts and activated immune cells are directly involved in the production and release of many pro-inflammatory cytokines that play a crucial role in the development and progression of RA [78].

In fact, the characteristic inflammatory process in RA is achieved by the abundance of inflammatory-promoting cytokines, in counterbalance with inhibitory cytokines, intercellular communication, immune responses, and boosting cell movement to territories of inflammatory, infectious, or post-traumatic conflict.

In RA, the cytokines of the immune network are classified into four groups: pro-inflammatory cytokines, inflammatory cytokines in the joints, anti-inflammatory cytokines, and natural cytokine antagonists [79].

After the onset of initial stimuli, the cytokines play an important role in communicating with the components of the immune system at each stage of the pathophysiology of RA.

The release of cytokines, particularly the TNF-α, IL-6, and IL-1, promotes the synovial inflammatory process.

IL-6 binds to cells via a specific receptor complex involving two proteins, IL-6 receptor α and gp130, in order to transmit information. IL-6 receptor α exists into two forms: a transmembrane IL-6 receptor α, or mIL-6R (membrane-bound form of IL-6R), and a soluble IL-6 receptor α, sIL-6R. After IL-6 binds to any IL-6 receptor, the complex formed will induce gp130 activation. All IL-6-type cytokines signal through the gp130/JAK/STAT pathway. The binding of IL-6 to mIL-6R induces anti-inflammatory classic signaling, whereas the binding of IL-6 to sIL-6R induces pro-inflammatory trans-signaling [80–82].

Recent clinical studies have shown that patients with RA (adults) or active polyarticular sJIA (children), who did not respond adequately to MTX (methotrexate) and TNF-alpha inhibitors, received an IL-6 inhibitor, for example, tocilizumab in children and sarilumab (in adults), which are biologics that can be more effective [83,84].

Among the pro-inflammatory cytokines at the synovial level, TNF-α is a pleiotropic cytokine produced by several cell types, such as T and B cells, but also by innate immune cells (dendritic, monocyte, neutrophil, mast cells) and has a very important role, because it participates as the main mediator in regulating and training other factors [85,86].

In addition to this role, it is known that TNF-α is associated with bone and cartilage destruction by activating chondrocytes and osteoclasts [87].

TNF-α induces the synthesis and secretion of MMPs (matrix metalloproteinases), which in turn affect the chemokine and cytokine action of MMP-2, MMP-3, MMP-7, and MMP-9, which release TGF beta (Transforming Growth Factor) from the matrix, thus enabling its activation [88].

Therefore, anti-TNF biological therapy has been considered a remarkable breakthrough in the treatment of chronic autoimmune diseases, such as RA and JIA [85].

The interleukin (IL)-1 (family) together with its members (IL-33, IL-36α, β, γ, IL-37, and IL-38), IL-6, and IL-12 superfamilies (IL-27, IL-35) together with the other key cytokines (IL-15, IL-16, IL-17 family IL-17A, IL-17B, IL-17C), the recently cloned cytokine IL-18, IL-32, IL-34, and interferon (IFN)-y, the granulocyte macrophage colony-stimulating factor, are detected in a high concentration in the synovial fluid, but also in the patient's serum, thus leading to the process of local joint destruction and systemic effects in the rheumatoid arthritis patient [79,89].

More explicitly, IL-1 has 11 pro-inflammatory and anti-inflammatory members, which are chronologically numbered based on their discovery, from the IL-1 first family member 1 (IL-1F1) to IL-1F11. More commonly, they are also known as receptor antagonist IL-1α, IL-1β, IL-1 (IL-1Ra), IL-18, IL-33, IL-36α, IL-36β, IL-36γ, IL-36Ra, IL-37, and IL-38 [90].

IL-33 has been detected in high serum concentrations in adult patients with rheumatoid arthritis, in contrast to those with osteoarthritis (OA) and psoriatic arthritis (PsA) and was associated with bone erosion and cardiovascular pathology, as a predictive factor for the evolution of atherosclerotic plaque [89]; however, the results are contradictory for its real role in the pathogenesis of RA, and as a consequence, specific drugs are not yet available [91–94].

Interleukin (IL)-17A is a pro-inflammatory cytokine that participates in the development of several autoimmune and inflammatory diseases [95].

IL-17A has a direct influence on the early pathogenesis and chronic stages of synovitis in rheumatoid and psoriatic arthritis, through systemic, but also local effects on keratinocytes [96].

The synovial membrane in RA is modified by inflammatory factors in the sense of the appearance of a local infiltrate of immune cells, hyperplasia, and angiogenesis tissue [97,98].

It has been shown that in the synovial lymphocyte infiltration and in the hyperplastic mucosa of RA, there are cells producing IL-17A and IL-17F; at the same time, there is a recruitment of Th17 cells that will interact with local cells and perpetuate chronic inflammation [99].

IL-17 is directly involved in the stimulation of vascular endothelial growth factor production in synovial fibroblasts, angiogenesis, and synovial pannus development [100,101].

The interaction between Th17 cells and synoviocytes is crucial, because as a result of this cooperation, IL-17 will be massively released [96].

TNF-alpha supports the effect of human IL-17A for the action of increasing the secretion of IL-6 and IL-8 from rheumatoid synoviocytes and vice versa, IL-17A and IL-17F induce TNFα receptor II expression and production [96,102,103].

Another particularly important role of IL-17 is to promote the expression of nuclear factor kappa-B (NF-κB) ligand receptor activator (RANKL) on osteoblasts and synoviocytes and to activate RANK signaling in osteoclasts [104–106].

Since 1999, it is known that IL-17 from human T cells activated in synovial tissues of patients with rheumatoid arthritis is a potent stimulator of osteoclastogenesis [107] and ultimately, the destruction of the bone [96].

The pro-inflammatory cytokines are also responsible for the synthesis of chemokines from MMPs, inducible nitric-oxide synthase, osteoclasts differentiation, and an increased expression of cell adhesion molecules. Disruption of MMP activity can lead to tissue degradation associated with inflammation in rheumatoid arthritis. Several inhibitors capable of modifying MMP activity are approved today, but unfortunately, they are associated with undesirable side effects [88].

Phytochemicals such as flavonoids, glycosides, lignans, and alkaloids are valuable natural sources for the development of new drugs with efficacy and safety in inhibiting upstream signaling molecules involved in MMP expression [88].

Helper T cells are deeply involved in the pathogenesis of autoimmune diseases, including RA; for example, it has been shown recently that Th17 can move into a "non-classical" class of Th1, with higher pathogenic activity, which is a phenomenon that further complicated the explanation of the pathogenic mechanisms of RA [108].

The same study has shown in patients with early-onset RA but without medication a higher ratio of Th17-derived Th1 cells comparatively to CD161 + Th17 cells, and an inverse correlation between interferon-γ (IFNγ) + Th17 cells, comparatively with the anti-CCP antibodies levels [108].

Today, it is known that Th17 produces the cytokine IL-17 [54], which activates inflammation by stimulating immune cells and at the same time activates osteoclasts by inducing kappa B ligand nuclear factor activator receptor (RANKL) in synovial fibroblasts. This fact opens new horizons for Th17-targeted therapies in order to stop the bone destruction associated with T cell activation [109].

At the same time, Foxp3 is essential for the suppressive function of Treg cells, and as a specific marker of Th17 cells, it accelerates osteoclasts differentiation. In RA, Foxp3(+)CD4(+) T cells are subjected to conversion into TH17 cells, which is mediated by synovial fibroblast-derived IL-6 [110], and meanwhile, IFN-gamma cytokines, IL-4, and cytotoxic T lymphocyte-associated protein 4 (CTLA-4), produced by Th1, Th2, and respectively, Treg, regulate osteoclast differentiation.

In RA, there is an imbalance in the Th17/Treg ratio, where Th17 is activated much more than Treg [111].

It is speculated that TNF inhibitors used in RA therapy reduce the passage of Th17 cells to non-classical Th1 cells, as well as direct inhibit the TNFα [85,108].

Inflammatory synovitis both in RA and JIA provides the image of an imbalance between pro-inflammatory and anti-inflammatory cytokines [IL-10, IL-11, and IL-13], which are insufficient to counterbalance the intensely active inflammatory process. Bone destruction in RA is caused by the effects of osteoclasts and not by the invasion of inflammatory factors directly into the synovium [112].

Synovial inflammatory cytokines [TNFα, IL-1, IL-6, and IL-17] promote excessive synthesis of (RANK)/RANKL (receptor activator of nuclear factor kappa-B ligand) on the membrane of synovial fibroblasts and/or osteoblasts and their differentiation [113,114].

Cartilage destruction is caused by MMPs or ADAMTS (a disinterring and metalloproteinase with thrombospondin motifs) that are produced by chondrocytes, synovial fibroblasts, and synovial macrophages. The JAK/STAT pathway is another signaling pathway for various cytokines and growth factors involved in the pathogenesis of rheumatoid arthritis. JAK is a tyrosine kinase receptor that mediates intracellular signaling through a transcription factor, STAT [115].

Currently, there is already experience with inhibitory drugs for the JAK receptor family; thus, tofacitinib for JAK1, JAK2, JAK3, and Tyk2; and baricitinib, which selectively act on JAK1 and JAK2 and are used in RA therapy [116,117].

Forty years after the discovery of IL-1, the "triggering agent" of the molecular and cellular mechanisms of the appearance and development of RA is constantly being sought as another fascinating field of intense investigation. In recent years, the range of pro- and anti-inflammatory cytokines has expanded rapidly with the identification of new members, and it has been proven to be involved to varying degrees in the pathogenesis of RA. Based on this knowledge, the therapeutic arsenal for RA patients includes monoclonal antibodies, fusion proteins, or antagonists against these molecules [89].

The treatment of rheumatoid arthritis in children and adults first benefits from methotrexate as "gold standard therapy", and if patients do not respond or experience complications and/or adverse reactions, TNF inhibitors will be given: infliximab, etanercept, adalimumab, golimumab, and certolizumab pegol (for adults). While TNF, IL-6, and JAK inhibitors directly regulate cytokine generation and bioactivity, a new biological product, abatacept (as a selective costimulation modulator), has been shown to inhibit T-cell activation by binding to CD80 and CD86, thereby blocking interaction with CD28. This results in the inhibition of autoimmune T-cell activation that is implicated in the pathogenesis of rheumatoid arthritis [118–120].

Although there are more and more biological agents with different mechanisms of action for the treatment of rheumatoid arthritis in children and adults, the results are not as we expected, because there are partial responses or non-responsive patients to these compounds, high therapeutic costs, side effects, and so on; therefore, we must turn our attention to other therapeutic modalities to induce disease remission.

4. New Introspections and Perspectives on Photobiomodulation in Arthritis

4.1. Photobiomodulation: Short History, Basic Concepts, and Current Applications

As an interdisciplinary field, photomedicine is growing in importance because of its relevance to light and laser therapies [121]. The whole spectrum of electromagnetic radiation is depicted in Figure 1.

Full-spectrum light or sunlight [122] covers the electromagnetic spectrum from infrared to near-ultraviolet, or all wavelengths that are useful to plant or animal life (Figure 2). Natural light is composed of various electromagnetic waves traveling in disoriented fashion, which is known as incoherent light.

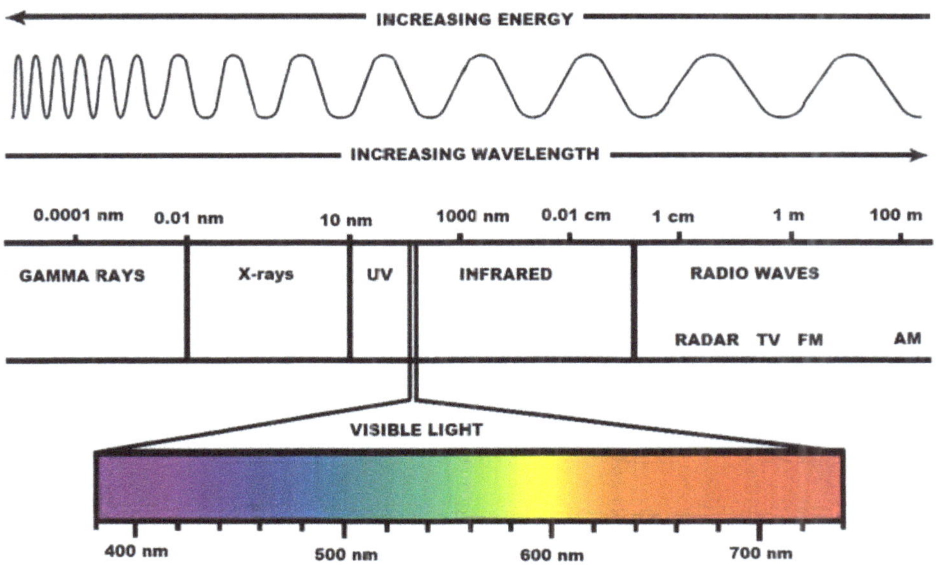

Figure 1. The aspect of the visible light spectrum within the electromagnetic radiation spectrum.

Phototherapy is rooted in the past when Egyptian, Indian, Chinese, and later Greek civilizations used light as a therapeutic agent to cure psoriasis, rickets, vitiligo, and even skin cancers [123].

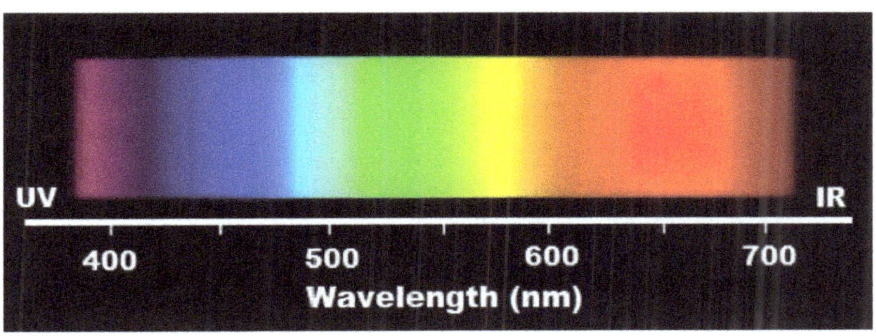

Figure 2. Wavelengths applied in photobiomodulation.

Since antiquity, we have known that the doctor's presence is needed where the Sun is missing. Although the therapeutic properties of light have been known for thousands of years, this therapy has been developed and applied extensively only in the last two centuries. For example, the Nobel Prize in Physiology or Medicine 1903 was awarded to Niels Ryberg Finsen "in recognition of his contribution to the treatment of diseases, especially lupus vulgaris, with concentrated light radiation, whereby he has opened a new avenue for medical science" [124].

Lighting with wavelengths ranging from near-ultraviolet to red and including near-infrared has demonstrated many beneficial effects of the stimulation, preservation, and regeneration in cells, tissues, and organs in animals and humans.

After the Nobel Prize was awarded in 1964 to researchers Townes, Basov, and Prohorov for their contributions to the development of laser-maser, applications of low-level laser therapy (LLLT) in multiple branches of medicine have spread around the world, and today, this method is called photobiomodulation (PBM).

LASER (the acronym for Light Amplification by Stimulated Emission of Radiation) was a pure invention of the human mind, which triggered a revolution.

Laser light differs from sunlight due to its three distinct properties: monochromaticity (extremely narrow wavelength range); collinearity (all quanta move into the same direction); and coherence (parallel phase run of the light waves). For example, the difference in the coherence of laser light compared to a lamp is shown in Figure 3.

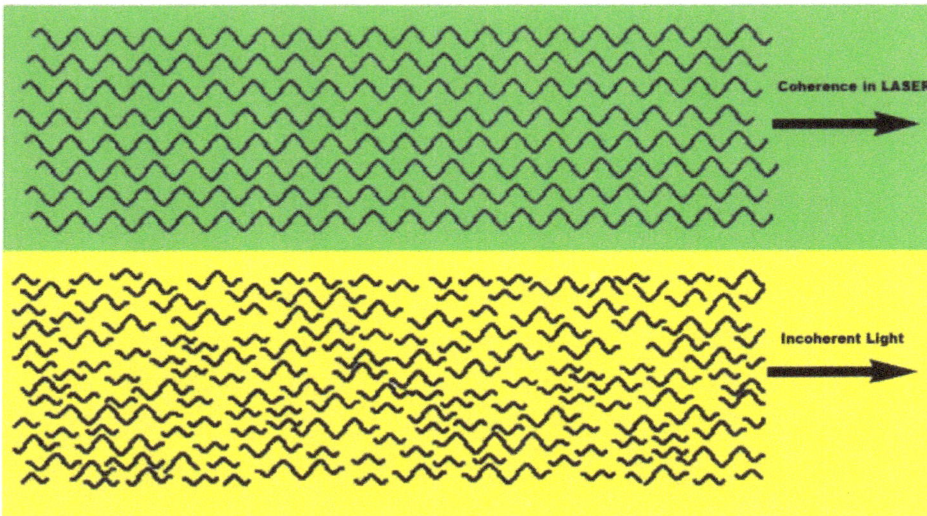

Figure 3. Coherent and incoherent light.

The most important and useful units of measurement in laser practice are: wavelength (nm, nanometer); power (W, watt or mW, milliwatt); energy (J, joule); power density (W/cm2), and energy density (J/cm^2).

Light-based treatment methods use lasers or other light sources, such as LEDs; lamps with polarized light, polychromatic, incoherent, and low energy; Super Luminous Diodes (SLD); flash lamps, etc.

These devices release energy into the irradiated tissue that will induce photophysical and photochemical reactions at different biological levels, implicating endogenous chromophores.

There are significant differences between lasers and other light sources, including the specificity of the wavelength and the physical characteristics of the generated beam.

The three unique properties of the LASER beam—monochromaticity, coherence, and collimation—which make it unique for stimulating chromophores in biological tissues that respond only to certain extremely specific wavelengths.

The depth of penetration is determined by the wavelength, the tissue composition, as well as forward and backscatter in the tissue. Coherence is very quickly lost, and the depth of penetration for a large spot (illumination area) can be substantially greater than for a smaller spot size with the same wavelength at the same irradiance (intensity) [125].

If we use PBM with LEDs, there are certain differences, among which we mention lower power delivered in a certain biological time window (for an optimal cellular response); longer wavelength band (approximately 20 nm width), compared to LASER (approximately 1 nm width); the beam is not collimated or coherent [126].

To obtain the desired photobiomodulation effect, a certain quantified amount of photonic energy is always required, and therefore, depending on the pathology, LASERs, LEDs, or other available lamps or devices can be used accordingly.

The success of therapy depends on the correct choice of a device for energy levels quantification targeting.

Today, PBM is widely used worldwide in a variety of pathologies in adult and pediatric medicine. It is a natural treatment that provides the living cells with an energy source in the form of photons. Many diseases or dysfunctional problems of a bodily system or organ can be successfully treated with this ingenious technology. Clinical practice and the scientific investigation had shown bright prospects for the further development of this trend. Lasers can be used to perform exceedingly small and delicate tasks inside the living organisms [127].

Photobiomodulation represents a good option, as it is highly effective in many children's and adult's disorders, offering cost-effective advantages over drug therapy, with a quicker more positive response to treatment and no side effects. Last but not least, PBM is painless and non-invasive [128].

For PBM, laser devices are used that have a low light emission power below 500 mW or less than 0.5 watts (class III), but also lasers with a high power of more than 500 mW (laser "therapeutic window" of approximately 650–1100 nm, class IV). The high-intensity laser (HIL) is used with great success especially for sports injuries (traumatic injuries, musculoskeletal strains, osteoarticular, and spine injuries—lumbar and cervical area) [129,130].

Apart from PBM, lasers with higher powers and low pulse widths are applied in surgery, ophthalmology, dermatology–cosmetology, gynecology, oncology, etc.

Figure 4 depicts some lasers applied in medicine.

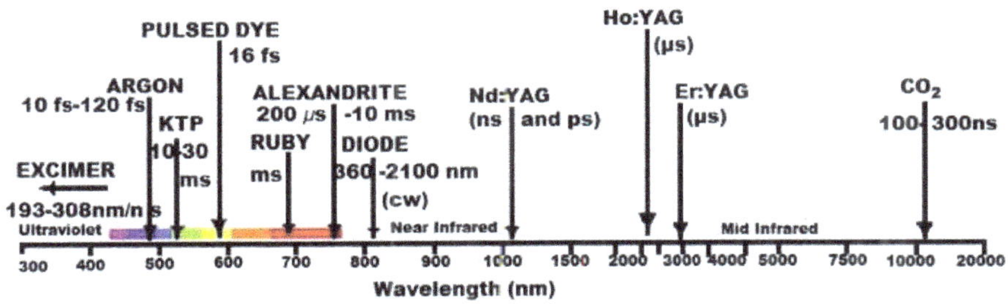

Figure 4. Types of lasers with applications in medicine.

In PBM, from light-emitting diodes or low-level energy lasers, the photonic fluxes enter the cells, penetrating the tissues quite well and initiating a cascade of photochemical reactions on specific signaling pathways due to the endogenous photoreceptors, triggering molecular mechanisms in the mitochondrial respiratory chain, reducing nitrite to nitric oxide, and enhancing the synthesis of the cytochrome c oxidase, which is involved in the electron transport chain in mitochondria [131,132].

Based on more than 30 years of research and treatments in our laboratory, we could really emphasize that PBM is a natural, non-invasive, effective, and well-proved method of treatment for many bodily disorders. Recently, the newest tested technologies such as intravenous, intra-nasal, or sublingual PBM appear to offer the best efficacy for many diseases, from depression to cancer, from acute to chronic pain, for infants and children, to the third age [121,133–135].

PBM, as original historical form of governing and influencing life, is able to reset all the body's self-organizing mechanisms starting from the nucleus to the cellular membranes, and even much more to the cortex and heart, to imprint with information from the millions and millions of the triggered cellular reactions per second in every cell, to balance the internal energy, to normalize the oxygen levels through the two enzymatic reactions of the cytochrome c oxidase, CcO/H_2O and CcO/NO, as well as to initiate life's intrinsic mechanisms and the inner biological clock. Even if the whole functional picture is very complex, and some would say that it is still unclear how this form of stimulation might work, we have to think of time in nanoseconds, and it is for sure that the future research will reveal all the cellular and molecular mechanisms underlying PBM [121,136,137].

All the important components of PBM, such as intensity, timing, duration, and wavelength are part of the mainstream process of recovery in a holistic attempt to maximize the benefits of the treatment [121,137].

Being non-invasive and painless, with very few side effects depending on the patient's health status, and with no known risks associated, PBM heightens the energy, triggering self-organizing phenomena and tissue repair, bringing relief of physical pain or symptoms, and governing the interplay of the oxidative stress by playing multiple roles; it can induce cell proliferation and enhance stem cell differentiation, assisting rejuvenation and normalizing the cellular functions [138,139].

PBM has been proven to target life itself at quantum levels, and so it brings hope for an innovative modulation of immunity, health, and youth. As a practical tool, PBM opens doors for unprecedented and fulminant advances in many nano-medical research fields, by providing the rediscovery of an energetic method for modulating life itself and allowing a systematic generation of data and knowledge through comparison, complementation, and connecting across different medical nanotechnologies [121].

The worldwide tendencies of the current medical fields of the 21st century are innovative energy-based devices and techniques that are highly effective, whether they are drug-free or combined with medication. If professionally managed, the impact on medical practice, especially in Pediatrics, can be revolutionary. The scientific confirmation of these methods is based on discoveries concerning energy and information exchange within living systems, which constitute a "quantum leap" in the understanding and use of light and its interaction with water and other relevant photoacceptors to restore physiologic function [140], cybernetics, biological theory of information, modern thermodynamic concepts, and self-organizing phenomena in complex systems [121].

The advantages of the new energy-based health-care models include the following benefits: they can address the biological processes at their energetic origins; they are able to regulate the biological processes with precision and flexibility; they bring up healing and prevent illness with interventions that can be readily, economically, and non-invasively applied; they include methods that strengthen the immune system; they tend to integrate the body, mind, and spirit, focusing not only on healing, but also on achieving a greater well-being state, especially in patients suffering from chronic diseases [121]; and in the future, they will benefit large, vulnerable population groups, including the elderly and the poor [140], and they will be utilized also at home.

The number of ill children is steadily growing, and they become resistant to some drug preparations starting even from infancy. As a result, new methods for fighting diseases should be figured out. Creative systems and devices, as well as new methods for performing PBM in children for enhanced immunity to fight specific diseases, as for example, juvenile arthritis, do have a great merit and medical value for their capacity to achieve fine-tuned applications, as further interventions for various pediatric diseases, as well as others [141].

4.2. Novel Therapeutics Using Photobiomodulation in Arthritis. Where Are We?

A generation ago, children with arthritis faced a lifetime of pain and disability. Juvenile idiopathic arthritis, an umbrella term covering multiple distinct categories, previously called juvenile rheumatoid arthritis until recent reclassification, is one of the most common chronic diseases of childhood, featuring arthritis of unknown etiology [142].

Arthritis with synovial proliferation, triggered by the secretion of pro-inflammatory factors and the formation of granular tissue with monocytes, macrophages, lymphocytes, and other immune cells, will lead to chronic pain and the progressive destruction of the articular structures and functional disability, both in children and in adults [143]. More than one-third of children have ongoing active disease into adulthood with sequelae from chronic inflammation [2,144].

Adult patients and children with moderate or severe forms of arthritis tend to have a worse prognosis, even with the early use of disease-modifying antirheumatic drugs (DMARDs). These patients have considerable morbidity from joint damage, osteoporosis, psychosocial morbidity, reduced quality of life, and educational or employment disadvantage [143,145].

Chronic pain has a large and wholly negative impact on the physical and psychological well-being of patients and their family. Most often, if the inflammation goes away after months or even years of inadequate treatment, the pain may persist for life, due to central sensitization. Childhood chronic pain is a modern public health disaster, which is only now coming to light [2].

In these cases, long-term drugs will induce moderate to severe side effects, so that PBM could be a potential non-invasive anti-inflammatory treatment with minimal side effects [143].

Although the mechanisms of photobiomodulation processes are still being debated, in order to interact with the living cell, light has to be absorbed and has to change the inner cellular state, leading to processes such as the activation of ATP and of protein (RNA, DNA) synthesis, the stimulation of enzyme synthesis, the modulation of prostaglandin synthesis, decrease in the lipid peroxidation rate, the stimulation of specific and non-specific immunity, antioxidant effects, etc. When correctly applied, PBM has the following main clinical effects: improvement of blood circulation and activation of microcirculation, enhancement of collagen synthesis, promotion of tissue regeneration, influence on skin receptors with the increase of pain threshold, improvement of nerve conductivity, acupuncture points stimulation, anti-inflammatory, antiallergic and antiseptic effects, and so on [146].

In children, it is especially valuable because it activates the immunocompetent systems and improves the neurohumoral and hormonal regulation of the metabolism. It must be applied properly and with greater care, because the health problems of children differ from those of adults, and the child's response to illness and stress varies with age. Each child reacts according to his or her development stage, and to provide the highest quality treatment, the physician requires a familiarity with age-appropriate intervention [126,128].

In certain situations, for an accurate diagnosis and the adequate treatment of infants, children, or adolescents, a multidisciplinary team with pediatric health care experts, as well as key facilities and specific protocols for PBM management of pediatric conditions are needed.

When treating a child with energy-based devices, the physician should have in mind the differences in metabolism, hormonal system, immune system (susceptible to generalized infections, allergic diseases, etc.), and central nervous system (generalization of the post-aggressive reactions in infants and little children). The unique needs of children should be considered by pediatricians and other personnel skilled at evaluating and treating children in such areas as advice, communication, prevention, and therapeutics.

The concept of patient management in infants and children is particularly important. Usually, children are afraid of the physician, or they seem to show a lack of trust toward the doctor and the consulting or treatment area. Furthermore, it is the doctor's job to cooperate with the child's parents and to have a supportive attitude to eliminate any kind of stress in the little patient. So, the model on which the doctor–child relation should be built is friendship.

The informed consent is especially important, both in adults and in children. PBM should never be performed on a child if parents or the legal guardians do not fully agree with that. It is even better to allow parents to be nearby the child during the treatment.

The physician should explain to the family and/or the patient that the disease has a chronic evolution, sometimes with little spectacular improvements.

In treating children's rheumatic conditions, one should have in mind that there are several studies affirming that the usage of PBM on growing articular cartilage may be harmful [147,148].

Consequently, in children's chronic rheumatic pathology, PBM should be applied by irradiating the blood sublingually, intranasal, venous transcutaneous, or intravenously [149–153]. Sublingual PBM is easy, non-invasive, and with high absorption on intensely vascularized buccal mucosa, triggering rapid systemic effects [134].

The initial approach to the management of patients with rheumatoid arthritis must be vigorous in all patients, to suppress articular inflammation, control systemic disease, prevent secondary deformities, and maintain muscle strength.

The primary aims of treatment in rheumatic pathology include pain relief, preservation of joint function, prevention of deformities, and avoiding drug toxicity. In the long term, minimizing side effects from disease and treatment as well as preserving vision and promoting normal growth and development should be major goals for which PBM can make an important contribution.

Therapy for patients with rheumatoid arthritis should focus on rapid suppression of the inflammatory disease.

The influence of PBM on the immune system has been documented in the medical literature; immunologic effects on leucocytes, T, B, and NK lymphocytes, macrophages, and other cells result in local and systemic effects through a complex mechanism of action that is not fully understood [154].

For a better understanding of concepts and effects, Table 1 presents PBM experimental studies [155–180].

Clinical studies [181–189] have also shown that PBM is a promising drug-free tool for inflammatory diseases and arthritis (Table 2).

Aimbire and Albertini et al. demonstrated in an animal model that depending on the dose of PBM, TNF release in acute lung lesions may decrease [190].

Albertini et al. in an experimental study of subplantar muscle in rats used a diode laser with an output power of 30 mW and wavelengths of 660 nm and 684 nm, with the laser beam covering an area of 0.785 cm^2, at an energy dose of 7.5 J/cm^2; they proved that COX-2 mRNA expression and edema decreased [191].

Chow R. et al. presented the results of the PBM effect in 16 randomized controlled trials, concluding a pain-reducing effect immediately after treatment in acute forms of neck pain, and up to 22 weeks after completion of treatment in patients with chronic neck pain [192].

Leal-Junior, Lopes-Martins, and Bjordal in a systematic review and meta-analysis of placebo-controlled studies or randomized PBM therapy show that despite growing evidence supporting the value of PBMT in improving and accelerating performance in patient recovery, sample quality needs to be improved to be sure of these effects. They recommend compliance with the Consolidated Test Reporting Guidelines (CONSORT) when designing a research study with PBMT, publishing the protocol with all recommended and used parameters, to allow replication of the study by other authors [193].

Stausholm et al. highlighted in a systematic review and meta-analysis of 22 randomized placebo-controlled trials in patients with pain and disability due to knee osteoarthritis that the pain was significantly reduced in PBM compared with *placebo* at the end of therapy and during follow-up 1–12 weeks later, compared to the placebo group. In addition, the pain decreased (significantly on VAS) at 2–4 weeks after completion of the recommended doses of PBM compared to placebo. There were no reported adverse events. In conclusion, PBM reduces pain and disability in knee osteoarthritis (KOA) at 4–8 J, 785–860 nm wavelength, and at 1–3 J at 904 nm wavelength per treatment site [194].

Following the retrospective evaluation of multiple experimental and clinical studies on the use of PBM on immune cells, appropriate signaling pathways, but also in clinical pathologies, we can support the immunomodulatory effect of PBM and that it is an important complementary and alternative method able to influence the evolution of arthritis and lead to the resolution of joint and systemic inflammatory phenomena through photobiomodulation.

PBM could directly control the autoimmune mechanism by reducing the local and systemic inflammatory response, as in the model we propose in Figure 5.

Table 1. Experimental photobiomodulation (PBM) studies applied to immune cells and signaling pathways. IL: interleukin, LLLT: low-level laser therapy, MMP: matrix metalloproteinases, NF-kB: nuclear factor kappa-B, TNF-α: tumor necrosis factor alpha.

No	References	Type of Study	PBM Properties	Immune Cells/Signaling Pathways	Brief Results
1.	Castano, A.P.; Dai, T.; Yaroslavsky, I. et al. Low-level laser therapy for zymosan-induced arthritis in rats: Importance of illumination time. *Lasers Surg Med.* **2007**, *39*, 543–550. doi:10.1002/lsm.20516 [155]	Animal Model	810 nm; 5 and 50 mW/cm^2; 3 and 30 J/cm^2	Pathway of prostanoids/PGE2	Light regimen (30 J/cm^2 at 50 mW/cm^2) effective in reducing swelling of the knees and a greater reduction in the serum PGE2.
2.	Chen, A.C.; Arany, P.R.; Huang, Y.Y. et al. Low-level laser therapy activates NF-kB via generation of reactive oxygen species in mouse embryonic fibroblasts. *PLoS ONE* **2011**, *6*, 22453. doi:10.1371/journal.pone.0022453 [156]	Animal Model	810 nm; different fluences (0.003, 0.03, 0.3, 3, and 30 J/cm^2); 1 mW/cm^2 to 30 mW/cm^2	Murine embryonic fibroblasts/NF-kB	Significant activation of NF-kB at fluences higher than 0.3 J/cm^2. NF-kB was activated earlier (1 h) by LLLT compared to conventional lipopolysaccharide treatment. Increase in ATP.
3.	Alves, A.C.; Vieira, R.; Leal-Junior, E. et al. Effect of low-level laser therapy on the expression of inflammatory mediators and on neutrophils and macrophages in acute joint inflammation. *Arthritis Res Ther.* **2013**, *15*, R116. doi:10.1186/ar4296 [157]	Animal Model	GaAlAs (808 nm); 50 mW; 0.028 cm^2 1.78 W/cm^2; 4 J; 142.4 J/cm^2; 80 s/point. 100 mW; GaAlAs (808 nm); 0.028 cm^2 3.57 W/cm^2; 4 J; 142.4 J/cm^2; 40 s/point	Inflammatory cells (macrophages and neutrophils); gene expression of IL-1β, IL-6, TNFα.	LLLT with 50 mW was more efficient in modulating inflammatory mediators (IL-1β, IL-6) and inflammatory cells (macrophages and neutrophils).
4.	Assis L.; Moretti, A.I.; Abrahão T.B.; de Souza, H.P.; Hamblin, M.R.; Parizotto, N.A. Low-level laser therapy (808 nm) contributes to muscle regeneration and prevents fibrosis in rat tibialis anterior muscle after cryolesion. *Lasers Med Sci.* **2013**, *28*, 947–955. doi:10.1007/s10103-012-1183-3 [158]	Experimental groups and freezing muscle injury (cryoinjury) Adult male Wistar rats were randomly divided.	808 nm; CW; 30 mW power output, 47 s irradiation time, 0.00785 cm^2 spot area, dose 180 J/cm^2, irradiance 3.8 W/cm^2 and 1.4 J total energy per point.	Myogenic regulatory factors (myoD and myogenin), vascular endothelial growth factor (VEGF), transforming growth factor-beta (TGF-β) 1 and type I collagen mRNA	LLLT improved skeletal muscle regeneration by reducing the injured area, increasing myoD, myogenin, and VECF gene expression and, simultaneously, reducing TGF-β mRNA and type I collagen deposition in the injured tissue. Therefore, LLLT can increase muscle regeneration markers and reduce scar tissue formation, which should favor tissue repair in muscle injuries.
5.	Hsieh, Y.L.; Cheng, Y.J.; Huang, F.C.; Yang, C.C. The fluence effects of low-level laser therapy on inflammation, fibroblast-like synoviocytes, and synovial apoptosis in rats with adjuvant-induced arthritis. *Photomed Laser Surg.* **2014**, *32*, 669–677. doi:10.1089/pho.2014.3821 [159]	Animal Model	780-nm GaAlAs, 30 mW; spot size 0.2 cm^2, power density 0.15 W/cm^2. 30 s and 3 min laser irradiation, total fluences at the lower and higher energy densities (power density×irradiation time) of 4.5 and 27 J/cm^2 were applied daily for five successive days. The accumulated energies delivered from all sessions were 0.9 and 5.4 J, respectively	β-endorphin (β-ep) and TNF-α; substance P and COX-2	This study determined that the fluence provided by LLLT is one of the factors affecting biochemicals related to pain in the treatment of myofascial pain. LLLT irradiation with fluences of 4.5 and 27 J/cm^2 at myofascial trigger spots can significantly reduce substance P level in dorsal root ganglion. LLLT with lower fluence of 4.5 J/cm^2 exerted lower levels of TNF-α and COX-2 expression in laser-treated muscle, but LLLT with a higher fluence of 27 J/cm^2 elevated the levels of β-ep in serum, DRG, and muscle.

Table 1. *Cont.*

No	References	Type of Study	PBM Properties	Immune Cells/Signaling Pathways	Brief Results
6.	dos Santos S.A.; Alves, A.C.; Leal-Junior, E.C. et al. Comparative analysis of two low-level laser doses on the expression of inflammatory mediators and on neutrophils and macrophages in acute joint inflammation. *Lasers Med Sci.* **2014**, *29*, 1051–1058. doi:10.1007/s10103-013-1467-2 [160]	Animal Model	AsGaAl-type diode laser with a wavelength (λ) of 808 nm LLLT at doses of 2 and 4 J on joint papain-induced inflammation in rats; Mean power output (mW = 50); 50; Spot size (cm^2) 0.028; Power density (W/cm^2) 1.78; 1.78; Energy (J); 2 and 4 Energy density (J/cm^2) 71.4; 142.8 Time per point (s) 40; 80.	Inflammatory cells (macrophages and neutrophils); gene expression of IL-1β, IL-6, and IL-10; and TNF-α	Dose of 2 J is more efficient in modulating inflammatory mediators (IL-1β, IL-6, TNF-α, and IL-10) and inflammatory cells (macrophages and neutrophils) and its effects can be observed by histological signs of attenuation of inflammatory processes.
7.	Torres-Silva, R.; Lopes-Martins, R.A.; Bjordal, J.M. et al. The low-level laser therapy (LLLT) operating in 660 nm reduce gene expression of inflammatory mediators in the experimental model of collagenase-induced rat tendinitis. *Lasers Med Sci.* **2015**, *30*, 1985–1990. doi:10.1007/s10103-014-1676-3 [161]	Animal Model	100 mW, 660 nm, 1 J or 3 J, comparatively.	Gene expression for COX-2; TNF-α; IL-6; and IL-10.	Reduction of important pro-inflammatory IL-6 and TNF-α, at 3 J.
8.	Fernandes, K.P.; Souza, N.H.; Mesquita-Ferrari, R.A.; Silva, D.; Rocha, L.A.; Alves, A.N.; Sousa, K.; Bussadori, S.K.; Hamblin, M.R.; Nunes, F.D. Photobiomodulation with 660-nm and 780-nm laser on activated J774 macrophage-like cells: Effect on M1 inflammatory markers. *Journal of photochemistry and photobiology. B, Biology*, **2015**, *153*, 344–351. doi:10.1016/j.jphotobiol.2015.10.015 [162]	Cells Culture J774 were derived from a BALB/c mouse.	660 nm (InGaAlP diode); 780 nm (GaAlAs diode) laser; CW. Average radiant power: 15 and 70 mW. Beam spot size at target: 0.04 cm^2. Total radiant energy 0.22 J and 0.16 J	Inflammatory cells (macrophages and neutrophils)/mRNA expression of TNF-α and iNOS; production of TNF-α and COX-2 proteins in M1 J774 cells.	660 nm and 780 nm lasers strongly reduced the mRNA expression of TNF-α and iNOS and down-regulated the production of TNF-α and COX-2 proteins in M1 J774 cells.
9.	Assis, L.; Milares, L.P.; Almeida, T.; Tim, C.; Magri, A.; Fernandes, K.R.; Medalha, C.; Muniz Renno, A.C. Aerobic exercise training and low-level laser therapy modulate inflammatory response and degenerative process in an experimental model of knee osteoarthritis in rats. *Osteoarthritis and Cartilage*, **2016**, *24*, 169–177. doi:10.1016/j.joca.2015.07.020 [163]	Animal Model	Diode laser (GaAlAs) 808 nm, cw, 50 mW output power, 28 s irradiation time, 0.028 cm^2 spot area, 50 J/cm^2, 1.7 W/cm^2, 1.4 J total energy per point/section. 3 days/week, at two points on left knee joint, contact technique, for 24 sessions (8 weeks).	IL-1, Caspase-3, and MMP-13 expression in nucleus of chondrocytes	808 nm laser prevented articular degenerative morphological modifications and modulated inflammatory process in OA rats.

Table 1. *Cont.*

No	References	Type of Study	PBM Properties	Immune Cells/Signaling Pathways	Brief Results
10.	Al Musawi, M.S.; Jaafar, M.S.; Al-Gailani, B.; et al. Effects of low-level laser irradiation on human blood lymphocytes in vitro. *Lasers Med Sci* **2017**, 32, 405–411. doi:10.1007/s10103-016-2134-1 [164]	Irradiation on human blood lymphocytes in vitro	Diode pump solid state (DPSS) laser, with wavelengths of 405, 589, and 780 nm, with an output power of 10 mW and irradiance rate fixed at 30 mW/cm^2.	Effect of laser at peripheral blood lymphocyte subsets	The effect of laser irradiation fluences of 36, 54, 72, and 90 J/cm^2 for each wavelength of 405, 589, or 780 nm, with an output power of 10 mW on human blood lymphocyte count in vitro are: no significant differences in lymphocyte count were observed before and after irradiation with the above fluences at wavelengths of 405 and 780 nm; however, a laser wavelength of 589 nm was associated with a significant increase in the lymphocyte count at a radiation fluence of 72 (by 1.6%) and increase in the NK cell lymphocyte subset.
11.	Baek, S.; Lee, K.P.; Cui, L.; et al. Low-power laser irradiation inhibits PDGF-BB-induced migration and proliferation via apoptotic cell death in vascular smooth muscle cells. *Lasers Med Sci* **2017**, 32, 2121–2127. doi:10.1007/s10103-017-2338-z [165]	Animal experiment In vivo vascular smooth muscle cells (VSMCs)	Low-power laser (LPL) green diode laser 532-nm pulsed wave of 300 mW at a spot diameter of 1 mm.	Apoptosis, migration, and proliferation in vascular smooth muscle cells (VSMCs)/ Caspase-3, Bax, and p38 mitogen-activated protein kinase in PDGF-BB-treated VSMCs.	The study demonstrated that 532 nm LPL irradiation inhibited VSMC proliferation and migration in response to platelet-derived growth factor (PDGF)-BB. LPL irradiation induced apoptosis and enhanced activation of caspase-3, Bax, and p38 mitogen-activated protein kinase in PDGF-BB-treated VSMCs. Based on these results, 532 nm LPL irradiation may inhibit PDGF-BB stimulated proliferation and migration, likely resulting from apoptosis associated with the interaction between 532 nm LPL irradiation and PDGF-BB in VSMCs. Therefore, this study provides a foundation for therapeutic strategies for vascular restenosis via 532 nm LPL irradiation as an alternative treatment against restenosis.
12.	Dos Anjos, L.M.J.; da Fonseca, A.S.; Gameiro, J.; de Paoli, F. Apoptosis induced by low-level laser in polymorphonuclear cells of acute joint inflammation: comparative analysis of two energy densities. *Lasers Med Sci.* **2017**, 32, 975–983. doi:10.1007/s10103-017-2196-8 [166]	Animal Model/randomly distributed	830 nm, output power 10 mW, 0.05 cm^2 laser beam area, power density 0.2 W/cm^2, energy densities:3 and 30 J/cm^2 (total energy of 150 and 1500 mJ were delivered after 15 and 150 s, respectively), in continuous wave emission mode.	Apoptotic cells in mouse ankle joint samples/DNA fragmentation rate of inflammatory cells Gene expression of proteins involved in apoptosis pathways Bcl2 protein and mRNA expression in PMN cells	The higher energy density (30 Jcm−2) can reduce the inflammatory process by PMN apoptosis induction, while the lower energy density (3 Jcm−2) could also induce apoptosis in PMN; however, this process seems to be slower. The results suggest that apoptosis in PMN cells comprises part of LLLT anti-inflammatory mechanisms and could be a consequence of the balance alteration between expression of proapoptotic (Bax and p53) and anti-apoptotic (Bcl-2) proteins in these cells.

Table 1. *Cont.*

No	References	Type of Study	PBM Properties	Immune Cells/Signaling Pathways	Brief Results
13.	Assis, L.; Tim, C.; Magri, A. et al. Interleukin-10 and collagen type II immunoexpression are modulated by photobiomodulation associated to aerobic and aquatic exercises in an experimental model of osteoarthritis. *Lasers Med Sci* **2018**, *33*, 1875–1882. doi:10.1007/s10103-018-2541-6 [167]	Study of the experimental animals. The degenerative process related to osteoarthritis (OA) in the articular cartilage in rats.	Diode laser GaAIAs 808 nm; CW; power output 50 mW; irradiance 1.7 W/cm^2; spot area 0.28 cm^2; dose 50 J/cm^2; total energy 1.4 J per point/section. Irradiation time: 28 s; local: 2 points (medial and lateral side of the left knee joint) Technique: punctual contact	Chondrocytes/IL-10 expression; transforming growth factor beta (TGF-β) expression; collagen type I (Col I) and II (Col II).	PBM associated with aerobic and aquatic exercise were effective in promoting chondroprotective effects and maintaining the integrity of the articular tissue in the knees of OA rats. PBM and aerobic exercises produced an increase in the expression of TGF-β, which is a member of a superfamily of cytokines; increased Col II and IL-10 expression, which may interfere in cell abnormal metabolism, preventing the matrix degradation and OA progression.
14.	Mergoni, G.; Vescovi, P.; Belletti, S. et al. Effects of 915 nm laser irradiation on human osteoblasts: a preliminary in vitro study. *Lasers Med Sci* **2018**, *33*, 1189–1195. doi:10.1007/s10103-018-2453-5 [168]	A primary culture of human osteoblasts was isolated from mandibular cortical bone of a young health donor.	915-nm GaAs diode laser in the different samples, was administered at 5, 15 and 45 J/cm^2 with a power output of 1.5 W in continuous wave. Using two different power densities: 0.12 and 1.25 W/cm^2. Irradiation time was 41.7, and 375 s using a power density of 0.12 W/cm^2 and 4, 12 and 36 s using a power density of 1.25 W/cm^2.	Osteoblast proliferation Osteoblast differentiation (bone nodule production)	Osteoblasts treated with a single irradiation per day for 3 days at doses of 5, 15, and 45 J/cm^2 (power density: 0.12 W/cm^2 showed no significant differences in terms of cell count compared to controls. PBM at parameters tested in the present study positively modulated the mineralization process in human osteoblasts, inducing the formation of a greater amount of bone nodules but did not increase cell proliferation.
15.	Shakir, E.A.; Rasheed Naji, N.A.; In vitro impact of laser irradiation on platelet aggregation. *Lasers Med Sci.* **2018**, *33*, 1717–1721. doi:10.1007/s10103-018-2527-4 [169]	In vitro blood platelets from 30 healthy volunteers	532 nm; power 100 mW; CW; 4-mm-diameter irradiation beam spot. Irradiation times: 1.8, 3.7, and 6.2 s giving doses of irradiation 1.5, 3, and 5 J/cm^2, respectively. The divergence was <1.5 m rad, the crystal type of this source was Nd:VYO4:KTP, the laser spot diameter was 0.4 cm, and the power density was 796.17 W/cm^2.	Platelet aggregation response to laser irradiation /ADP/ATP	Low laser irradiation induced significant changes in platelet aggregation in the presence of weak agonists such as adenosine diphosphate (ADP) and epinephrine. PBM has no influence on platelet count; however, it promotes platelet aggregation in response to weak agonists, specifically ADP and epinephrine.
16.	De Souza Costa, M.; Teles, R.H.G.; Dutra, Y.M. et al. Photobiomodulation reduces neutrophil migration and oxidative stress in mice with carrageenan-induced peritonitis. *Lasers Med Sci.* **2018**, *33*, 1983–1990. doi:10.1007/s10103-018-2569-7 [170]	Animal Model (28 animals were randomly divided)	904 nm ± 5% Operating mode Pulsed. Frequency 1000 Hz; Pulse duration 100 ns; Peak radiant power 50 W; Average radiant power 50 mW.	Cell migration and oxidative stress, in a model of carrageenan-induced inflammation	Treatment with laser decreased the number of leukocytes, especially the neutrophils, in the PBM group and reduced the concentrations of MDA (malondialdehyde), GSH (glutathione), and NO_3/NO_2 (nitrate/nitrite) in the peritoneal fluid.

Table 1. *Cont.*

No	References	Type of Study	PBM Properties	Immune Cells/Signaling Pathways	Brief Results
17.	Amaroli, A.; Ravera, S.; Baldini, F. et al. Photobiomodulation with 808-nm diode laser light promotes wound healing of human endothelial cells through increased reactive oxygen species production stimulating mitochondrial oxidative phosphorylation. *Lasers Med Sci* 2019, *34*, 495–504. doi:10.1007/s10103-018-2623-5 [171]	In vitro Human Endothelial Cells (HECV)	808-nm diode laser light emitted by the flat-top handpiece using 1 W of power energy, 1 W/cm^2 of power density, single dose of 60 J, irradiation of 60 s, fluence of 60 J/cm^2, mode CW (corresponding to the measured laser therapy of 0.95 W, 0.95 W/cm^2, 57 J, 60 s, 57 J/cm^2). To assess the effect of 808-nm laser light irradiation on cell viability, also longer irradiations were performed (100 s and 150 s) corresponding to a final fluences of 100 J/cm^2 and 150 J/cm^2, respectively.	HECV/Oxidative phosphorylation aerobic metabolism of HECV, NF-κB/ROS and NO production in endothelial cells.	The present report demonstrated that the short irradiation of 60 s, by the laser setup of 1 W, 1 W/cm^2, 60 J, 60 J/cm^2, CW (real measured energy = 0.95 W, 0.95 W/cm^2, 57 J, 57 J/cm^2, CW), of HECV in vitro with 808-nm diode laser light was able to stimulate endothelial cell proliferation and oxidative metabolism, which resulted in a more efficient wound repair ability; increase in NO; activate NF-κB; NIR treatment is able to increase the aerobic metabolism, enhancing the O2 consumption and the aerobic ATP synthesis.
18.	Felizatti, A.L.; do Bomfim, F.R.C.; Bovo, J.L. et al. Effects of low-level laser therapy on the organization of articular cartilage in an experimental microcrystalline arthritis model. *Lasers Med Sci.* **2019**, *34*, 1401–1412. doi:10.1007/s10103-019-02740-5 [172]	Animal Model	The gallium arsenide laser device AsGa (λ = 830 nm), CW, fluence = 18 J/cm^2, power = 40 mW, total energy = 0.36 J, beam area = 0.02 cm^2, by 9 s. The therapies were applied punctually in the right knee patellar region. After 7, 14, and 21 days of treatment, the animals from the three groups were euthanized (xylazine = 20 mg/kg/ketamine = 40 mg/kg associated with cardiac exsanguination) and the knees were removed and processed for structural and biochemical analysis (*n* = 4/experimental time/analysis) of the AC of the femur and tibia.	Morphometric parameters evaluated in the articular cartilage in male rats. Biochemical parameters evaluated in the articular cartilage (Glycosaminoglycans, Hydroxyproline, Non-collagen proteins) Non-collagen proteins	The present study shows that the phototherapy protocol, using AsGa (λ = 830 nm) in the experimental period employed, was able to revert tissue injuries produced by the microcrystalline arthritis (MA) model in young adult rats.
19.	Han, B.; Fan, J.; Liu, L. et al. Adipose-derived mesenchymal stem cells treatments for fibroblasts of fibrotic scar via downregulating TGF-β1 and Notch-1 expression enhanced by photobiomodulation therapy. *Lasers Med Sci.* **2019**, *34*, 1–10. doi:10.1007/s10103-018-2567-9 [173]	Culture of cells	The total surface of the culture dishes was irradiated for 152 s each time; the energy density of the laser was 4 J/cm^2. The dual model device emitted florida 6 laser beams (beam diameter <5 mm) at a wavelength of 655 nm (± 5%) and 6 laser beams at a wavelength of 635 nm.	Fibroblasts/TGF-β1 and Notch-1 expression Cell proliferation (CCK-8), cell apoptosis (MUSE), and cytotoxicity (LDH) assays	Results obtained from experiments showed that cell culture supernatant of post-PBM, adipose-derived mesenchymal stem cells (ADSCs) has much more potential as a fibrotic treatment of keloid fibroblasts (KFs) and hypertrophic scar fibroblasts (HSFs), and acting by inhibition of the proliferation, migration, and profibrotic genes synthesis via downregulating TGF-β1 and Notch-1 expression.

Table 1. *Cont.*

No	References	Type of Study	PBM Properties	Immune Cells/Signaling Pathways	Brief Results
20.	Tsuka, Y.; Kunimatsu, R.; Gunji, H. et al. Effects of Nd:YAG low-level laser irradiation on cultured human osteoblasts migration and ATP production: in vitro study. *Lasers Med Sci* **2019**, *34*, 55–60. doi:10.1007/s10103-018-2586-6 [174]	In vivo and In vitro was studied a variety of cell types	Nd:YAG laser (wavelength of 1064 nm) for 60 s at 0.3 W (10 pps, 30 mJ). The total energy density was about 10.34 J/cm^2.	Migration of cultured human osteoblasts; ATP synthesis	This study showed that Nd:YAG laser irradiation (wavelength of 1064 nm, 0.3W, 10 pps, 30 mJ, 10.34 J/cm^2, irradiation time 60 s) may contribute to the regeneration of bone tissues owing to enhanced osteoblast cell migration. ATP synthesis was significantly increased in the laser irradiation group compared to the control group.
21.	Cardoso, L.M.; Pansani, T.N.; Hebling, J.; de Souza Costa C.A.; Basso, F.G. Photobiomodulation of inflammatory-cytokine-related effects in a 3-D culture model with gingival fibroblasts. *Lasers Med Sci.* **2020**, *35*, 1205–1212. doi:10.1007/s10103-020-02974-8 [175]	Primary cell culture Gingival fibroblast isolation	12 units of laser diode DL-7140-201S, InGaAsP laser. Center wavelength (nm) 780 nm; spectral band width 780 nm ± 5 nm; Operating mode Continuous wave Frequency 1012 Hz to 1015 Hz; Pulse on duration 40 s; Pulse of duration or duty cycle 40 s; Energy per pulse 0.5 J Peak radiant power 0.07 W; Average radiant power 0.025 W. Number and frequency of treatment sessions 1 irradiation per day, over 3 days. Total radiant energy 1.5 J	Cytokine exposure Cell viability Gene expression of collagen type I and vascular endothelial growth factor (VEGF); Synthesis of VEGF, TNF-α, IL-1β	PBM on the selected parameters (0.5 J/cm^2, 0.025 W, 780 nm) was capable of adequately penetrating the collagen matrix and positively stimulating human gingival fibroblasts (HGF) wound healing-related functions and decreasing TNF-α synthesis, even in the presence of inflammatory challenge. IL-6 and IL-8 decreased cell viability, the synthesis of VEGF, and gene expression of collagen type I. PBM enhanced cell density in the matrices and stimulated VEGF expression, even after IL-6 challenge.
22.	Katagiri, W.; Lee, G.; Tanushi, A.; Tsukada, K.; Choi, H.S.; Kashiwagi, S. High-throughput single-cell live imaging of photobiomodulation with multispectral near-infrared lasers in cultured T cells. *Journal of biomedical optics*, **2020**, *25*, 1–18. doi:10.1117/1.JBO.25.3.036003 [176]	In vitro T cells culture	Two lasers were adjusted from 200 to 400 mW/cm^2 for 1064 nm and 50 to 100 mW/cm^2 for 1270 nm at the focal plane. Dual laser irradiation at an irradiance of 400 mW/cm^2 for 1064 nm and 100 mW/cm^2 for 1270 nm was monitored using an IR camera (FLIR Systems).	T cells/PBM on T cells and imaging of intracellular calcium levels and ROS generation nitric oxide binding to cytochrome c oxidase/mitochondrial retrograde signaling	A specific combination of wavelengths at low irradiances (250 to 400 mW/cm^2 for 1064 nm and 55 to 65 mW/cm^2 for 1270 nm) modulates mitochondrial retrograde signaling, including intracellular calcium and reactive oxygen species in T cells. The time-dependent density functional theory computation of binding of nitric oxide (NO) to cytochrome c oxidase indicates that the illumination with NIR light could result in the NO release, which might be involved in these changes.
23.	Lemos, G.A., Batista, A.U.D., da Silva, P.L.P. et al. Photobiostimulation activity of different low-level laser dosage on masticatory muscles and temporomandibular joint in an induced arthritis rat model. *Lasers Med Sci.* **2020**, *35*, 1129–1139. doi:10.1007/s10103-019-02933-y [177]	Animal Model	(GaAlAs), 830 nm, 30 mW, 0.116 cm^2, irradiance 0.259 W/cm^2, CW, divided as follows: LG5: 5 J/cm^2, 0.6 J, 20 s/session LG10: 10 J/cm^2, 1.2 J, 40 s /session LG20: 20 J/cm^2, 2.4 J, 80 s /session Ten sessions, with 48-h intervals.	Pro-inflammatory cells/IL-1β and TNF-α/ Matrix metalloproteinases (MMPs) family MMP 9 and MMP 2 activity	Results suggest that in this experimental model of joint inflammation, PBM can modulate pro-inflammatory mediators, reducing IL-1β and TNF-α concentrations in affected tissues. LLLT doses promoted better organization of articular disc collagen fibers, a greater number of proteoglycans in articular cartilage, increased area and diameter of left lateral pterygoid fibers, reduced latent and active MMP 9 and 2 activity, and lower IL-1β concentration.

Table 1. *Cont.*

No	References	Type of Study	PBM Properties	Immune Cells/Signaling Pathways	Brief Results
24.	Li, K., Liang, Z., Zhang, J. et al. Attenuation of the inflammatory response and polarization of macrophages by photobiomodulation. *Lasers Med Sci.* **2020**, *35*, 1509–1518. [178]	Culture bone marrow-derived macrophages (BMDMs)	GaAlAs; 810 nm, 2 mW/cm^2, 4 J and 10 J.	Inflammatory cells (macrophages and neutrophils)/NF-κB p65	PBM suppressed the expression of a marker of classically activated macrophages, inducible nitric oxide synthase; decreased the mRNA expression and secretion of pro-inflammatory cytokines, TNF-α, iNOS, and IL-1β; increased the secretion of monocyte chemotactic protein 1; significantly decreased NF-κB p65 expression in the 4J and 10 J PBM groups.
25.	Moreira, S.H.; Pazzini, J.M.; Álvarez, J.L.G. et al. Evaluation of angiogenesis, inflammation, and healing on irradiated skin graft with low-level laser therapy in rats (Rattus norvegicus albinus wistar). *Lasers Med Sci.* **2020**. *35*, 1103–1109 doi:10.1007/s10103-019-02917-y [179]	Animal Model	AlGaInP 660 nm, 30 mW; its local action area of 2 cm^2. The laser tip was positioned at a 90° angle in contact with the skin at each predetermined point of the graft, and it was kept for 12 s/point in 6 J/cm^2 dose and 20 s/point in 10 J/cm^2 dose. The animals were seen for 15 days, being the sessions performed every 3 or 5 days with 6 J/cm^2 or 10 J/cm^2 dose. The groups were G1—control; G2—6 J/cm^2 every 3 days; G3—10 J/cm^2 every 3 days; G4—6 J/cm^2 every 5 days; and G5—10 J/cm^2 every 5 days.	Fibroblasts/skin grafts/the expression of collagen type III the inflammatory response/COX-2 expression/CD31 expression	It is concluded the exhibition of the skin grafts to 6 J/cm^2 or 10 J/cm^2 dose every 5 days improved the healing and the modulation of the local inflammation. The results showed the LLLT may modulate the COX-2 expression in G3, when it has lower average; a greater trend of CD31 expression in G1 was observed as well as less expression in G2. The greater collagen type III–green expression was observed in grafts from G4 in association with greater fibroblasts count. However, in grafts from G5, the collagen type I–red expression was better seen. It was possible to deduce the 10 J/cm^2 dose every 5 days in G5 resulted in the collagen ripeness.
26.	da Silva, J.G.F.; dos Santos, S.S.; de Almeida, P. et al. Effect of systemic photobiomodulation in the course of acute lung injury in rats. *Lasers Med Sci.* **2020**. doi:10.1007/s10103-020-03119-7 [180]	Animal Model	Red light-emitting diode (LED) (660 nm) 100 mW; 5 J/cm; Energy density 5.35 J/cm^2; Power density = 33.3 mW/cm^2; Area = 2.8 cm^2; total energy= 15 J; time= 150 sec.	Inflammatory cells (macrophages and neutrophils)/ myeloperoxidase activity/ (IL) 1β, IL-6, and IL-17.	PBM on the systemic lipopolysaccharide induced acute lung injury, as it reduced the number of neutrophils recruited into the bronchoalveolar lavage, myeloperoxidase activity, and reduced interleukins (IL) 1β, IL-6, and IL-17 in the lung.

Table 2. Clinical effects of PBM on various inflammatory pathologies and associated pain.

Authors/year	Type of Clinical Pathology	Type of Laser/ Wavelength (nm)	Mean Output Power (mW)	Energy Density (J/cm^2)	Power Density mW/cm^2/Beam Spot Size (cm^2)	Area/Pulse (ns)	Time (s or min)	Total E (J)	Results
Bjordal, J.M.; Lopes-Martins, R.A.; Iversen, V.V. A randomized, placebo controlled trial of low-level laser therapy for activated achilles tendinitis with microdialysis measurement of peritendinous prostaglandin E2 concentrations. *Br J Sports Med.* **2006**, *40*, 76–80. [181]	Bilateral Achilles tendinitis	GaAs Infrared 904 nm	Peak power 10 W/Freq. 5000 Hz	20 mW/cm^2	Fluence 20 mW/cm^2/0.5 cm^2	1.8 J for each of 3 points along the tendon	200 ns	In total 5.4 J per tendon	LLLT at a dose of 5.4 J per point can reduce inflammation and pain in activated Achilles tendinitis. LLLT may have potential in the management of diseases with an inflammatory component.
Nakamura, T.; Ebihara, S.; Ohkuni, I. et al. Low Level Laser Therapy for chronic knee joint pain patients. *Laser therapy* **2014**, *23*, 273–277. doi:10.5978/islsm.14-OR-21 [182]	35 subjects with of chronic knee joint pain caused by OA- induced degenerative meniscal tear.	Ga-Al-AS: 830 nm ± 15 nm; CW	1000 mW ± 20%	20.1 J/cm^2/point	-	20.1 J/cm^2/point	30 s/point	-	This study confirmed that 830 nm diode laser LLLT was an effective treatment for pain related to knee osteoarthritis.
Soleimanpour, H.; Gahramani, K.; Taheri, R. et al. The effect of low-level laser therapy on knee osteoarthritis: prospective, descriptive study. *Lasers Med Sci.* **2014**; *29*, 1695-1700. doi:10.1007/s10103-014-1576-6 [183]	18 patients with knee osteoarthritis	Gal-Al-As: 810 nm; 50 mW pulse; radiation mode F = 3000 Hz, Δt = 200 ns.	80 W	6 J/cm^2	0.05 W/cm^2	1 cm^2	120 s	36 J	Significant reduction of the nocturnal pain, pain on walking and ascending the steps, knee circumference, distance between the hip and heel, and knee to horizontal hip to heel distance at the end of the treatment course.
		890 nm; 30 mW; F = 3000 Hz Δt = 200 ns	peak power = 50 W	10 J/cm^2	17 mW /cm^2	1.765 cm^2	588 s	53.6 J	
Youssef, E.F.; Muaidi, Q.I.; Shanb, A.A. Effect of Laser Therapy on Chronic Osteoarthritis of the Knee in Older Subjects. *J Lasers Med Sci.* **2016**, *7*, 112–119. doi:10.15171/jlms.2016.19 [184]	Patients with OA, Group 1 (*n* = 18)	880 nm, 2 times/ week for 8 weeks = 16 sessions;	50 mW, CW	-	-	-	6 J/point for 60 s, for 8 points	48 J in each session	LLLT to exercise training program is more effective than exercise training alone in the treatment of patients with chronic knee OA and the rate of improvements may be dose dependent, as with 6 J/cm^2 or 3 J/cm^2.
	Group 2 (n = 18)	904 nm, frequency 700 Hz; 2 times/ week for 8 weeks = 16 sessions-	60 mW	3 J/cm^2	Peak power 20 WSpot: 0.5 cm^2	Pulse duration 4.3 ms	50 s per point	27 J per session	
	Group 3 (*placebo* laser) (*n* = 15)	-	-	-	-	-	-	-	
Nambi, S.G.; Kamal, W.; George, J.; Manssor, E. Radiological and biochemical effects (CTX-II, MMP-3, 8, and 13) of low-level laser therapy (LLLT) in chronic osteoarthritis in Al-Kharj, Saudi Arabia. *Lasers Med Sci.* **2017**, *32*, 297–303. doi:10.1007/s10103-016-2114-5 [185]	Thirty-four subjects with knee OA were randomized into two groups: active group (n = 17) and	GaAs super pulsed laser: 905 nm	25 mW	1.5 J per point for 8 points in total.	-	1 cm^2	60 s	Total dose 12 J	This study provides the evidence of PBM in reduction of pain and the therapy's ability to inhibit the proliferation of collagen type II C-telopeptide and other proteins MMP-3 (stromelysin), MMP-8 (collagenase-2), and MMP-13 (collagenase-3), making it an ideal treatment for subjects in the later stages of OA.
	Placebo (*n* = 17).	-	-	-	-	-	-	-	

Table 2. *Cont.*

Authors/year	Type of Clinical Pathology	Type of Laser/ Wavelength (nm)	Mean Output Power (mW)	Energy Density (J/cm²)	Power Density mW/cm²/Beam Spot Size (cm²)	Area/Pulse (ns)	Time (s or min)	Total E (J)	Results
Alayat, M.S.; Ali, M.M. Efficacy of class IV diode laser on pain and dysfunction in patients with knee osteoarthritis: a randomized placebo-control trial. *Bull Fac Phys Ther* **2017**, *22*, 40–5. doi:10.4103/1110-6611.209880 [186]	Randomized blinded placebo-controlled trial 50 patients with knee OA	Ga–Al–Ar 808 nm CW 3 sessions /week/for 4 consecutive weeks	1000 mW	Mean power 500 mW	Spot diam = 2 cm; Aria= 3.14 cm²	2.14 J/cm²	6 min and 17 s per session	150 J	Class IV diode laser combined with exercise was more effective than exercise alone in the treatment of knee OA. PBM combined with exercise effectively decreased pain and WOMAC index (Western Ontario and McMaster Universities Osteoarthritis Index), as compared with exercise alone.
		905 nm pulsed emission, frequency: 1500 Hz. 3 sessions /week/for 4 consecutive weeks	Peak power 25 W	Mean power 54 mW	Spot diam = 2 cm; Aria= 3.14 cm²	Scan on 100 cm²; Trigg. Points 6.175 J on each point in an average time of 16 s	9 min.	214 J	
Tomazoni, S.S.; Costa, L.; Joensen, J.; Stausholm, M.B.; Naterstad, I.F.; Leal-Junior, E.; Bjordal, J.M. Effects of photobiomodulation therapy on inflammatory mediators in patients with chronic non-specific low back pain: Protocol for a randomized placebo-controlled trial. *Medicine* **2019**, *98*, e15177. doi:10.1097/MD.0000000000015177 [187]	Randomized placebo-controlled trial PBMT with 5 lasers, skin contact	905 ± 1 nm, Super pulsed infrared 3000 Hz	25 W	1,35 J	17.05 mW/cm² 0.44 cm² (spot)	3.07 J/cm²	-		This is the first study that will investigate a possible biological mechanism behind the positive clinical effects of PBMT on non-specific chronic low back pain. We strongly believe that this investigation can be helpful in the management of this condition.
		905 ± 1 nm, Super pulsed infrared1000 Hz	Laser shower 12.5 W	0.225 J	2.84 mW/cm² 0.44 cm² (spot)	0.511 J/cm²	-		
		640 ± 10 nm,2 Hz	15 mW	2.7 J	0.9 cm²	-	-	4 LEDs Red 24.75 J	
		640 ± 10 nm, 2 Hz2 Hz	15 mW	2.7 J	0.9 cm²	-	-	4 LEDs Red 24.30 J	
		875 ± 10 nm,16 Hz	17.5 mW	3.15 J	0.9 cm²	-	180 s	4 LEDs Infrared	
		875 ± 10 nm,16 Hz	17.5 mW	3.15 J	0.9 cm²	-	180 s	idem	
Isuk, S.; Lev, Y.H., Fox, O.; Caracco, R.; Dunsky, A. Does Photobiomodulation Therapy Enhance Maximal Muscle Strength and Muscle Recovery? *J Hum Kinet*. **2020**, *73*, 135–144. Published 2020 Jul 21. doi:10.2478/hukin-2019-0138 [188]	Randomized double-blinded placebo-controlled trial	GaAlAs: 808 nm, Pulse frequency: 13 kHz	250 mW	-	Average power: 84.5 mW, Beam size: 1 × 4,5 cm² on 3 quadriceps points located in parallel	Pulse width26 µs	Dose rate: 5.07 J/min (1.13 J/cm²/ min)	~150 J overall treatment	Photobiomodulation protocol of irradiation that was used (20 min, 808 nm, energy of 150 J) did not show beneficial effects on quadriceps muscle performance or recovery after induction of fatigue, when applied immediately after exercise.
Tomazoni, S.S.; Costa, L.O.P.; Joensen, J.; Stausholm, M.B.; Naterstad, I.F.; Ernberg, M.; Leal-Junior, E.C.P. and Bjordal, J.M. Photobiomodulation Therapy is Able to Modulate PGE2 Levels in Patients With Chronic Non-Specific Low Back Pain: A Randomized Placebo-Controlled Trial. *Lasers Surg Med*. **2020**, doi:10.1002/lsm.23255 [189]	Randomized placebo-controlled trial PBMT with multiple lasers, skin contact	SE 25TM Super pulsed infrared: 905 ± 1 nm, 3000 Hz	Peak power 25 W	7.5 mW	0.44 cm² (spot)	17.05 mW/cm²	3.07 J/cm²	1.35 J	Our results suggest that PBMT was able to modulate PGE2 levels. Results are compatible with the hypothesis that modulating inflammation by decreasing PGE2 levels may be one of the mechanisms involved in the effects of PBMT in patients with LBP.
		Laser Shower 4 Super pulsed infrared: 905 ± 1 nm, 1000 Hz	12.5 W	1.25 mW	0.44 cm² (spot)	2.84 mW/cm²	0.51 J/cm²	0.225 J	
		SE 25TM 4 RED LEDs (nm): 640 ± 10 nm, 2 Hz	-	15 mW	0.9 cm² (spot)	16.67 mW/cm²	3 J/cm²	2.7 J	
		Laser Shower 640 ± 10 nm, 2 Hz	-	15 mW	0.9 cm²	16.67 mW/cm²	3 J/cm²	2.7 J	
		SE 25TM 4 Infrared LEDs (nm): 875 ± 10 nm, 16 Hz; Magnetic field: 35 mT	-	17.5 mW	0.9 cm²/spot	19.44 mW/cm²	3.5 J/cm²/ 180 s	Total dose/site 24.75 J	
		Laser Shower 4 Infrared LEDs (nm): 875 ± 10 nm, 16 Hz	-	17.5 mW	0.9 cm²/spot	19.44 mW/cm²	3.5 J/cm²/180 s	Total dose/site 24.3 J	

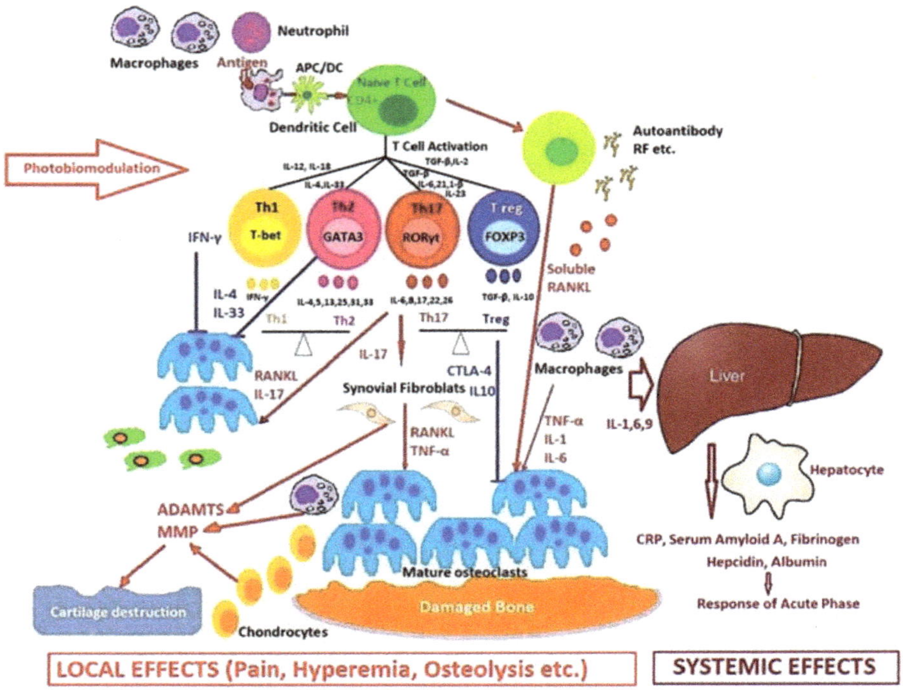

Figure 5. How photobiomodulation could regulate the immune response in arthritis. Possible mechanisms of action on excessive T cell immune response, regulation of pro- and anti-inflammatory cytokines balance, and the process of stopping the proliferative synovium and the osteocartilaginous destruction.

Figure 5 shows many cells and the resulting cytokines, which participate with different roles in the occurrence and evolution of rheumatoid arthritis. The synovial membrane is penetrated by cells of the immune system (innate and adaptative), and in the synovial fluid appear pro-inflammatory mediators that trigger an inflammatory cascade, activating fibroblast-like synoviocytes and dendritic cells, monocytes, macrophages, mast cells, as well as the T cells and the B cells. An extensive network of new blood vessels is formed, which will lead to the appearance of a synovial hyperplasia, osteocartilaginous erosion, and all the secondary systemic effects.

PBM can very gently modulate the balance between Treg and Th17 cells, i.e., between physiological regulation and the stimulation of the inflammatory process.

An established philosophy in the management of a patient with rheumatoid arthritis is to begin with the safest and simplest therapy judged to be effective. PBM applied in different stages of rheumatoid arthritis is safe, effective, and free of side effects. PBM exerts a positive influence on the synovial membrane and the immune system.

In the inflammatory phase of rheumatoid arthritis, PBM improves the macrophages and lymphocytes activity, decreases the level of immune complexes, and regulates the level of immunoglobulins A (IgA), immunoglobulins M (IgM), immunoglobulins G (IgG), and the balance between pro-inflammatory and anti-inflammatory cytokines [195–200].

Photobiomodulation activates the non-specific cellular immune mechanisms, improves the microcirculation of the central and peripheral nervous system, adjusts the functional activity of the hypothalamus and all marginal systems, activates the energetic metabolism, and modulates the immune and vegetative responses. The anti-inflammatory, anti-nociceptive (which elude peripheral and central sensitivity that is the cause for psychological chronic pain) and immunomodulatory effects of PBM allow the reduction, even up to elimination, of the pharmacological drugs and promote the disease remission [201,202].

In recent years, photobiomodulation has become an increasingly mainstream modality, especially in the areas of physical medicine and rehabilitation [130].

Moreover, despite the best efforts of "big pharma," distrust of pharmaceuticals is growing in general because of uncertain efficacy and troublesome adverse effects. Photobiomodulation has no reported adverse effects, and no reports of adverse events can be directly attributed to laser or light therapy. The high benefit/risk ratio of photobiomodulation should be better appreciated by medical professionals in the rehabilitation and physical medicine specialties [203–206].

Every patient is unique, and the medical doctor must treat him in an integrative manner for the mind, soul, and physical body.

In the situation of chronic arthritis as in other pathological conditions, a clinician should have a solid knowledge of the disease to be addressed, be up-to-date with its pathogenesis, the modern therapies, and their mode of action, and consider alternatives and complementary therapies that are much older than the pharmacological ones. Only these data should be the basis of the attitude he would have when deciding whether to turn to PBM.

The successful management of PBM in arthritis is based on the clinician's ability to evaluate correctly the inflammatory status of the patient, to seek the optimal solution, to choose the best technology with the best physical parameters and mode of action, so that the treatment can target very precisely the immune system and the molecular signaling pathways at the molecular level with the exact amount of quantum light energy in order to obtain the desired immune modulation and the remission of the disease.

5. Conclusions

Applied PBM could be a safe and an exceptionally good option in the multidisciplinary management of rheumatoid arthritis and chronic pain in children and adults.

To achieve the desired effect of photobiomodulation, a certain quantified amount of photonic energy is always required to target the cells and the immune signaling pathways, to modulate the immune system, and LASERS, LEDs or other available light devices can be used accordingly.

There is currently no consensus on the effective PBM treatment method in improving symptoms and remission of chronic rheumatic diseases.

Successful management of PBM in arthritis is based on the clinician's ability to evaluate correctly the inflammatory status of the patient, to seek the optimal solution, to choose the best technology with the best physical parameters and mode of action, so that at molecular level the treatment can target very precisely the immune system and the molecular signaling pathways with the exact amount of quantum light energy in order to obtain the desired immune modulation and the remission of the disease.

Light is a very powerful tool in medicine because it can simultaneously target many cascades of immune system activation in comparison with drugs, so PBM can perform very delicate tasks inside our cells to modulate cellular dysfunctions, helping to initiate self-organization phenomena and finally healing the disease.

A lot of information can be stored or transmitted using light.

The near future will be focused on state-of-the-art laser therapy, in an atmosphere concentrated not only on reducing pain and inflammation, but also early healing of the disease.

Interdisciplinary teams should work diligently to meet these needs by also using single-cell imaging devices for multispectral laser photobiomodulation on immune cells.

A new field of innovative research with multiple treatment options in immune-mediated inflammatory diseases opens up by the application of PBM with important clinical implications for the future.

Author Contributions: Conceptualization, L.M.A.; writing and original draft preparation, L.M.A.; review and editing, G.L., L.M.A. Both authors have read and agreed to the published version of the manuscript. All authors have read and agreed to the published version of the manuscript.

Funding: This project is funded by the Ministry of Research and Innovation within Program 1—Development of the national RD system, Subprogram 1.2—Institutional Performance—RDI excellence funding projects, Contract no.34PFE/19.10.2018, Romania.

Conflicts of Interest: The authors declare no conflict of interest.

References

1. Sherry, D.D.; Bhaskar, R.S.A.; Poduval, M.; Rabinovich, C.L.; Myones, B.L. Juvenile Idiopathic Arthritis. Available online: https://emedicine.medscape.com/article/1007276-overview (accessed on 24 August 2020).
2. Ailioaie, C.; Ailioaie, L.M. Juvenile idiopathic arthritis. In *Management of Chronic Rheumatic Pain*; PIM Publishing House: Iaşi, Romania, 2008; pp. 129–146.
3. Haasnoot, A.J.W.; Sint Jago, N.F.M.; Tekstra, J.; de Boer, J.H. Impact of Uveitis on Quality of Life in Adult Patients with Juvenile Idiopathic Arthritis. *Arthritis Care Res.* **2017**, *69*, 1895–1902. [CrossRef]
4. Petty, R.E.; Southwood, T.R.; Manners, P.; Baum, J.; Glass, D.N.; Goldenberg, J.; He, X.; Maldonado-Cocco, J.; Orozco-Alcala, J.; Prieur, A.M.; et al. International League of Associations for Rheumatology Classification of Juvenile Idiopathic Arthritis: Second Revision, Edmonton, 2001. *J. Rheumatol.* **2004**, *31*, 390–392.
5. Cassidy, J.T.; Kivlin, J.; Lindsley, C.; Nocton, J. Ophthalmologic Examinations in Children with Juvenile Rheumatoid Arthritis. *Pediatrics* **2006**, *117*, 1843–1845. [CrossRef] [PubMed]
6. World Health Organization. Chronic rheumatic conditions. Available online: https://www.who.int/chp/topics/rheumatic/en/ (accessed on 19 August 2020).
7. Systemic juvenile idiopathic arthritis: Clinical manifestations and diagnosis. Available online: https://www.uptodate.com/contents/systemic-juvenile-idiopathic-arthritis-clinical-manifestations-and-diagnosis (accessed on 19 August 2020).
8. Angelis, A.; Kanavos, P.; López-Bastida, J.; Linertová, R.; Serrano-Aguilar, P.; BURQOL-RD Research Network. Socioeconomic costs and health-related quality of life in juvenile idiopathic arthritis: A cost-of-illness study in the United Kingdom. *BMC Musculoskelet. Disord.* **2016**, *17*, 321. [CrossRef] [PubMed]
9. Aggarwal, R.; Ringold, S.; Khanna, D.; Neogi, T.; Johnson, S.R.; Miller, A.; Brunner, H.I.; Ogawa, R.; Felson, D.; Ogdie, A.; et al. Distinctions between diagnostic and classification criteria? *Arthritis Care Res.* **2015**, *67*, 891–897. [CrossRef] [PubMed]
10. Dewint, P.; Hoffman, I.E.A.; Rogge, S.; Joos, R.; Union, A.; Dehoorne, J.; Delanghe, J.; Veys, E.M.; De Keyser, F.; Elewaut, D. Effect of age on prevalence of anticitrullinated protein/peptide antibodies in polyarticular juvenile idiopathic arthritis. *Rheumatology* **2006**, *45*, 204–208. [CrossRef]
11. Packham, J.C.; Hall, M.A.; Pimm, T.J. Long-term follow-up of 246 adults with juvenile idiopathic arthritis: Predictive factors for mood and pain. *Rheumatol. (Oxf.)* **2002**, *41*, 1444–1449. [CrossRef]
12. Gotia, S.; Ailioaie, C.; Ailioaie, L.M. *Rheumatic Diseases and Physical Therapy in Children*; Tehnopress: Iaşi, Romania, 2004; pp. 140–152.
13. Barut, K.; Adrovic, A.; Şahin, S.; Kasapçopur, ö. Juvenile Idiopathic Arthritis. *Balkan Med. J.* **2017**, *34*, 90–101. [CrossRef]
14. Prieur, A.M.; Deslandre, C.J. Les arthrites juvéniles idiopathiques Maladies: Aspects nosologiques actuels. *Presse med.* **2000**, *29*, 499–501.
15. Ailioaie, C. Contributions to the treatment of juvenile chronic arthritis. Ph.D. Thesis, University of Medicine and Pharmacy, Iaşi, Publishing House, Iaşi, Romania, 1996; pp. 102–127.
16. Chkirate, B.; Aitouamar, H.; Bentahila, A.; Rouichi, A.; Belhadi Mouhid, A. Actualités dans les rheumatismes inflammatoires de l'enfant. *Rev. Maghr Pediatr.* **2001**, *11*, 3–8.
17. Ailioaie, C.; Burdea, M.; Tansanu, I. Evolutionary considerations on juvenile chronic arthritis systemic form at onset. In *Recent Advances in Pediatrics*; Romanian Society of Pediatrics, Curtea Veche Publishing House: Bucharest, Romania, 1996; p. 603.
18. Prieur, A.M. Progrès récents en rhumatologie pédiatrique. À propos des formes systèmiques d'arthrite chronique juvénile. *Arch. Fr. Pediatr.* **1991**, *48*, 287–289. [PubMed]

19. Martini, A.; Ravelli, A.; Avcin, T.; Beresford, M.W.; Burgos-Vargas, R.; Cuttica, R.; Ilowite, N.T.; Khubchandani, R.; Laxer, R.M.; Lovell, D.J.; et al. Toward New Classification Criteria for Juvenile Idiopathic Arthritis: First Steps, Pediatric Rheumatology International Trials Organization International Consensus. For the Pediatric Rheumatology International Trials Organization (PRINTO). *J. Rheumatol.* **2019**, *46*, 190–197. [CrossRef] [PubMed]
20. Van der Linden, S.; Valkenburg, H.A.; Cats, A. Evaluation of diagnostic criteria for ankylosing spondylitis. A proposal for modification of the New York criteria. *Arthritis Rheum.* **1984**, *27*, 361–368. [CrossRef] [PubMed]
21. Lambert, R.G.; Bakker, P.A.; Van der Heijde, D.; Weber, U.; Rudwaleit, M.; Hermann, K.G.; Sieper, J.; Baraliakos, X.; Bennett, A.; Braun, J.; et al. Defining active sacroiliitis on MRI for classification of axial spondyloarthritis: Update by the ASAS MRI working group. *Ann. Rheum. Dis.* **2016**, *75*, 1958–1963. [CrossRef]
22. Cassidy, J.T.; Petty, R.E. Chronic Arthritis in Childhood. In *Textbook of Pediatric Rheumatology*, 5th ed.; Cassidy, J.T., Petty, R.E., Laxer, R., Lindlsy, C., Eds.; Elsevier Saunders: Philadelphia, PA, USA, 2005; pp. 206–321.
23. Kim, K.H.; Kim, D.S. Juvenile idiopathic arthritis: Diagnosis and differential diagnosis. *Korean J. Pediatr.* **2010**, *53*, 931–935. [CrossRef]
24. Martini, A. It is time to rethink juvenile idiopathic arthritis classification and nomenclature. *Ann. Rheum. Dis.* **2012**, *71*, 1437–1479. [CrossRef]
25. Moretti, D.; Cianchi, I.; Vannucci, G.; Cimaz, R.; Simonini, G. Psoriatic Juvenile Idiopathic Arthritis Associated with Uveitis: A Case Report. *Case Rep. Rheumatol.* **2013**, 595890. [CrossRef]
26. Ravelli, A.; Varnier, G.C.; Oliveira, S.; Castell, E.; Arguedas, O.; Magnani, A.; Pistorio, A.; Ruperto, N.; Magni-Manzoni, S.; Galasso, R.; et al. Antinuclear antibody-positive patients should be grouped as a separate category in the classification of juvenile idiopathic arthritis. *Arthritis Rheum.* **2011**, *63*, 267–275. [CrossRef]
27. Ailioaie, C.; Ailioaie, L.M. Progresses and perspectives in chronic arthritis in children. *Rev. Med. Chir. Soc. Med. Nat.* **2004**, *108*, 415–423.
28. Merino, R.; de Inocencio, J.; García-Consuegra, J. Evaluation of revised International League of Associations for Rheumatology classification criteria for juvenile idiopathic arthritis in Spanish children (Edmonton 2001). *J. Rheumatol.* **2005**, *32*, 559–561.
29. Ailioaie, C. *Idiopathic Juvenile Arthritis Family Guide*; CERMI Technical, Scientific and Didactic Publishing House: Iaşi, Romania, 2005; pp. 36–41. ISBN 973-667-109-7.
30. Pascual, V.; Allantaz, F.; Arce, E.; Punaro, M.; Banchereau, J. Role of interleukin-1 (IL-1) in the pathogenesis of systemic onset juvenile idiopathic arthritis and clinical response to IL-1 blockade. *J. Exp. Med.* **2005**, *201*, 1479–1486. [CrossRef] [PubMed]
31. Woo, P. Systemic juvenile idiopathic arthritis: Diagnosis, management, and outcome. *Nat. Clin. Pract. Rheumatol.* **2006**, *2*, 28–34. [CrossRef]
32. Mellins, E.D.; Macaubas, C.; Grom, A.A. Pathogenesis of systemic juvenile idiopathic arthritis: Some answers, more questions. *Nat. Rev. Rheumatol.* **2011**, *7*, 416–426. [CrossRef]
33. Prakken, B.; Albani, S.; Martini, A. Juvenile idiopathic arthritis. *Lancet* **2011**, *377*, 2138–2149. [CrossRef]
34. Nigrovic, P.A.; Schneider, R. Systemic Juvenile Idiopathic Arthritis and Adult Onset Still Disease. In *Textbook of Autoinflammation*; Hashkes, P., Laxer, R., Simon, A., Eds.; Springer: Cham, Switzerland, 2019; pp. 587–616. [CrossRef]
35. Singh-Grewal, D.; Schneider, R.; Bayer, N.; Feldman, B.M. Predictors of disease course and remission in systemic juvenile idiopathic arthritis: Significance of early clinical and laboratory features. *Arthritis Rheum.* **2006**, *54*, 1595–1601. [CrossRef] [PubMed]
36. Kelly, A.; Ramanan, A.V. Recognition and management of macrophage activation syndrome in juvenile arthritis. *Curr. Opin. Rheumatol.* **2007**, *19*, 477–481. [CrossRef] [PubMed]
37. Weaver, L.K.; Behrens, E.M. Hyperinflammation, rather than hemophagocytosis, is the common link between macrophage activation syndrome and hemophagocytic lymphohistiocytosis. *Curr. Opin. Rheumatol.* **2014**, *26*, 562–569. [CrossRef]

38. Put, K.; Avau, A.; Brisse, E.; Mitera, T.; Put, S.; Proost, P.; Bader-Meunier, B.; Westhovens, R.; Van den Eynde, B.J.; Orabona, C.; et al. Cytokines in systemic juvenile idiopathic arthritis and haemophagocytic lymphohistiocytosis: Tipping the balance between interleukin-18 and interferon-γ. *Rheumatol. (Oxf. Engl.)* **2015**, *54*, 1507–1517. [CrossRef]
39. Ramanan, A.V.; Grom, A.A. Does systemic-onset juvenile idiopathic arthritis belong under juvenile idiopathic arthritis? *Rheumatol. (Oxf.)* **2005**, *44*, 1350–1353. [CrossRef]
40. Barnes, M.G.; Grom, A.A.; Thompson, S.D.; Griffin, T.A.; Pavlidis, P.; Itert, L.; Fall, N.; Sowders, D.P.; Hinze, C.H.; Aronow, B.J.; et al. Subtype-specific peripheral blood gene expression profiles in recent-onset juvenile idiopathic arthritis. *Arthritis Rheum.* **2009**, *60*, 2101–2112. [CrossRef]
41. Fishman, D.; Faulds, G.; Jeffery, R.; Mohamed-Ali, V.; Yudkin, J.S.; Humphries, S.; Woo, P. The effect of novel polymorphisms in the interleukin-6 (IL-6) gene on IL-6 transcription and plasma IL-6 levels, and an association with systemic-onset juvenile chronic arthritis. *J. Clin. Invest.* **1998**, *102*, 1369–1376. [CrossRef] [PubMed]
42. Ogilvie, E.M.; Fife, M.S.; Thompson, S.D.; Twine, N.; Tsoras, M.; Moroldo, M.; Fisher, S.A.; Lewis, C.M.; Prieur, A.-M.; Glass, D.N.; et al. The -174G allele of the interleukin-6 gene confers susceptibility to systemic arthritis in children: A multicenter study using simplex and multiplex juvenile idiopathic arthritis families. *Arthritis Rheum.* **2003**, *48*, 3202–3206. [CrossRef] [PubMed]
43. Fife, M.S.; Gutierrez, A.; Ogilvie, E.M.; Stock, C.J.; Samuel, J.M.; Thomson, W.; Mack, L.F.; Lewis, G.M.; Woo, P. Novel IL10 gene family associations with systemic juvenile idiopathic arthritis. *Arthritis Res. Ther.* **2006**, *8*, R148. [CrossRef] [PubMed]
44. Möller, J.C.; Paul, D.; Ganser, G.; Range, U.; Gahr, M.; Kelsch, R.; Rösen-Wolff, A.; Hedrich, C.M. IL10 promoter polymorphisms are associated with systemic onset juvenile idiopathic arthritis (SoJIA). *Clin. Exp. Rheumatol.* **2010**, *28*, 912–918. [PubMed]
45. Fall, N.; Barnes, M.G.; Thornton, S.; Luyrink, L.; Olson, J.; Ilowite, N.T.; Gottlieb, B.S.; Griffin, T.; Sherry, D.D.; Thompson, S.; et al. Gene expression profiling of peripheral blood from patients with untreated new-onset systemic juvenile idiopathic arthritis reveals molecular heterogeneity that may predict macrophage activation syndrome. *Arthritis Rheum.* **2007**, *56*, 3793–3804. [CrossRef]
46. Gabay, C.; Lamacchia, C.; Palmer, G. IL-1 pathways in inflammation and human diseases. *Nat. Rev. Rheumatol.* **2010**, *6*, 232–241. [CrossRef] [PubMed]
47. Nigrovic, P.A. Review: Is there a window of opportunity for treatment of systemic juvenile idiopathic arthritis? *Arthritis Rheumatol.* **2014**, *66*, 1405–1413. [CrossRef]
48. Verbsky, J.; White, A. Effective use of the recombinant interleukin 1 receptor antagonist anakinra in therapy resistant systemic onset juvenile rheumatoid arthritis. *J. Rheumatol.* **2004**, *31*, 2071–2075.
49. Irigoyen, P.I.; Olson, J.; Hom, C.; Ilowite, N.T. Treatment of systemic onset juvenile rheumatoid arthritis with anakinra. *Arthritis Rheum.* **2004**, *50*, S437.
50. Henrickson, M. Efficacy of anakinra in refractory systemic arthritis. *Arthritis Rheum.* **2004**, *50*, S438.
51. Sikora, K.A.; Grom, A.A. Update on the pathogenesis and treatment of systemic idiopathic arthritis. *Curr. Opin. Pediatr.* **2011**, *23*, 640–646. [CrossRef] [PubMed]
52. Toplak, N.; Blazina, Š.; Avčin, T. The role of IL-1 inhibition in systemic juvenile idiopathic arthritis: Current status and future perspectives. *Drug Des. Devel Ther.* **2018**, *12*, 1633–1643. [CrossRef] [PubMed]
53. De Benedetti, F.; Massa, M.; Robbioni, P.; Ravelli, A.; Burgio, G.R.; Martini, A. Correlation of serum interleukin-6 levels with joint involvement and thrombocytosis in systemic juvenile rheumatoid arthritis. *Arthritis Rheum.* **1991**, *34*, 1158–1163. [CrossRef] [PubMed]
54. Tateiwa, D.; Yoshikawa, H.; Kaito, T. Cartilage and Bone Destruction in Arthritis: Pathogenesis and Treatment Strategy: A Literature Review. *Cells* **2019**, *8*, 818. [CrossRef] [PubMed]
55. Heinrich, P.C.; Castell, J.V.; Andus, T. Interleukin-6 and the acute phase response. *Biochem. J.* **1990**, *265*, 621–636. [CrossRef]
56. Korn, T.; Bettelli, E.; Oukka, M.; Kuchroo, V.K. IL-17 and Th17 Cells. *Annu. Rev. Immunol.* **2009**, *27*, 485–517. [CrossRef]
57. Muller, K.; Herner, E.B.; Stagg, A.; Bendtzen, K.; Woo, P. Inflammatory cytokines and cytokine antagonists in whole blood cultures of patients with systemic juvenile chronic arthritis. *Br. J. Rheumatol.* **1998**, *37*, 562–569. [CrossRef]

58. Imbrechts, M.; Avau, A.; Vandenhaute, J.; Malengier-Devlies, B.; Put, K.; Mitera, T.; Berghmans, N.; Burton, O.; Junius, S.; Liston, A.; et al. Insufficient IL-10 Production as a Mechanism Underlying the Pathogenesis of Systemic Juvenile Idiopathic Arthritis. *J. Immunol.* **2018**, *201*, 2654–2663. [CrossRef]
59. Vandenhaute, J.; Avau, A.; Filtjens, J.; Malengier-Devlies, B.; Imbrechts, M.; Van den Berghe, N.; Ahmadzadeh, K.; Mitera, T.; Boon, L.; Leclercq, G.; et al. Regulatory Role for NK Cells in a Mouse Model of Systemic Juvenile Idiopathic Arthritis. *J. Immunol.* **2019**, *203*, 3339–3348. [CrossRef]
60. Put, K. Interferon-Gamma en 'Natural Killer' Cellen in Systemische Juveniele Idiopathische Artritis en Macrofaagactivatiesyndroom. Ph.D. Thesis, KU Leuven, Leuven, Belgium, 2015. Available online: https://limo.libis.be/primo-explore/fulldisplay?docid=LIRIAS1907034&context=L&vid=Lirias&search_scope=Lirias&tab=default_tab&lang=en_US&fromSitemap=1 (accessed on 24 August 2020).
61. Put, K.; Vandenhaute, J.; Avau, A.; Van Nieuwenhuijze, A.; Brisse, E.; Dierckx, T.; Rutgeerts, O.; Garcia-Perez, J.; Toelen, J.; Waer, M.; et al. Inflammatory gene expression profile and defective IFN-gamma and granzyme K in natural killer cells of systemic juvenile idiopathic arthritis patients. *Arthritis Rheumatol.* **2017**, *69*, 213–224. [CrossRef]
62. Lerkvaleekul, B.; Vilaiyuk, S. Macrophage activation syndrome: Early diagnosis is key. *Open Access Rheumatol.* **2018**, *10*, 117–128. [CrossRef] [PubMed]
63. Ruscitti, P.; Rago, C.; Breda, L.; Cipriani, P.; Liakouli, V.; Berardicurti, O.; Carubbi, F.; Di Battista, C.; Verrotti, A.; Giacomelli, R. Macrophage activation syndrome in Still's disease: Analysis of clinical characteristics and survival in paediatric and adult patients. *Clin. Rheumatol.* **2017**, *36*, 2839–2845. [CrossRef] [PubMed]
64. Behrens, E.M.; Beukelman, T.; Paessler, M.; Cron, R.Q. Occult macrophage activation syndrome in patients with systemic juvenile idiopathic arthritis. *J. Rheumatol.* **2007**, *34*, 1133–1138.
65. Ravelli, A.; Davi, S.; Minoia, F.; Martini, A.; Cron, R.Q. Macrophage activation syndrome. *Hematol. Oncol. Clin. N. Am.* **2015**, *29*, 927–941. [CrossRef]
66. Grom, A.A.; Horne, A.; De Benedetti, F. Macrophage activation syndrome in the era of biologic therapy. *Nat. Rev. Rheumatol.* **2016**, *12*, 259–268. [CrossRef]
67. Zhang, K.; Biroschak, J.; Glass, D.N.; Thompson, S.D.; Finkel, T.; Passo, M.H.; Binstadt, B.A.; Filipovich, A.; Grom, A.A. Macrophage activation syndrome in patients with systemic juvenile idiopathic arthritis is associated with MUNC13-4 polymorphisms. *Arthritis Rheum.* **2008**, *58*, 2892–2896. [CrossRef] [PubMed]
68. Vastert, S.J.; van Wijk, R.; D'Urbano, L.E.; de Vooght, K.M.; de Jager, W.; Ravelli, A.; Magni-Manzoni, S.; Insalaco, A.; Cortis, E.; van Solinge, W.W.; et al. Mutations in the perforin gene can be linked to macrophage activation syndrome in patients with systemic onset juvenile idiopathic arthritis. *Rheumatol. (Oxf.)* **2010**, *49*, 441–449. [CrossRef]
69. Zhang, M.; Behrens, E.M.; Atkinson, T.P.; Shakocry, B.; Grom, A.A.; Cron, R.Q. Genetic defects in cytolysis in macrophage activation syndrome. *Curr. Rheumatol. Rep.* **2014**, *16*, 439. [CrossRef]
70. Davì, S.; Consolaro, A.; Guseinova, D.; Pistorio, A.; Ruperto, N.; Martini, A.; Cron, R.Q.; Ravelli, A.; MAS Study Group. An international consensus survey of diagnostic criteria for macrophage activation syndrome in systemic juvenile idiopathic arthritis. *J. Rheumatol.* **2011**, *38*, 764–768. [CrossRef]
71. Minoia, F.; Davì, S.; Horne, A.C.; Demirkaya, E.; Bovis, F.; Li, C.; Lehmberg, K.; Weitzman, S.; Insalaco, A.; Wouters, C.; et al. Clinical features, treatment, and outcome of macrophage activation syndrome complicating systemic juvenile idiopathic arthritis: A multinational, multicenter study of 362 patients. *Arthritis Rheumatol.* **2014**, *66*, 3160–3169. [CrossRef]
72. Ravelli, A.; Minoia, F.; Davì, S.; Horne, A.C.; Bovis, F.; Pistorio, A.; Aricò, M.; Avcin, T.; Behrens, E.M.; De Benedetti, F.; et al. 2016 Classification Criteria for Macrophage Activation Syndrome Complicating Systemic Juvenile Idiopathic Arthritis: A European League Against Rheumatism/American College of Rheumatology/Paediatric Rheumatology International Trials Organisation Collaborative Initiative. *Ann. Rheum. Dis.* **2016**, *68*, 566–576. [CrossRef]
73. Fournier, C. Where do T cells stand in rheumatoid arthritis? *Joint Bone Spine* **2005**, *72*, 527–532. [CrossRef]
74. Pennock, D.N.; White, J.T.; Cross, E.W.; Cheney, E.E.; Tamburini, B.A.; Kedl, R.M. T cell responses: Naïve to memory and everything in between. *Adv. Physiol. Educ.* **2013**, *37*, 273–283. [CrossRef] [PubMed]
75. Iwasaki, A.; Medzhitov, R. Toll-like receptor control of the adaptive immune responses. *Nat. Immunol.* **2004**, *5*, 987–995. [CrossRef] [PubMed]
76. Kasama, T.; Isozaki, T.; Takahashi, R.; Miwa, Y. Clinical effects of tocilizumab on cytokines and immunological factors in patients with rheumatoid arthritis. *Int. Immunopharmacol.* **2016**, *35*, 301–306. [CrossRef] [PubMed]

77. Burmester, G.R.; Feist, E.; Dörner, T. Emerging cell and cytokine targets in rheumatoid arthritis. *Nat. Rev. Rheumatol.* **2014**, *10*, 77–88. [CrossRef] [PubMed]
78. Ponchel, F.; Goëb, V.; Parmar, R.; El-Sherbiny, Y.; Boissinot, M.; El Jawhari, J.; Burska, A.; Vital, E.M.; Harrison, S.; Conaghan, P.G.; et al. An immunological biomarker to predict MTX response in early RA. *Ann. Rheum. Dis.* **2014**, *73*, 2047–2053. [CrossRef]
79. Nalbant, S.; Birlik, A.M. Cytokines in Rheumatoid Arthritis (RA). In *New Developments in the Pathogenesis of Rheumatoid Arthritis*; Sakkas, L.I., Ed.; IntechOpen: Rijeka, Croatia, 2017; Available online: https://www.intechopen.com/books/new-developments-in-the-pathogenesis-of-rheumatoid-arthritis/cytokines-in-rheumatoid-arthritis-ra- (accessed on 25 August 2020).
80. Hibi, M.; Murakami, M.; Saito, M.; Hirano, T.; Taga, T.; Kishimoto, T. Molecular cloning and expression of an IL-6 signal transducer, gp130. *Cell* **1990**, *63*, 1149–1157. [CrossRef]
81. Mihara, M.; Hashizume, M.; Yoshida, H.; Suzuki, M.; Shiina, M. IL-6/IL-6 receptor system and its role in physiological and pathological conditions. *Clin. Sci. (Lond.)* **2012**, *122*, 143–159. [CrossRef]
82. Reeh, H.; Rudolph, N.; Billing, U.; Christen, H.; Streif, S.; Bullinger, E.; Schliemann-Bullinger, M.; Findeisen, R.; Schaper, F.; Huber, H.J.; et al. Response to IL-6 trans- and IL-6 classic signaling is determined by the ratio of the IL-6 receptor α to gp130 expression: Fusing experimental insights and dynamic modelling. *Cell Commun. Signal.* **2019**, *17*, 46. [CrossRef]
83. Yokota, S.; Tanaka, T.; Kishimoto, T. Efficacy, safety and tolerability of tocilizumab in patients with systemic juvenile idiopathic arthritis. *Ther. Adv. Musculoskelet. Dis.* **2012**, *4*, 387–397. [CrossRef] [PubMed]
84. Gabay, C.; Msihid, J.; Zilberstein, M.; Paccard, C.; Lin, Y.; Graham, N.M.H.; Boyapati, A. Identification of sarilumab pharmacodynamic and predictive markers in patients with inadequate response to TNF inhibition: A biomarker substudy of the phase 3 TARGET study. *RMD Open* **2018**, *4*, e000607. [CrossRef] [PubMed]
85. Davignon, J.; Rauwel, B.; Degboé, Y.; Constantin, A.; Boyer, J.F.; Kruglov, A.; Cantagrel, A. Modulation of T-cell responses by anti-tumor necrosis factor treatments in rheumatoid arthritis: A review. *Arthritis Res. Ther.* **2018**, *20*, 229. [CrossRef] [PubMed]
86. Choy, E. Understanding the dynamics: Pathways involved in the pathogenesis of rheumatoid arthritis. *Rheumatology* **2012**, *51*, 3–11. [CrossRef]
87. Jimenez-Boj, E.; Redlich, K.; Türk, B.; Hanslik-Schnabel, B.; Wanivenhaus, A.; Chott, A.; Ramiro, S.; Schett, G. Interaction between synovial inflammatory tissue and bone marrow in rheumatoid arthritis. *J. Immunol.* **2005**, *175*, 2579–2588. [CrossRef] [PubMed]
88. Alamgeer, H.U.; Uttra, A.M.; Qasim, S.; Ikram, J.; Saleem, M.; Niazi, Z.R. Phytochemicals targeting matrix metalloproteinases regulating tissue degradation in inflammation and rheumatoid arthritis. *Phytomedicine* **2020**, *66*, 153134. [CrossRef] [PubMed]
89. Alunno, A.; Carubbi, F.; Giacomelli, R.; Gerli, R. Cytokines in the pathogenesis of rheumatoid arthritis: New players and therapeutic targets. *BMC Rheumatol.* **2017**, *1*, 3. [CrossRef]
90. Dinarello, C.; Arend, W.; Sims, J.; Smith, D.; Blumberg, H.; O'Neill, L.; Goldbach-Mansky, R.; Pizarro, T.; Hoffman, H.; Bufler, P.; et al. IL-1 family nomenclature. *Nat. Immunol.* **2010**, *11*, 973. [CrossRef]
91. Matsuyama, Y.; Okazaki, H.; Tamemoto, H.; Kimura, H.; Kamata, Y.; Nagatani, K.; Yoshio, T.; Nagashima, T.; Iwamoto, M.; Hayakawa, M.; et al. Increased levels of interleukin 33 in sera and synovial fluid from patients with active rheumatoid arthritis. *J. Rheumatol.* **2010**, *37*, 18–25. [CrossRef]
92. Hong, Y.S.; Moon, S.J.; Joo, Y.B.; Jeon, C.H.; Cho, M.L.; Ju, J.H.; Oh, H.J.; Heo, Y.J.; Park, S.H.; Kim, H.Y.; et al. Measurement of interleukin-33 (IL-33) and IL-33 receptors (sST2 and ST2L) in patients with rheumatoid arthritis. *J. Korean Med. Sci.* **2011**, *26*, 1132–1139. [CrossRef]
93. Xiangyang, Z.; Lutian, Y.; Lin, Z.; Liping, X.; Hui, S.; Jing, L. Increased levels of interleukin-33 associated with bone erosion and interstitial lung diseases in patients with rheumatoid arthritis. *Cytokine* **2012**, *58*, 6–9. [CrossRef] [PubMed]
94. Talabot-Ayer, D.; McKee, T.; Gindre, P.; Bas, S.; Baeten, D.L.; Gabay, C.; Palmer, G. Distinct serum and synovial fluid interleukin (IL)-33 levels in rheumatoid arthritis, psoriatic arthritis and osteoarthritis. *Joint Bone Spine* **2012**, *79*, 32–37. [CrossRef] [PubMed]
95. Miossec, P.; Kolls, J.K. Targeting IL-17 and TH17 cells in chronic inflammation. *Nat. Rev. Drug Discov.* **2012**, *11*, 763–776. [CrossRef] [PubMed]
96. Robert, M.; Miossec, P. IL-17 in Rheumatoid Arthritis and Precision Medicine: From Synovitis Expression to Circulating Bioactive Levels. *Front. Med.* **2019**, *5*, 364. [CrossRef]

97. Sweeney, S.E.; Firestein, G.S. Rheumatoid arthritis: Regulation of synovial inflammation. *Int J. Biochem. Cell Biol.* **2004**, *36*, 372–378. [CrossRef]
98. Bottini, N.; Firestein, G.S. Duality of fibroblast-like synoviocytes in RA: Passive responders and imprinted aggressors. *Nat. Rev. Rheumatol.* **2013**, *9*, 24–33. [CrossRef]
99. Eljaafari, A.; Tartelin, M.L.; Aissaoui, H.; Chevrel, G.; Osta, B.; Lavocat, F.; Miossec, P. Bone marrow-derived and synovium-derived mesenchymal cells promote Th17 cell expansion and activation through caspase 1 activation: Contribution to the chronicity of rheumatoid arthritis. *Arthritis Rheum.* **2012**, *64*, 2147–2157. [CrossRef]
100. Honorati, M.C.; Neri, S.; Cattini, L.; Facchini, A. Interleukin-17, a regulator of angiogenic factor release by synovial fibroblasts. *Osteoarthritis Cartilage* **2006**, *14*, 345–352. [CrossRef]
101. Daoussis, D.; Andonopoulos, A.P.; Liossis, S.N. Wnt pathway and IL-17: Novel regulators of joint remodeling in rheumatic diseases. Looking beyond the RANK-RANKL-OPG axis. *Semin. Arthritis Rheum.* **2010**, *39*, 369–383. [CrossRef]
102. Hot, A.; Miossec, P. Effects of interleukin (IL)-17A and IL-17F in human rheumatoid arthritis synoviocytes. *Ann. Rheum. Dis.* **2011**, *70*, 727–732. [CrossRef]
103. Hot, A.; Zrioual, S.; Toh, M.L.; Lenief, V.; Miossec, P. IL-17A- versus IL-17F-induced intracellular signal transduction pathways and modulation by IL-17RA and IL-17RC RNA interference in rheumatoid synoviocytes. *Ann. Rheum. Dis.* **2011**, *70*, 341–348. [CrossRef]
104. Park, J.H.; Lee, N.K.; Lee, S.Y. Current Understanding of RANK Signaling in Osteoclast Differentiation and Maturation. *Mol. Cells* **2017**, *40*, 706–713. [CrossRef] [PubMed]
105. Van Bezooijen, R.L.; Papapoulos, S.E.; Löwik, C.W. Effect of interleukin-17 on nitric oxide production and osteoclastic bone resorption: Is there dependency on nuclear factor-kappaB and receptor activator of nuclear factor kappaB (RANK)/RANK ligand signaling? *Bone* **2001**, *28*, 378–386. [CrossRef]
106. Lavocat, F.; Maggi, L.; Annunziato, F.; Miossec, P. T-cell clones from Th1, Th17 or Th1/17 lineages and their signature cytokines have different capacity to activate endothelial cells or synoviocytes. *Cytokine* **2016**, *88*, 241–250. [CrossRef]
107. Kotake, S.; Udagawa, N.; Takahashi, N.; Matsuzaki, K.; Itoh, K.; Ishiyama, S.; Saito, S.; Inoue, K.; Kamatani, N.; Gillespie, M.T.; et al. IL-17 in synovial fluids from patients with rheumatoid arthritis is a potent stimulator of osteoclastogenesis. *J. Clin. Investig.* **1999**, *103*, 1345–1352. [CrossRef] [PubMed]
108. Kotake, S.; Yago, T.; Kobashigawa, T.; Nanke, Y. The Plasticity of Th17 Cells in the Pathogenesis of Rheumatoid Arthritis. *J. Clin Med.* **2017**, *6*, 67. [CrossRef]
109. Sato, K.; Suematsu, A.; Okamoto, K.; Yamaguchi, A.; Morishita, Y.; Kadono, Y.; Tanaka, S.; Kodama, T.; Akira, S.; Iwakura, Y.; et al. Th17 functions as an osteoclastogenic helper T cell subset that links T cell activation and bone destruction. *J. Exp. Med.* **2006**, *203*, 2673–2682. [CrossRef]
110. Komatsu, N.; Okamoto, K.; Sawa, S.; Nakashima, T.; Oh-hora, M.; Kodama, T.; Tanaka, S.; Bluestone, J.A.; Takayanagi, H. Pathogenic conversion of Foxp3+ T cells into TH17 cells in autoimmune arthritis. *Nat. Med.* **2014**, *20*, 62–68. [CrossRef]
111. Takayanagi, H. Osteoimmunology and the effects of the immune system on bone. *Nat. Rev. Rheumatol.* **2009**, *5*, 667–676. [CrossRef]
112. Gravallese, E.M.; Harada, Y.; Wang, J.T.; Gorn, A.H.; Thornhill, T.S.; Goldring, S.R. Identification of cell types responsible for bone resorption in rheumatoid arthritis and juvenile rheumatoid arthritis. *Am. J. Pathol.* **1998**, *152*, 943–951.
113. Yasuda, H.; Shima, N.; Nakagawa, N.; Yamaguchi, K.; Kinosaki, M.; Mochizuki, S.; Tomoyasu, A.; Yano, K.; Goto, M.; Murakami, A.; et al. Osteoclast differentiation factor is a ligand for osteoprotegerin/osteoclastogenesis-inhibitory factor and is identical to TRANCE/RANKL. *Proc. Natl. Acad. Sci. USA* **1998**, *95*, 3597–3602. [CrossRef] [PubMed]
114. Braun, T.; Zwerina, J. Positive regulators of osteoclastogenesis and bone resorption in rheumatoid arthritis. *Arthritis Res. Ther.* **2011**, *13*, 235. [CrossRef] [PubMed]
115. Heinrich, P.C.; Behrmann, I.; Muller-Newen, G.; Schaper, F.; Graeve, L. Interleukin-6-type cytokine signaling through the gp130/Jak/STAT pathway. *Biochem. J.* **1998**, *334*, 297–314. [CrossRef]
116. Yamaoka, K.; Saharinen, P.; Pesu, M.; Holt III, V.E.T.; Silvennoinen, O.; O'Shea, J.J. The Janus kinases (Jaks). *Genome Biol.* **2004**, *5*, 253. [CrossRef] [PubMed]

117. Fridman, J.S.; Scherle, P.A.; Collins, R.; Burn, T.C.; Li, Y.; Li, J.; Covington, M.B.; Thomas, B.; Collier, P.; Favata, M.F.; et al. Selective inhibition of JAK1 and JAK2 is efficacious in rodent models of arthritis: Preclinical characterization of INCB028050. *J. Immunol.* **2010**, *184*, 5298–5307. [CrossRef]
118. Kremer, J.M. Selective costimulation modulators: A novel approach for the treatment of rheumatoid arthritis. *J. Clin. Rheumatol.* **2005**, *11*, S55–S62. [CrossRef]
119. Abatacept. DrugBank. Available online: https://www.drugbank.ca/drugs/DB01281 (accessed on 24 August 2020).
120. Fukuyo, S.; Nakayamada, S.; Iwata, S.; Kubo, S.; Saito, K.; Tanaka, Y. Abatacept therapy reduces CD28+CXCR5+ follicular helper-like T cells in patients with rheumatoid arthritis. *Clin. Exp. Rheumatol.* **2017**, *35*, 562–570.
121. Ailioaie, L.M.; Ailioaie, C. Photobiomodulation—Targeting the quantum life. Newest implications for immunity, health, and youth. Invited Lecture. In Proceedings of the 11th International ISLA Congress for Medical Laser Applications, Lauenförde-Beverungen, Germany, 10–11 June 2016.
122. Full-spectrum light. Available online: https://en.wikipedia.org/wiki/Full-spectrum_light (accessed on 23 August 2020).
123. Dolmans, D.E.; Fukumura, D.; Jain, R.K. Photodynamic therapy for cancer. *Nat. Rev. Cancer* **2003**, *3*, 380–387. [CrossRef]
124. NobelPrize.org; Nobel Media AB 2020. The Nobel Prize in Physiology or Medicine 1903. Available online: https://www.nobelprize.org/prizes/medicine/1903/summary/ (accessed on 3 August 2020).
125. Keijzer, M.; Jacques, S.L.; Prahl, S.A.; Welch, A.J. Light distributions in artery tissue: Monte Carlo simulations for finite-diameter laser beams. *Lasers Surg. Med.* **1989**, *9*, 148–154. [CrossRef]
126. Understanding the Differences between LED and Laser Therapy. Available online: https://www.lightforcemedical.com/understanding-the-differences-between-led-and-laser-therapy/ (accessed on 23 August 2020).
127. Ailioaie, L.M. New clinical results in intravenous laser therapy. Invited lecture. In Proceedings of the 9th International ISLA Congress for Medical Laser Applications, Lauenförde-Beverungen, Germany, 27–29 June 2014.
128. Ailioaie, C.; Ailioaie, L.M. Laser photobiostimulation and safety in pediatric diseases. In *Lasers in Medicine, Science and Praxis*; Simunovic, Z., Ed.; Printery Publishing House: Cakovec, Croatia, 2009; Chapter 32; pp. 467–504.
129. All about High Intensity Laser. BTL High Intensity Laser. Available online: https://www.high-intensity-laser.com/subpage (accessed on 4 August 2020).
130. Overman, D. Treating Pain with Low vs. High-Power Lasers: What is the Difference? *Rehab Managagement*, 4 April 2019. Available online: https://www.rehabpub.com/pain-management/products/treating-pain-low-vs-high-power-lasers-difference/ (accessed on 4 August 2020).
131. Moskvin, S.V.; Kisselev, S.B. *Laser Therapy for Joint and Muscle Pain*; OOO Izdatelstvo "Triada": Moscow/Tver, Russia, 2017; pp. 10, 169, 175–176. ISBN 978-5-94789-787-6.
132. Moskvin, S.V.; Khadartsev, A.A. *Basic Techniques of Low Level Laser Therapy*; OOO Izdatelstvo "Triada": Moscow/Tver, Russia, 2017; pp. 11–12. ISBN 978-5-94789-772-2.
133. Chiran, D.A.; Litscher, G.; Weber, M.; Ailioaie, L.M.; Ailioaie, C.; Litscher, D. Intravenous laser blood irradiation increases efficacy of etanercept in selected subtypes of juvenile idiopathic arthritis: An innovative clinical research approach. *Evid. Based Complement. Alternat. Med.* **2013**, *2013*, 168134. [CrossRef] [PubMed]
134. Ailioaie, L.M.; Litscher, G.; Weber, M.; Ailioaie, C.; Litscher, D.; Chiran, D.A. Innovations and challenges by applying sublingual laser blood irradiation in juvenile idiopathic arthritis. *Int. J. Photoenergy* **2014**, *2014*, 130417. [CrossRef]
135. Chiran, D.A.; Weber, M.; Ailioaie, L.M.; Moraru, E.; Ailioaie, C.; Litscher, D.; Litscher, G. Intravenous laser blood irradiation and tocilizumab in a patient with juvenile arthritis. *Case Rep. Med.* **2014**, *2014*, 923496. [CrossRef]
136. Srinivasan, S.; Avadhani, N.G. Cytochrome c oxidase dysfunction in oxidative stress. *Free Radic. Biol. Med.* **2012**, *53*, 1252–1263. [CrossRef]
137. Photobiomodulation. Available online: http://www.appliedbiophotonics.com/photobiomodulation/ (accessed on 4 August 2020).
138. Cotler, H.B.; Chow, R.T.; Hamblin, M.R.; Carroll, J. The use of Low-Level Laser Therapy (LLLT) for musculoskeletal pain. *MOJ Orthop. Rheumatol.* **2015**, *2*, 188–194. [CrossRef]

139. Dompe, C.; Moncrieff, L.; Matys, J.; Grzech-Leśniak K.; Kocherova, I.; Bryja, A.; Bruska, M.; Dominiak, M.; Mozdziak, P.; Skiba, T.H.I.; et al. Photobiomodulation—Underlying Mechanism and Clinical Applications. *J. Clin. Med.* **2020**, *9*, 1724. [CrossRef]
140. Santana-Blank, L.; Rodríguez-Santana, E.; Santana-Rodríguez, K.E.; Reyes, H. "Quantum Leap" in Photobiomodulation Therapy Ushers in a New Generation of Light-Based Treatments for Cancer and Other Complex Diseases: Perspective and Mini-Review. *Photomed. Laser Surg.* **2016**, *34*, 93–101. [CrossRef]
141. Chiran, D.A.; Ailioaie, L.M.; Ailioaie, C. New challenges in treating pediatric rheumatic diseases with lasers in the age of biologic therapy. In Proceedings of the 9th World Association for Laser Therapy, Gold Coast, Australia, 28–30 September 2012; Laakso, E.L., Young, C., Eds.; World Association for Laser Therapy Congress (WALT): Gold Coast, Australia, 2013; pp. 25–27.
142. Stoll, M.L.; Cron, R.Q. Treatment of juvenile idiopathic arthritis: A revolution in care. *Pediatr. Rheumatol. Online J.* **2014**, *12*, 13. [CrossRef]
143. Wickenheisser, V.A.; Zywot, E.M.; Rabjohns, E.M.; Lee, H.H.; Lawrence, D.S.; Tarrant, T.K. Laser Light Therapy in Inflammatory, Musculoskeletal, and Autoimmune Disease. *Curr. Allergy Asthma Rep.* **2019**, *19*, 37. [CrossRef]
144. Zak, M.; Pedersen, F.K. Juvenile chronic arthritis into adulthood: A long-term follow-up study. *Rheumatology* **2000**, *39*, 198–204. [CrossRef]
145. Prieur, A.M.; Chèdeville, G. Prognostic factors in juvenile idiopathic arthritis. *Curr. Rheumatol. Rep.* **2001**, *3*, 371–378. [CrossRef] [PubMed]
146. Ailioaie, C.; Ailioaie, L.M. Beneficial effects of laser therapy in the early stages of rheumatoid arthritis onset. *J. Laser Ther.* **1999**, *11*, 79–87. [CrossRef]
147. Tuner, J.; Hode, L. The Laser Therapy Handbook. *Prima Books. Sweden.* **2007**, 292.
148. Contraindications for Use of Therapeutic Laser. Available online: https://www.practicalpainmanagement.com/treatments/complementary/lasers/contraindications-use-therapeutic-laser (accessed on 4 August 2020).
149. Meesters, A.A.; Pitassi, L.H.; Campos, V.; Wolkerstorfer, A.; Dierickx, C.C. Transcutaneous laser treatment of leg veins. *Lasers Med. Sci.* **2014**, *29*, 481–492. [CrossRef]
150. Liu, T.C.Y.; Wu, D.F.; Gu, Z.Q.; Wu, M. Applications of intranasal low intensity laser therapy in sports medicine. *J. Innov. Opt. Health Sci.* **2010**, *3*, 1–16. [CrossRef]
151. Wirz-Ridolfi, A. Comparison between Intravenous and Various Types of Transcutaneous Laser Blood Irradiation. *Internet J. Laserneedle Med.* **2013**, *3*. Available online: http://ispub.com/IJLNM/3/1/14462 (accessed on 4 August 2020).
152. Mikhaylov, V.A. The use of Intravenous Laser Blood Irradiation (ILBI) at 630–640 nm to prevent vascular diseases and to increase life expectancy. *Laser Ther.* **2015**, *24*, 15–26. [CrossRef]
153. Amjadi, A.; Mirmiranpor, H.; Khandani, S.; Sobhani, S.O.; Shafaee, Y. Intravenous laser wavelength irradiation effect on interleukins: IL-1α, IL-1β, IL6 in diabetic rats. *Laser Ther.* **2019**, *28*, 267–273.
154. Hamblin, M.R. Mechanisms and applications of the anti-inflammatory effects of photobiomodulation. *AIMS Biophys.* **2017**, *4*, 337–361. [CrossRef]
155. Castano, A.P.; Dai, T.; Yaroslavsky, I.; Cohen, R. Apruzzese, W.A.; Smotrich, M.H.; Hamblin, M.R. Low-level laser therapy for zymosan-induced arthritis in rats: Importance of illumination time. *Lasers Surg. Med.* **2007**, *39*, 543–550. [CrossRef] [PubMed]
156. Chen, A.C.; Arany, P.R.; Huang, Y.Y.; Tomkinson, E.M.; Sharma, S.K.; Kharkwal, G.B.; Saleem, T.; Mooney, D. Yull, F.E.; Blackwell, T.S.; et al. Low-level laser therapy activates NF-kB via generation of reactive oxygen species in mouse embryonic fibroblasts. *PLoS ONE* **2011**, *6*, e22453. [CrossRef]
157. Alves, A.C.; Vieira, R.; Leal-Junior, E.; dos Santos, S.; Ligeiro, A.P.; Albertini, R.; Junior, J.; de Carvalho, P. Effect of low-level laser therapy on the expression of inflammatory mediators and on neutrophils and macrophages in acute joint inflammation. *Arthritis Res. Ther.* **2013**, *15*, R116. [CrossRef] [PubMed]
158. Assis, L.; Moretti, A.I.; Abrahão, T.B.; de Souza, H.P.; Hamblin, M.R.; Parizotto, N.A. Low-level laser therapy (808 nm) contributes to muscle regeneration and prevents fibrosis in rat tibialis anterior muscle after cryolesion. *Lasers Med. Sci.* **2013**, *28*, 947–955. [CrossRef]
159. Hsieh, Y.L.; Cheng, Y.J.; Huang, F.C.; Yang, C.C. The fluence effects of low-level laser therapy on inflammation, fibroblast-like synoviocytes, and synovial apoptosis in rats with adjuvant-induced arthritis. *Photomed. Laser Surg.* **2014**, *32*, 669–677. [CrossRef]

160. dos Santos, S.A.; Alves, A.C.; Leal-Junior, E.C.; Albertini, R.; de Paula Vieira, R.; Ligeiro, A.P.; Silva Junior, J.A.; de Carvalho, P. Comparative analysis of two low-level laser doses on the expression of inflammatory mediators and on neutrophils and macrophages in acute joint inflammation. *Lasers Med. Sci.* **2014**, *29*, 1051–1058. [CrossRef]
161. Torres-Silva, R.; Lopes-Martins, R.A.B.; Bjordal, J.M.; Frigo, L.; Rahouadj, R.; Arnold, G.; Leal-Junior, E.C.P.; Magdalou, J.; Pallotta, R.; Marcos, R.L. The low-level laser therapy (LLLT) operating in 660 nm reduce gene expression of inflammatory mediators in the experimental model of collagenase-induced rat tendinitis. *Lasers Med. Sci.* **2015**, *30*, 1985–1990. [CrossRef]
162. Fernandes, K.P.; Souza, N.H.; Mesquita-Ferrari, R.A.; Silva, D.; Rocha, L.A.; Alves, A.N.; Sousa, K.; Bussadori, S.K.; Hamblin, M.R.; Nunes, F.D. Photobiomodulation with 660-nm and 780-nm laser on activated J774 macrophage-like cells: Effect on M1 inflammatory markers. *J. Photochem. Photobiol. B Biol.* **2015**, *153*, 344–351. [CrossRef]
163. Assis, L.; Milares, L.P.; Almeida, T.; Tim, C.; Magri, A.; Fernandes, K.R.; Medalha, C.; Muniz Renno, A.C. Aerobic exercise training and low-level laser therapy modulate inflammatory response and degenerative process in an experimental model of knee osteoarthritis in rats. *Osteoarthr. Cartil.* **2016**, *24*, 169–177. [CrossRef]
164. Al Musawi, M.S.; Jaafar, M.S.; Al-Gailani, B.; Ahmed, N.M.; Suhaimi, F.M.; Suardi, N. Effects of low-level laser irradiation on human blood lymphocytes in vitro. *Lasers Med. Sci.* **2017**, *32*, 405–411. [CrossRef]
165. Baek, S.; Lee, K.P.; Cui, L.; Ryu, Y.; Hong, J.M.; Kim, J.; Jung, S.H.; Bae, Y.M.; Won, K.J.; Kim, B. Low-power laser irradiation inhibits PDGF-BB-induced migration and proliferation via apoptotic cell death in vascular smooth muscle cells. *Lasers Med. Sci.* **2017**, *32*, 2121–2127. [CrossRef] [PubMed]
166. Dos Anjos, L.M.J.; da Fonseca, A.S.; Gameiro, J.; de Paoli, F. Apoptosis induced by low-level laser in polymorphonuclear cells of acute joint inflammation: Comparative analysis of two energy densities. *Lasers Med. Sci.* **2017**, *32*, 975–983. [CrossRef] [PubMed]
167. Assis, L.; Tim, C.; Magri, A.; Fernandes, K.R.; Vassão, P.G.; Renno, A.C.M. Interleukin-10 and collagen type II immunoexpression are modulated by photobiomodulation associated to aerobic and aquatic exercises in an experimental model of osteoarthritis. *Lasers Med. Sci* **2018**, *33*, 1875–1882. [CrossRef] [PubMed]
168. Mergoni, G.; Vescovi, P.; Belletti, S.; Uggeri, J.; Nammour, S.; Gatti, R. Effects of 915 nm laser irradiation on human osteoblasts: A preliminary in vitro study. *Lasers Med. Sci* **2018**, *33*, 1189–1195. [CrossRef] [PubMed]
169. Shakir, E.A.; Rasheed Naji, N.A. In vitro impact of laser irradiation on platelet aggregation. *Lasers Med. Sci.* **2018**, *33*, 1717–1721. [CrossRef]
170. De Souza Costa, M.; Teles, R.H.G.; Dutra, Y.M.; Neto, J.C.R.M.; de Brito, T.V.; Queiroz, F.F.S.N.; do Vale, D.B.N.; de Souza, L.K.M.; Silva, I.S.; Barbosa, A.L.D.R.; et al. Photobiomodulation reduces neutrophil migration and oxidative stress in mice with carrageenan-induced peritonitis. *Lasers Med. Sci.* **2018**, *33*, 1983–1990. [CrossRef]
171. Amaroli, A.; Ravera, S.; Baldini, F.; Benedicenti, S.; Panfoli, I.; Vergani, L. Photobiomodulation with 808-nm diode laser light promotes wound healing of human endothelial cells through increased reactive oxygen species production stimulating mitochondrial oxidative phosphorylation. *Lasers Med. Sci.* **2019**, *34*, 495–504. [CrossRef]
172. Felizatti, A.L.; do Bomfim, F.R.C.; Bovo, J.L.; de Aro, A.A.; do Amaral, M.E.C.; Esquisatto, M.A.M. Effects of low-level laser therapy on the organization of articular cartilage in an experimental microcrystalline arthritis model. *Lasers Med. Sci.* **2019**, *34*, 1401–1412. [CrossRef]
173. Han, B.; Fan, J.; Liu, L.; Tian, J.; Gan, C.; Yang, Z.; Jiao, H.; Zhang, T.; Liu, Z.; Zhang, H. Adipose-derived mesenchymal stem cells treatments for fibroblasts of fibrtic scar via downregulating TGF-β1 and Notch-1 expression enhanced by photobiomodulation therapy. *Lasers Med. Sci.* **2019**, *34*, 1–10. [CrossRef]
174. Tsuka, Y.; Kunimatsu, R.; Gunji, H.; Nakajima, K.; Kimura, A.; Hiraki, T.; Nakatani, A.; Tanimoto, K. Effects of Nd:YAG low-level laser irradiation on cultured human osteoblasts migration and ATP production: In vitro study. *Lasers Med. Sci.* **2019**, *34*, 55–60. [CrossRef]
175. Cardoso, L.M.; Pansani, T.N.; Hebling, J.; de Souza Costa, C.A.; Basso, F.G. Photobiomodulation of inflammatory-cytokine-related effects in a 3-D culture model with gingival fibroblasts. *Lasers Med. Sci.* **2020**, *35*, 1205–1212. [CrossRef] [PubMed]

176. Katagiri, W.; Lee, G.; Tanushi, A.; Tsukada, K.; Choi, H.S.; Kashiwagi, S. High-throughput single-cell live imaging of photobiomodulation with multispectral near-infrared lasers in cultured T cells. *J. Biomed. Opt.* **2020**, *25*, 1–18. [CrossRef] [PubMed]
177. Lemos, A.U.D.; Batista, G.A.; da Silva, P.L.P.; Araújo, D.N.; Sarmento, W.E.A.; Palomari, E.T. Photobiostimulation activity of different low-level laser dosage on masticatory muscles and temporomandibular joint in an induced arthritis rat model. *Lasers Med. Sci.* **2020**, *35*, 1129–1139. [CrossRef] [PubMed]
178. Li, K.; Liang, Z.; Zhang, J.; Zuo, X.; Sun, J.; Zheng, Q.; Song, J.; Ding, T.; Hu, X.; Wang, Z. Attenuation of the inflammatory response and polarization of macrophages by photobiomodulation. *Lasers Med. Sci.* **2020**, *35*, 1509–1518. [CrossRef]
179. Moreira, S.H.; Pazzini, J.M.; Álvarez, J.L.G.; Cassino, P.C.; Bustamante, C.C.; Bernardes, F.J.L.; Kajiura, C.Y.; De Nardi, A.B. Evaluation of angiogenesis, inflammation, and healing on irradiated skin graft with low-level laser therapy in rats (Rattus norvegicus albinus wistar). *Lasers Med. Sci.* **2020**, *35*, 1103–1109. [CrossRef]
180. da Silva, J.G.F.; dos Santos, S.S.; de Almeida, P.; Marcos, R.L.; Lino-Dos-Santos-Franco, A. Effect of systemic photobiomodulation in the course of acute lung injury in rats. *Lasers Med. Sci.* **2020**. [CrossRef] [PubMed]
181. Bjordal, J.M.; Lopes-Martins, R.A.; Iversen, V.V. A randomised, placebo-controlled trial of low-level laser therapy for activated achilles tendinitis with microdialysis measurement of peritendinous prostaglandin E2 concentrations. *Br. J. Sports Med.* **2006**, *40*, 76–80. [CrossRef]
182. Nakamura, T.; Ebihara, S.; Ohkuni, I.; Izukura, H.; Harada, T.; Ushigome, N.; Ohshiro, T.; Musha, Y.; Nakamura, T.; Takahashi, H.; et al. Low Level Laser Therapy for chronic knee joint pain patients. *Laser Ther.* **2014**, *23*, 273–277. [CrossRef]
183. Soleimanpour, H.; Gahramani, K.; Taheri, R.; Golzari, S.E.; Safari, S.; Esfanjani, R.M.; Iranpour, A. The effect of low-level laser therapy on knee osteoarthritis: Prospective, descriptive study. *Lasers Med. Sci.* **2014**, *29*, 1695–1700. [CrossRef]
184. Youssef, E.F.; Muaidi, Q.I.; Shanb, A.A. Effect of Laser Therapy on Chronic Osteoarthritis of the Knee in Older Subjects. *J. Lasers Med. Sci.* **2016**, *7*, 112–119. [CrossRef]
185. Nambi, S.G.; Kamal, W.; George, J.; Manssor, E. Radiological and biochemical effects (CTX-II, MMP-3, 8, and 13) of low-level laser therapy (LLLT) in chronic osteoarthritis in Al-Kharj, Saudi Arabia. *Lasers Med. Sci.* **2017**, *32*, 297–303. [CrossRef]
186. Alayat, M.S.; Ali, M.M. Efficacy of class IV diode laser on pain and dysfunction in patients with knee osteoarthritis: A randomized placebo-control trial. *Bull. Fac. Phys. Ther.* **2017**, *22*, 40–45. [CrossRef]
187. Tomazoni, S.S.; Costa, L.; Joensen, J.; Stausholm, M.B.; Naterstad, I.F.; Leal-Junior, E.; Bjordal, J.M. Effects of photobiomodulation therapy on inflammatory mediators in patients with chronic non-specific low back pain: Protocol for a randomized placebo-controlled trial. *Medicine* **2019**, *98*, e15177. [CrossRef] [PubMed]
188. Tsuk, S.; Lev, Y.H.; Fox, O.; Carasso, R.; Dunsky, A. Does Photobiomodulation Therapy Enhance Maximal Muscle Strength and Muscle Recovery? *J. Hum. Kinet.* **2020**, *73*, 135–144. [CrossRef] [PubMed]
189. Tomazoni, S.S.; Costa, L.O.P.; Joensen, J.; Stausholm, M.B.; Naterstad, I.F.; Ernberg, M.; Leal-Junior, E.C.P.; Bjordal, J.M. Photobiomodulation Therapy is Able to Modulate PGE2 Levels in Patients With Chronic Non-Specific Low Back Pain: A Randomized Placebo-Controlled Trial. *Lasers Surg. Med.* **2020**. [CrossRef]
190. Aimbire, F.; Albertini, R.; Pacheco, M.T.; Castro-Faria-Neto, H.C.; Leonardo, P.S.L.M.; Iversen, V.V.; Lopes-Martins, R.A.B.; Bjordal, J.M. Low-level laser therapy induces dose-dependent reduction of TNFalpha levels in acute inflammation. *Photomed. Laser Surg.* **2006**, *24*, 33–37. [CrossRef]
191. Albertini, R.; Aimbire, F.; Villaverde, A.B.; Silva, J.A., Jr.; Costa, M.S. COX-2 mRNA expression decreases in the subplantar muscle of rat paw subjected to carrageenan-induced inflammation after low level laser therapy. *Inflamm. Res.* **2007**, *56*, 228–229. [CrossRef]
192. Chow, R.T.; Johnson, M.I.; Lopes-Martins, R.A.B.; Bjordal, J.M. Efficacy of low-level laser therapy in the management of neck pain: A systematic review and meta-analysis of randomised placebo or active-treatment controlled trials. *Lancet* **2009**, *374*, 1897–1908. [CrossRef]
193. Leal-Junior, E.; Lopes-Martins, R.; Bjordal, J.M. Clinical and scientific recommendations for the use of photobiomodulation therapy in exercise performance enhancement and post-exercise recovery: Current evidence and future directions. *Braz. J. Physic. Ther.* **2019**, *23*, 71–75. [CrossRef]
194. Stausholm, M.B.; Naterstad, I.F.; Lopes-Martins, R.A.B.; Sæbø, H.; Lund, H.; Fersum, K.V.; Bjordal, J.M. Efficacy of low-level laser therapy on pain and disability in knee osteoarthritis: Systematic review and meta-analysis of randomised placebo-controlled trials. *BMJ Open* **2019**, *9*, e031142. [CrossRef]

195. Weber, M.H.; Fussgänger-May, T.; Wolf, T. The intravenous laser blood irradiation - introduction of a new therapy. *Dt. Ztschr. f Akup.* **2007**, *50*, 12–23. [CrossRef]
196. Dube, A.; Bansal, H.; Gupta, P.K. Modulation of macrophage structure and function by low level He-Ne laser irradiation. *Photochem. Photobiol. Sci.* **2003**, 851–855. [CrossRef] [PubMed]
197. Agaiby, A.D.; Ghali, L.R.; Wilson, R.; Dyson, M. Laser modulation of angiogenic factor production by T-lymphocytes. *Lasers Surg. Med.* **2000**, *26*, 357–363. [CrossRef]
198. Momenzadeh, S.; Abbasi, M.; Ebadifar, A.; Aryani, M.; Bayrami, J.; Nematollahi, F. The intravenous laser blood irradiation in chronic pain and fibromyalgia. *J. Lasers Med. Sci.* **2015**, *6*, 6. [PubMed]
199. Yamaura, M.; Yao, M.; Yaroslavsky, I.; Cohen, R.; Smotrich, M.; Kochevar, I.E. Low-level light effects on inflammatory cytokine production by rheumatoid arthritis synoviocytes. *Lasers Surg. Med.* **2009**, *41*, 282–290. [CrossRef] [PubMed]
200. Funk, J.O.; Kruse, A.; Kirchner, H. Cytokine production after helium neon laser irradiation in cultures of human peripheral blood mononuclear cells. *J. Photochem. Photobiol. B.* **1992**, *16*, 347–355. [CrossRef]
201. Hashmi, J.T.; Huang, Y.Y.; Osmani, B.Z.; Sharma, S.K.; Naeser, M.A.; Hamblin, M.R. Role of low-level laser therapy in neurorehabilitation. *PM & R: J. Injury Func. Rehabil.* **2010**, *2*, S292–S305. [CrossRef]
202. Ailioaie, L.M.; Ailioaie, C.; Chiran, D.A. Laser therapy in neurophatic pain. In Proceedings of the Annual Symposium on Mathematics Applied in Biology & Biophisics, Iaşi, Romania, 28–29 May 2004; Volume XL VII, pp. 303–308.
203. Sobol, E.; Baum, O.; Shekhter, A.; Wachsmann-Hogiu, S.; Shnirelman, A.; Alexandrovskaya, Y.; Sadovskyy, I.; Vinokur, V. Laser-induced micropore formation and modification of cartilage structure in osteoarthritis healing. *J. Biomed. Opt.* **2017**, *22*, 091515. [CrossRef]
204. Ip, D. Does addition of low-level laser therapy (LLLT) in conservative care of knee arthritis successfully postpone the need for joint replacement? *Lasers Med. Sci.* **2015**, *30*, 2335–2339. [CrossRef]
205. Brosseau, L.; Robinson, V.; Wells, G.; Debie, R.; Gam, A.; Harman, K.; Morin, M.; Shea, B.; Tugwell, P. Withdrawn: Low-level laser therapy (Classes III) for treating osteoarthritis. *Cochrane Database Syst. Rev.* **2007**, *1*, CD002046. [CrossRef] [PubMed]
206. Brosseau, L.; Robinson, V.; Wells, G.; Debie, R.; Gam, A.; Harman, K.; Morin, M.; Shea, B.; Tugwell, P. Low-level laser therapy (Classes I, II and III) for treating rheumatoid arthritis. *Cochrane Database Syst. Rev.* **2005**, *19*, CD002049. [CrossRef] [PubMed]

International Journal of
Molecular Sciences

MDPI

Review

The Role of the IL-23/IL-17 Pathway in the Pathogenesis of Spondyloarthritis

Hiroyuki Tsukazaki and Takashi Kaito *

Department of Orthopedic Surgery, Osaka University Graduate School of Medicine, 2-2 Yamadaoka, Suita, Osaka 565-0871, Japan; tsukazaki.hiroyuki@gmail.com

* Correspondence: takashikaito@ort.med.osaka-u.ac.jp; Tel.: +81-(6)-6879-3552

Received: 4 August 2020; Accepted: 2 September 2020; Published: 3 September 2020

Abstract: Spondyloarthritis (SpA) is a subset of seronegative rheumatic-related autoimmune diseases that consist of ankylosing spondylitis (AS), psoriatic spondylitis (PsA), reactive spondylitis (re-SpA), inflammatory bowel disease (IBD)-associated spondylitis, and unclassifiable spondylitis. These subsets share clinical phenotypes such as joint inflammation and extra-articular manifestations (uveitis, IBD, and psoriasis [Ps]). Inflammation at the enthesis, where ligaments and tendons attach to bones, characterizes and distinguishes SpA from other types of arthritis. Over the past several years, genetic, experimental, and clinical studies have accumulated evidence showing that the IL-23/IL-17 axis plays a critical role in the pathogenesis of SpA. These discoveries include genetic association and the identification of IL-23- and IL-17-producing cells in the tissue of mouse models and human patients. In this review, we summarize the current knowledge of the pathomechanism by focusing on the IL-23/IL-17 pathway and examine the recent clinical studies of biological agents targeting IL-23 and IL-17 in the treatment of SpA.

Keywords: Spondyloarthritis; ankylosing arthritis; psoriatic arthritis; interleukin-17; interleukin-23

1. Introduction

In 1974, the concept of a group that was termed seronegative spondarthritides was first introduced [1] and is now known as Spondyloarthritis (SpA). These heterogeneous rheumatoid-related diseases consist of ankylosing spondylitis (AS), psoriatic spondylitis (PsA), reactive spondylitis (re-SpA), inflammatory bowel disease (IBD)-associated spondylitis, and unclassifiable spondylitis. These diseases share various clinical manifestations including sacroiliac arthritis, spinal arthritis, peripheral arthritis, enthesitis, and extra-articular forms (uveitis, inflammatory bowel disease, and psoriasis [Ps]), and the clinical commonality led to the grouping of these diseases. In addition, after the discovery of IL-23 and IL-17-producing Th17, it was revealed that molecular pathomechanisms were also shared among the different types of SpA.

The pro-inflammatory cytokines IL-23 and IL-17 play an important role in activating the immune response in the host defense against pathogens and maintaining barrier functions of mucosal surfaces. Over the past several years, genetic, experimental, and clinical evidence that SpA was triggered by pathological activation of the IL-23/IL-17 axis has accumulated. Inflammation at the sites of tendon insertion into bone is one of the characteristics of SpA, and it distinguishes SpA from other rheumatoid diseases. Recent studies have suggested the involvement of IL-23 and IL-17 in producing cells with enthesitis. In this review, we focus on the current knowledge of the role of the IL-23/IL-17 pathway in the pathogenesis of SpA and summarize the results of recent clinical trials targeting IL-23 and IL-17 in the treatment of SpA.

2. The Concept of SpA

In the 1970s, several diagnostic criteria were proposed to define patients with a specific subtype of SpA, such as the modified New York criteria for AS [2,3]. However, these criteria had inherent limitations since they focused on only spinal symptoms. In 1990, Amor et al. proposed the first set of comprehensive classification criteria for the entire group of SpA conditions, which enables patients to be diagnosed with SpA through peripheral manifestations [4]. Comprehensive criteria similar to those established by Amor et al. were also proposed by the European Spondyloarthropathy Study Group (ESSG) in 1991 [5].

Currently, SpA patients are divided into two subtypes based on their predominant clinical presentation: axial SpA and peripheral SpA. Spinal symptoms are predominant in the former subtype, whereas peripheral arthritis is predominant in the latter subtype, with some overlap between these two groups. In addition, the term axial-SpA includes both patients who have already developed structural damage (radiographic axial SpA, also termed ankylosing spondylitis [AS]) and patients who have experienced only inflammation without bone changes, termed non-radiographic axial SpA, which may be detectable by magnetic resonance imaging (MRI) (Figure 1). To meet the need to establish new criteria for classifying non-radiographic axial SpA, the Assessment of SpondyloArthritis International Society (ASAS) conducted a large cross-sectional study, resulting in the ASAS criteria for axial SpA and peripheral SpA [6,7]. Important advances in the ASAS criteria included the use of MRI capable of detecting sacroiliac inflammation before radiographic changes could be confirmed with plain radiographs.

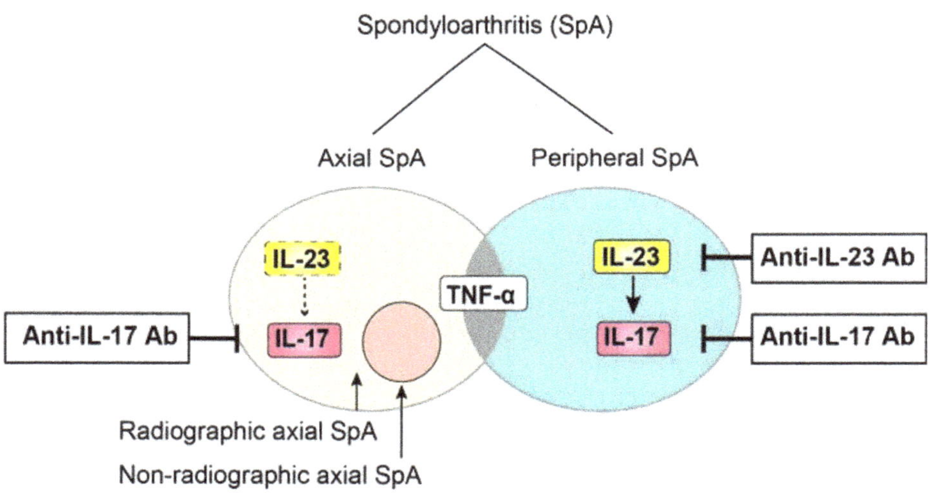

Figure 1. Schematic classification of SpA. SpA patients are mainly classified into two groups (axial SpA and peripheral SpA) based on their predominant clinical manifestation, with some overlap between these two groups. Axial SpA are further divided into two subtypes depending on whether there is radiographical bone destruction.

3. Pathogenesis

3.1. Genetic Background

Human MHC class I, also referred to as HLA, belongs to the cell surface proteins that are present on all nucleated cells and platelets. MHC class I presents small antigen peptides to the T cell receptor (TCR) of cytotoxic T lymphocytes (CTLs), playing a pivotal role in the immune system [8].

HLA-B27, one of the proteins belonging to MHC class I, was first reported to associate with AS in 1973 and is now considered the essential genetic factor in the pathogenesis of SpA [9]. The varying prevalence of HLA-B27-positive populations among ethnicities seems to contribute to the different epidemiology of SpA [10]. The high HLA-B27 positivity (90–95%) in AS patients suggests that HLA-B27 is strongly related to axial SpA. In contrast, the positivity is lower (22–36%) in PsA in which peripheral joints are mainly affected [11,12]. In addition, HLA-B27-positive PsA patients had a higher risk of axial involvement than did HLA-B27 negative PsA patients [13]. However, the fact that only 2–10% of an HLA-B27-positive population develops AS [11] suggests that the disease-developing mechanisms other than HLA-B27 contribute to the pathogenesis of axial SpA.

In the past decade, genome-wide association studies (GWAS) identified *ERAP1* (coding for endoplasmic reticulum aminopeptidase1 [ERAP1]) as a risk factor for AS and PsA [14,15]. ERAP1 is one of the aminopeptidases expressed on the endoplasmic reticulum. ERAP1 takes part in the process of trimming peptides in the endoplasmic reticulum (ER) to 8–10 amino acids to present an antigen by MHC class I molecules, such as HLA-B27 [16]. It is presumed that ER stress caused by HLA-B27 and ERAP1 may trigger the activation of the IL-23/IL-17 pathway [17]. HLA-B27 has a predisposition for misfolding, and the accumulation of the improperly folded HLA-B27 in the ER interferes with ER function, which can lead to ER stress. ERAP1 polymorphisms can also affect the function of antigen presentation by the ER, resulting in ER stress.

Additionally, the SNP of the IL-23 receptor (IL-23R) has been reported to be a risk factor for AS and PsA in GWAS studies [14,18]. In addition, variants of STAT3 and Tyk2, which are downstream targets of IL-23, have also been reported to be associated with AS and PsA [14,19,20].

3.2. Mechanical Stress

Both animal and clinical studies suggest the involvement of mechanical strain in the development of inflammation and bone formation at the enthesis.

Higher involvement of the lower limbs than the upper limbs for enthesitis [21,22] suggests that a higher load in the lower limbs may be related to the development of enthesitis [21,23]. Primarily in the spine of patients with AS, entheseal inflammation and subsequent new bone formation often occur at the anterior longitudinal ligament, which bears a higher load. In support of this concept, tail suspension in the collagen antibody-induced arthritis (CAIA) model mice attenuated Achilles tendon enthesitis and led to a decrease in osteophyte formation [24]. These results suggest the involvement of mechanical stress on the development and/or progression of AS though the exact molecular mechanisms have not been clarified.

3.3. Dysbiosis

The microbiome that is resident in the intestine of mammals plays an important role not only in the regulation of nutrition but also in the adjustment of immune systems. Gut microbiota influences the balance between Th1, Th2, and Th17, which are essential in the host defense [25]. Once some environmental- or host-related factors alter the configuration of the Th cells, abnormal microbiome structure, referred to as dysbiosis, can induce several autoimmune diseases [26,27]. The HLA-B27 transgenic rat, which is a model of SpA, remains healthy in a germ-free environment due to the absence of IL-17-producing Th17 cells [28]. However, they developed SpA when exposed to commensal bacteria, such as segmental filamentous bacteria (SFB) [28,29]. The results suggest that the interactions between HLA-B27 and the microbiome are relevant to the pathogenesis of SpA. Clinical evidence has also been reported. Colonoscopies identified microscopic gut inflammation in 46.2% of the patients with SpA. Histological gut inflammation was correlated with the disease activity [30] and bone marrow edema in sacroiliac joints [31], supporting the involvement of dysbiosis in SpA. Interestingly, the effects on bacterial diversity differ between PsA and AS; the bacterial diversity decreases in PsA [32] and increases in AS [33].

4. IL-23

IL-23, consisting of a heterodimeric protein that contains subunits p19 and p40, was first cloned in 2000 [34]. IL-23 is produced by antigen-presenting cells (APCs) such as dendric cells (DCs), monocytes, and macrophages. Although IL-23 and IL-12 share subunit p40, only IL-12 can induce IFN-γ-producing Th1 cells. The increased production of IL-17 in response to IL-23 by CD4+ T cells was reported [35], and the novel population of IL-17-producing CD4+ T cells (Th17), clearly distinct from Th1 and Th2 cells, was identified in 2005 [36]. This discovery of the IL-23/Th17 pathway led to the clarification of the pathogenesis of autoimmune and autoinflammatory diseases that cannot be adequately explained by the Th1–Th2 concept [37]. Experimental evidence has demonstrated that the pathological activation of IL-23 and IL-17 triggers chronic inflammatory diseases, including SpA [38–41].

IL-23 in SpA Patients

The upregulated presence of IL-23 in SpA patients confirms the involvement of the IL-23/IL-17 pathway. In AS, the elevated serum level of IL-17 and the expression of IL-23 p19 in peripheral blood mononuclear cells were demonstrated [42,43]. Additionally, increased expression of IL-23 in regional skin in patients with Ps and in synovial tissue in patients with PsA has been reported [44,45]. Despite the elevation of IL-23 levels in the synovial fluid in rheumatoid arthritis (RA) and PsA patients, only the disease activity parameters in RA patients correlated with IL-23 expression. These results suggest the existence of a different immunoregulation process for SpA and RA [46].

One question that arises here is where IL-23 originates. Two studies have reported the involvement of the intestine. Ciccia et al. found the upregulation of IL-23 expression, but not IL-17, in the terminal ileum in patients with AS and identified resident Paneth cells as a pivotal source of IL-23 production [47]. Furthermore, they found IL-23-responsive type 3 innate lymphoid cells (ILC3) in the gut and that IL-17+ ILC3 derived from the gut is expanded in the peripheral blood. These studies suggest that the intestine is at least one of the main producers of IL-23 [48].

5. IL-17

IL-17 is a pro-inflammatory cytokine that was first identified in 1993 [49]. The IL-17 cytokine family consists of six members, from IL-17A to IL-17F. IL-17A is the prototypical member, and IL-17A and IL-17F have the highest homology and overlap in many functions. There are five members of the IL-17 receptor family: IL17-RA, IL-17RB, IL-17RC, IL17-RD, and IL-17RE. IL-17 receptors exist as heterodimers, and IL-17RA is a common subunit. The IL-17 RA and IL-17RC heterodimer is the receptor of IL-17A, IL-17F, and the heterodimer of IL-17A and IL-17F. IL-17RA is ubiquitously expressed, whereas IL-17RC is mainly expressed on non-hematopoietic cells [50].

IL-17 plays an important role in acute inflammation by accumulating neutrophils through IL-6 [37]. IL-17R knockout mice displayed a significant delay in neutrophil recruitment and an attenuated host defense against bacterial infection [51,52], supporting the essential role of IL-17 in the inflammatory response. IL-17 targets various cells such as endothelial cells, fibroblasts, and macrophages, leading to the production of inflammatory cytokines [53,54] (Figure 2). The key role of IL-17 in the pathogenesis of chronic inflammatory diseases including SpA as well as in host defense has also been reported [54,55]. In addition to arthritis, IL-17 has been shown to affect bone metabolism by activating the production of matrix metalloproteinases by macrophages and the receptor activator of NF-κB ligand (RANKL) presented by osteoblasts [54,56]. Furthermore, IL-17 has direct effects on osteoclasts and activates osteoclastogenesis [56]. Thus, IL-17 has been demonstrated to be involved with the pathogenesis of SpA.

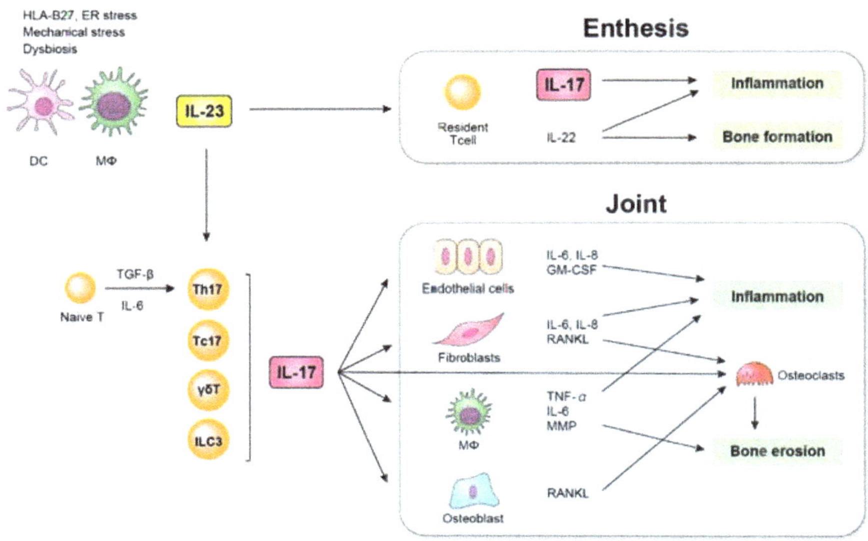

Figure 2. Schematic overview of the role of IL-23 and IL-17 in SpA. Dendric cells (DCs) and macrophages (MΦs) produce IL-23. IL-23 induces the production of IL-17 by various cells and contributes to inflammation by upregulating the production of inflammatory cytokines such as IL-6 and TNF-α, which induces inflammation in the enthesis and joint.

5.1. IL-17 in SpA Patients

Many studies have demonstrated the increased IL-17 production and mRNA expression in the serum, synovium, or tissue in RA patients [57]. These results indicate the importance of IL-17 in the development of arthritis. The increased IL-17 level was also reported in patients with SpA [43,58–64]. The serum levels of IL-17 were significantly higher in SpA patients (AS, re-SpA, and undifferentiated Spondyloarthritis [uSpA]) than in healthy controls [58,59] and were positively correlated to the disease activity measured by the Bath Ankylosing Spondylitis Disease Activity Index (BASDAI) [60,61]. In addition, the strong positive correlation between the serum levels of IL-17 and IL-23 in AS patients suggests the close relationship between these two cytokines [43].

As for the IL-17 levels in the patients' tissues, a higher concentration of IL-17 in synovial fluid was reported in patients with PsA, re-SpA, and uSpA compared to patients with RA [62,63]. Furthermore, mRNA and protein levels of IL-17 receptor A were elevated in the synoviocytes of patients with PsA and RA compared to patients with osteoarthritis (OA) [64].

5.2. IL-17-Producing Cells

5.2.1. Th17 Cells (IL-17+ CD4+ T Cells)

In 2005, a novel population of CD4+ T cells that secretes IL-17, clearly distinguished from Th1 and Th2, was identified [65,66]. IL-17 was initially recognized as a product of Th17 cells, but IL-17 production from other immune cells was also demonstrated [55].

IL-23 was thought to regulate the differentiation from CD4+ naive T cells to Th17 cells. But three independent studies revealed that IL-6 and TGF-β required to induce IL-17 in naïve T cells do not express IL-23 receptors [67–69]. Activation of STAT3 by IL-6 and TGF-β induces the master regulator of Th-17 cells, the transcription factor retinoid-related orphan receptor-γ (RORC), which expresses IL-23 receptor on the surface of Th 17 cells and enables them to secrete IL-17 in response to IL-23 [35]. IL-23 has now been shown to contribute to the lineage maintenance and proliferation of Th17.

The increased presence of Th17 in SpA patients has been reported. The serum levels of Th17 were higher in the peripheral blood in AS and PsA patients than in healthy controls [70,71]. Furthermore, several studies demonstrated the increased existence of Th17 in the inflamed tissue. The increase of Th17 cells in the synovial fluid in patients with PsA and reactive SpA has been reported [63,72,73]. As well as in SpA, the increased number of Th17 cells has also been identified in the skin of Ps patients, suggesting the involvement of local inflammation induced by Th17-derived IL-17 [74]. Immunohistological analysis of the facet joint in AS patients also revealed a higher expression of IL-17+ T cells [75].

In terms of the contribution of Th17 in the disease activity, correlations between the number of Th17 cells and disease activity score (BASDAI score) in AS [61] and the correlation between the number of Th17 cells in synovial fluid and C-reactive protein (CRP) level, erythrocyte sedimentation rate (ESR), and disease activity score (DAS) 28 in PsA were reported [72].

5.2.2. γδT Cells

γδT cells, a subset of T cells that expresses γδTCR, account for a minor portion (3–5%) of all circulating T cells, but they are much more prevalent at mucosal and epithelial sites, where they account for approximately 50% of the intraepithelial lymphocyte population [76]. γδT cells play an important role in the mucosal defense against bacterial infection and antitumor immunity [77,78]. Among them, a subset of IL-17-producing γδT cells also play an especially pathological role in SpA [79]. In Ps patients, dermal γδT cells that produce IL-17 in response to IL-23 were increased in the affected skin, leading to disease progression [80,81]. In addition, the enrichment of circulating IL-17-secreting γδT cells was identified in patients with PsA and AS [82,83]. Cuthbert et al. identified tissue-resident γδT cells in the spinal enthesis, which were divided into two subsets: Vδ1 and Vδ2. While Vδ2 cells expressed IL-23/IL-17 axis-associated transcripts including IL-23R, Vδ1 completely lacked IL-23R expression and produced IL-17 in an IL-23-independent manner [84].

5.2.3. Mucosa-Associated Invariant T (MAIT) Cells

Mucosal-associated invariant T (MAIT) cells are one of the subsets of innate-like cells, abundantly enriched in mucosal tissue, liver, and blood. MAIT cells act at the intersection of the innate and adaptive immune system and play an important role against bacterial infections. MAIT cells express the TCR αchain, and their activation depends on a restriction by a nonpolymorphic MHC-related molecule-1 (MR1) [85]. Through MR1 activation, MAIT cells produce pro-inflammatory cytokines such as IL-17, IL-22, and IFN-γ. Recent evidence has indicated the involvement of MAIT cells in the derivation of IL-17 in the Spondyloarthritis. IL-17-producing CD8+ MAIT cells were identified in psoriatic skin and blood in Ps patients [86] and were also identified in the synovial fluid in patients with PsA [72]. In addition, MAIT cells were found to be involved in AS. Although the frequency of circulating MAIT cells was lower than in healthy controls, the proportion of IL-17+ MAIT cells in the blood of patients with AS was elevated [87–89]. Higher proportions of MAIT cells were found in the synovial fluid than in the circulation. Hayashi et al. also demonstrated the correlation between the expression of CD69 on MAIT cells with the Ankylosing Spondylitis Disease Activity Score (ASDAS) in patients with AS. These results suggest that the upregulation of IL-17 by MAIT cells contributes to the pathogenesis of SpA.

5.2.4. Type 3 Innate Lymphoid Cells (ILC3)

Innate lymphoid cells (ILCs) are immune cells that belong to the family of lymphoid effector cells and that play a pivotal role in immune defense, inflammation, and tissue remodeling [90]. ILCs are divided into three lineages based on their distinct production of cytokines: ILC1 produces IFN-γ; ILC2 is the predominant source of IL-4, IL-5, and IL-9; and ILC3 produces IL-17 and IL-22 in response to IL-23 [91].

Increased levels of IL-17-producing ILC3s, a lineage-negative cell population, have been identified in the peripheral blood of patients with PsA compared with healthy controls, and the levels of ILC3 correlated with the disease activity [92]. In AS patients, Cuthbert et al. identified ILC3s in the human enthesis [93] and Ciccia et al. demonstrated that gut-derived IL-17-producing ILC3s were expanded in the peripheral blood and synovial fluid [48].

5.2.5. Other IL-17-Producing Cells

In 2005, a novel population of CD4+ T cells that secretes IL-17, clearly distinguished from Th1 and Th2, was identified [65,66]. IL-17 is initially recognized as a product of Th17 cells, but IL-17 production from other immune cells was also demonstrated [55].

The presence of IL-17-producing CD8+ T cells (also referred to as Tc17) has been identified in SpA patients. Increased levels of Tc17 were present in the peripheral blood of patients with AS, and the proportion of Tc17 positively correlated with the disease severity [94]. In addition, the increased number of Tc17 was identified in the synovial fluid in patients with PsA or AS [72,95].

Other IL-17-producing cells such as tissue-resident memory T cells, CD3-CD56+NK cells, and mast cells were also demonstrated in the skin, peripheral blood, or synovial fluid of patients with SpA [96–98]. However, further studies are needed to confirm the role of these cells in the pathogenesis of SpA.

6. IL-23/IL-17 Axis-Targeting Therapies

New targeted therapies using cytokine-specific monoclonal antibodies provide some of the most compelling evidence for the important roles of IL-23/IL-17 pathways in the pathogenesis of SpA. Various drugs along with IL-23 and IL-17 are summarized here (Table 1) and illustrated in Figure 3.

Table 1. Agents targeting IL-23/IL-17 pathway.

Name	Target Cytokine	AS	PsA	Other Autoinflammatory Diseases
Ustekinumab	IL-12-p40 and IL-23-p40	Phase 3	Marketed	CD,UC (Marketed)
Guselkumab	IL-23-p19	-	Marketed	CD,UC (Phase 3)
Tildrakizumab	IL-23-p19	Phase 2	Marketed	-
Risankizumab	IL-23-p19	Phase 2	Marketed	CD,UC (Phase 3)
Secukinumab	IL-17A	Marketed	Marketed	-
Ixekizumab	IL-17A	Marketed	Marketed	-
Netakimab	IL-17A	Phase 3	Phase 3	-
Brodalumab	IL-17RA	Phase 3	Phase 3	CD (Phase 2)
Bimekizumab	IL-17A/F	Phase 2	Phase 3	-
ABT-122	IL-17A and TNF-α	-	Phase 2	-

CD; Crohn's disease, UC; Ulcerative colitis.

6.1. Anti IL-23

6.1.1. Ustekinumab

Ustekinumab is a human monoclonal antibody that binds to the p40 subunit that is shared by both IL-12 and IL-23 and inhibits the functions of both IL-12 and IL-23. In three clinical trials in patients with PsA, ustekinumab treatment demonstrated higher improvement of the disease activity [99–101]. Following these results, ustekinumab received FDA approval for the treatment of PsA in 2013. On the other hand, there is no evidence of the efficacy of ustekinumab in the treatment of AS. Three placebo-controlled clinical trials of ustekinumab were conducted for AS. However, after the insufficient effectiveness of the first clinical trial the following two trials were discontinued before full patient enrollment [102].

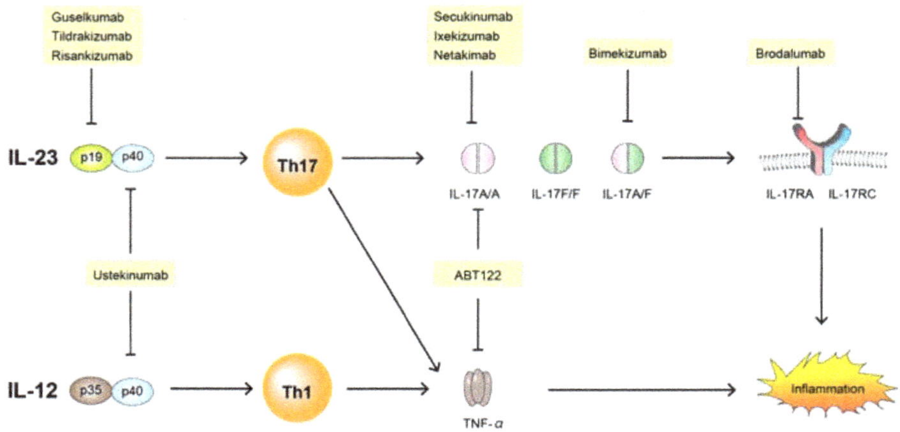

Figure 3. Targeting the IL-23/IL-17 pathway. IL-23, interleukin-23; IL-12, interleukin-12; p19, p19 subunit of interleukin-23; p35, p35 subunit of interleukin-12; p40, p40 subunit of interleukin-12 or of interleukin-23; IL-17A, interleukin-17A; IL-17F, interleukin17F; IL-17RA, interleukin-17 receptor A; IL-17RC, interleukin-17 receptor C; Th1, T helper cell 1; Th17, T helper cell 17; TNF-α, tumor necrosis factor-α.

6.1.2. Guselkumab

Guselkumab targets the p19 subunit that is shared between IL-23 and IL-39 [103]. While ustekinumab targets both IL-12 and IL-23 via binding to the p40 subunit, guselkumab inhibits IL-23 specifically. The results of two phase 3 clinical trials demonstrated the efficacy of guselkumab in the treatment of PsA [104,105]. The DISCOVER-1 trial aimed to assess the effects of guselkumab in patients with various levels of disease activity, while the DISCOVER-2 trial targeted biologic-naïve patients with active PsA. Guselkumab demonstrated greater improvement in the primary endpoint (American College of Rheumatology 20% improvement [ACR20] response at week 24) in both trials. These trials are being extended (DISCOVER-1 for 1 year and DISCOVER-2 for 2 years) to accumulate additional data related to the efficacy and safety of guselkumab [106].

6.1.3. Tildrakizumab

Tildrakizumab is a high-affinity humanized antibody targeting IL-23 p19 and the second selective IL-23 antagonist and has been approved for the treatment of Ps by the FDA [107]. A phase 2b study for PsA reported the significant improvement of joint and skin manifestations. At week 24, patients receiving tildrakizumab achieved superior improvement in ACR20 and on the Psoriasis Area and Severity Index (PASI) 95 [108]. Furthermore, phase 3 trials are underway for PsA (NCT04314531 and NCT04314544) and AS (NCT-0355276). The most common treatment-emergent adverse events reported through week 24 were nasopharyngitis (tildrakizumab: 5.4%, placebo: 6.3%) and diarrhea (tildrakizumab: 1.3%, placebo: 0%).

6.1.4. Risankizumab

Risankizumab is expected to have quick efficacy, based on the results of the phase 1 trial during which rapid and durable clearing of skin lesions was demonstrated in Ps patients [109]. Risankizumab is a humanized IgG1 monoclonal antibody that selectively inhibits the IL-23 p19 subunit. In the head-to-head trial of risankizumab and ustekinumab for Ps patients, risankizumab demonstrated significantly greater improvement in the PASI score at week 12, and this efficacy was maintained up to week 48 [110]. In this study, a 50% reduction of VAS score caused by arthritis was also reported in both the ustekinumab and risankizumab groups.

As for PsA, a phase 2 trial demonstrated the primary end point of ACR20 response at week 16 was superior in the risankizumab-treated patients, and this efficacy was maintained at week 24 [111].

On the other hand, risankizumab demonstrated no significant effectiveness against active AS. A total of 159 patients with untreated active AS were included in the study. A roughly 40% improvement in Assessment in SpondyloArthritis International Society (ASAS40) score at week 12 was attained in 25.5%, 20.5%, and 15.0% of subjects in the 18 mg, 90 mg, and 180 mg risankizumab groups, respectively, compared with 17.5% of subjects in the placebo group [112].

6.2. *Anti IL-17*

6.2.1. Secukinumab

Secukinumab is a fully human monoclonal IgG1 antibody that selectively inhibits IL-17A. After the phase 3 studies demonstrated its significant efficacy in 2015 [113,114], secukinumab received FDA approval for the treatment of AS and PsA in 2016. In other phase 3 trials, secukinumab also showed efficacy in delaying radiographic changes in AS patients whose illness was unable to be controlled by or was contraindicated by TNF-inhibitors [115], and a sustained, long-time efficacy in patients with AS was also reported [116,117]. With an extension of the phase 3 trial (FUTURE 2) [114], the long-term effects of secukinumab in PsA were also demonstrated [118,119]. In addition, a head-to-head comparison study of secukinumab and adalimumab involving a first-line biological monotherapy (EXCEED) trial demonstrated that the ACR 20 response at week 52 was 67% in the secukinumab group and 62% in the adalimumab group (OR, 1.30; 95%CI, 0.98–1.72; $p = 0.0719$). Although the difference was not statistically significant in terms of the ACR20 response, a higher treatment retention rate and better improvement in PASI was reported, which suggests that secukinumab is a useful option for the treatment of AS [120].

6.2.2. Ixekizumab

Ixekizumab is a humanized IgG4 monoclonal antibody that neutralizes IL-17A in contrast to secukinumab, which is an IgG1 monoclonal antibody. This structural difference characterizes the higher affinity of ixekizumab to IL-17 [121]. For the treatment of Ps, ixekizumab showed a superior short-term outcome compared to secukinumab [122,123]. In a phase 3 clinical trial (SPRIT-P1) [124], ACR20 response at week 24 was superior in the ixekizumab group (60.3%) compared to placebo (30.1%), and an extension of the study revealed the long-term persistent efficacy, safety, and inhibition of radiographic progression [125]. As for the treatment of AS, ixekizumab also demonstrated a superior response of ASAS40 at week 16 compared to placebo (ixekizumab: 52%, placebo: 18%) [126]. Ixekizumab received approval by the FDA for the treatment of PsA in 2017, radiographic axial SpA in 2019, and non-radiographic axial SpA in 2020. The comparison between ixekizumab and adalimumab in the treatment of PsA demonstrated that the effects related to joint improvement in ACR20/50/70 response were comparable, but ixekizumab had a greater response for skin manifestations (PASI) [127].

6.2.3. Netakimab

Netakimab (BCD-085) is a novel recombinant IgG1 anti-IL-17 monoclonal antibody with a modified complementarity determining region (CDR) and Fc-fragment, which results in a higher affinity of IL-17 to the Fab fragment of netakimab [128,129].

A phase 3 trial for PsA (NCT03598751: PATERA study) [130,131] is in progress and is expected to generate new evidence in support of the use of netakimab in SpA treatment.

6.2.4. Brodalumab

IL-17 receptor (IL-17R) is a heterodimer of IL17-RA and IL-17RC. Brodalumab is a humanized IgG2 monoclonal antibody that binds to IL-17RA and inhibits IL-17A, IL-17A/F, IL-17F/F, and IL-17E [132]. A phase 2 clinical study on PsA patients demonstrated that ACR20 response rates at week 12 in the

140 mg and 280 mg brodalumab groups were 37% and 39%, respectively, as compared with 18% among the placebo group [133]. A study with brodalumab for AS was discontinued because of suicidality being one of the adverse events that developed during the trial [134] although no causal relationship between suicidality and brodalumab treatment was confirmed [135].

6.2.5. Bimekizumab

Bimekizumab is a humanized IgG1 monoclonal antibody with dual neutralization effects of both IL-17A and IL-17F [136]. A phase 2b dose-ranging trial (BE ACTIVE study) [137] and one for AS (BE AGILE study) [138] demonstrated the short-term efficacy of bimekizumab for PsA. In the BE ACTIVE study, the ACR50 response at week 12 was greater in the 16 mg (27%), 160 mg (41%), and 320 mg bimekizumab (24%) groups than in the placebo group (7%) [137]. In addition, the primary end point (ASAS40 at week 12) was achieved in all of the bimekizumab-treated groups (16 mg: 29.5%, 64 mg: 42.6%, 160 mg: 46.7%, and 320 mg: 45.9%) compared with placebo (13.3%) [138].

6.3. Bispecific TNF/IL-17A Inhibitor

ABT-122

ABT-122 is an IgG1 dual-variable domain immunoglobulin (DVD-Ig) that was engineered to bind to and neutralize human TNF and IL-17A. It is built on an adalimumab backbone by adding IL-17A binding domains [139–141]. Although the dual inhibition of TNF and IL-17A was expected to provide greater effects compared to adalimumab, which targets only TNF, two phase 2 clinical studies have failed to demonstrate the superiority of ABT-122 for the treatment of PsA compared to adalimumab at 12 weeks [141,142].

7. Future Prospective

While the targeting IL-23 and IL-17 have shown good results for the patients with AS and PsA, it was also effective in the treatment of IBD [143,144]. This finding suggests that the IL-23/ IL-17 pathway isn't specific in the development of SpA

There remains an unclear mechanism that is not fully explained by only IL-23 and IL-17 in the pathogenesis of SpA. According to the results of clinical trials, anti-IL-23 antibody showed significant efficacy in the patients with peripheral SpA, but not in the patients with AS. Besides, only IL-23 and IL-17 cannot explain the different sites of manifestations between axial SpA and peripheral SpA, implying the contribution of the mechanisms that are independent of the IL-23/IL-17 pathway. However, different action mechanisms of IL-23/IL-17 pathway between axial SpA and peripheral SpA remains unknown.

The evidence has been insufficient about the efficacy of targeting IL-23 and IL-17 for the patients with other subtypes of SpA, such as re-SpA, IBD-associated spondylitis, and unclassifiable spondylitis.

Further research is required to elucidate underlying mechanism for the difference between axial SpA and peripheral SpA including the mechanism other than IL-23/IL-17 pathway and to evaluate the therapeutic effects of targeting the IL-23/IL-17 in each subtype of SpA.

8. Conclusions

Recent studies have clarified the essential roles of IL-23 and IL-17 in SpA. Although clinical and genetic evidence has demonstrated the involvement of IL-23 and IL-17 in the various tissues from patients with SpA, this IL-23/IL-17 pathway cannot explain the whole range of pathogenic conditions in SpA, which suggests the involvement of unknown pathways or mechanisms for the development of SpA. IL-17 originally acts only during an immune response, yet genetic and environmental conditions such as HLA-B27, mechanical stress, and dysbiosis can cause a pathological up-regulation of IL-23 and/or IL-17 and lead to the development of SpA. Indeed, specific inhibition of IL-23 and/or IL-17 by monoclonal antibodies have shown the effects on the control of the disease activity of SpA.

The IL-17-producing cells such as Th17, Tc17, and γδT cells and ILC3 were newly identified. However, whether the IL-17 from different cellular sources exerts a different immunopathological response remains to be determined. Further understanding of cellular and molecular regulatory mechanisms of the IL-23/IL-17 axis and other inflammatory cytokines may provide a promising strategy in the treatment of SpA.

Author Contributions: H.T. provided overall direction, final editing, and contributed to original writing. T.K. provided overall direction and final editing and supervised this work. All authors have read and agreed to the published version of the manuscript.

Funding: This research received no external funding

Conflicts of Interest: The authors declare no conflict of interest.

Abbreviations

SpA	Spondyloarthritis
AS	Ankylosing spondylitis
PsA	Psoriatic spondylitis
re-SpA	Reactive spondylitis
uSpA	Undifferentiated arthritis
IBD	Inflammatory bowel disease
Ps	Psoriasis
RA	Rheumatoid arthritis
IL-23	Interleukin-23
IL-17	Interleukin-17
IL-17R	Interleukin-17 receptor
Th1	Type 1 helper T cell
Th2	Type 2 helper T cell
Th17	Type 17 helper T cell
TCR	T cell receptor
CTL	Cytotoxic T lymphocyte
HLA	Human leukocyte antigen
MHC	Major histocompatibility complex
ERAP1	Endoplasmic reticulum aminopeptidase 1
ER	Endoplasmic reticulum
SFB	Segmental filamentous bacteria
APC	Antigen presenting cells
DC	Dendric dell
RANKL	Receptor activator of NF-κB ligand
NF-kB	Nuclear factor kappa-light-chain-enhancer of activated B cells
TNF-α	Tumor necrosis factor α
ILC3	Type 3 innate lymphoid cells
MAIT	Mucosa-associated invariant T (MAIT) cells

References

1. Moll, J.M.H.; Haslock, I.; Macrae, I.F.; Wright, V. Associations between ankylosing spondylitis, psoriatic arthritis, Reiter's disease, the intestinal arthropathies, and Behcet's syndrome. *Medicine* **1974**, *53*, 343–364. [CrossRef] [PubMed]
2. Kellgren, J.H. Epidemiology of Chronic Rheumatism. In *Atlas of Standard Radiographs of Arthritis*; Blackwell Science Ltd.: Oxford, UK, 1963.
3. Van Der Linden, S.; Valkenburg, H.A.; Cats, A. Evaluation of Diagnostic Criteria for Ankylosing Spondylitis. *Arthritis Rheum.* **1984**, *27*, 361–368. [CrossRef] [PubMed]
4. Amor, B.; Dougados, M.; Mijiyawa, M. Criteria of the classification of spondylarthropathies. *Rev. Rhum. Mal. Osteoartic.* **1990**, *57*, 85–89. [PubMed]

5. Dougados, M.; Van Der Linden, S.; Juhlin, R.; Huitfeldt, B.; Amor, B.; Calin, A.; Cats, A.; Dijkmans, B.; Olivieri, I.; Pasero, G.; et al. The European Spondylarthropathy Study Group Preliminary Criteria for the Classification of Spondylarthropathy. *Arthritis Rheum.* **1991**, *34*, 1218–1227. [CrossRef]
6. Rudwaleit, M.; Van Der Heijde, D.; Landewé, R.; Listing, J.; Akkoc, N.; Brandt, J.; Braun, J.; Chou, C.T.; Collantes-Estévez, E.; Dougados, M.; et al. The development of Assessment of SpondyloArthritis international Society classification criteria for axial spondyloarthritis (part II): Validation and final selection. *Ann. Rheum. Dis.* **2009**, *68*, 777–783. [CrossRef]
7. Rudwaleit, M.; Van Der Heijde, D.; Landewe, R.; Akkoc, N.; Brandt, J.; Chou, C.T.; Dougados, M.; Huang, F.; Gu, J.; Kirazli, Y.; et al. The Assessment of SpondyloArthritis international Society classification criteria for peripheral spondyloarthritis and for spondyloarthritis in general. *Ann. Rheum. Dis.* **2010**, *70*, 25–31. [CrossRef]
8. Norment, A.M.; Salter, R.D.; Parham, P.; Engelhard, V.H.; Littman, D.R. Cell-cell adhesion mediated by CD8 and MHC class I molecules. *Nature* **1988**, *336*, 79–81. [CrossRef]
9. Schlosstein, L.; Terasaki, P.I.; Bluestone, R.; Pearson, C.M. High Association of an HL-A Antigen, W27, with Ankylosing Spondylitis. *N. Engl. J. Med.* **1973**, *288*, 704–706. [CrossRef]
10. Zhu, W.; He, X.; Cheng, K.; Zhang, L.; Chen, D.; Wang, X.; Qiu, G.; Cao, X.; Weng, X. Ankylosing spondylitis: Etiology, pathogenesis, and treatments. *Bone Res.* **2019**, *7*, 22. [CrossRef]
11. Taurog, J.D.; Chhabra, A.; Colbert, R.A. Ankylosing Spondylitis and Axial Spondyloarthritis. *N. Engl. J. Med.* **2016**, *374*, 2563–2574. [CrossRef]
12. Ruiz, D.G.; De Azevedo, M.N.L.; Lupi, O. HLA-B27 frequency in a group of patients with psoriatic arthritis. *An. Bras. Dermatol.* **2012**, *87*, 847–850. [CrossRef] [PubMed]
13. Baraliakos, X.; Coates, L.C.; Braun, J. The involvement of the spine in psoriatic arthritis. *Clin. Exp. Rheumatol.* **2015**, *33* (Suppl. 93), S31–S35. [PubMed]
14. Burton, P.R.; Clayton, D.G.; Cardon, L.R.; Craddock, N.; Deloukas, P.; Duncanson, A.; Kwiatkowski, D.P.; McCarthy, M.I.; Ouwehand, W.H.; Samani, N.J.; et al. Association scan of 14,500 nonsynonymous SNPs in four diseases identifies autoimmunity variants. *Nat. Genet.* **2007**, *39*, 1329–1337. [PubMed]
15. Strange, A.; Capon, F.; Spencer, C.C.A.; Knight, J.; Weale, M.E.; Allen, M.H.; Barton, A.; Band, G.; Bellenguez, C.; Bergboer, J.G.M.; et al. A genome-wide association study identifies new psoriasis susceptibility loci and an interaction between HLA-C and ERAP1. *Nat. Genet.* **2010**, *42*, 985–990.
16. York, I.A.; Chang, S.-C.; Saric, T.; Keys, J.A.; Favreau, J.M.; Goldberg, A.L.; Rock, K.L. The ER aminopeptidase ERAP1 enhances or limits antigen presentation by trimming epitopes to 8–9 residues. *Nat. Immunol.* **2002**, *3*, 1177–1184. [CrossRef]
17. DeLay, M.L.; Turner, M.J.; Klenk, E.I.; Smith, J.A.; Sowders, D.P.; Colbert, R.A. HLA-B27 misfolding and the unfolded protein response augment interleukin-23 production and are associated with Th17 activation in transgenic rats. *Arthritis Rheum.* **2009**, *60*, 2633–2643. [CrossRef]
18. Cargill, M.; Schrodi, S.J.; Chang, M.; Garcia, V.E.; Brandon, R.; Callis, K.P.; Matsunami, N.; Ardlie, K.G.; Civello, D.; Catanese, J.J.; et al. A Large-Scale Genetic Association Study Confirms IL12B and Leads to the Identification of IL23R as Psoriasis-Risk Genes. *Am. J. Hum. Genet.* **2007**, *80*, 273–290. [CrossRef]
19. Cenit, M.C.; Ortego-Centeno, N.; Raya, E.; Callejas, J.L.; García-Hernández, F.J.; Castillo-Palma, M.J.; Fernández-Sueiro, J.; Magro, C.; Solans, R.; Castañeda, S.; et al. Influence of the STAT3 genetic variants in the susceptibility to psoriatic arthritis and Behcet's disease. *Hum. Immunol.* **2013**, *74*, 230–233. [CrossRef]
20. Ellinghaus, D.; The International IBD Genetics Consortium (IIBDGC); Jostins, L.; Spain, S.L.; Cortes, A.; Bethune, J.; Han, B.; Park, Y.R.; Raychaudhuri, S.; Pouget, J.G.; et al. Analysis of five chronic inflammatory diseases identifies 27 new associations and highlights disease-specific patterns at shared loci. *Nat. Genet.* **2016**, *48*, 510–518. [CrossRef]
21. Jacques, P.; McGonagle, D. The role of mechanical stress in the pathogenesis of spondyloarthritis and how to combat it. *Best Pract. Res. Clin. Rheumatol.* **2014**, *28*, 703–710. [CrossRef]
22. Schett, G.; Lories, R.J.; D'Agostino, M.-A.; Elewaut, D.; Kirkham, B.; Soriano, E.R.; McGonagle, D. Enthesitis: From pathophysiology to treatment. *Nat. Rev. Rheumatol.* **2017**, *13*, 731–741. [CrossRef] [PubMed]
23. Ruff, C.B. Mechanical determinants of bone form: Insights from skeletal remains. *J. Musculoskelet. Neuronal Interact.* **2005**, *5*, 202. [PubMed]

24. Jacques, P.; Lambrecht, S.; Verheugen, E.; Pauwels, E.; Kollias, G.; Armaka, M.; Verhoye, M.; Van Der Linden, A.M.; Achten, R.; Lories, R.J.; et al. Proof of concept: Enthesitis and new bone formation in spondyloarthritis are driven by mechanical strain and stromal cells. *Ann. Rheum. Dis.* **2013**, *73*, 437–445. [CrossRef] [PubMed]
25. Levy, M.; Kolodziejczyk, A.A.; Thaiss, C.A.; Elinav, E. Dysbiosis and the immune system. *Nat. Rev. Immunol.* **2017**, *17*, 219–232. [CrossRef]
26. Manichanh, C.; Borruel, N.; Casellas, F.; Guarner, F. The gut microbiota in IBD. *Nat. Rev. Gastroenterol. Hepatol.* **2012**, *9*, 599–608. [CrossRef]
27. Scher, J.U.; Littman, D.R.; Abramson, S.B. Microbiome in Inflammatory Arthritis and Human Rheumatic Diseases. *Arthritis Rheumatol.* **2016**, *68*, 35–45. [CrossRef]
28. Taurog, J.D.; Richardson, J.A.; Croft, J.T.; Simmons, W.A.; Zhou, M.; Fernández-Sueiro, J.L.; Balish, E.; Hammer, R.E. The germfree state prevents development of gut and joint inflammatory disease in HLA-B27 transgenic rats. *J. Exp. Med.* **1994**, *180*, 2359–2364. [CrossRef]
29. Cua, D.J.; Sherlock, J.P. Autoimmunity's collateral damage: Gut microbiota strikes "back". *Nat. Med.* **2011**, *17*, 1055–1056. [CrossRef]
30. Van Praet, L.; Bosch, F.E.V.D.; Jacques, P.; Carron, P.; Jans, L.; Colman, R.; Glorieus, E.; Peeters, H.; Mielants, H.; De Vos, M.; et al. Microscopic gut inflammation in axial spondyloarthritis: A multiparametric predictive model. *Ann. Rheum. Dis.* **2012**, *72*, 414–417. [CrossRef]
31. Van Praet, L.; Jans, L.; Carron, P.; Jacques, P.; Glorieus, E.; Colman, R.; Cypers, H.; Mielants, H.; De Vos, M.; Cuvelier, C.; et al. Degree of bone marrow oedema in sacroiliac joints of patients with axial spondyloarthritis is linked to gut inflammation and male sex: Results from the GIANT cohort. *Ann. Rheum. Dis.* **2013**, *73*, 1186–1189. [CrossRef]
32. Scher, J.U.; Ubeda, C.; Artacho, A.; Attur, M.; Isaac, S.; Reddy, S.M.; Marmon, S.; Neimann, A.; Brusca, S.B.; Patel, T.; et al. Decreased bacterial diversity characterizes the altered gut microbiota in patients with psoriatic arthritis, resembling dysbiosis in inflammatory bowel disease. *Arthritis Rheumatol.* **2015**, *67*, 128–139. [CrossRef] [PubMed]
33. Costello, M.-E.; Ciccia, F.; Willner, D.; Warrington, N.M.; Robinson, P.C.; Gardiner, B.; Marshall, M.; Kenna, T.J.; Triolo, G.; Brown, M.A. Brief Report: Intestinal Dysbiosis in Ankylosing Spondylitis. *Arthritis Rheumatol.* **2015**, *67*, 686–691. [CrossRef] [PubMed]
34. Oppmann, B.; Lesley, R.; Blom, B.; Timans, J.C.; Xu, Y.; Hunte, B.; Vega, F.; Yu, N.; Wang, J.; Singh, K.; et al. Novel p19 Protein Engages IL-12p40 to Form a Cytokine, IL-23, with Biological Activities Similar as Well as Distinct from IL-12. *Immunology* **2000**, *13*, 715–725. [CrossRef]
35. Aggarwal, S.; Ghilardi, N.; Xie, M.-H.; De Sauvage, F.J.; Gurney, A.L. Interleukin-23 Promotes a Distinct CD4 T Cell Activation State Characterized by the Production of Interleukin-17. *J. Biol. Chem.* **2002**, *278*, 1910–1914. [CrossRef]
36. Langrish, C.L.; Chen, Y.; Blumenschein, W.M.; Mattson, J.; Basham, B.; Sedgwick, J.D.; McClanahan, T.; Kastelein, R.A.; Cua, D.J. IL-23 drives a pathogenic T cell population that induces autoimmune inflammation. *J. Exp. Med.* **2005**, *201*, 233–240. [CrossRef]
37. Lubberts, E. The IL-23–IL-17 axis in inflammatory arthritis. *Nat. Rev. Rheumatol.* **2015**, *11*, 415–429. [CrossRef]
38. Duvallet, E.; Semerano, L.; Assier, E.; Falgarone, G.; Boissier, M.-C. Interleukin-23: A key cytokine in inflammatory diseases. *Ann. Med.* **2011**, *43*, 503–511. [CrossRef]
39. Tang, C.; Chen, S.; Qian, H.; Huang, W. Interleukin-23: As a drug target for autoimmune inflammatory diseases. *Immunology* **2012**, *135*, 112–124. [CrossRef]
40. Teng, M.W.; Bowman, E.P.; McElwee, J.J.; Smyth, M.J.; Casanova, J.-L.; Cooper, A.M.; Cua, D.J. IL-12 and IL-23 cytokines: From discovery to targeted therapies for immune-mediated inflammatory diseases. *Nat. Med.* **2015**, *21*, 719–729. [CrossRef]
41. Abraham, C.; Cho, J. Interleukin-23/Th17 pathways and inflammatory bowel disease. *Inflamm. Bowel Dis.* **2009**, *15*, 1090–1100. [CrossRef]
42. Wang, X.-W.; Lin, Z.; Wei, Q.; Jiang, Y.; Gu, J. Expression of IL-23 and IL-17 and effect of IL-23 on IL-17 production in ankylosing spondylitis. *Rheumatol. Int.* **2009**, *29*, 1343–1347. [CrossRef] [PubMed]
43. Mei, Y.; Pan, F.; Gao, J.; Ge, R.; Duan, Z.; Zeng, Z.; Liao, F.; Xia, G.; Wang, S.; Xu, S.; et al. Increased serum IL-17 and IL-23 in the patient with ankylosing spondylitis. *Clin. Rheumatol.* **2010**, *30*, 269–273. [CrossRef] [PubMed]

44. Lee, E.; Trepicchio, W.L.; Oestreicher, J.L.; Pittman, D.; Wang, F.; Chamian, F.; Dhodapkar, M.; Krueger, J.G. Increased Expression of Interleukin 23 p19 and p40 in Lesional Skin of Patients with Psoriasis Vulgaris. *J. Exp. Med.* **2004**, *199*, 125–130. [CrossRef] [PubMed]
45. Celis, R.; Planell, N.; Fernandez-Sueiro, J.L.; Sanmartí, R.; Ramirez, J.; González-Álvaro, I.; Pablos, J.L.; Cañete, J.D. Synovial cytokine expression in psoriatic arthritis and associations with lymphoid neogenesis and clinical features. *Arthritis Res. Ther.* **2012**, *14*, R93. [CrossRef] [PubMed]
46. Melis, L.; Vandooren, B.; Kruithof, E.; Jacques, P.; De Vos, M.; Mielants, H.; Verbruggen, G.; De Keyser, F.; Elewaut, D. Systemic levels of IL-23 are strongly associated with disease activity in rheumatoid arthritis but not spondyloarthritis. *Ann. Rheum. Dis.* **2010**, *69*, 618–623.
47. Ciccia, F.; Bombardieri, M.; Principato, A.; Giardina, A.; Tripodo, C.; Porcasi, R.; Peralta, S.; Franco, V.; Giardina, E.; Craxi, A.; et al. Overexpression of interleukin-23, but not interleukin-17, as an immunologic signature of subclinical intestinal inflammation in ankylosing spondylitis. *Arthritis Rheum.* **2009**, *60*, 955–965. [CrossRef] [PubMed]
48. Ciccia, F.; Guggino, G.; Rizzo, A.; Saieva, L.; Peralta, S.; Giardina, A.; Cannizzaro, A.; Sireci, G.; De Leo, G.; Alessandro, R.; et al. Type 3 innate lymphoid cells producing IL-17 and IL-22 are expanded in the gut, in the peripheral blood, synovial fluid and bone marrow of patients with ankylosing spondylitis. *Ann. Rheum. Dis.* **2015**, *74*, 1739–1747. [CrossRef]
49. Rouvier, E.; Luciani, M.F.; Mattéi, M.G.; Denizot, F.; Golstein, P. CTLA-8, cloned from an activated T cell, bearing AU-rich messenger RNA instability sequences, and homologous to a herpesvirus saimiri gene. *J. Immunol.* **1993**, *150*, 5445–5456.
50. Gaffen, S.L. Structure and signalling in the IL-17 receptor family. *Nat. Rev. Immunol.* **2009**, *9*, 556–567. [CrossRef]
51. Ye, P.; Rodriguez, F.H.; Kanaly, S.; Stocking, K.L.; Schurr, J.; Schwarzenberger, P.; Oliver, P.; Huang, W.; Zhang, P.; Zhang, J.; et al. Requirement of Interleukin 17 Receptor Signaling for Lung Cxc Chemokine and Granulocyte Colony-Stimulating Factor Expression, Neutrophil Recruitment, and Host Defense. *J. Exp. Med.* **2001**, *194*, 519–528. [CrossRef]
52. Huang, W.; Na, L.; Fidel, P.L.; Schwarzenberger, P. Requirement of Interleukin-17A for Systemic Anti–Candida albicans Host Defense in Mice. *J. Infect. Dis.* **2004**, *190*, 624–631. [CrossRef] [PubMed]
53. Korn, T.; Bettelli, E.; Oukka, M.; Kuchroo, V.K. IL-17 and Th17 Cells. *Annu. Rev. Immunol.* **2009**, *27*, 485–517. [CrossRef] [PubMed]
54. Miossec, P.; Kolls, J.K. Targeting IL-17 and TH17 cells in chronic inflammation. *Nat. Rev. Drug Discov.* **2012**, *11*, 763–776. [CrossRef] [PubMed]
55. Taams, L.S.; Steel, K.J.A.; Srenathan, U.; Burns, L.A.; Kirkham, B.W. IL-17 in the immunopathogenesis of spondyloarthritis. *Nat. Rev. Rheumatol.* **2018**, *14*, 453–466. [CrossRef]
56. Gravallese, E.M.; Schett, G. Effects of the IL-23–IL-17 pathway on bone in spondyloarthritis. *Nat. Rev. Rheumatol.* **2018**, *14*, 631–640. [CrossRef] [PubMed]
57. Gaffen, S.L. The role of interleukin-17 in the pathogenesis of rheumatoid arthritis. *Curr. Rheumatol. Rep.* **2009**, *11*, 365–370. [CrossRef]
58. Romero-Sanchez, C.; Jaimes, D.A.; Londoño, J.; De Avila, J.; Castellanos, J.E.; Bello, J.M.; Bautista, W.; Valle-Oñate, R. Association between Th-17 cytokine profile and clinical features in patients with spondyloarthritis. *Clin. Exp. Rheumatol.* **2011**, *29*, 828–834.
59. Wendling, D.; Cedoz, J.-P.; Racadot, E.; Dumoulin, G. Serum IL-17, BMP-7, and bone turnover markers in patients with ankylosing spondylitis. *Jt. Bone Spine* **2007**, *74*, 304–305. [CrossRef]
60. Chen, W.-S.; Chang, Y.-S.; Lin, K.-C.; Lai, C.-C.; Wang, S.-H.; Hsiao, K.-H.; Lee, H.-T.; Chen, M.-H.; Tsai, C.-Y.; Chou, C.-T. Association of serum interleukin-17 and interleukin-23 levels with disease activity in Chinese patients with ankylosing spondylitis. *J. Chin. Med Assoc.* **2012**, *75*, 303–308. [CrossRef]
61. Xueyi, L.; Lina, C.; Zhenbiao, W.; Qing, H.; Qiang, L.; Zhu, P. Levels of Circulating Th17 Cells and Regulatory T Cells in Ankylosing Spondylitis Patients with an Inadequate Response to Anti−TNF-α Therapy. *J. Clin. Immunol.* **2012**, *33*, 151–161. [CrossRef]
62. Singh, R.; Aggarwal, A.; Misra, R. Th1/Th17 cytokine profiles in patients with reactive arthritis/undifferentiated spondyloarthropathy. *J. Rheumatol.* **2007**, *34*, 2285–2290. [PubMed]
63. Leipe, J.; Grunke, M.; DeChant, C.; Reindl, C.; Kerzendorf, U.; Skapenko, A.; Schulze-Koops, H. Role of Th17 cells in human autoimmune arthritis. *Arthritis Rheum.* **2010**, *62*, 2876–2885. [CrossRef] [PubMed]

64. Raychaudhuri, S.P.; Raychaudhuri, S.K.; Genovese, M.C. IL-17 receptor and its functional significance in psoriatic arthritis. *Mol. Cell. Biochem.* **2011**, *359*, 419–429. [CrossRef] [PubMed]
65. Park, H.; Li, Z.; Yang, X.O.; Chang, S.H.; Nurieva, R.; Wang, Y.-H.; Wang, Y.; Hood, L.; Zhu, Z.; Tian, Q.; et al. A distinct lineage of CD4 T cells regulates tissue inflammation by producing interleukin 17. *Nat. Immunol.* **2005**, *6*, 1133–1141. [CrossRef] [PubMed]
66. Harrington, L.E.; Hatton, R.D.; Mangan, P.R.; Turner, H.; Murphy, T.L.; Murphy, K.M.; Weaver, C.T. Interleukin 17–producing CD4+ effector T cells develop via a lineage distinct from the T helper type 1 and 2 lineages. *Nat. Immunol.* **2005**, *6*, 1123–1132. [CrossRef]
67. Bettelli, E.; Carrier, Y.; Gao, W.; Korn, T.; Strom, T.B.; Oukka, M.; Weiner, H.L.; Kuchroo, V.K. Reciprocal developmental pathways for the generation of pathogenic effector TH17 and regulatory T cells. *Nature* **2006**, *441*, 235–238. [CrossRef]
68. Mangan, P.R.; Harrington, L.E.; O'Quinn, D.B.; Helms, W.S.; Bullard, D.C.; Elson, C.O.; Hatton, R.D.; Wahl, S.M.; Schoeb, T.R.; Weaver, C.T. Transforming growth factor-β induces development of the TH17 lineage. *Nature* **2006**, *441*, 231–234. [CrossRef]
69. Veldhoen, M.; Hocking, R.J.; Atkins, C.J.; Locksley, R.M.; Stockinger, B. TGFbeta in the context of an inflammatory cytokine milieu supports de novo differentiation of IL-17-producing T cells. *Immunity* **2006**, *24*, 179–189. [CrossRef]
70. Jandus, C.; Bioley, G.; Rivals, J.-P.; Dudler, J.; Speiser, D.E.; Romero, P. Increased numbers of circulating polyfunctional Th17 memory cells in patients with seronegative spondylarthritides. *Arthritis Rheum.* **2008**, *58*, 2307–2317. [CrossRef]
71. Shen, H.; Goodall, J.C.; Gaston, H. Frequency and phenotype of peripheral blood Th17 cells in ankylosing spondylitis and rheumatoid arthritis. *Arthritis Rheum.* **2009**, *60*, 1647–1656. [CrossRef]
72. Menon, B.; Gullick, N.J.; Walter, G.J.; Rajasekhar, M.; Garrood, T.; Evans, H.G.; Taams, L.S.; Kirkham, B.W. Interleukin-17+CD8+ T Cells Are Enriched in the Joints of Patients With Psoriatic Arthritis and Correlate With Disease Activity and Joint Damage Progression. *Arthritis Rheumatol.* **2014**, *66*, 1272–1281. [CrossRef] [PubMed]
73. Shen, H.; Goodall, J.C.; Gaston, J.H. Frequency and Phenotype of T Helper 17 Cells in Peripheral Blood and Synovial Fluid of Patients with Reactive Arthritis. *J. Rheumatol.* **2010**, *37*, 2096–2099. [CrossRef] [PubMed]
74. Benham, H.; Norris, P.; Goodall, J.C.; Wechalekar, M.D.; Fitzgerald, O.; Szenpetery, A.; Smith, M.; Thomas, R.; Gaston, H. Th17 and Th22 cells in psoriatic arthritis and psoriasis. *Arthritis Res. Ther.* **2013**, *15*, R136. [CrossRef] [PubMed]
75. Appel, H.; Heydrich, R.; Wu, P.; Scheer, R.; Hempfing, A.; Kayser, R.; Thiel, A.; Radbruch, A.; Loddenkemper, C.; Sieper, J. Analysis of IL-17+ cells in facet joints of patients with spondyloarthritis suggests that the innate immune pathway might be of greater relevance than the Th17-mediated adaptive immune response. *Arthritis Res. Ther.* **2011**, *13*, R95. [CrossRef] [PubMed]
76. Sutton, C.E.; Mielke, L.A.; Mills, K.H.G. IL-17-producing γδ T cells and innate lymphoid cells. *Eur. J. Immunol.* **2012**, *42*, 2221–2231. [CrossRef]
77. Hamada, S.; Umemura, M.; Shiono, T.; Tanaka, K.; Yahagi, A.; Begum, M.D.; Oshiro, K.; Okamoto, Y.; Watanabe, H.; Kawakami, K.; et al. IL-17A Produced by γδ T Cells Plays a Critical Role in Innate Immunity against *Listeria monocytogenes* Infection in the Liver. *J. Immunol.* **2008**, *181*, 3456–3463. [CrossRef]
78. Nielsen, M.M.; Witherden, D.A.; Havran, W.L. γδ T cells in homeostasis and host defence of epithelial barrier tissues. *Nat. Rev. Immunol.* **2017**, *17*, 733–745. [CrossRef]
79. Roark, C.L.; Simonian, P.L.; Fontenot, A.P.; Born, W.K.; O'Brien, R.L. γδ T cells: An important source of IL-17. *Curr. Opin. Immunol.* **2008**, *20*, 353–357. [CrossRef]
80. Sutton, C.E.; Lalor, S.J.; Sweeney, C.M.; Brereton, C.F.; Lavelle, E.C.; Mills, K.H.G. Interleukin-1 and IL-23 Induce Innate IL-17 Production from γδ T Cells, Amplifying Th17 Responses and Autoimmunity. *Immunity* **2009**, *31*, 331–341. [CrossRef]
81. Cai, Y.; Shen, X.; Ding, C.; Qi, C.; Li, K.; Li, X.; Jala, V.R.; Zhang, H.G.; Wang, T.; Zheng, J.; et al. Pivotal role of dermal IL-17-producing γδ T cells in skin inflammation. *Immunity* **2011**, *35*, 596–610. [CrossRef]
82. Kenna, T.J.; Davidson, S.I.; Duan, R.; Bradbury, L.A.; McFarlane, J.; Smith, M.; Weedon, H.; Street, S.; Thomas, R.; Thomas, G.P.; et al. Enrichment of circulating interleukin-17-secreting interleukin-23 receptor-positive gamma/delta T cells in patients with active ankylosing spondylitis. *Arthritis Rheum.* **2012**, *64*, 1420–1429. [CrossRef]

83. Guggino, G.; Ciccia, F.; Di Liberto, D.; Lo Pizzo, M.; Ruscitti, P.; Cipriani, P.; Ferrante, A.; Sireci, G.; Dieli, F.; Fourniè, J.J. Interleukin (IL)-9/IL-9R axis drives γδ T cells activation in psoriatic arthritis patients. *Clin. Exp. Immunol.* **2016**, *186*, 277–283. [CrossRef] [PubMed]
84. Cuthbert, R.J.; Watad, A.; Fragkakis, E.M.; Dunsmuir, R.; Loughenbury, P.; Khan, A.; Millner, P.A.; Davison, A.; Marzo-Ortega, H.; Newton, D.; et al. Evidence that tissue resident human enthesis γδT-cells can produce IL-17A independently of IL-23R transcript expression. *Ann. Rheum. Dis.* **2019**, *78*, 1559–1565. [CrossRef] [PubMed]
85. Martin, E.; Treiner, E.; Duban, L.; Guerri, L.; Laude, H.; Toly, C.; Prémel, V.; Devys, A.; Moura, I.C.; Tilloy, F.; et al. Stepwise development of MAIT cells in mouse and human. *PLoS Biol.* **2009**, *7*, e54. [CrossRef]
86. Teunissen, M.B.M.; Yeremenko, N.; Baeten, D.L.P.; Chielie, S.; Spuls, P.I.; De Rie, M.A.; Lantz, O.; Res, P.C. The IL-17A-Producing CD8 + T-Cell Population in Psoriatic Lesional Skin Comprises Mucosa-Associated Invariant T Cells and Conventional T Cells. *J. Investig. Dermatol.* **2014**, *134*, 2898–2907. [CrossRef] [PubMed]
87. Gracey, E.; Qaiyum, Z.; Almaghlouth, I.; Lawson, D.O.; Karki, S.; Avvaru, N.; Zhang, Z.; Yao, Y.; Ranganathan, V.; Baglaenko, Y.; et al. IL-7 primes IL-17 in mucosal-associated invariant T (MAIT) cells, which contribute to the Th17-axis in ankylosing spondylitis. *Ann. Rheum. Dis.* **2016**, *75*, 2124–2132. [CrossRef] [PubMed]
88. Hayashi, E.; Chiba, A.; Tada, K.; Haga, K.; Kitagaichi, M.; Nakajima, S.; Kusaoi, M.; Sekiya, F.; Ogasawara, M.; Yamaji, K.; et al. Involvement of Mucosal-associated Invariant T cells in Ankylosing Spondylitis. *J. Rheumatol.* **2016**, *43*, 1695–1703. [CrossRef]
89. Toussirot, É.; Laheurte, C.; Gaugler, B.; Gabriel, D.; Saas, P. Increased IL-22- and IL-17A-Producing Mucosal-Associated Invariant T Cells in the Peripheral Blood of Patients With Ankylosing Spondylitis. *Front. Immunol.* **2018**, *9*. [CrossRef]
90. Spits, H.; Artis, D.; Colonna, M.; Diefenbach, A.; Di Santo, J.P.; Eberl, G.; Koyasu, S.; Locksley, R.M.; McKenzie, A.N.J.; Mebius, R.E.; et al. Innate lymphoid cells—A proposal for uniform nomenclature. *Nat. Rev. Immunol.* **2013**, *13*, 145–149. [CrossRef]
91. Serafini, N.; Vosshenrich, C.A.J.; Di Santo, J.P. Transcriptional regulation of innate lymphoid cell fate. *Nat. Rev. Immunol.* **2015**, *15*, 415–428. [CrossRef]
92. Soare, A.; Weber, S.; Maul, L.; Rauber, S.; Gheorghiu, A.M.; Luber, M.; Houssni, I.; Kleyer, A.; Von Pickardt, G.; Gado, M.; et al. Cutting Edge: Homeostasis of Innate Lymphoid Cells Is Imbalanced in Psoriatic Arthritis. *J. Immunol.* **2018**, *200*, 1249–1254. [CrossRef] [PubMed]
93. Cuthbert, R.J.R.J.; Fragkakis, E.M.; Dunsmuir, R.; Li, Z.; Coles, M.; Marzo-Ortega, H.; Giannoudis, P.V.; Jones, E.; El-Sherbiny, Y.; McGonagle, D. Brief Report: Group 3 Innate Lymphoid Cells in Human Enthesis. *Arthritis Rheumatol.* **2017**, *69*, 1816–1822. [CrossRef] [PubMed]
94. Wang, C.; Liao, Q.; Hu, Y.; Zhong, D. T lymphocyte subset imbalances in patients contribute to ankylosing spondylitis. *Exp. Ther. Med.* **2014**, *9*, 250–256. [CrossRef] [PubMed]
95. Al-Mossawi, M.H.; Chen, L.; Fang, H.; Ridley, A.; De Wit, J.; Yager, N.; Hammitzsch, A.; Pulyakhina, I.; Fairfax, B.P.; Simone, D.; et al. Unique transcriptome signatures and GM-CSF expression in lymphocytes from patients with spondyloarthritis. *Nat. Commun.* **2017**, *8*, 1510. [CrossRef]
96. Chowdhury, A.C.; Chaurasia, S.; Mishra, S.K.; Aggarwal, A.; Misra, R. IL-17 and IFN-γ producing NK and γδ-T cells are preferentially expanded in synovial fluid of patients with reactive arthritis and undifferentiated spondyloarthritis. *Clin. Immunol.* **2017**, *183*, 207–212. [CrossRef]
97. Noordenbos, T.; Yeremenko, N.; Gofita, I.; Van De Sande, M.; Tak, P.P.; Cañete, J.D.; Baeten, D. Interleukin-17-positive mast cells contribute to synovial inflammation in spondylarthritis. *Arthritis Rheum.* **2011**, *64*, 99–109. [CrossRef]
98. Steel, K.; Wu, S.-Y.; Srenathan, U.; Chan, E.; Kirkham, B.; Taams, L. O016 Synovial IL-17+ CD8+ T cells are a pro-inflammatory tissue resident population enriched in spondyloarthritis. *Ann. Rheum. Dis.* **2018**, *77* (Suppl. 1), A8–A9.
99. Gottlieb, A.B.; Menter, A.; Mendelsohn, A.; Shen, Y.-K.; Li, S.; Guzzo, C.; Fretzin, S.; Kunynetz, R.; Kavanaugh, A. Ustekinumab, a human interleukin 12/23 monoclonal antibody, for psoriatic arthritis: Randomised, double-blind, placebo-controlled, crossover trial. *Lancet* **2009**, *373*, 633–640. [CrossRef]

100. McInnes, I.B.; Kavanaugh, A.; Gottlieb, A.B.; Puig, L.; Rahman, P.; Ritchlin, C.; Brodmerkel, C.; Li, S.; Wang, Y.; Mendelsohn, A.M.; et al. Efficacy and safety of ustekinumab in patients with active psoriatic arthritis: 1 year results of the phase 3, multicentre, double-blind, placebo-controlled PSUMMIT 1 trial. *Lancet* **2013**, *382*, 780–789. [CrossRef]
101. Helliwell, P.S.; Gladman, D.D.; Chakravarty, S.D.; Kafka, S.; Karyekar, C.S.; You, Y.; Campbell, K.; Sweet, K.; Kavanaugh, A.; Gensler, L.S. Effects of ustekinumab on spondylitis-associated endpoints in TNFi-naïve active psoriatic arthritis patients with physician-reported spondylitis: Pooled results from two phase 3, randomised, controlled trials. *RMD Open* **2020**, *6*, e001149. [CrossRef]
102. Deodhar, A.; Gensler, L.S.; Sieper, J.; Clark, M.; Calderon, C.; Wang, Y.; Zhou, Y.; Leu, J.H.; Campbell, K.; Sweet, K.; et al. Three Multicenter, Randomized, Double-Blind, Placebo-Controlled Studies Evaluating the Efficacy and Safety of Ustekinumab in Axial Spondyloarthritis. *Arthritis Rheumatol.* **2019**, *71*, 258–270. [CrossRef] [PubMed]
103. Gaffen, S.L.; Jain, R.; Garg, A.V.; Cua, D.J. The IL-23–IL-17 immune axis: From mechanisms to therapeutic testing. *Nat. Rev. Immunol.* **2014**, *14*, 585–600. [CrossRef] [PubMed]
104. Deodhar, A.; Helliwell, P.S.; Boehncke, W.-H.; Kollmeier, A.P.; Hsia, E.C.; Subramanian, R.A.; Xu, X.L.; Sheng, S.; Agarwal, P.; Zhou, B.; et al. Guselkumab in patients with active psoriatic arthritis who were biologic-naive or had previously received TNFα inhibitor treatment (DISCOVER-1): A double-blind, randomised, placebo-controlled phase 3 trial. *Lancet* **2020**, *395*, 1115–1125. [CrossRef]
105. Mease, P.J.; Rahman, P.; Gottlieb, A.B.; Kollmeier, A.P.; Hsia, E.C.; Xu, X.L.; Sheng, S.; Agarwal, P.; Zhou, B.; Zhuang, Y.; et al. Guselkumab in biologic-naive patients with active psoriatic arthritis (DISCOVER-2): A double-blind, randomised, placebo-controlled phase 3 trial. *Lancet* **2020**, *395*, 1126–1136. [CrossRef]
106. McHugh, J. IL-23 inhibitor guselkumab shows promise for PsA. *Nat. Rev. Rheumatol.* **2020**, *16*, 247. [CrossRef]
107. Banaszczyk, K. Tildrakizumab in the treatment of psoriasis—literature review. *Reumatologia* **2019**, *57*, 234–238. [CrossRef]
108. Mease, P.J.; Chohan, S.; Fructuoso, F.J.G.; Chou, R.C.; Nograles, K.E.; Mendelsohn, A.M.; Luggen, M.E. Lb0002 Randomised, Double-blind, Placebo-controlled, Multiple-dose, Phase 2b Study to Demonstrate the Safety and Efficacy Of Tildrakizumab, a High-affinity Anti-interleukin-23p19 Monoclonal Antibody, un Patients with Active Psoriatic Arthritis. *Ann. Rheum. Dis.* **2019**, *78* (Suppl. 2), 78–79.
109. Krueger, J.G.; Ferris, L.K.; Menter, A.; Wagner, F.; White, A.; Visvanathan, S.; Lalovic, B.; Aslanyan, S.; Wang, E.E.; Hall, D.; et al. Anti–IL-23A mAb BI 655066 for treatment of moderate-to-severe psoriasis: Safety, efficacy, pharmacokinetics, and biomarker results of a single-rising-dose, randomized, double-blind, placebo-controlled trial. *J. Allergy Clin. Immunol.* **2015**, *136*, 116–124. [CrossRef]
110. Papp, K.A.; Blauvelt, A.; Bukhalo, M.; Gooderham, M.; Krueger, J.G.; Lacour, J.; Menter, A.; Philipp, S.; Sofen, H.; Tyring, S.; et al. Risankizumab versus Ustekinumab for Moderate-to-Severe Plaque Psoriasis. *N. Engl. J. Med.* **2017**, *376*, 1551–1560. [CrossRef]
111. Mease, P.J.; Kellner, H.; Morita, A.; Kivitz, A.; Papp, K.; Aslanyan, S.; Berner, B.; Chen, S.; Eldred, A.; Behrens, F. OP0307 Efficacy and safety of risankizumab, a selective il-23p19 inhibitor, in patients with active psoriatic arthritis over 24 weeks: Results from a phase 2 trial. *Ann. Rheum. Dis.* **2018**, *77* (Suppl. 2), 200–201.
112. Baeten, D.; Østergaard, M.; Wei, J.C.-C.; Sieper, J.; Järvinen, P.; Tam, L.-S.; Salvarani, C.; Kim, T.-H.; Solinger, A.; Datsenko, Y.; et al. Risankizumab, an IL-23 inhibitor, for ankylosing spondylitis: Results of a randomised double-blind, placebo-controlled, proof-of-concept, dose-finding phase 2 study. *Ann. Rheum. Dis.* **2018**, *77*, 1295–1302. [CrossRef] [PubMed]
113. Mease, P.J.; McInnes, I.B.; Kirkham, B.; Kavanaugh, A.; Rahman, P.; Van Der Heijde, D.; Landewé, R.; Nash, P.; Pricop, L.; Yuan, J.; et al. Secukinumab Inhibition of Interleukin-17A in Patients with Psoriatic Arthritis. *N. Engl. J. Med.* **2015**, *373*, 1329–1339. [CrossRef] [PubMed]
114. McInnes, I.B.; Mease, P.J.; Kirkham, B.; Kavanaugh, A.; Ritchlin, C.T.; Rahman, P.; Van Der Heijde, D.; Landewé, R.; Conaghan, P.G.; Gottlieb, A.B.; et al. Secukinumab, a human anti-interleukin-17A monoclonal antibody, in patients with psoriatic arthritis (FUTURE 2): A randomised, double-blind, placebo-controlled, phase 3 trial. *Lancet* **2015**, *386*, 1137–1146. [CrossRef]
115. Braun, J.; Baraliakos, X.; Deodhar, A.; Baeten, M.; Sieper, J.; Emery, P.; Readie, A.; Martin, R.; Mpofu, S.; Richards, H.B. Effect of secukinumab on clinical and radiographic outcomes in ankylosing spondylitis: 2-year results from the randomised phase III MEASURE 1 study. *Ann. Rheum. Dis.* **2016**, *76*, 1070–1077. [CrossRef]

116. Pavelka, K.; Kivitz, A.; Dokoupilova, E.; Blanco, R.; Maradiaga, M.; Tahir, H.; Pricop, L.; Andersson, M.; Readie, A.; Porter, B. Efficacy, safety, and tolerability of secukinumab in patients with active ankylosing spondylitis: A randomized, double-blind phase 3 study, MEASURE 3. *Arthritis Res. Ther.* **2017**, *19*, 285. [CrossRef]
117. Baraliakos, X.; Kivitz, A.J.; Deodhar, A.A.; Braun, J.; Wei, J.C.; Delicha, E.M.; Tolloczy, Z.; Porter, B. Long-term effects of interleukin-17A inhibition with secukinumab in active ankylosing spondylitis: 3-year efficacy and safety results from an extension of the Phase 3 MEASURE 1 trial. *Clin. Exp. Rheumatol.* **2018**, *36*, 50–55.
118. Coates, L.C.; Gladman, D.D.; Nash, P.; Fitzgerald, O.; Kavanaugh, A.; Kvien, T.K.; Gossec, L.; Strand, V.; Rasouliyan, L.; Pricop, L.; et al. Secukinumab provides sustained PASDAS-defined remission in psoriatic arthritis and improves health-related quality of life in patients achieving remission: 2-year results from the phase III FUTURE 2 study. *Arthritis Res.* **2018**, *20*, 272. [CrossRef]
119. McInnes, I.B.; Mease, P.J.; Kivitz, A.J.; Nash, P.; Rahman, P.; Rech, J.; Conaghan, P.G.; Kirkham, B.; Navarra, S.; Belsare, A.D.; et al. Long-term efficacy and safety of secukinumab in patients with psoriatic arthritis: 5-year (end-of-study) results from the phase 3 FUTURE 2 study. *Lancet Rheumatol.* **2020**, *2*, e227–e235. [CrossRef]
120. McInnes, I.B.; Behrens, F.; Mease, P.J.; Kavanaugh, A.; Ritchlin, C.; Nash, P.; Masmitja, J.G.; Goupille, P.; Korotaeva, T.; Gottlieb, A.B.; et al. Secukinumab versus adalimumab for treatment of active psoriatic arthritis (EXCEED): A double-blind, parallel-group, randomised, active-controlled, phase 3b trial. *Lancet* **2020**, *395*, 1496–1505. [CrossRef]
121. Liu, L.; Lu, J.; Allan, B.W.; Tang, Y.; Tetreault, J.; Chow, C.-K.; Barmettler, B.; Nelson, J.; Bina, H.; Huang, L.; et al. Generation and characterization of ixekizumab, a humanized monoclonal antibody that neutralizes interleukin-17A. *J. Inflamm. Res.* **2016**, *9*, 39–50. [CrossRef]
122. Paul, C. Ixekizumab or secukinumab in psoriasis: What difference does it make? *Br. J. Dermatol.* **2018**, *178*, 1003–1005. [CrossRef] [PubMed]
123. Warren, R.; Brnabic, A.; Saure, D.; Langley, R.G.; See, K.; Wu, J.J.; Schacht, A.; Mallbris, L.; Nast, A. Matching-adjusted indirect comparison of efficacy in patients with moderate-to-severe plaque psoriasis treated with ixekizumab vs. *secukinumab. Br. J. Dermatol.* **2018**, *178*, 1064–1071. [CrossRef]
124. Mease, P.J.; Van Der Heijde, D.; Ritchlin, C.T.; Okada, M.; Cuchacovich, R.S.; Shuler, C.L.; Lin, C.-Y.; Braun, D.K.; Lee, C.H.; Gladman, D.D.; et al. Ixekizumab, an interleukin-17A specific monoclonal antibody, for the treatment of biologic-naive patients with active psoriatic arthritis: Results from the 24-week randomised, double-blind, placebo-controlled and active (adalimumab)-controlled period of the phase III trial SPIRIT-P1. *Ann. Rheum. Dis.* **2016**, *76*, 79–87. [PubMed]
125. Chandran, V.; Van Der Heijde, D.; Fleischmann, R.M.; Lespessailles, E.; Helliwell, P.S.; Kameda, H.; Burgos-Vargas, R.; Erickson, J.S.; Rathmann, S.S.; Sprabery, A.T.; et al. Ixekizumab treatment of biologic-naïve patients with active psoriatic arthritis: 3-year results from a phase III clinical trial (SPIRIT-P1). *Rheumatology* **2020**. [CrossRef] [PubMed]
126. Van Der Heijde, D.; Wei, J.C.-C.; Dougados, M.; Mease, P.J.; Deodhar, A.; Maksymowych, W.P.; Bosch, F.V.D.; Sieper, J.; Tomita, T.; Landewé, R.; et al. Ixekizumab, an interleukin-17A antagonist in the treatment of ankylosing spondylitis or radiographic axial spondyloarthritis in patients previously untreated with biological disease-modifying anti-rheumatic drugs (COAST-V): 16 week results of a phase 3 randomised, double-blind, active-controlled and placebo-controlled trial. *Lancet* **2018**, *392*, 2441–2451. [PubMed]
127. Mease, P.J.; Smolen, J.S.; Behrens, F.; Nash, P.; Leage, S.L.; Li, L.; Tahir, H.; Gooderham, M.; Krishnan, E.; Liu-Seifert, H.; et al. A head-to-head comparison of the efficacy and safety of ixekizumab and adalimumab in biological-naïve patients with active psoriatic arthritis: 24-week results of a randomised, open-label, blinded-assessor trial. *Ann. Rheum. Dis.* **2019**, *79*, 123–131. [CrossRef]
128. Kostareva, O.S.; Kolyadenko, I.; Ulitin, A.; Ekimova, V.; Evdokimov, S.; Garber, M.; Tishchenko, S.V.; Gabdoulkhakov, A. Fab Fragment of VHH-Based Antibody Netakimab: Crystal Structure and Modeling Interaction with Cytokine IL-17A. *Crystals* **2019**, *9*, 177. [CrossRef]
129. Erdes, S.; Nasonov, E.; Kunder, E.; Pristrom, A.; Soroka, N.; Shesternya, P.; Dubinina, T.; Smakotina, S.; Raskina, T.; Krechikova, D.; et al. Primary efficacy of netakimab, a novel interleukin-17 inhibitor, in the treatment of active ankylosing spondylitis in adults. *Clin. Exp. Rheumatol.* **2019**, *38*, 27–34.

130. Korotaeva, T.; Gaydukova, I.; Mazurov, V.; Samtsov, A.; Khayrutdinov, V.; Bakulev, A.; Kokhan, M.; Kundzer, A.; Soroka, N.; Dokukina, E.; et al. AB0791 Netakimab Reduces Skin Manifestations of Psoriatic Arthritis: Results of Subanalysis From a Double-blind Randomized Phase 3 Study (Patera). *Ann. Rheum. Dis.* **2020**, *79* (Suppl. 1), 1690–1691.

131. Gaydukova, I.; Mazurov, V.; Erdes, S.; Dubinina, T.; Nesmeyanova, O.; Ilivanova, E.; Kundzer, A.; Soroka, N.; Kastanayan, A.; Povarova, T.; et al. OP0232 Netakimab Reduces the Disease Activity of Radiographic Axial Spondyloarthritis. *Results of Astera Study. Ann. Rheum. Dis.* **2019**, *78* (Suppl. 2), 193–194.

132. Papp, K.A.; Reid, C.; Foley, P.; Sinclair, R.; Salinger, D.H.; Williams, G.; Dong, H.; Krueger, J.G.; Russell, C.B.; Martin, D.A.; et al. Anti-IL-17 Receptor Antibody AMG 827 Leads to Rapid Clinical Response in Subjects with Moderate to Severe Psoriasis: Results from a Phase I, Randomized, Placebo-Controlled Trial. *J. Investig. Dermatol.* **2012**, *132*, 2466–2469. [CrossRef]

133. Mease, P.J.; Genovese, M.C.; Greenwald, M.W.; Ritchlin, C.T.; Beaulieu, A.D.; Deodhar, A.; Newmark, R.; Feng, J.; Erondu, N.; Nirula, A. Brodalumab, an Anti-IL17RA Monoclonal Antibody, in Psoriatic Arthritis. *N. Engl. J. Med.* **2014**, *370*, 2295–2306. [CrossRef] [PubMed]

134. Wendling, D.; Verhoeven, F.; Prati, C. Anti-IL-17 monoclonal antibodies for the treatment of ankylosing spondylitis. *Expert Opin. Boil. Ther.* **2018**, *19*, 55–64. [CrossRef] [PubMed]

135. Lebwohl, M.G.; Papp, K.A.; Marangell, L.B.; Koo, J.; Blauvelt, A.; Gooderham, M.; Wu, J.J.; Rastogi, S.; Harris, S.; Pillai, R.; et al. Psychiatric adverse events during treatment with brodalumab: Analysis of psoriasis clinical trials. *J. Am. Acad. Dermatol.* **2018**, *78*, 81–89. [CrossRef] [PubMed]

136. Nash, P. Inhibition of interleukins 17A and 17F in psoriatic arthritis. *Lancet* **2020**, *395*, 395–396. [CrossRef]

137. Ritchlin, C.T.; Kavanaugh, A.; Merola, J.F.; Schett, G.; Scher, J.U.; Warren, R.B.; Gottlieb, A.B.; Assudani, D.; Bedford-Rice, K.; Coarse, J.; et al. Bimekizumab in patients with active psoriatic arthritis: Results from a 48-week, randomised, double-blind, placebo-controlled, dose-ranging phase 2b trial. *Lancet* **2020**, *395*, 427–440. [CrossRef]

138. Van Der Heijde, D.; Gensler, L.S.; Deodhar, A.; Baraliakos, X.; Poddubnyy, D.; Kivitz, A.; Farmer, M.K.; Baeten, D.; Goldammer, N.; Coarse, J.; et al. Dual neutralisation of interleukin-17A and interleukin-17F with bimekizumab in patients with active ankylosing spondylitis: Results from a 48-week phase IIb, randomised, double-blind, placebo-controlled, dose-ranging study. *Ann. Rheum. Dis.* **2020**, *79*, 595–604. [CrossRef]

139. Hsieh, C.-M.; Cuff, C.; Tarcsa, E.; Hugunin, M. FRI0303 Discovery and Characterization of Abt-122, an Anti-TNF/IL-17 Dvd-Ig™ Molecule as A Potential Therapeutic Candidate for Rheumatoid Arthritis. *Ann. Rheum. Dis.* **2014**, *73*, 495. [CrossRef]

140. Genovese, M.C.; Weinblatt, M.E.; Mease, P.J.; Aelion, J.A.; Peloso, P.M.; Chen, K.; Li, Y.; Liu, J.; Othman, A.A.; Khatri, A.; et al. Dual inhibition of tumour necrosis factor and interleukin-17A with ABT-122: Open-label long-term extension studies in rheumatoid arthritis or psoriatic arthritis. *Rheumatology* **2018**, *57*, 1972–1981. [CrossRef]

141. Mease, P.J.; Genovese, M.C.; Weinblatt, M.E.; Peloso, P.M.; Chen, K.; Othman, A.A.; Li, Y.; Mansikka, H.T.; Khatri, A.; Wishart, N.; et al. Phase II Study of ABT-122, a Tumor Necrosis Factor- and Interleukin-17A-Targeted Dual Variable Domain Immunoglobulin, in Patients With Psoriatic Arthritis With an Inadequate Response to Methotrexate. *Arthritis Rheumatol.* **2018**, *70*, 1778–1789. [CrossRef]

142. Khatri, A.; Klünder, B.; Peloso, P.M.; Othman, A.A. Exposure-response analyses demonstrate no evidence of interleukin 17A contribution to efficacy of ABT-122 in rheumatoid or psoriatic arthritis. *Rheumatology* **2019**, *58*, 352–360. [CrossRef] [PubMed]

143. Sandborn, W.J.; Gasink, C.; Gao, L.-L.; Blank, M.A.; Johanns, J.; Guzzo, C.; Sands, B.E.; Hanauer, S.B.; Targan, S.; Rutgeerts, P.; et al. Ustekinumab Induction and Maintenance Therapy in Refractory Crohn's Disease. *N. Engl. J. Med.* **2012**, *367*, 1519–1528. [CrossRef] [PubMed]

144. Sands, B.E.; Sandborn, W.J.; Panaccione, R.; O'Brien, C.D.; Zhang, H.; Johanns, J.; Adedokun, O.J.; Roblin, X.; Peyrin-Biroulet, L.; Van Assche, G.; et al. Ustekinumab as Induction and Maintenance Therapy for Ulcerative Colitis. *N. Engl. J. Med.* **2019**, *381*, 1201–1214. [CrossRef] [PubMed]

International Journal of
Molecular Sciences

MDPI

Review

Emerging Gene-Editing Modalities for Osteoarthritis

Alekya S. Tanikella [1], Makenna J. Hardy [1,2,3], Stephanie M. Frahs [1,2,3], Aidan G. Cormier [4], Kalin D. Gibbons [4], Clare K. Fitzpatrick [4] and Julia Thom Oxford [1,2,3,*]

1 Biomolecular Research Center, Boise State University, Boise, ID 83725, USA; atlearning2014@gmail.com (A.S.T.); makennahardy@u.boisestate.edu (M.J.H.); StephanieTuft@boisestate.edu (S.M.F.)
2 Department of Biological Sciences, Boise State University, Boise, ID 83725, USA
3 Biomolecular Sciences Graduate Programs, Boise State University, Boise, ID 83725, USA
4 Mechanical and Biomedical Engineering, Boise State University, Boise, ID 83725, USA; aidancormier@u.boisestate.edu (A.G.C.); kalingibbons@u.boisestate.edu (K.D.G.); clarefitzpatrick@boisestate.edu (C.K.F.)
* Correspondence: joxford@boisestate.edu; Tel.: +1-208-426-2395

Received: 11 July 2020; Accepted: 19 August 2020; Published: 22 August 2020

Abstract: Osteoarthritis (OA) is a pathological degenerative condition of the joints that is widely prevalent worldwide, resulting in significant pain, disability, and impaired quality of life. The diverse etiology and pathogenesis of OA can explain the paucity of viable preventive and disease-modifying strategies to counter it. Advances in genome-editing techniques may improve disease-modifying solutions by addressing inherited predisposing risk factors and the activity of inflammatory modulators. Recent progress on technologies such as CRISPR/Cas9 and cell-based genome-editing therapies targeting the genetic and epigenetic alternations in OA offer promising avenues for early diagnosis and the development of personalized therapies. The purpose of this literature review was to concisely summarize the genome-editing options against chronic degenerative joint conditions such as OA with a focus on the more recently emerging modalities, especially CRISPR/Cas9. Future advancements in novel genome-editing therapies may improve the efficacy of such targeted treatments.

Keywords: osteoarthritis; CRISPR/Cas9; miRNA; genome editing

1. Introduction

Osteoarthritis (OA) is a chronic disease affecting the joints of the body, especially the weight-bearing joints, chiefly the knees, hips, shoulders, and spine. OA is the most common type of degenerative arthritis, affecting over 30 million Americans [1]. It is also the second most expensive disease to treat in the US, costing $139.8 billion in 2013 [2]. As the fifth leading cause of disability in the US, OA has a significant impact on the quality of life.

In 2017, the Centers for Disease Control (CDC) published results on the prevalence of doctor-diagnosed arthritis from 2013 to 2015, including 54.4 million adults, nearly half of whom had activity limitations attributable to arthritis [3]. More alarmingly, as our US population ages, the number of cases is projected to increase to 78.4 million, or 25.9% of the population, by 2040 [4]. According to the World Health Organization (WHO), the United Nations has categorized OA as a priority disease in need of research into potential therapies. Given that between 2015 and 2050, the proportion of the world's population over 60 years old will nearly double from 12% to 22%, an estimated 130 million people will suffer from OA worldwide (WHO, 2018).

The progression of OA includes the degradation of the hyaline articular cartilage at the ends of the articulating bones of the synovial joints. The articular cartilage, when healthy, functions to resist compression, prevent bone–bone contact, and maintain a low-friction surface [5]. Damaged joint articular cartilage, on the other hand, cannot perform the necessary functions [6]. Additionally, the repair of the damaged articular cartilage is a challenging issue, due in part to its avascular nature and its limited ability to heal by itself [5–7]. This often results in the formation of fibrocartilage, which lacks the ideal biomechanical characteristics needed to withstand the compressive stress imposed on the synovial joints during articulation and load-bearing [8,9].

Normally, synovial joints in the body move effortlessly, gliding across each other [10]. This is due in part to the unique properties of the synovial fluid secreted by the cells of the inner lining of the joint capsule and its ability to reduce the friction that is generated by movement at the joint surfaces [5,10,11]. The articular hyaline cartilage at the joint surfaces maintains the proper structure, function, and stability of the synovial joints [10]. Unfortunately, chondrocytes have limited potential for replication, a factor that contributes to the limited intrinsic healing capacity of cartilage in response to injury. Chondrocyte survival depends on an optimal biochemical and mechanical environment [5,12], Localized stress, wear, and tear lead to degeneration of the cartilage and may also lead to the activation of osteoblasts, resulting in new anomalous bone formation [13,14] (Figure 1). Opportunities for prevention or slowing the progression of degradation may exist if the disease is detected during its early stages. If left untreated, however, OA can lead to complete loss of joint cartilage, severe pain, restricted range of joint and limb movement, and altered reshaping of the bones within the joint [15–17].

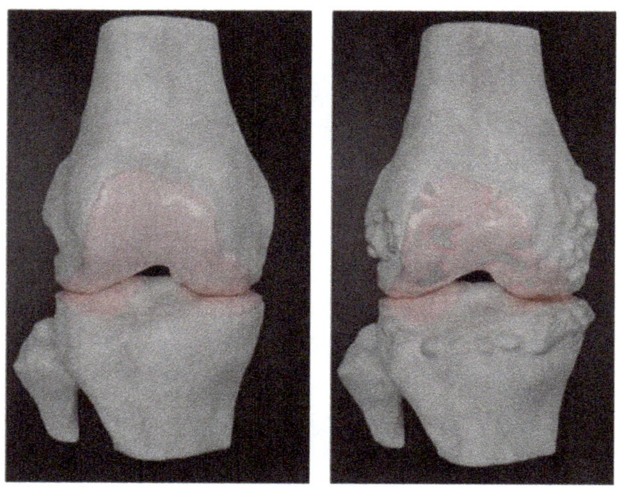

(a) (b)

Figure 1. Articular joint structure. (**a**) Bone and cartilage of a healthy tibiofemoral joint (**b**) Simulation of cartilage degeneration and bone spur formation in an osteoarthritic knee.

OA, characterized by joint stiffness, tenderness, swelling, and pain, is not a single disease per se [14]. It is, rather, a complex disease consisting of a group of conditions with multiple pathways that all result ultimately in progressive, irreversible joint failure as the outcome. Many susceptibility factors play a part in the pathogenesis of OA, such as age, gender, and weight [18–20]. Old age, female gender, repetitive joint stress, injury, joint laxity, high body weight, and osteoporosis all contribute to OA [21,22]. With the increasing life span of the population in addition to the epidemic of obesity, the number of people affected by joint degeneration is expected to increase substantially [23–25]. Severe OA can prevent a person from being able to work, especially if their work involves putting stress on a specific joint for an extended duration. OA can result in significant physical, mental, emotional, and social challenges as well [26–28].

Despite nonsurgical and surgical interventions, there is currently neither a cure for this disease nor a means to halt its inevitable progression [22,29]. Autologous chondrocyte transplantation has shown promise in clinical treatment, however, the process involves the harvest, culture, and transplant of cells grown in a monolayer (2D culture) [30–33]. Under these culture conditions, the risk of dedifferentiation of the chondrocytes and an altered phenotype is a major concern of tissue engineering [34].

2. Current Treatment Options and Limitations

The progressive erosion of articular cartilage is a prevalent symptom of OA [35]. Articular cartilage is made up of chondrocytes embedded within a collagenous extracellular matrix (ECM) [36]. Disruption of the articular cartilage prevents pain-free movement and affects the load-bearing abilities of the joint. Current treatments for OA can include intra-articular joint injections of steroids and arthroscopic lavage with debridement; however, these may have short-term benefits without long-term benefit to the cartilage [22,37,38]. Anti-inflammatory and analgesic drugs may help to address some of the symptoms of OA, but they do not tackle the fundamental pathologies involved in the inexorable degenerative process, in addition to having significant side effects associated with prolonged use [39–42]. Surgery and joint replacement, if possible in the early stages of OA, are expensive and may need to be performed multiple times during an individual's life [22,43]. Alternative modalities of treatment may well be helpful in the short term, but may not be a sustainable strategy for OA treatment and potential prevention [44,45].

The best way to combat the root cause of joint degeneration in OA may be through the exploration of the various possibilities that genome editing offers [46,47]. There is increasing evidence that genetic and epigenetic modifications play a substantive role in OA; however, it has been difficult to separate the individual effects from the combined effects of genetic and environmental factors acting together to cause progressive joint degeneration [48–51]. Characterizing and analyzing the genetic factors underpinning the pathology of OA may provide viable options for the diagnosis, prognosis, and development of novel treatment targets for future personalized biological therapies.

3. CRISPR/Cas

Several gene therapy systems such as viral, engineered scaffold, and other approaches hold promise [52]. However, while such systems hold promise, the advantages are offset by some potential disadvantages. Here we focus on the CRISPR/Cas9 system, a very powerful gene therapy tool.

CRISPR/Cas is a novel, versatile, and promising genome-editing technique that is opening up new avenues and possibilities in the effective treatment of OA [53] and other degenerative joint diseases [54,55]. CRISPR is an acronym for "clustered regularly interspaced short palindromic repeats", discovered through investigation of the prokaryotic adaptive immune system. It was identified as an effective system used by bacteria and archaea to remember infecting agents such as phage viruses and destroy them upon subsequent exposure, similarly to the memory cells in the human immune system. When paired with different proteins, specifically enzymes such as Cas, that are produced naturally by the prokaryotic cells, the CRISPR system can be used to make deletions, insertions, substitutions, or other changes at specific sites of the prokaryotic and eukaryotic genome [56,57]. From finding a cure for cancer, to treating sickle-cell disease, to growing drought- and pest-resistant crops, CRISPR has many exciting possibilities and potential in several fields [58].

The prokaryotic CRISPR/Cas system has three main components: a Cas nuclease, a crRNA (CRISPR RNA), and a tracrRNA (trans-activating crRNA). In bacterial cells, the CRISPR/Cas system works by recognizing the invading bacteriophage DNA, chopping it up into several pieces, and incorporating them into its DNA. These CRISPR pieces are then transcribed, generating a crRNA and a tracrRNA to create a double-stranded RNA structure that can recruit the Cas proteins. When the offending phage is encountered again, the CRISPR/Cas system is directed to a specific location on the foreign DNA because of a protospacer adjacent motif (PAM) short nucleotide base sequence which is upstream of the crRNA targeted sequence. The Cas protein is programmed to be the "molecular scissors" of the system which carries out the cutting, splicing, and any other editing that is desired [59–61]. The therapeutic application of CRISPR/Cas is illustrated in Figure 2.

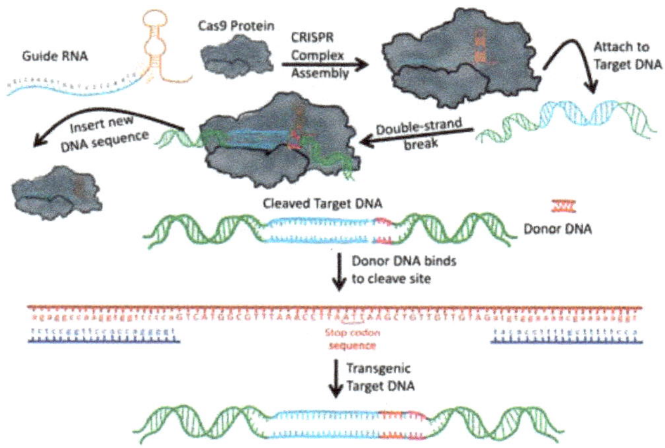

Figure 2. CRISPR/Cas mechanism. Trans-activating RNA (orange) with CRISPR RNA (blue) the guide RNA. The guide RNA assembles with the Cas9 protein to form the CRISPR complex. Using the guide RNA for specificity, the CRISPR complex binds to the target DNA. Transgenic DNA can be inserted using homology arm inserts.

The most widely used of the six major types of CRISPR/Cas system, the Type II system, is derived from the *Streptococcus pyogenes* bacteria. It uses the Cas9 protein because of its wide working range and efficiency [62]. The CRISPR/Cas9 system that is used currently by researchers and scientists worldwide consists of a single guide RNA (sgRNA) with a binding end (analogous to tracrRNA) for the Cas9 nuclease to attach and a targeting end (similar to crRNA) with nucleotide base pairs that are complementary to the DNA sequence that is meant to be edited (Figure 2). Only the targeting end of the sgRNA needs to be synthesized for any specific targeting sequence, while the binding end does not need to be redesigned every time, thus reducing the time needed to get the tool ready for editing. Cas9 recruitment to the exact DNA target sequence is mediated by the sgRNA. Cas9-induced double-stranded breaks (DSBs) are repaired either by spontaneously nonhomologous end joining (NHEJ) or by homology-directed repair (HDR) using a synthetic donor DNA template [63]. CRISPR/Cas RNA-guided DNA endonuclease genome targeting is much easier to design and apply when compared to other available site-specific editing tools using engineered nucleases such as transcription activator-like effector nuclease (TALENS) and zinc finger nucleases (ZFNs), which are controlled by protein–DNA interactions. CRISPR/Cas is also much more cost- and time-effective because researchers only need to code for a small section of sgRNA [64].

4. Mesenchymal Stem Cells and Tissue Regeneration

Tissue regeneration and self-renewal of articular cartilage, in general, is a very limited process [65]. The avascularity of articular cartilage may hinder progenitor cells access to the site of injured cartilage [66]). It may also limit molecular factors that are vital to extracellular matrix repair and homeostasis [67–70].

Chondrocytes originate from mesenchymal stem cells [71,72]. Bone-marrow-derived MSCs (BM-MSCs) have much promise in aiding articular cartilage repair due to their proximity to the joint, high differentiation capability, and ability to secrete different growth, anti-inflammatory, and immunomodulatory factors [73–77]. They could affect a clinically relevant improvement in joint pain and function. Additional studies are needed, however, to demonstrate the efficacy of cultured versus noncultured BM-MSCs and the best ways to deliver them into the joint. MSCs derived from fetal cells also have therapeutic properties, but ethical concerns have been raised about using them for treatment and therapeutic applications [78,79]. Additional challenges arise due to the potential of fetal MSCs to differentiate into several different types of cells, which might be more difficult to control and direct [76,80,81]. The capabilities of MSCs are usually age-dependent. MSCs have a short lifespan but can secrete paracrine factors that may be beneficial in tissue regeneration [81,82]. In addition to BM-MSCs, MSCs derived from other sites such as adipose tissue can be isolated, expanded, characterized, and used to regenerate cartilage [83,84]. However, MSCs tend to form mechanically inferior fibrocartilage instead of the glassy, hyaline cartilage that covers the ends of bones at articulating joints [85].

5. Extracellular Vesicles

Genome-editing factors, packaged in engineered CRISPR/Cas9 complexes, can be enclosed in extracellular vesicles (EVs), for delivery to specific target cells [86,87]. EVs are composed of cellular constituents such as lipids, proteins, RNA, and DNA [86,88]. EVs may cross the blood–brain barrier, target cells in vivo, and protect their components from degradation in the circulatory system [87,89]. Their function is dependent upon their origin, and EVs derived from MSCs could have the potential to deliver contents to OA cells [90–93], as shown in Figure 3 [85,94,95]. The use of exosomes as a nonselective cell system may have limitations, including the delivery of contents to unintended cell targets. Possible solutions to this challenge include the design of targeted exosomes, as suggested by Bellavia and colleagues [96].

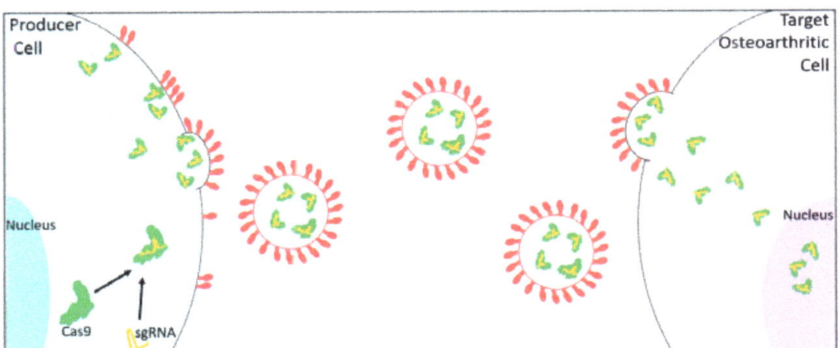

Figure 3. Extracellular vesicle delivery of CRISPR/Cas9 in the treatment of OA. Inside a producer cell (**left**), engineered OA-targeted sgRNA transcription may occur. SgRNA combines with Cas9 to form CRISPR/Cas9 sgRNA complexes. CRISPR/Cas9 complexes load into extracellular vesicles with fluorescent tags containing a dimerization domain compatible with a dimerization domain in engineered CRISPR/Cas9 complexes. These fluorescent tags also contain targets for the target osteoarthritic cell (**right**). Loaded EVs attach to target cells and unload the CRISPR/Cas9 complexes, which are then transported to the nucleus to perform gene modification.

Exogenous-cell-based therapy is gaining traction for the regeneration of articular cartilage over stimulation therapy such as electric stimulation of endogenous cartilage growth factors [97]. Exogenous cell therapy can be done through the delivery of chondrocytes (either autologous or allogeneic), mesenchymal stem cells (MSCs), or extracellular vesicles [98]. MSCs are used for regenerative medicine due to their ability to promote regeneration based on environmental signals at sites of injury. As inhibitors of the immune system and multilineage differentiators, MSCs are an important alternative cell source for articular cartilage repair and regeneration [97]. MSCs derived from the synovial membranes of joints have been shown to be more effective in terms of articular cartilage formation in in vitro studies when compared to MSCs from other tissues, joint and nonjoint [99,100].

In vitro studies performed in mice showed that microparticles and exosomes, which are EVs derived from MSCs, exerted similar chondroprotective and anti-inflammatory functions, protecting mice from developing osteoarthritis and reproducing the main therapeutic effect of reducing symptoms [101, 102]. Thus, a combinatorial approach to the treatment of OA may be feasible.

6. Potential CRISPR/Cas9 Molecular Targets for the Treatment of Osteoarthritis

Cell therapy has great potential to help treat OA, but inflammation can prevent new articular cartilage from forming after the introduction of stem cells. Inflammation and inflammatory modulators must be addressed in the treatment of OA, and these inflammatory modulators may serve as targets for CRISPR/Cas9 strategies [103]. Table 1 identifies potential targets for CRISPR/Cas9 editing and the laboratories that are making progress in the use of CRISPR/Cas9 techniques in OA treatment.

IL-1β is a pro-inflammatory cytokine secreted primarily by neutrophils. IL-1β induces the expression of many OA-related genes and other cytokines, including tumor necrosis factor-alpha (TNFα) [104]. Current OA therapies target TNFα, however, deleterious side effects occur due to TNFα's role in facilitating many other functions [105,106]. Human articular cartilage (hAC) exposed to TNFα displays increased levels of expression of interleukin IL-1β [105,106]. Karlsen and colleagues, in their 2016 study, were able to silence the IL-1β cytokine receptor (IL1-R1) in hACs to determine its effect on inflammation and the redifferentiation potential of the hACs after exposure to the interleukin IL-1β. The hACs were isolated from cartilage, and CRISPR/Cas9 was used to knock out the IL1-R1 receptor and insert a puromycin-resistance gene to allow the selection of the knockout cells. The colonies of knockout cells were expanded and exposed to recombinant IL-1β and TNFα to assess their response. The results showed that the addition of recombinant IL-1β increased inflammation to high levels in the control group, as expected. However, in the knockout group, exposure to recombinant IL-1β did not cause measurable inflammation. Therefore, the therapeutic knockdown of IL1-R1 in articular cartilage cells in vitro prior to re-injection into the body may improve cell-therapy results [106].

Table 1. Potential CRISPR/Cas9 molecular targets for CRISPR/Cas treatment of osteoarthritis.

Gene Symbol	Gene Name	Function	Reference
IL1-β	*Interleukin 1 beta*	Inflammation	Karlsen, 2016 [106] Zhao, 2019 [53] Guilak [73]
IL1-R1	*Interleukin 1 beta receptor*	Inflammation	Karlsen, 2016 [106]
BGLAP	*Osteocalcin*	Trabecular bone formation	Lambert, 2016 [107]
miR-140	*Micro RNA 140*	Chondrocyte homeostasis	Asahara, 2016 [108]
Has2	*Hyaluronan synthase 2*	Chondrocyte accumulation of aggrecan	Huang, 2016 [109]
sTNFR1α	*Soluble Tumor necrosis factor receptor 1*	TNF antagonist	Brunger, 2017 [110]
IL1RA	*Interleukin 1 bets receptor antagonist*	IL-1 beta antagonist	Brunger, 2017 [110]
PRG4	*Lubricin*	Joint lubrication	Khakshooy, 2017 [111]
Runx2	*Runt Related Transcription Factor 2*	Osteoblast differentiation	Rice, 2018 [112]
Hrdl	*E3 ubiquitin-protein ligase hrd-like protein 1*	Protein turnover and proteasomal degradation	Ye, 2018 [113]
Mmp13	*Matrix metalloprotein 13*	Tissue degradation	Seidl, 2019 [114] Zhao, 2019 [53]
Cx43	*Connexin 43*	Gap junction protein	Varela-Eirín M, 2018 [115]
NGF	*Nerve growth factor*	Pain sensitivity	Zhao, 2019 [53]
Cbx4	*Chromobox 4*	Nucleolar homeostasis	Ren, 2019 [116]
Foxd1	*Forkhead box D1*	Transcription factor	Fu, 2019 [117]
YAP	*Yes-associated protein 1*	Mechanosensing transcription factor	Fu, 2019 [117]

Recent gene-editing efforts have targeted cellular senescence. Ren and colleagues found that by targeting CBX4, cellular senescence could be alleviated, with positive outcomes for OA [116]. FOXD1 is a transcription factor that can be regulated by YAP. Recent research indicates that the upregulation of FOXD1 by YAP may hold promise for OA treatment by alleviating senescence [117]. Further studies that focused on connexin 43 modulation were able to demonstrate that the attenuation of cellular senescence could promote the regenerative capacity of cells and improve tissue quality in OA [115].

Degradative enzymes such as matrix metalloproteinases (MMP) play important roles in joint health. Seidl and colleagues utilized CRISPR/Cas9 to modify the MMP13 levels in human chondrocytes and found that by reducing the level of MMP activity, cells were able to accumulate higher levels of the beneficial type II collagen to strengthen the extracellular matrix of the articular cartilage [114].

7. Additional Emerging Targets for the Treatment of Osteoarthritis Using CRISPR/Cas9

While a significant focus is placed on cartilage and the chondrocytes that maintain articular cartilage, there is wide agreement that OA is not simply a disease of the cartilage, but rather of the entire joint, and all of the specific tissue types within the joint play essential roles. Osteocalcin, a small protein hormone secreted by the osteoblasts of the bone, has been studied recently for its endocrine functions, which impact several physiological processes. Lambert and colleagues found in their 2016 study that by applying CRISPR/Cas9 technologies to osteocalcin expression, they were able to improve bone biomechanics and increase the trabecular bone in a rat model system [107].

Additional potential targets for therapy have been identified using CRISPR/Cas9 technology. For example, CRISPR/Cas9 knockout of hyaluronan synthase 2 (HAS2) in rat chondrocytes demonstrated the importance of the glycosaminoglycan hyaluronan, for the retention of aggrecan, a proteoglycan necessary for the functional integrity of the articular cartilage [109]. CRISPR/Cas9 can, therefore, provide fundamental information about the molecular mechanisms required for healthy joint tissue in addition to potential use as a direct treatment.

8. Limitations and Future Considerations

The CRISPR/Cas9 system is being used in a wide range of applications and many studies. However, notwithstanding its meteoric rise in a short period of time and its potential applications in medicine and beyond, it, like other genome-editing tools, does come with limitations and concerns, ethical and otherwise. One of these limitations is the effective targeting range, as the sgRNA can only bind to a region near a specific PAM sequence on the DNA. The PAM sequence for Cas9 is 5′-NGG-3′, where "N" can be any nucleotide base, but the third base must be G. This can greatly reduce the potential target locations available to make DNA edits such as insertions or deletions. In experiments conducted by Nishimasu and colleagues, a Cas9 with a more relaxed preference for the PAM third base resulted in the recognition of an NGD PAM instead of an NGG PAM requirement. This effectively increased the potential targets for Cas9 nuclease, as the NGD sequence occurs more frequently in human DNA than NGG sequences. The engineered Cas9 in this instance had a wider range and increased cleavage specificity, reducing instances of off-target incisions. The new Cas, termed SpCas9-NG, can bind to A, G, or T in the 3rd base of the PAM sequence [118].

MicroRNAs (miRNAs), small, non-coding RNA molecules, may help to regulate inflammation, promote MSC differentiation, and ensure the homeostasis of cartilage [119]. As a key factor in epigenetic regulation, miRNAs can change the gene expression without modifying the sequence of the DNA that encodes proteins [120]. This may be a much safer way to modulate gene expression since the genome sequence does not change, and the gene expression pattern may still be inheritable from one cell generation to the next [85]. miRNAs may be used in combination with CRISPR/Cas9 and EVs to design patient-specific approaches to the treatment of OA [103].

9. Conclusions

Investigators and practitioners the world over are working toward a better understanding of the basis of degenerative joint diseases such as OA. Devising ways to alter or modify the relevant genes impacting the joint articular cartilage may lead to the development of successful, safe, and effective therapies to halt the progress, treat, or even prevent the occurrence of OA and other debilitating joint disorders in humans. CRISPR/Cas9, MSCs, EVs, and miRNAs may all play key roles in future treatments.

Author Contributions: Conceptualization, A.S.T. and J.T.O.; methodology, A.S.T. and J.T.O.; investigation, A.S.T.; writing—original draft preparation, A.S.T. and J.T.O.; writing—review and editing, C.K.F., A.G.C., J.T.O.; illustrations, S.M.F., M.J.H., A.G.C., and K.D.G.; supervision, J.T.O.; funding acquisition, J.T.O. All authors have read and agreed to the published version of the manuscript.

Funding: This research was funded by NIH NIGMS, grant number P20GM109095 and P20GM103408.

Acknowledgments: Authors wish to acknowledge support from the Institutional Development Awards (IDeA) from the National Institute of General Medical Sciences of the National Institutes of Health under Grants #P20GM103408, P20GM109095, and 1C06RR020533. We also acknowledge support from The Biomolecular Research Center at Boise State with funding from the National Science Foundation, Grants #0619793 and #0923535; the M. J. Murdock Charitable Trust; Lori and Duane Stueckle, and the Idaho State Board of Education.

Conflicts of Interest: The authors declare no conflict of interest. The funders had no role in the design of the study; in the collection, analyses, or interpretation of data; in the writing of the manuscript, or in the decision to publish the results.

Abbreviations

OA	Osteoarthritis
CRISPR	Clustered Regularly Interspaced Short Palindromic Repeats
Cas	Cas nuclease
crRNA	CRISPR RNA
tracrRNA	trans-activating crRNA
PAM	protospacer adjacent motif
sgRNA	single guide RNA
MSC	Mesenchymal stem cells
miRNA	Micro RNA
EV	Extracellular vesicles
IL-1β	Interleukin 1 beta
TNFα	Tumor Necrosis Factor
Hac	Human articular cartilage
IL1-R1	IL-1β cytokine receptor 1
BGLAP	Osteocalcin
Has2	Hyaluronan synthase 2
PRG4	Lubricin
Runx2	Runt Related Transcription Factor 2
Hrdl	E3 ubiquitin-protein ligase hrd-like protein 1
Mmp13	Matrix metalloprotein 13
Cx43	Connexin 43
Cbx4	Chromobox 4
Foxd1	Forkhead box D1
YAP	Yes-associated protein 1
NHEJ	Non-homologous end joining
HDR	Homology Directed Repair
TALENs	Transcription activator-like effector nucleases
ZFN	Zinc finger nucleases

References

1. Bitton, R. The economic burden of osteoarthritis. *Am. J. Manag. Care* **2009**, *15*, S230–S235. [PubMed]

2. Murphy, L.B.; Cisternas, M.G.; Pasta, D.J.; Helmick, C.G.; Yelin, E.H. Medical Expenditures and Earnings Losses Among US Adults with Arthritis in 2013. *Arthritis Care Res.* **2018**, *70*, 869–876. [CrossRef] [PubMed]
3. Barbour, K.E.; Helmick, C.G.; Boring, M.; Brady, T.J. Vital Signs: Prevalence of Doctor-Diagnosed Arthritis and Arthritis-Attributable Activity Limitation-United States, 2013–2015. *MMWR. Morb. Mortal. Wkly. Rep.* **2017**, *66*, 246–253. [CrossRef] [PubMed]
4. Hootman, J.M.; Helmick, C.G.; Barbour, K.E.; Theis, K.A.; Boring, M.A. Updated Projected Prevalence of Self-Reported Doctor-Diagnosed Arthritis and Arthritis-Attributable Activity Limitation Among US Adults, 2015–2040. *Arthritis Rheumatol.* **2016**, *68*, 1582–1587. [CrossRef]
5. Sophia Fox, A.J.; Bedi, A.; Rodeo, S.A. The basic science of articular cartilage: Structure, composition, and function. *Sports Health* **2009**, *1*, 461–468. [CrossRef]
6. Medvedeva, E.V.; Grebenik, E.A.; Gornostaeva, S.N.; Telpuhov, V.I.; Lychagin, A.V.; Timashev, P.S.; Chagin, A.S. Repair of damaged articular cartilage: Current approaches and future directions. *Int. J. Mol. Sci.* **2018**, *19*, 2366. [CrossRef] [PubMed]
7. Karuppal, R. Current concepts in the articular cartilage repair and regeneration. *J. Orthop.* **2017**, *14*, A1–A3. [CrossRef]
8. Kreuz, P.C.; Steinwachs, M.R.; Erggelet, C.; Krause, S.J.; Konrad, G.; Uhl, M.; Südkamp, N. Results after microfracture of full-thickness chondral defects in different compartments in the knee. *Osteoarthr. Cartil.* **2006**, *14*, 1119–1125. [CrossRef]
9. Armiento, A.R.; Alini, M.; Stoddart, M.J. Articular fibrocartilage—Why does hyaline cartilage fail to repair? *Adv. Drug Deliv. Rev.* **2019**, *146*, 289–305. [CrossRef]
10. Tamer, T.M. Hyaluronan and synovial joint: Function, distribution and healing. *Interdiscip. Toxicol.* **2013**, *6*, 111–125. [CrossRef]
11. Seror, J.; Zhu, L.; Goldberg, R.; Day, A.J.; Klein, J. Supramolecular synergy in the boundary lubrication of synovial joints. *Nat. Commun.* **2015**, *6*, 1–7. [CrossRef] [PubMed]
12. Odgren, P.R.; Witwicka, H.; Reyes-Gutierrez, P. The cast of clasts: Catabolism and vascular invasion during bone growth, repair, and disease by osteoclasts, chondroclasts, and septoclasts. *Connect. Tissue Res.* **2016**, *57*, 161–174. [CrossRef] [PubMed]
13. Buckwalter, J.A.; Mankin, H.J. Articular cartilage: Degeneration and osteoarthritis, repair, regeneration, and transplantation. *Instr. Course Lect.* **1998**, *47*, 487–504. [PubMed]
14. Harrell, C.R.; Markovic, B.S.; Fellabaum, C.; Arsenijevic, A.; Volarevic, V. Mesenchymal stem cell-based therapy of osteoarthritis: Current knowledge and future perspectives. *Biomed. Pharmacother.* **2019**, *109*, 2318–2326. [CrossRef]
15. Sandell, L.J.; Aigner, T. Articular cartilage and changes in arthritis. An introduction: Cell biology of osteoarthritis. *Arthritis Res.* **2001**, *3*, 107–113. [CrossRef]
16. Berenbaum, F. Osteoarthritis as an inflammatory disease (osteoarthritis is not osteoarthrosis!). *Osteoarthr. Cartil.* **2013**, *21*, 16–21. [CrossRef]
17. Fukui, N.; Purple, C.R.; Sandell, L.J. Cell biology of osteoarthritis: The chondrocyte's response to injury. *Curr. Rheumatol. Rep.* **2001**, *3*, 496–505. [CrossRef]
18. Andriacchi, T.P.; Mündermann, A.; Smith, R.L.; Alexander, E.J.; Dyrby, C.O.; Koo, S. A framework for the in vivo pathomechanics of osteoarthritis at the knee. *Ann. Biomed. Eng.* **2004**, *32*, 447–457. [CrossRef]
19. DeFrate, L.E.; Kim-Wang, S.Y.; Englander, Z.A.; McNulty, A.L. Osteoarthritis year in review 2018: Mechanics. *Osteoarthr. Cartil.* **2019**, *27*, 392–400. [CrossRef]
20. Musumeci, G.; Aiello, F.C.; Szychlinska, M.A.; Di Rosa, M.; Castrogiovanni, P.; Mobasheri, A. Osteoarthritis in the XXIst century: Risk factors and behaviours that influence disease onset and progression. *Int. J. Mol. Sci.* **2015**, *16*, 6093–6112. [CrossRef]
21. Qin, Y.X.; Lam, H.Y. Intramedullary pressure and matrix strain induced by oscillatory skeletal muscle stimulation and its potential in adaptation. *J. Biomech.* **2009**, *42*, 140–145. [CrossRef] [PubMed]
22. Anandacoomarasamy, A.; March, L. Current evidence for osteoarthritis treatments. *Ther. Adv. Musculoskelet Dis.* **2010**, *2*, 17–28. [CrossRef] [PubMed]
23. Songer, T.J.; LaPorte, R.E. Disabilities due to injury in the military. *Am. J. Prev. Med.* **2000**, *18*, 33–40. [CrossRef]
24. Ma, V.Y.; Chan, L.; Carruthers, K.J. Incidence, prevalence, costs, and impact on disability of common conditions requiring rehabilitation in the united states: Stroke, spinal cord injury, traumatic brain injury,

multiple sclerosis, osteoarthritis, rheumatoid arthritis, limb loss, and back pa. *Arch. Phys. Med. Rehabil.* **2014**, *95*, 986–995. [CrossRef]
25. Losina, E.; Walensky, R.P.; Reichmann, W.M.; Holt, H.L.; Gerlovin, H.; Solomon, D.H.; Jordan, J.M.; Hunter, D.J.; Suter, L.G.; Weinstein, A.M.; et al. Impact of obesity and knee osteoarthritis on morbidity and mortality in older Americans. *Ann. Intern. Med.* **2011**, *154*, 217–226. [CrossRef]
26. Park, H.M.; Kim, H.S.; Lee, Y.J. Knee osteoarthritis and its association with mental health and health-related quality of life: A nationwide cross-sectional study. *Geriatr. Gerontol. Int.* **2020**, *20*, 379–383. [CrossRef]
27. Sharma, M.; Jamieson, C.; Johnson, M.; Molloy, M.P.; Henderson, B.R. Specific Armadillo Repeat Sequences Facilitate β-Catenin Nuclear Transport in Live Cells via Direct Binding to Nucleoporins Nup62, Nup153, and RanBP2/Nup358. *J. Biol. Chem.* **2012**, *287*, 819–831. [CrossRef]
28. Luong, M.L.N.; Cleveland, R.J.; Nyrop, K.A.; Callahan, L.F. Social determinants and osteoarthritis outcomes. *Aging Health* **2012**, *8*, 413–437. [CrossRef]
29. Grässel, S.; Muschter, D. Recent advances in the treatment of osteoarthritis. *F1000Research* **2020**, *9*, 325. [CrossRef]
30. Brittberg, M.; Lindahl, A.; Nilsson, A.; Ohlsson, C.; Isaksson, O.; Peterson, L. Treatment of deep cartilage defects in the knee with autologous chondrocyte transplantation. *N. Engl. J. Med.* **1994**, *331*, 889–895. [CrossRef]
31. Dozin, B.; Malpeli, M.; Cancedda, R.; Bruzzi, P.; Calcagno, S.; Molfetta, L.; Priano, F.; Kon, E.; Marcacci, M. Comparative evaluation of autologous chondrocyte implantation and mosaicplasty: A multicentered randomized clinical trial. *Clin. J. Sport Med.* **2005**, *15*, 220–226. [CrossRef] [PubMed]
32. Dewan, A.K.; Gibson, M.A.; Elisseeff, J.H.; Trice, M.E. Evolution of autologous chondrocyte repair and comparison to other cartilage repair techniques. *Biomed Res. Int.* **2014**, *2014*, 272481. [CrossRef] [PubMed]
33. Stein, S.; Strauss, E.; Bosco, J. Advances in the Surgical Management of Articular Cartilage Defects: Autologous Chondrocyte Implantation Techniques in the Pipeline. *Cartilage* **2013**, *4*, 12–19. [CrossRef] [PubMed]
34. Hubka, K.M.; Dahlin, R.L.; Meretoja, V.V.; Kasper, F.K.; Mikos, A.G. Enhancing Chondrogenic Phenotype for Cartilage Tissue Engineering: Monoculture and Coculture of Articular Chondrocytes and Mesenchymal Stem Cells. *Tissue Eng. Part B Rev.* **2014**, *20*, 641–654. [CrossRef]
35. Goldring, M.B. Articular Cartilage Degradation in Osteoarthritis. *HSS J.* **2012**, *8*, 7–9. [CrossRef]
36. Gao, Y.; Liu, S.; Huang, J.; Guo, W.; Chen, J.; Zhang, L.; Zhao, B.; Peng, J.; Wang, A.; Wang, Y.; et al. The ECM-Cell Interaction of Cartilage Extracellular Matrix on Chondrocytes. *Biomed Res. Int.* **2014**, *2014*, 648459. [CrossRef]
37. Gesslein, M.; Merkl, C.; Bail, H.J.; Krutsch, V.; Biber, R.; Schuster, P. Refixation of Large Osteochondral Fractures After Patella Dislocation Shows Better Mid- to Long-Term Outcome Compared with Debridement. *Cartilage* **2019**, *13*. [CrossRef]
38. Ravaud, P.; Moulinier, L.; Giraudeau, B.; Ayral, X.; Guerin, C.; Noel, E.; Thomas, P.; Fautrel, B.; Mazieres, B.; Dougados, M. Effects of joint lavage and steroid injection in patients with osteoarthritis of the knee: Results of a multicenter, randomized, controlled trial. *Arthritis Rheum.* **1999**, *42*, 475–482. [CrossRef]
39. Ghouri, A.; Conaghan, P.G. Treating osteoarthritis pain: Recent approaches using pharmacological therapies. *Clin. Exp. Rheumatol.* **2019**, *37*, 124–129.
40. Jaswal, A.P.; Bandyopadhyay, A. Re-examining osteoarthritis therapy from a developmental biologist's perspective. *Biochem. Pharmacol.* **2019**, *165*, 17–23. [CrossRef]
41. Honvo, G.; Leclercq, V.; Geerinck, A.; Thomas, T.; Veronese, N.; Charles, A.; Rabenda, V.; Beaudart, C.; Cooper, C.; Reginster, J.Y.; et al. Safety of Topical Non-steroidal Anti-Inflammatory Drugs in Osteoarthritis: Outcomes of a Systematic Review and Meta-Analysis. *Drugs Aging* **2019**, *36*, 45–64. [CrossRef] [PubMed]
42. Zhang, W.; Robertson, W.B.; Zhao, J.; Chen, W.; Xu, J. Emerging trend in the pharmacotherapy of osteoarthritis. *Front. Endocrinol.* **2019**, *10*, 431. [CrossRef] [PubMed]
43. Palsis, J.A.; Brehmer, T.S.; Pellegrini, V.D.; Drew, J.M.; Sachs, B.L. The cost of joint replacement comparing two approaches to evaluating costs of total hip and knee arthroplasty. *J. Bone Jt. Surg.-Am. Vol.* **2018**, *100*, 326–333. [CrossRef] [PubMed]
44. DeRogatis, M.; Anis, H.K.; Sodhi, N.; Ehiorobo, J.O.; Chughtai, M.; Bhave, A.; Mont, M.A. Non-operative treatment options for knee osteoarthritis. *Ann. Transl. Med.* **2019**, *7* (Suppl 7), S245. [CrossRef]

45. Deyle, G.D.; Allen, C.S.; Allison, S.C.; Gill, N.W.; Hando, B.R.; Petersen, E.J.; Dusenberry, D.I.; Rhon, D.I. Physical therapy versus glucocorticoid injection for osteoarthritis of the knee. *N. Engl. J. Med.* **2020**, *382*, 1420–1429. [CrossRef] [PubMed]
46. Hermann, W.; Lambova, S.; Müller- Ladner, U. Current Treatment Options for Osteoarthritis. *Curr. Rheumatol. Rev.* **2018**, *14*, 108–116. [CrossRef]
47. Choi, Y.R.; Collins, K.H.; Lee, J.W.; Kang, H.J.; Guilak, F. Genome Engineering for Osteoarthritis: From Designer Cells to Disease-Modifying Drugs. *Tissue Eng. Regen. Med.* **2019**, *1*, 1–9. [CrossRef]
48. Shen, J.; Abu-Amer, Y.; O'Keefe, R.J.; McAlinden, A. Inflammation and epigenetic regulation in osteoarthritis. *Connect. Tissue Res.* **2017**, *58*, 49–63. [CrossRef]
49. Im, G.-I.; Choi, Y.-J. Epigenetics in osteoarthritis and its implication for future therapeutics. *Expert Opin. Biol. Ther.* **2013**, *13*, 713–721. [CrossRef]
50. García-Ibarbia, C.; Delgado-Calle, J.; Casafont, I.; Velasco, J.; Arozamena, J.; Pérez-Núñez, M.I.; Alonso, M.A.; Berciano, M.T.; Ortiz, F.; Pérez-Castrillón, J.L.; et al. Contribution of genetic and epigenetic mechanisms to Wnt pathway activity in prevalent skeletal disorders. *Gene* **2013**, *532*, 165–172. [CrossRef]
51. Simon, T.C.; Jeffries, M.A. The Epigenomic Landscape in Osteoarthritis. *Curr. Rheumatol. Rep.* **2017**, *19*, 30. [CrossRef] [PubMed]
52. Bellavia, D.; Veronesi, F.; Carina, V.; Costa, V.; Raimondi, L.; De Luca, A.; Alessandro, R.; Fini, M.; Giavaresi, G. Gene therapy for chondral and osteochondral regeneration: Is the future now? *Cell. Mol. Life Sci.* **2018**, *75*, 649–667. [CrossRef] [PubMed]
53. Zhao, L.; Huang, J.; Fan, Y.; Li, J.; You, T.; He, S.; Xiao, G.; Chen, D. Exploration of CRISPR/Cas9-based gene editing as therapy for osteoarthritis. *Ann. Rheum. Dis.* **2019**, *78*, 676–682. [CrossRef] [PubMed]
54. Adkar, S.S.; Brunger, J.M.; Willard, V.P.; Wu, C.-L.; Gersbach, C.A.; Guilak, F. Genome Engineering for Personalized Arthritis Therapeutics. *Trends Mol. Med.* **2017**, *23*, 917–931. [CrossRef] [PubMed]
55. Mali, P.; Esvelt, K.M.; Church, G.M. Cas9 for engineering biology. *Nat. Methods* **2013**, *10*, 957–963. [CrossRef]
56. Karimian, A.; Azizian, K.; Parsian, H.; Rafieian, S.; Shafiei-Irannejad, V.; Kheyrollah, M.; Yousefi, M.; Majidinia, M.; Yousefi, B. CRISPR/Cas9 technology as a potent molecular tool for gene therapy. *J. Cell. Physiol.* **2019**, *234*, 12267–12277. [CrossRef]
57. Magee, C.L.; Kleyn, P.W.; Monks, B.M.; Betz, U.; Basnet, S. Pre-existing technological core and roots for the CRISPR breakthrough. *PLoS ONE* **2018**, *13*, e0198541. [CrossRef]
58. Broeders, M.; Herrero-Hernandez, P.; Ernst, M.P.T.; van der Ploeg, A.T.; Pijnappel, W.W.M.P. Sharpening the Molecular Scissors: Advances in Gene-Editing Technology. *Iscience* **2020**, *23*, 100789. [CrossRef]
59. Ratan, Z.A.; Son, Y.J.; Haidere, M.F.; Uddin, B.M.M.; Yusuf, M.A.; Zaman, S.B.; Kim, J.H.; Banu, L.A.; Cho, J.Y. CRISPR-Cas9: A promising genetic engineering approach in cancer research. *Ther. Adv. Med. Oncol.* **2018**, *10*, 1758834018755089. [CrossRef]
60. Adli, M. The CRISPR tool kit for genome editing and beyond. *Nat. Commun.* **2018**, *9*, 1–3. [CrossRef]
61. Khan, S.; Mahmood, M.S.; Rahman, S.U.; Zafar, H.; Habibullah, S.; Khan, Z.; Ahmad, A. CRISPR/Cas9: The Jedi against the dark empire of diseases. *J. Biomed. Sci.* **2018**, *25*, 29. [CrossRef] [PubMed]
62. Mei, Y.; Wang, Y.; Chen, H.; Sun, Z.S.; Ju, X.-D. Recent Progress in CRISPR/Cas9 Technology. *J. Genet. Genom.* **2016**, *43*, 63–75. [CrossRef] [PubMed]
63. Sahel, D.K.; Mittal, A.; Chitkara, D. CRISPR/Cas System for Genome Editing: Progress and Prospects as a Therapeutic Tool. *J. Pharmacol. Exp. Ther.* **2019**, *370*, 725–735. [CrossRef] [PubMed]
64. Doench, J.G.; Fusi, N.; Sullender, M.; Hegde, M.; Vaimberg, E.W.; Donovan, K.F.; Smith, I.; Tothova, Z.; Wilen, C.; Orchard, R.; et al. Optimized sgRNA design to maximize activity and minimize off-target effects of CRISPR-Cas9. *Nat. Biotechnol.* **2016**, *34*, 184–191. [CrossRef]
65. Iwamoto, M.; Ohta, Y.; Larmour, C.; Enomoto-Iwamoto, M. Toward regeneration of articular cartilage. *Birth Defects Res. Part C-Embryo Today Rev.* **2013**, *99*, 192–202. [CrossRef]
66. Grimaud, E.; Blanchard, F.; Charrier, C.; Gouin, F.; Redini, F.; Heymann, D. Leukaemia inhibitory factor (lif) is expressed in hypertrophic chondrocytes and vascular sprouts during osteogenesis. *Cytokine* **2002**, *20*, 224–230. [CrossRef]
67. Loeser, R.F. Aging and osteoarthritis: The role of chondrocyte senescence and aging changes in the cartilage matrix. *Osteoarthr. Cartil.* **2009**, *17*, 971–979. [CrossRef]

68. Shi, Y.; Hu, X.; Cheng, J.; Zhang, X.; Zhao, F.; Shi, W.; Ren, B.; Yu, H.; Yang, P.; Li, Z.; et al. A small molecule promotes cartilage extracellular matrix generation and inhibits osteoarthritis development. *Nat. Commun.* **2019**, *10*, 1–4. [CrossRef]
69. Akkiraju, H.; Nohe, A. Role of chondrocytes in cartilage formation, progression of osteoarthritis and cartilage regeneration. *J. Dev. Biol.* **2015**, *3*, 177–192. [CrossRef]
70. Chittiboyina, S.; Bai, Y.; Lelièvre, S.A. Microenvironment-cell nucleus relationship in the context of oxidative stress. *Front. Cell Dev. Biol.* **2018**, *6*, 23. [CrossRef]
71. Jiang, Y.; Tuan, R.S. Origin and function of cartilage stem/progenitor cells in osteoarthritis. *Nat. Rev. Rheumatol.* **2015**, *11*, 206. [CrossRef] [PubMed]
72. de Crombrugghe, B.; Lefebvre, V.; Nakashima, K. Regulatory mechanisms in the pathways of cartilage and bone formation. *Curr. Opin. Cell Biol.* **2001**, *13*, 721–727. [CrossRef]
73. Guilak, F.; Pferdehirt, L.; Ross, A.K.; Choi, Y.; Collins, K.; Nims, R.J.; Katz, D.B.; Klimak, M.; Tabbaa, S.; Pham, C.T.N. Designer Stem Cells: Genome Engineering and the Next Generation of Cell-Based Therapies. *J. Orthop. Res.* **2019**, *37*, 1287–1293. [CrossRef] [PubMed]
74. García-Álvarez, F.; Alegre-Aguarón, E.; Desportes, P.; Royo-Cañas, M.; Castiella, T.; Larrad, L.; Martínez-Lorenzo, M.J. Chondrogenic differentiation in femoral bone marrow-derived mesenchymal cells (MSC) from elderly patients suffering osteoarthritis or femoral fracture. *Arch. Gerontol. Geriatr.* **2011**, *52*, 239–242. [CrossRef]
75. Tuan, R.S.; Boland, G.; Tuli, R. Adult mesenchymal stem cells and cell-based tissue engineering. *Arthritis Res. Ther.* **2003**, *5*, 1–4. [CrossRef]
76. Fellows, C.R.; Matta, C.; Zakany, R.; Khan, I.M.; Mobasheri, A. Adipose, bone marrow and synovial joint-derived mesenchymal stem cells for cartilage repair. *Front. Genet.* **2016**, *7*, 213. [CrossRef]
77. Wang, H.; Leng, Y.; Gong, Y. Bone Marrow Fat and Hematopoiesis. *Front. Endocrinol.* **2018**, *9*, 694. [CrossRef]
78. O'Donoghue, K.; Fisk, N.M. Fetal stem cells. *Best Pract. Res. Clin. Obstet. Gynaecol.* **2004**, *18*, 853–875. [CrossRef]
79. Choi, W.H.; Kim, H.R.; Lee, S.J.; Jeong, N.; Park, S.R.; Choi, B.H.; Min, B.H. Fetal cartilage-derived cells have stem cell properties and are a highly potent cell source for cartilage regeneration. *Cell Transpl.* **2016**, *25*, 449–461. [CrossRef]
80. Park, D.Y.; Min, B.H.; Park, S.R.; Oh, H.J.; Truong, M.D.; Kim, M.; Choi, J.Y.; Park, I.S.; Choi, B.H. Engineered cartilage utilizing fetal cartilage-derived progenitor cells for cartilage repair. *Sci. Rep.* **2020**, *10*, 5722. [CrossRef]
81. Zhang, R.; Ma, J.; Han, J.; Zhang, W.; Ma, J. Mesenchymal stem cell related therapies for cartilage lesions and osteoarthritis. *Am. J. Transl. Res.* **2019**, *11*, 6275. [PubMed]
82. McGonagle, D.; Baboolal, T.G.; Jones, E. Native joint-resident mesenchymal stem cells for cartilage repair in osteoarthritis. *Nat. Rev. Rheumatol.* **2017**, *13*, 719–730. [CrossRef] [PubMed]
83. Jo, C.H.; Lee, Y.G.; Shin, W.H.; Kim, H.; Chai, J.W.; Jeong, E.C.; Kim, J.E.; Shim, H.; Shin, J.S.; Shin, I.S.; et al. Intra-articular injection of mesenchymal stem cells for the treatment of osteoarthritis of the knee: A proof-of-concept clinical trial. *Stem Cells* **2014**, *32*, 1254–1266. [CrossRef] [PubMed]
84. Damia, E.; Chicharro, D.; Lopez, S.; Cuervo, B.; Rubio, M.; Sopena, J.J.; Vilar, J.M.; Carrillo, J.M. Adipose-derived mesenchymal stem cells: Are they a good therapeutic strategy for osteoarthritis? *Int. J. Mol. Sci.* **2018**, *19*, 1926. [CrossRef]
85. Lee, W.Y.-w.; Wang, B. Cartilage repair by mesenchymal stem cells: Clinical trial update and perspectives. *J. Orthop. Transl.* **2017**, *9*, 76–88. [CrossRef]
86. Gee, P.; Lung, M.S.Y.; Okuzaki, Y.; Sasakawa, N.; Iguchi, T.; Makita, Y.; Hozumi, H.; Miura, Y.; Yang, L.F.; Iwasaki, M.; et al. Extracellular nanovesicles for packaging of CRISPR-Cas9 protein and sgRNA to induce therapeutic exon skipping. *Nat. Commun.* **2020**, *11*, 1–18. [CrossRef]
87. de Jong, O.G.; Murphy, D.E.; Mäger, I.; Willms, E.; Garcia-Guerra, A.; Gitz-Francois, J.J.; Lefferts, J.; Gupta, D.; Steenbeek, S.C.; van Rheenen, J.; et al. A CRISPR-Cas9-based reporter system for single-cell detection of extracellular vesicle-mediated functional transfer of RNA. *Nat. Commun.* **2020**, *11*, 1–3.
88. Campbell, L.A.; Coke, L.M.; Richie, C.T.; Fortuno, L.V.; Park, A.Y.; Harvey, B.K. Gesicle-Mediated Delivery of CRISPR/Cas9 Ribonucleoprotein Complex for Inactivating the HIV Provirus. *Mol. Ther.* **2019**, *27*, 151–163. [CrossRef]

89. Murphy, D.E.; de Jong, O.G.; Brouwer, M.; Wood, M.J.; Lavieu, G.; Schiffelers, R.M.; Vader, P. Extracellular vesicle-based therapeutics: Natural versus engineered targeting and trafficking. *Exp. Mol. Med.* **2019**, *51*, 1–2. [CrossRef]
90. Ramirez, S.H.; Andrews, A.M.; Paul, D.; Pachter, J.S. Extracellular vesicles: Mediators and biomarkers of pathology along CNS barriers. *Fluids Barriers CNS* **2018**, *15*, 19. [CrossRef]
91. Levy, O.; Zhao, W.; Mortensen, L.J.; LeBlanc, S.; Tsang, K.; Fu, M.; Phillips, J.A.; Sagar, V.; Anandakumaran, P.; Ngai, J.; et al. MRNA-engineered mesenchymal stem cells for targeted delivery of interleukin-10 to sites of inflammation. *Blood* **2013**, *122*, e23–e32. [CrossRef] [PubMed]
92. Ragni, E.; Banfi, F.; Barilani, M.; Cherubini, A.; Parazzi, V.; Larghi, P.; Dolo, V.; Bollati, V.; Lazzari, L. Extracellular Vesicle-Shuttled mRNA in Mesenchymal Stem Cell Communication. *Stem Cells* **2017**, *35*, 1093–1105. [CrossRef] [PubMed]
93. Martin-Rufino, J.D.; Espinosa-Lara, N.; Osugui, L.; Sanchez-Guijo, F. Targeting the Immune System with Mesenchymal Stromal Cell-Derived Extracellular Vesicles: What Is the Cargo's Mechanism of Action? *Front. Bioeng. Biotechnol.* **2019**, *7*, 308. [CrossRef] [PubMed]
94. Wang, Y.; Yu, D.; Liu, Z.; Zhou, F.; Dai, J.; Wu, B.; Zhou, J.; Heng, B.C.; Zou, X.H.; Ouyang, H.; et al. Exosomes from embryonic mesenchymal stem cells alleviate osteoarthritis through balancing synthesis and degradation of cartilage extracellular matrix. *Stem Cell Res. Ther.* **2017**, *8*, 189. [CrossRef] [PubMed]
95. Murphy, C.; Withrow, J.; Hunter, M.; Liu, Y.; Tang, Y.L.; Fulzele, S.; Hamrick, M.W. Emerging role of extracellular vesicles in musculoskeletal diseases. *Mol. Aspects Med.* **2018**, *60*, 123–128. [CrossRef]
96. Bellavia, D.; Raimondi, L.; Costa, V.; De Luca, A.; Carina, V.; Maglio, M.; Fini, M.; Alessandro, R.; Giavaresi, G. Engineered exosomes: A new promise for the management of musculoskeletal diseases. *Biochim. Biophys. Acta-Gen. Subj.* **2018**, *1862*, 1893–1901. [CrossRef]
97. Hiemer, B.; Krogull, M.; Bender, T.; Ziebart, J.; Krueger, S.; Bader, R.; Jonitz-Heincke, A. Effect of electric stimulation on human chondrocytes and mesenchymal stem cells under normoxia and hypoxia. *Mol. Med. Rep.* **2018**, *18*, 2133–2141. [CrossRef]
98. Lo Monaco, M.; Merckx, G.; Ratajczak, J.; Gervois, P.; Hilkens, P.; Clegg, P.; Bronckaers, A.; Vandeweerd, J.M.; Lambrichts, I. Stem Cells for Cartilage Repair: Preclinical Studies and Insights in Translational Animal Models and Outcome Measures. *Stem Cells Int.* **2018**, *2018*. [CrossRef]
99. De Bari, C.; Roelofs, A.J. Stem cell-based therapeutic strategies for cartilage defects and osteoarthritis. *Curr. Opin. Pharmacol.* **2018**, *40*, 74–80. [CrossRef]
100. Fernandes, T.L.; Kimura, H.A.; Pinheiro, C.C.G.; Shimomura, K.; Nakamura, N.; Ferreira, J.R.; Gomoll, A.H.; Hernandez, A.J.; Bueno, D.F. Human synovial mesenchymal stem cells good manufacturing practices for articular cartilage regeneration. *Tissue Eng.-Part C Methods* **2018**, *24*, 709–716. [CrossRef]
101. Cosenza, S.; Ruiz, M.; Toupet, K.; Jorgensen, C.; Noël, D. Mesenchymal stem cells derived exosomes and microparticles protect cartilage and bone from degradation in osteoarthritis. *Sci. Rep.* **2017**, *7*, 1–2. [CrossRef] [PubMed]
102. Cosenza, S.; Ruiz, M.; Toupet, K.; Bony, C.; Jorgensen, C.; Noel, D. Mesenchymal stem cells produced exosomes and microparticles that exert a similar chondroprotective effect in osteoarthritis. *Osteoarthr. Cartil.* **2018**, *26*, S297. [CrossRef]
103. Farhang, N.; Brunger, J.M.; Stover, J.D.; Thakore, P.I.; Lawrence, B.; Guilak, F.; Gersbach, C.A.; Setton, L.A.; Bowles, R.D. CRISPR-Based Epigenome Editing of Cytokine Receptors for the Promotion of Cell Survival and Tissue Deposition in Inflammatory Environments. *Tissue Eng. Part A* **2017**, *23*, 738–749. [CrossRef] [PubMed]
104. Matsukawa, A.; Yoshinaga, M. Sequential generation of cytokines during the initiative phase of inflammation, with reference to neutrophils. *Inflammation Reearchs* **1998**, *47* (Suppl. 3), S137–S144. [CrossRef]
105. Cigan, A.D.; Roach, B.L.; Nims, R.J.; Tan, A.R.; Albro, M.B.; Stoker, A.M.; Cook, J.L.; Vunjak-Novakovic, G.; Hung, C.T.; Ateshian, G.A. High seeding density of human chondrocytes in agarose produces tissue-engineered cartilage approaching native mechanical and biochemical properties. *J. Biomech.* **2016**, *49*, 1909–1917. [CrossRef]
106. Karlsen, T.A.; Pernas, P.F.; Staerk, J.; Caglayan, S.; Brinchmann, J.E. Generation of IL1β-resistant chondrocytes using CRISPR-CAS genome editing. *Osteoarthr. Cartil.* **2016**, *24*, S325. [CrossRef]

107. Lambert, L.J.; Challa, A.K.; Niu, A.; Zhou, L.; Tucholski, J.; Johnson, M.S.; Nagy, T.R.; Eberhardt, A.W.; Estep, P.N.; Kesterson, R.A.; et al. Increased trabecular bone and improved biomechanics in an osteocalcin-null rat model created by CRISPR/Cas9 technology. *DMM Dis. Model. Mech.* **2016**, *9*, 1169–1179. [CrossRef]
108. Asahara, H. Current Status and Strategy of microRNA Research for Cartilage Development and Osteoarthritis Pathogenesis. *J. Bone Metab.* **2016**, *23*, 121–127. [CrossRef]
109. Huang, Y.; Askew, E.B.; Knudson, C.B.; Knudson, W. CRISPR/Cas9 knockout of HAS2 in rat chondrosarcoma chondrocytes demonstrates the requirement of hyaluronan for aggrecan retention. *Matrix Biol.* **2016**, *56*, 74–94. [CrossRef]
110. Brunger, J.M.; Zutshi, A.; Willard, V.P.; Gersbach, C.A.; Guilak, F. Genome Engineering of Stem Cells for Autonomously Regulated, Closed-Loop Delivery of Biologic Drugs. *Stem Cell Rep.* **2017**, *8*, 1202–1213. [CrossRef]
111. Khakshooy, A.; Balenton, N.; Chiappelli, F. Lubricin: A Principal Modulator of the Psychoneuroendocrine-Osteoimmune Interactome-Implications for Novel Treatments of Osteoarthritic Pathologies. *Bioinformation* **2017**, *13*, 343–346. [CrossRef] [PubMed]
112. Rice, S.J.; Aubourg, G.; Sorial, A.K.; Almarza, D.; Tselepi, M.; Deehan, D.J.; Reynard, L.N.; Loughlin, J. Identification of a novel, methylation-dependent, RUNX2 regulatory region associated with osteoarthritis risk. *Hum. Mol. Genet.* **2018**, *27*, 3464–3474. [CrossRef] [PubMed]
113. Ye, Y.; Baek, S.-H.; Ye, Y.; Zhang, T. Proteomic characterization of endogenous substrates of mammalian ubiquitin ligase Hrd1. *Cell Biosci.* **2018**, *8*, 46. [CrossRef] [PubMed]
114. Seidl, C.I.; Fulga, T.A.; Murphy, C.L. CRISPR-Cas9 targeting of MMP13 in human chondrocytes leads to significantly reduced levels of the metalloproteinase and enhanced type II collagen accumulation. *Osteoarthr. Cartil.* **2019**, *27*, 140–147. [CrossRef]
115. Varela-Eirín, M.; Varela-Vázquez, A.; Guitián-Caamaño, A.; Paíno, C.L.; Mato, V.; Largo, R.; Aasen, T.; Tabernero, A.; Fonseca, E.; Kandouz, M.; et al. Targeting of chondrocyte plasticity via connexin43 modulation attenuates cellular senescence and fosters a pro-regenerative environment in osteoarthritis. *Cell Death Dis.* **2018**, *9*, 1–6. [CrossRef] [PubMed]
116. Ren, X.; Hu, B.; Song, M.; Ding, Z.; Dang, Y.; Liu, Z.; Zhang, W.; Ji, Q.; Ren, R.; Ding, J.; et al. Maintenance of Nucleolar Homeostasis by CBX4 Alleviates Senescence and Osteoarthritis. *Cell Rep.* **2019**, *26*, 3643–3656. [CrossRef] [PubMed]
117. Fu, L.; Hu, Y.; Song, M.; Liu, Z.; Zhang, W.; Yu, F.X.; Wu, J.; Wang, S.; Belmonte, J.C.I.; Chan, P.; et al. Up-regulation of FOXD1 by yap alleviates senescence and osteoarthritis. *PLoS Biol.* **2019**, *17*, e3000201. [CrossRef]
118. Nishimasu, H.; Shi, X.; Ishiguro, S.; Gao, L.; Hirano, S.; Okazaki, S.; Noda, T.; Abudayyeh, O.O.; Gootenberg, J.S.; Mori, H.; et al. Engineered CRISPR-Cas9 nuclease with expanded targeting space. *Science* **2018**, *361*, 1259–1262. [CrossRef]
119. O'Brien, J.; Hayder, H.; Zayed, Y.; Peng, C. Overview of microRNA biogenesis, mechanisms of actions, and circulation. *Front. Endocrinol.* **2018**, *9*, 402. [CrossRef]
120. Ramos, Y.F.M.; Meulenbelt, I. The role of epigenetics in osteoarthritis: Current perspective. *Curr. Opin. Rheumatol.* **2017**, *29*, 119–129. [CrossRef]

International Journal of
Molecular Sciences

MDPI

Review

Genetic Polymorphisms Associated with Rheumatoid Arthritis Development and Antirheumatic Therapy Response

Dmitry S. Mikhaylenko [1,2,*], Marina V. Nemtsova [1,2], Irina V. Bure [1], Ekaterina B. Kuznetsova [1,2], Ekaterina A. Alekseeva [1,2], Vadim V. Tarasov [3], Alexander N. Lukashev [1,4], Marina I. Beloukhova [1], Andrei A. Deviatkin [1] and Andrey A. Zamyatnin, Jr. [1,5,*]

1 Institute of Molecular Medicine, Sechenov First Moscow State Medical University (Sechenov University), 119991 Moscow, Russia; nemtsova_m_v@mail.ru (M.V.N.); bureira@mail.ru (I.V.B.); kuznetsova.k@bk.ru (E.B.K.); ekater.alekseeva@gmail.com (E.A.A.); alexander_lukashev@hotmail.com (A.N.L.); beloukhovamarina@gmail.com (M.I.B.); andreideviatkin@gmail.com (A.A.D.)

2 Laboratory of Epigenetics, Research Centre for Medical Genetics, 115478 Moscow, Russia

3 Department of Pharmacology and Pharmacy, Sechenov First Moscow State Medical University, 119991 Moscow, Russia; tarasov-v-v@mail.ru

4 Martsinovsky Institute of Medical Parasitology, Tropical and Vector Borne Diseases, Sechenov First Moscow State Medical University, 119435 Moscow, Russia

5 Belozersky Institute of Physico-Chemical Biology, Lomonosov Moscow State University, 119992 Moscow, Russia

* Correspondence: dimserg@mail.ru (D.S.M.); zamyat@belozersky.msu.ru (A.A.Z.J.)

Received: 17 June 2020; Accepted: 9 July 2020; Published: 11 July 2020

Abstract: Rheumatoid arthritis (RA) is the most common inflammatory arthropathy worldwide. Possible manifestations of RA can be represented by a wide variability of symptoms, clinical forms, and course options. This multifactorial disease is triggered by a genetic predisposition and environmental factors. Both clinical and genealogical studies have demonstrated disease case accumulation in families. Revealing the impact of candidate gene missense variants on the disease course elucidates understanding of RA molecular pathogenesis. A multivariate genomewide association study (GWAS) based analysis identified the genes and signalling pathways involved in the pathogenesis of the disease. However, these identified RA candidate gene variants only explain 30% of familial disease cases. The genetic causes for a significant proportion of familial RA have not been determined until now. Therefore, it is important to identify RA risk groups in different populations, as well as the possible prognostic value of some genetic variants for disease development, progression, and treatment. Our review has two purposes. First, to summarise the data on RA candidate genes and the increased disease risk associated with these alleles in various populations. Second, to describe how the genetic variants can be used in the selection of drugs for the treatment of RA.

Keywords: rheumatoid arthritis; polymorphism; genetic predisposition; mutation; methotrexate; interleukin; targeted therapy

1. Introduction

Rheumatoid arthritis (RA) is a chronic autoinflammatory disease affecting connective tissue, characterised by progressive joint damage and specific systemic disorders. To date, the number of patients with autoimmune arthritis is almost 1% of the world's population, establishing an urgent problem for healthcare systems worldwide. An evident feature of RA is clinical polymorphism, represented by a wide variability of symptoms, clinical forms, and progression rates. RA is considered to be a multifactorial disease triggered by a genetic predisposition and environmental factors. Both clinical and genealogical studies have shown that the disease can accumulate in families. This relationship has been confirmed by modern molecular genetics. The opportunity to identify RA risk groups in different populations, as well as the possible prognostic value of some genetic variants for disease development, progression, and treatment, including a personalised antirheumatic therapy response, has promoted new studies of germline genetic variants in RA patients [1,2]. This review has two purposes. First, to summarise the data on the RA candidate genes in various populations and the increased disease risk associated with those alleles. Second, to describe how the genetic variants can be used in the selection of drugs such as methotrexate, interleukin-6 signalling pathway inhibitors or TNF (tumor necrosis factor) inhibitors for the treatment of RA. Papers in the PubMed and Scopus databases published in 2010–2020, as well as clinical recommendations and information materials from the American College of Rheumatology and the European League Against Rheumatism, were analysed to understand the current state in this field. A total of 125 sources were selected, of which 96 are mentioned in this review.

2. Genetic Predisposition for Rheumatoid Arthritis

The mechanisms for RA development are similar to those of other autoimmune diseases—an immune response to the patient's self-proteins develops, which drives a cascade of proinflammatory signalling pathways and activates the production of corresponding cytokines and chemokines. In some cases, rheumatoid factor (RF) and anticitrullinated protein antibodies (ACPAs) can be found in patients before any clinical manifestations of RA. Proposed in 2010, the RA classification is based on the presence of ACPAs, found in 90% of patients. These antibodies are considered as more distinctive immunological markers of RA than others, while citrulline compounds seem to play an important role in the disease pathogenesis [3,4].

Unfavourable alleles of various genes have a relatively small influence on the disease risk when they appear individually, but in combination, they genetically predispose an individual to RA development. Currently, more than 100 loci associated with RA have been described [5]. These changes can also be found in genes whose products are not directly involved in immune reactions. The variants associated with RA pathogenesis can be found in a wide range of genes that mediate cell signalling pathways.

2.1. *Role of HLA Genes in Rheumatoid Arthritis Development*

Based on data from the genomewide association study (GWAS), the main genes for RA predisposition belong to the major histocompatibility complex (MHC) locus. This locus, spanning 4 Mbp, occurs in the 6p21.3 region and contains about 250 genes coding the antigen proteins for T-cell recognition. Up to 60% of possible polymorphisms (genetic variants) responsible for RA susceptibility are considered to arise from the MHC locus [6]. For instance, HLA-DRB1 alleles encode unfavourable variants of the shared epitope (SE), which is critical for the correct T-cell antigen presentation process. Eighteen percent of the ACPA-positive and 2.4% of the ACPA-negative RA hereditary component is associated with these alleles. Predisposing HLA-DRB1 SE alleles are found in 64–70% of RA patients and 55% of their healthy relatives, while only being found in 35% of the average population [7].

Sequencing of the HLA-DRB1 alleles encoding the polymorphic β-chain of the DR molecule shows a prevalence of *04:01 and *04:04 alleles in RA patients in Europe and the *04:05 allele in East Asia. Alleles *04:02 and *04:03 are shown to be protective. Based on these data, the hypothesis of the importance of the conserved epitope structure, which forms the third β-chain hypervariable region (positions p.70-74) for RA development, was postulated: whether it contains the unfavourable variants, i.e., QKRAA, QQRAA, KKRAA, QRRAA, RRRAA, or, on the contrary, the protective structure of DERAA. Moreover, amino acid substitutions at positions 11 and 13 of DR4 are also associated with RA (alleles *04:01/*04:04/*04:05 compared to DR1 *01:01) [1,8,9]. Association of the ACPAs and the hypervariable epitope alleles indicates the role of these variants in the T-cell presentation of citrullinated proteins and the further development of autoreactivity. In addition, some of the specific positions of amino acid residues suggest their participation in HLA-DR intracellular transport. Citrulline residues are located inside the DRB1*04:01/04 positively charged P4 pocket of the peptides but not in the negatively charged P4 pocket (encoded by the protective allele *04:02), as shown by model experiments and crystal structure analysis. Namely, the P4 amino acid residues at positions 13 and 71 directly interact with the citrulline, so their alterations are believed to be the most relevant for RA development [10,11].

As noted above, polymorphisms leading to substitutions of amino acid residues at positions 11, 13, 71, and 74 of HLA-DRB1, as well as at position 9 in HLA-B and HLA-DPB1, have the greatest association with RA development. These residues are faced towards the protein pocket to bind the antigen in HLA molecules. These relations are more evident in African Americans and Asians compared to Caucasians. In contrast, HLA-DR3 associations, mainly the protective role of the HLA-DRB1*13 haplotype (five amino acid residues of the "wildtype" DERAA at positions 70–74), are shown in European populations. Individuals of such a haplotype have a decreased number of autoreactive T-cells, presumably due to their negative thymus selection [6]. Associations with HLA-DRB1 alleles at position 57 rather than 71–74 are shown in African populations [12]. Thus, the main critical site related to RA development in different populations of both Caucasians and Asians is the 13th amino acid residue. This position substitution increases its pathogenic effect as follows: Ser < Gly ≤ Tyr < Arg < Phe < His [8]

The observed data explain the hypervariable epitope and its polymorphism roles in the development of RA with ACPA formation. However, HLA-RA associations are shown in the absence of ACPAs as well. The DRB1*03:01 allele associated with ACRA-negative RA was found in Europeans, but not Japanese, in whom HLA-DR8 and DR14 homozygotes are associated with the disease. In addition, DRB1*03 (serine at position 11) and HLA-B*08 (aspartic acid at position 9) alleles are associated with ACPA-negative RA regardless of population. Hence, RA is not only clinically but also genetically a heterogeneous disease [13].

In general, RA-associated amino acid positions are located in the middle of the HLA molecules epitope-binding pockets; thus, the substitutions can directly affect antigenic specificity and result in protein binding to the citrulline residues. In discrepancy with the Hardy–Weinberg ratio, heterozygotes are more common in patients with RA (they have a greater predisposition to ACPA-positive RA). This could be due to a wider range of exposed autoantigens compared to homozygotes [14]. Citrullinated proteins are seen as foreign antigens. This complies with the confirmed hypotheses of neoantigens (i.e., peptides with citrulline residues), as well as with the assumption that the calreticulin signalling pathway and the low-affinity HLA-DR molecules carrying SE epitopes for class II-associated invariant chain peptides (CLIPs) are involved in RA pathogenesis [10,15].

In addition to the HLA-DRB1 alleles, other loci have also been associated with RA development, particularly the *04 allele of the DQB1 locus, as revealed by meta-analysis [16]. It is not only the polymorphisms predisposed to RA that are of interest to professionals in rheumatology, but also those associated with disease prognosis and the severity of the disease. Thus, the HLA-DRB1*08, HLA-DRB1*11, and HLA-DPB1*02:01 alleles are associated with oligoarticular RA—no more than 4 points, according to the International League of Associations for Rheumatology (ILAR) classification. Polyarticular RA (5 points or more) is associated with the HLA-DRB1*11:01 and HLA-DRB1*11:04 alleles [10]. At the same time, a meta-analysis of 2775 RA cases showed the association between HLA-DRB1*04:01 polymorphism and the degree of joint damage [17]. The combination of HLA gene alleles predisposed to RA predetermines the genetic component for the development of this disease. At the same time, many other genes encoding enzymes, receptors, and auxiliary proteins may affect the severity of the clinical manifestations and the development of RA [18].

2.2. Polymorphisms of Non-HLA Genes Associated with Rheumatoid Arthritis

Genes for the predisposition to RA can be conditionally divided into groups of cytokines and their receptors, chemokines and their receptors, key components of intracellular signalling pathways and auxiliary (costimulating) factors.

2.2.1. Cytokines and Cytokine Receptors

A significant number of RA-associated genetic variants have been identified in the interleukins (ILs) and their receptor genes. Interleukins are cytokines that stimulate hematopoietic cell development and T- and B-lymphocyte differentiation. There are seven interleukin families characterised by significant variability in both ligand forms and receptors. The key mediator of inflammation, IL1, is represented by two isoforms and is combined with another nine interleukins in one family. Its expression is affected by the –511A/G (rs16944) polymorphism in the promoter (associated with RA in Caucasians) and the +3953C/T polymorphism in exon 5 (RA-associated in some Asian populations). According to meta-analyses, RA-associated alleles in Caucasians include –174G/C and –572G/C of the *IL6* gene, rs1800896 in the *IL10* gene, rs13151961 and rs6822844 located near the *IL2* and *IL21* genes, rs7530511 and rs11209026 in the *IL23R* gene, and some others. A significant number of RA-associated polymorphic loci included in the meta-analyses are unique to Asian populations. The polymorphism found at rs1946518 of the *IL18* gene is found in Egyptian populations, and the polymorphism found at rs549908 is found in the Taiwanese population. Thus the candidate genes for assessing genetic RA predisposition need to be thoroughly selected [19–22].

Another candidate gene is *IL2RA*, which encodes the interleukin 2 (IL2) receptor α-subunit. The rs12722495 polymorphism of this gene correlates with its mRNA and protein expression in stimulated monocytes, naive T-cells, and memory T-cells [6]. Additionally, according to a meta-analysis of 37 studies, a minor allele A of the rs1343151 polymorphism in the IL23R gene, which encodes the receptor for interleukin 23, is associated with a risk of developing RA [23].

2.2.2. Chemokines and Chemokine Receptors

Changes in the *CCR6* gene can affect the development of RA. This gene encodes the chemokine receptor, which is the surface marker of Th17 cells. Dinucleotide polymorphism rs3093024 in the 5′ regulatory sequence of CCR6 binds nuclear proteins. This polymorphism is associated with expression levels of the chemokine receptor and increased plasma concentration of IL17 cytokine in RA patients. The role of the CCR6 receptor in RA development appears to be more significant than previously known due to its expression on different subtypes of T-cells involved in the regulation of inflammation. According to a meta-analysis, rs3093024 and several other SNPs (single nucleotide polymorphism) in *CCR6* are associated with RA in European and Asian populations [6,24]. At the same time, a 32-bp deletion in another chemokine receptor gene, *CCR5*, has a protective effect, according to a case–control study in Brazil with samples of 740 RA patients and 676 controls [25].

The *CCL2* gene encodes the chemoattractant protein, which recruits monocytes and T-cells during inflammation. A meta-analysis of the functionally significant 2518A/G polymorphism of this gene promoter on chromosome 17 was performed. This polymorphism was studied for associations with various autoimmune diseases (systemic lupus erythematosus, RA, systemic sclerosis, nephropathy with Ig-A, Crohn's disease) in different populations. The unfavourable allele A showed the most pronounced association with RA in Asian populations, as well as with Crohn's disease in Europeans [26].

2.2.3. Components of Intracellular Pathways That Regulate Proliferation

A number of RA candidate genes are involved in the NF-κB signalling pathway. One of the *CD40* alleles, which is also an RA candidate gene, is associated with increased expression of CD40 molecules on the surface of B-cells and intensified NF-κB signalling. Another RA candidate gene is *TNFAIP3*, which encodes a component of the NF-κB signalling pathway—the A20 ubiquitin-modifying enzyme. These independent gene polymorphisms associated with RA were identified by meta-analyses. One of them—the TT > A substitution located a 42-kb distance from the promoter—reduces the binding avidity of NF-κB signalling pathway transcription factors, leading to decreased TNFAIP3 and A20 protein expression. Another possible SNP is the replacement of phenylalanine with cysteine at the 127 position, which disturbs the A20 function. Interestingly, A20 is often inactivated due to somatic mutations in B-cell lymphoma. The *TNFAIP3* gene is located in the 6q23 region. Besides the *TNFAIP3* gene, this region contains plenty of autoimmune disease candidate genes: *IL20RA*, *IFNGR*, *OLIG3* and others [27,28].

Involved in the JAK/STAT pathway, the *STAT4* gene was identified as a candidate gene for RA and other autoimmune diseases as a result of GWAS. *STAT4* encodes the signal transducer and activator of transcription protein 4 (STAT4). The rs7574865 polymorphism of the *STAT4* gene is associated with RA in different ethnic populations. The STAT family proteins act as JAK-activated transcription factors and are important in many cytokines signalling pathways, primarily the interferon pathways. Detected unfavourable rs7574865 alleles were associated with STAT4 overexpression and increased production of interferon-α [29]. STAT4 transcription factors are also involved in the regulation of proinflammatory helper T-cell (Th1, Th2, Th17) differentiation, of which Th1 and Th17 are directly involved in autoimmune reactions [6,19,29].

2.2.4. Genes That Encode Costimulatory Molecules

Some of the most significant RA candidate genes are enzymes or costimulating auxiliary proteins that are important for the metabolism of immunocompetent cells, although not directly involved in the formation of the immune response. For instance, a missense mutation in exon 14 of the *PTPN22* gene leads to the arginine/tryptophan replacement at the 620 position of the polypeptide chain (p. R620W, rs2476601) [30]. This R620W substitution is localised in the motif responsible for the interaction of cofactor proteins and could mediate an increase in autoreactive B-cell numbers during the experiment. This replacement is not only associated with RA but other autoimmune diseases as well, namely, systemic lupus erythematosus, type 1 diabetes, and Graves' disease (European populations only; the site is usually not polymorphic in Asians). The *PTPN22* gene encodes lymphocyte tyrosine phosphatase, and the mentioned substitution acts as a gain of function mutation. A detailed study of the normal and mutant alleles' functions in model experiments revealed unexpected difficulties—the homologous 619W mutation in mice acts as a loss of function mutation that is identical to the full knockout of the orthologous gene [6,19,30]. According to a recent meta-analysis of 53 original case–control studies, the polymorphism rs2476601 is associated with RA development in homozygous and heterozygous models in Caucasians and Africans [31]. In addition, the C allele of rs2488457 is associated with RA progress in Caucasians but not in Asians [32]. PTPN22 interacts with the product of *PADI4*, another RA candidate gene encoding peptidyl arginine deaminase. This enzyme converts arginine amino acid residues into citrulline, and a disturbance of this process can contribute to anticitrulline antibody formation. Increased PADI4 activity leading to abnormal citrullination of fibrin strands is noted in inflammatory infiltrate. In addition, it is known that PADI enzyme expression is increased and citrullinated peptides are found in the bronchoalveolar lavage cells of smokers compared to nonsmokers. Smoking is considered an RA-provoking environmental factor that contributes to the multifactorial basis for disease development [33]. The *PADI4* gene located in the 1p36 region was the first RA candidate gene identified in the Asian population. Unfavourable substitutions of the *PADI4* codons—G55S, V82A and G112A—do not significantly affect the activity of the enzyme itself but reduces the gene's mRNA stability. A meta-analysis of the SNP gene in 20,000 RA patients and 25,000 controls determined the associations of the disease with the –94G/A polymorphism in Asian populations, the –92C/G polymorphism in African populations, and the —90C/T polymorphism in Latin populations. Interestingly, the PTPN22 and PADI4 interaction most likely has a functional significance since PTPN22 deficiency leads to an increased production of citrulline compounds and the formation of extracellular neutrophilic traps [6,27,34].

The autoimmune regulator transcription factor (AIRE), with its 11 polymorphic variants studied in autoimmune diseases, should also be noted. The association of rs2075876 and rs760426 of *AIRE* gene polymorphisms with RA was shown by the meta-analysis, which included a total of 6696 RA patients and 8164 controls. The polymorphisms were localised in the gene promoter; the presence of unfavourable alleles reduced gene expression. A lack of AIRE protein led to the failure of naive T-cell specific selection in the thymus, resulting in autoimmune T-cell survival [35]. Thus, specific polymorphisms associated with the disease as predisposition factors in various populations and heterogeneous clinical groups, according to a number of meta-analyses, could be distinguished among the large number of genetic variants related to RA. The main RA-predisposing polymorphisms are presented in Table 1.

Table 1. Polymorphisms (non-HLA genes) associated with rheumatoid arthritis (RA) in mixed populations according to meta-analyses data.

Protein Product	Gene	Polymorphism	Allele/Genotype Associated with RA	Reference
Protein tyrosine phosphatase, nonreceptor type 22	*PTPN22*	rs2476601 rs2488457	T C	[30–32,36]
Peptidyl arginine deiminase 4	*PADI4*	rs11203367 rs884871 rs2240340	T G A	[37]
Tumor necrosis factor, alpha-induced protein 3 (A20)	*TNFAIP3*	rs2230926 rs5029937	G T	[28]
Cytotoxic T-lymphocyte associated protein 4	*CTLA4*	rs231775	GG	[38]
Signal transducer and activator of transcription 4	*STAT4*	rs7574865	T	[29]
C-C motif chemokine receptor 6	*CCR6*	rs3093024	A	[24]
C-C motif chemokine ligand 2 (monocytes chemo-attractant)	*CCL2*	rs1024611	G	[39]
Autoimmune regulator (transcription factor)	*AIRE*	rs2075876 rs760426	A G	[35]
Methylene tetrahydrofolate reductase	*MTHFR*	rs1801133 rs1801131	T CC	[40,41]
Interleukin 10	*IL10*	rs1800896 rs3021097 rs1800872	AA TT AA	[42]
Interleukin 23 receptor	*IL23R*	rs11209026 rs10489629 rs1343151	AA G A	[23,43]
Interleukin 17	*IL17*	rs2275913	AA	[44]
Tumour necrosis factor receptor type 2	*TNFR2*	rs1061622	GG	[45]
Transforming growth factor beta and its receptors	*TGFB*	rs1800470 rs1800469	TT TT	[46]

Some of the candidate genes and polymorphic variants are not directly related to cytokines and intracellular signalling pathways that enhance inflammatory processes. However, polymorphisms in such genes may change the activity of the protein product, which leads to the accumulation of certain metabolites and the subsequent overproduction of proinflammatory cytokines. For example, a meta-analysis shows the association of intron SNP in the *SLC8A3* gene encoding a Na^+/Ca^+ transmembrane transfer protein with ACPA-positive RA. However, there is evidence that this carrier protein hyperactivity may be accompanied by an increased level of tumour necrosis factor alpha (TNFα) [47]. The *MTHFR* gene encodes methylenetetrahydrofolate reductase, promoting the homocysteine to methionine conversion that is important for folate metabolism and the synthesis of nucleic acids. According to the meta-analysis, the T-allele of the C677T polymorphism (rs1801133) is associated with RA in Caucasians. This allele encodes an enzyme with reduced activity that leads to hyperhomocysteinemia in homozygotes, which results in an increase in proinflammatory cytokine concentration [40]. Moreover, according to a meta-analysis of 16 original studies published in 2020, C677T is associated with RA in the dominant and recessive models in Caucasians and Africans, and in the recessive model in Asians [41]. In addition, a meta-analysis of eight papers demonstrated the association of TIM3 with RA development. This gene encodes the auxiliary factor expressed by dendritic cells, macrophages, type 1 T-helper, and type 2 T-helper cells. TIM3 modulates the differentiation of type 1 T-helper and type 17 T-helper cells, which suppress autoimmune processes. The polymorphism rs1036199 in TIM3 is associated with RA development [48].

3. Predisposition to RA Depends on the Method of Analysis of Genes and Population Characteristics

Candidate gene missense variant impact studies have led to a greater understanding of the molecular pathogenesis of RA. A multivariate GWAS-based analysis identified the genes and signalling pathways involved in the pathogenesis of the disease. However, these identified RA candidate gene variants only explain 30% of the disease cases with family accumulation, while the actual family prevalence among all RA patients reaches 65% [1,14,18]. The genetic causes of a significant proportion of familial RA have not been identified until now. Perhaps high-performance sequencing technology—high-throughput sequencing (HTS)—will help to solve this problem in the near future. The list of unfavourable alleles has already been supplemented with missense variants of the *IL2RA* and *IL2RB* genes by the first HTS experiments. By the in-silico constructing of an interactome between the already known RA candidate genes, about 160 other presumptive candidates were identified. Subsequently, a number of them were considered RA-associated according to the GWAS results: the *NOTCH4* gene, the *TNXB* gene located near the MHC class III genes, the *BTNL2* gene (especially rs3817963; also associated with systemic sarcoidosis), as well as the insufficiently characterised sequence C6orf10, expressed in autoimmune and some other diseases [49].

The population genetics characteristic, as well as the results of previous meta-analyses, need to be taken into account when using GWAS and HTS technologies. A list of the main predisposing RA genes identified in Latin American populations is an example of such research. The list was mostly formed based on the results of studies done between 2003 and 2013, and it is consistent with similar lists of European populations. This could be explained by a significant proportion of Spanish origin RA patients amongst all of the examined patients. At the same time, the RA candidate genes attributable to Latin American populations have only been described in recent years, such as *ENOX1* on chromosome 13 and *NNA25* on chromosome 12 [7].

SNPs occur in no more than 1% of the coding part of the genome; most of them are localised in noncoding DNA. Single RA-associated nucleotide substitutions have been detected near the noncoding regions of 40–50 genes. At least some of them are suggested to increase RA risk by means of the activation of tissue-specific superenhancers. Thus, polymorphic variants associated with RA are mainly localised in the T-cell and natural killer enhancers compared to the other cell types, according to the FANTOM5 consortium (contains information for 71 cell type tissue-specific enhancers). In addition, SNPs associated with RA and other autoimmune diseases are more likely to occur in superenhancers than in "regular" enhancer regions of $CD4^{+}$ T-cells [50]. These superenhancers are associated with 27 of the 100 major RA candidate genes. Moreover, 12 loci have shown an association with RA according to GWAS and contained long noncoding RNA genes that regulate the expression of other candidate genes. RA-associated SNPs of noncoding regions are often found in candidate gene enhancer regions. Therefore, a number of functionally significant polymorphisms could be identified by reverse genetics methods. Some authors have searched for SNPs in regulatory regions of genes using data on its expression changes. The RA association of rs2013109 in the *RNASE2* gene was shown this way [51]. Currently, the search for RA candidate genes is performed by bioinformatic analysis of published expression profiles obtained with high-density microchip technology (for instance, Affymetrix) [52–55]. Whole-genome or whole-exome sequencing, utilising high-performance HTS platforms, could also help to identify rare and population-specific pathogenic genetic variants. In particular, rare RA-associated germline variants were identified in the *NCR3LG1*, *RAP1GAP*, *CHCHD5*, *HIPK2*, and *DIAPH2* genes by whole-exome sequencing with Illumina HiSeq in a Han (Chinese ethnic group) patient cohort [56].

The data presented in this section indicate the significant experimental and bioinformatic work performed by researchers in countries all over the world to elucidate the genetic causes of RA development. However, whether the genetic determinants can help in personalising and increasing the effectiveness of RA treatment remains an important question for clinical rheumatology.

4. Genetic Factors are Prognostic Markers Associated with RA Clinical Manifestations

There are currently many genes and loci associated with a predisposition to RA. The identification of genetic markers associated with the clinical prognosis of RA is more difficult than identifying predisposition markers. This is because the severity of the disease depends not only on genetic factors but also on epigenetic changes, as well as the action of provoking environmental factors.

Some genetic factors predisposing to RA can be associated with the intensity of the course of the disease. As such, the genetic variants HLA-DRB1 alleles were identified as associated with radiologically determined joint damage, which is one of the main manifestations of the severity of the disease. Sixteen HLA-DRB1 haplotypes are associated with an increased risk of RA, erosive joint damage, and the patient's lifespan [57]. Valine at position 11 of HLA-DRB1 is a predictor of joint erosion and an unfavourable outcome, whereas serine at the same position is associated with a less severe clinical course of the disease [58]. Besides such modifications, the rs112112734 polymorphism of the HLA-DRB1 gene is also connected with radiologically determined joint damage [17]. In addition, this study showed that rs112112734 is also associated with the presence of rheumatoid factor and ACPAs, which are serological markers of RA.

The IL6 signalling pathway is an important participant in the proinflammatory network of cytokines, which contributes to the destruction of articular tissues. A study of the IL6R gene polymorphism and the extent of joint erosion in RA revealed an association between SNP rs4845618, located in the first intron of the *IL6R* gene, and joint damage. It was shown that rs4845618 is significant for the expression of IL6R in the study of whole blood samples. Using the latest data from the Roadmap Epigenomics Project epigenetic consortia, it has been demonstrated that the SNP rs4845618 localisation region is associated with the regulation of gene activity in more than 50 different types of human cells, including T-cells. This suggests an association between joint damage and the regulatory sequence of the *IL6R* gene [59].

The serum level of another interleukin, IL37, which is one of the key modulators of RA, correlates with disease activity. An analysis of the *IL37* gene rs3811047 polymorphism in patients with RA in the Egyptian Arab population showed that patients with the GG genotype had a higher severity score of lesions on the DAS28 clinical scale than patients with genotypes AA or AG [60]. In another study, the polymorphism rs911263 located inside the *RAD51B* gene was presented as a genetic factor associated with joint erosion and the severity of RA. Allele C rs911263 is associated with a lower incidence of joint erosion in patients with RA [61]. This polymorphism demonstrated a strong protective effect on RA [61]. RAD51B is a member of the RAD51 family of proteins that are required for DNA repair through recombination. It is currently not known how this polymorphism is functionally related to the severity of the clinical manifestations of RA.

Associated with the development of RA in the Korean population and Caucasians, the *UBASH3A* gene [62] is also associated with the intensity of the course of the disease. The C allele of the rs1893592 polymorphism of the *UBASH3A* gene was shown to be protective with respect to RA activity (scores according to DAS28, C-reactive protein level and bone erosion). At the same time, this may be caused by population specificity [63]. The *UBASH3A* gene encodes a protein involved in the degradation of receptor tyrosine kinases, with proapoptotic properties in T-cells, which may explain its involvement in the pathogenesis of RA. It is noteworthy that AA homozygotes at position −308 of the *TNFA* gene also have a pronounced association with both the risk of developing RA and the severity of the clinical picture of this disease [64].

The above examples show that polymorphic variants of RA candidate genes can not only increase the risk of developing a disease but also increase the likelihood of a more severe course of the disease, ceteris paribus. Although their use in clinical practice as markers is impractical due to low penetrance and, in some cases, population specificity, polymorphisms associated with RA activity indicate the molecular pathways underlying the intensive development of RA and the possibilities of targeted therapy of this disease.

5. Genetic Predictors of Response to Rheumatoid Arthritis Drug Therapy

5.1. Therapy of RA with the Use of Antirheumatic Drugs

RA treatment aims to achieve clinical remission and minimal disease activity. The classes of drugs used in RA therapy are known under the common name disease-modifying antirheumatic drugs (DMARDs). Synthetic DMARDs are divided into conventional synthetic DMARDs (csDMARD, for example, methotrexate, leflunomide, sulfasalazine, hydroxychloroquine, and others) and targeted synthetic DMARDs (tsDMARD, for example, baricitinib, tofacitinib, upadacitinib). Biological DMARDs (bDMARDs) comprise the second group of drugs. bDMARDs may be subdivided into distinct classes depending on their targets: TNF inhibitors (adalimumab, certolizumab, etanercept, golimumab, infliximab), IL6 inhibitors (sarilumab, tocilizumab), inhibitor of B-cells harboring CD20 (rituximab), and costimulating factors (abatacept). According to the recommendations of The European League Against Rheumatism (EULAR), updated in 2019, some basic rules should be followed in the treatment of RA. DMARD treatment should be started immediately after a diagnosis of RA. The first line of therapy uses methotrexate, which is the most widely used csDMARD. Methotrexate can be effective both in mono mode and in combination with other csDMARDs, tsDMARDs, and bDMARDs. If the patient has methotrexate intolerance, then leflunomide or sulfasalazine may be used instead. Glucocorticoids are prescribed only to a small number of patients for a short period in the first line of therapy. If during the first three months of treatment with methotrexate, there is no improvement, and clinical remission is not achieved after six months, then the second line of RA therapy should be used. In the absence of unfavourable prognosis factors (high levels of ACPAs, rheumatoid factor, high activity of the disease according to clinical scales and early damage to joints, ineffective use of two csDMARDs), another csDMARD is added to methotrexate. Another possible option is to replace methotrexate with another csDMARD. In the presence of unfavourable prognostic factors, bDMARDs or JAK inhibitors may be used instead of methotrexate. If after some time (for example, three months), it is not possible to achieve an improvement in the condition and clinical remission, then another bDMARD is prescribed as a third-line drug. If remission is achieved as a result of using any of the described lines of therapy, the dose of DMARD is reduced and the optimal period of visits to the rheumatologist is established to control the activity of the disease [65]. Similar recommendations for the treatment of RA were previously published by the American College of Rheumatology (ACR) [66]. It should be noted that maybe in the future, the characteristics of the patient's genome would determine the sensitivity and resistance to various DMARDs.

5.2. Genetic Variants Affecting csDMARD Effectiveness

Methotrexate-sensitivity pharmacogenetic studies are quite numerous as it is the first-line therapy drug of choice. The main genetic variants associated with methotrexate treatment response determined by separate original works, multicenter studies, and meta-analyses are summarised in Table 2; similar loci associated with the effectiveness of targeted DMARD therapy are also shown. A better methotrexate response is noted in the presence of 3435C > T polymorphism's T-allele in *ABCB1* gene exon 26. In contrast, del28-bp TSER*3/*3 homozygotes of the thymidyl synthase gene (*TYMS*) require a higher dose of the drug. Finally, a C > G substitution at position 347 of the *ATIC* gene is associated with methotrexate toxicity. As a less often used first-line drug for RA treatment, leflunomide has a lower response rate among 19AA homozygotes of the *DHODH* gene, encoding an enzyme of the de novo pyrimidine synthesis chain [67]. According to recent meta-analyses and earlier original works, sensitivity to methotrexate is associated with 34C/T substitutions in the *AMPD1* gene, 675T/C in the *ATIC* gene, and 80G/A in the *SLC19A1* gene in Caucasians, while 3435C/T in the *ABCB1* gene in this population and 28-bp 2R/3R in the *TYMS* gene in representatives of other races are associated with resistance. Polymorphisms in the *MTHFR* (C677T and A1298C) and *TYMS* (1494 del6 and 28-bp 2R/3R) genes were associated with the severity of side effects in various populations [11,68–70]. The *FPGS* gene encoding the transfer protein has rs10987742 and rs10106 SNPs associated with methotrexate sensitivity in RA [71]. Among the genes encoding other transfer proteins, methotrexate resistance in RA was associated with the *SLC22A11* gene (rs11231809, T-allele), the *ABCC1* gene (rs246240, G-allele; rs3784864, G-allele), and its CGG-(rs35592, rs2074087 and rs3784864) and CGG-haplotypes (rs35592, rs246240 and rs3784864), as well as with substitutions in the *SLC19A1*, *SLC46A1*, and *SLCO1B1* genes [72,73]. However, the last two mentioned studies were performed in a Portuguese population only and may not reflect associations in other Caucasoid groups. It is preferable to focus on meta-analyses that include dozens of original works with Caucasians as an object of study. Thus, the association of the methotrexate toxicity and 80G/A polymorphism in the *RFC1* gene, encoding a transfer protein involved in the folate cycle, was shown [11,74].

Table 2. Polymorphisms (non-HLA genes) associated with disease-modifying antirheumatic drugs (DMARD) efficacy, according to meta-analyses and multicenter studies data.

Drug Class	Gene	Polymorphism	Association	Reference
Cytostatic agents	*MTHFR*	rs1801133	T-allele–MTX toxicity	[75,76]
	ATIC	rs7563206 rs2372536	T-allele G allele–MTX nonresponders	[77,78]
	TYMS	rs2244500 rs2847153 rs3786362	AA genotype A-allele G-allele–MTX efficacy	[78]
	RFC1	rs1051266	AA genotype–MTX efficacy	[70]
	ABCB1	rs1045642	C-allele–MTX efficacy	[79]
	DHODH	rs3213422	AA genotype–leflunomide efficacy	[67]
IL6 inhibitors	*IL6R*	rs12083537 rs11265618	AA genotype CC genotype–tocilizumab better response	[80,81]
Glucocorticoids	*GLCCI1* *GR*	rs37972 rs41423247 rs6195	T-allele–decreased sensitivity G-allele–increased sensitivity to transition therapy	[82]
TNF inhibitors	*TNFRSF1B*	rs1061622	G-allele–increased sensitivity	[83]
	TNFA	rs1800629 rs361525	A-alleles–anti-TNF agent efficacy	[11]
	FCGR2A	rs1801274	HH + HR genotype–adalimumab efficacy	[84]
	PTPRC	rs10919563	A-allele–decreased sensitivity	[84]
	TLR1 *TLR5*	rs4833095 rs5744174	CC genotype; C-allele–anti-TNF agent efficacy	[85]
	NUBPL	rs2378945	Minor allele–decreased etanercept sensitivity	[86]

MTX—methotrexate, IL6 – interleukine 6, TNF—tumor necrosis factor.

Patients could also be prescribed transitional therapy with glucocorticoids, anti-inflammatory drugs that suppress the immune system (prednisone, dexamethasone, methylprednisolone), before the maximum effect of DMARDs is reached. Subsequently, corticoid dose is gradually reduced, and the therapy is transferred completely to DMARDs. The rs37972 polymorphism minor allele of the glucocorticoid-induced transcript 1 gene (*GLCCI1*) was shown to be associated with reduced glucocorticoid sensitivity in men [82]. Polymorphisms associated with these anti-inflammatory drug sensitivity panels include the GLCCI1-C allele, glucocorticoid receptor gene (*GR*) BclI-G (rs41423247) and N363S-G (rs6195) alleles, and the G2677A/T replacement in the multidrug resistance factor (MDR1) *ABCB1* gene [82,87].

5.3. Polymorphic Genetic Variants Associated with the Biological and Targeted DMARD Effectiveness

About 45% of patients with RA develop resistance to methotrexate by the end of the second year of treatment. In such cases, the therapy should be switched to targeted drugs. Such second line DMARDs may be inhibitors of the TNFα-signalling pathway, which reduce inflammation and include infliximab, adalimumab, golimumab, etanercept, and certolizumab. These drugs interfere with the binding of TNFα with its receptor. Second-line therapy is quite expensive, while drug resistance occurs in 30–40% of cases. Rituximab, affecting B-cells, or recently developed targeted drugs such as tocilizumab or sarilumab (blocking the IL6-signalling pathway) could be used as a treatment of choice [49,88,89].

Some of the polymorphisms associated with RA affect gene expression or the function of its protein product; hence, the search for targeted drugs based on genetic data is possible. To date, there are specific FDA-approved (Food and Drug Administration) drugs for autoimmune disease treatment targeted against 18 known proteins encoded by RA-associated genes. Among them are abatacept and tocilizumab, which interfere with the *CTLA4* and *IL6R* gene products, respectively. Abatacept, a recombinant protein consisting of the CTLA-4 extracellular domain and the human IgG1 Fc-domain, interacts with the CTLA-4 molecule (CD28) and thereby inhibits T-cell activities. Tocilizumab is a monoclonal antibody blocking the IL6 receptor (IL6R) in soluble form as well as in membrane-bound form.

Since the IL6 signalling pathway is one of the main proinflammatory cascades in RA, its inhibition leads to a pronounced therapeutic effect However, sensitivity to tocilizumab may vary; for instance, the replacement of asparagine with alanine in the 358 codon of the *IL6R* gene increases the relative concentration of the soluble receptor form by 35%. According to an original RA study in Spain, patients with the AA rs12083537 and CC rs11265618 genotypes respond better to targeted tocilizumab therapy [80]. Tocilizumab efficacy is associated with the *IL6R* gene polymorphisms rs12083537, rs2228145, and rs4329505, as shown by various sources [11]. Tofacitinib, which has been approved by the FDA and EMA (European Medical Agency) to treat RA, could also be considered as a drug of choice. It regulates the inflammatory process in RA by blocking JAK1-3 [13,14]. Other possible options are anakinra, an IL1R inhibitor, or secukinumab, directed against the cytokine IL17. The association of HLA-DRB1*SE (unfavourable alleles in the RA-critical epitope) and HLA-DRB1*pos11 V/L with secukinumab therapy effectiveness was shown during a pharmacogenetic study [90].

Expanding the list of treatment options for RA is important for personalised therapy assignment. Thus, the use of anti-TNF antibodies led to a revolution in RA treatment. However, up to 40% of patients remain resistant to this therapy, as estimated by various authors, although it has been shown to date that some of them may respond to anti-IL6R therapy. This is where the analysis of gene networks in RA can contribute. In particular, rituximab, initially developed as an antitumour agent, has specificity for CD20 molecules and suppresses $CD20^+$ B-cell function. As CD20 is encoded by one of the candidate genes associated with RA, therapy with rituximab results in the reduction of disease symptom intensity. Rituximab's effectiveness is associated with polymorphisms *FCGR3A* rs396991, *IL6* rs1800795, and *BAFF* rs9514828. Moreover, rs4810485 of the *CD40* gene's allelic variants is associated with increased gene expression. Such CD40 overexpression results in an increased concentration of TNF superfamily receptor type 5 on the blood mononuclear cells' surface, which makes them targets for TNF inhibitors in this particular cohort of patients [11,14]. Polymorphic variants of the genes encoding TNF and its receptor (*TNFA*), namely, –875T, –308G/A (rs1800629), 238G/A (rs361525), and TNFR1A 36A, are also associated with TNF inhibitor (etanercept, infliximab, and adalimumab) sensitivity [11,91]. Increased anti-TNF therapy sensitivity has also been shown in women with HLA-E*01:03:01/01:03:01 alleles (Polish population only) [92]. *MED15* and *MAFB* genes polymorphisms are associated with etanercept and infliximab sensitivity according to the results of GWAS in Spain [93]. As was shown in a meta-analysis, tyrosine phosphatase receptor type C (*CD45*) and Fc-γ receptor type 2A gene polymorphisms are also associated with anti-TNF drug sensitivity. Thus, the HH + HR genotype of the *FCGR2A* gene is associated with adalimumab efficacy in patients with RA, while the polymorphism rs10919563 allele A of the *PTPRC* gene is related to the sensitivity of three anti-TNF drugs [84,94]. Polymorphisms of the Toll-like receptor genes, which are initial units in proinflammatory intracellular signalling pathways, such as *TLR5* (rs5744174) and *TLR1* (rs4833095), are shown to be associated with the effectiveness of anti-TNF therapy as well [95]. According to the other meta-analyses, more than 20 SNPs associated with the targeted anti-TNF therapy response in patients with RA could be identified in the genes involved in T-cell functioning, NFκB and TNFα signalling pathways, as well as in *CTCN5*, *TEC*, *PTPRC*, *FCGR2A*, *NFKBIB*, *FCGR2A*, *IRAK325*, and other genes [85]. A recently published review summarised data on various polymorphisms of 12 genes, best studied as predictive factors for the response to RA drug therapy: methotrexate (HLA-G, MTHFR, ABCB1, TNFA, TYMS), leflunomide

(CYP1A2, CYP2C19), etanercept (IL10, TNFA), infliximab (TNFRSF1B, TNFA, FCGR2A/3A), and other drugs [83]. In other words, today, it is possible to choose about 10–15 genes, the polymorphisms of which can serve as a prognostic criterion for Caucasians in RA therapy.

6. Conclusions

Recently, the results of a GWAS—a study aimed to determine personalised RA therapy based on the genetic polymorphisms associated with sensitivity to FDA-approved antirheumatic drugs—have been published. Moreover, epigenetic changes (including microRNA polymorphism and expression) altering the disease complication risk and response to treatment should be taken to account, along with the germline variants assessment for RA predisposition and therapy response [96,97]. In that way, researchers are striving to develop a genetic testing algorithm for DMARD therapy personalisation to make RA treatment more clinically- and cost-effective. Thus, the published results of original scientific studies, reviews, and meta-analyses allow us to characterise the genetic component of RA predisposition in various populations and emphasise specific variants to be analysed for the most effective treatment regimens.

Author Contributions: Conceptualization, D.S.M., M.V.N., I.V.B., V.V.T., A.N.L., E.A.A. and A.A.Z.J.; writing—original draft preparation, D.S.M, I.V.B., E.B.K., M.I.B. and A.A.D.; writing—review and editing, D.S.M., M.V.N., E.B.K. and A.A.Z.J.; project administration, A.A.Z.J.; funding acquisition, A.A.Z.J. All authors have read and agreed to the published version of the manuscript.

Funding: The authors received funding from the Ministry of Science and Higher Education of the Russian Federation, Ref. No. RFMEFI60518X0003, for this work.

Conflicts of Interest: The authors declare no conflict of interest.

References

1. Karami:, J.; Aslani, S.; Jamshidi, A.; Garshasbi, M.; Mahmoudi, M. Genetic implications in the pathogenesis of rheumatoid arthritis; an updated review. *Gene* **2019**, *702*, 8–16. [CrossRef] [PubMed]
2. Sparks, J.A.; Costenbader, K.H. Genetics, Environment, and Gene-Environment Interactions in the Development of Systemic Rheumatic Diseases. *Rheum. Dis. Clin. N. Am.* **2014**, *40*, 637–657. [CrossRef] [PubMed]
3. Aletaha, D.; Neogi, T.; Silman, A.J.; Funovits, J.; Felson, D.T.; Bingham, C.O.; Birnbaum, N.S.; Burmester, G.R.; Bykerk, V.P.; Cohen, M.D.; et al. 2010 Rheumatoid arthritis classification criteria: An American College of Rheumatology/European League Against Rheumatism collaborative initiative. *Arthritis Rheum.* **2010**, *62*, 2569–2581. [CrossRef] [PubMed]
4. Scherer, H.U.; Häupl, T.; Burmester, G.R. The etiology of rheumatoid arthritis. *J. Autoimmun.* **2020**, *110*, 102400. [CrossRef] [PubMed]
5. Suzuki, A.; Terao, C.; Yamamoto, K. Linking of genetic risk variants to disease-specific gene expression via multi-omics studies in rheumatoid arthritis. *Semin. Arthritis Rheum.* **2019**, *49*, S49–S53. [CrossRef] [PubMed]
6. Messemaker, T.C.; Huizinga, T.W.; Kurreeman, F. Immunogenetics of rheumatoid arthritis: Understanding functional implications. *J. Autoimmun.* **2015**, *64*, 74–81. [CrossRef] [PubMed]
7. Castro-Santos, P.; Díaz-Peña, R. Genetics of rheumatoid arthritis: A new boost is needed in Latin American populations. *Rev. Bras. Reum. Engl. Ed.* **2016**, *56*, 171–177. [CrossRef]
8. Okada, Y.; Kim, K.; Han, B.; Pillai, N.E.; Ong, R.T.-H.; Saw, W.-Y.; Luo, M.; Jiang, L.; Yin, J.; Bang, S.-Y.; et al. Risk for ACPA-positive rheumatoid arthritis is driven by shared HLA amino acid polymorphisms in Asian and European populations. *Hum. Mol. Genet.* **2014**, *23*, 6916–6926. [CrossRef]
9. Raslan, H.M.; Attia, H.R.; Hamed Ibrahim, M.; Mahmoud Hassan, E.; Salama, I.I.; Ismail, S.; Abdelmotaleb, E.; El Menyawi, M.M.; Amr, K.S. Association of anti-cyclic citrullinated peptide antibodies and rheumatoid factor isotypes with HLA-DRB1 shared epitope alleles in Egyptian rheumatoid arthritis patients. *Int. J. Rheum. Dis.* **2020**, *23*, 647–653. [CrossRef]

10. Busch, R.; Kollnberger, S.; Mellins, E.D. HLA associations in inflammatory arthritis: Emerging mechanisms and clinical implications. *Nat. Rev. Rheumatol.* **2019**, *15*, 364–381. [CrossRef]
11. Machaj, F.; Rosik, J.; Szostak, B.; Pawlik, A. The evolution in our understanding of the genetics of rheumatoid arthritis and the impact on novel drug discovery. *Expert Opin. Drug Discov.* **2020**, *15*, 85–99. [CrossRef] [PubMed]
12. Reynolds, R.J.; Ahmed, A.F.; Danila, M.I.; Hughes, L.B.; Gregersen, P.K.; Raychaudhuri, S.; Plenge, R.M.; Bridges, S.L. HLA-DRB1-associated rheumatoid arthritis risk at multiple levels in African Americans: Hierarchical classification systems, amino acid positions, and residues. *Arthritis Rheumatol.* **2014**, *66*, 3274–3282. [CrossRef] [PubMed]
13. Kochi, Y.; Suzuki, A.; Yamamoto, K. Genetic basis of rheumatoid arthritis: A current review. *Biochem. Biophys. Res. Commun.* **2014**, *452*, 254–262. [CrossRef] [PubMed]
14. Kim, K.; Bang, S.Y.; Lee, H.S.; Bae, S.C. Update on the genetic architecture of rheumatoid arthritis. *Nat. Rev. Rheumatol.* **2017**, *13*, 13–24. [CrossRef] [PubMed]
15. Law, S.; Street, S.; Yu, C.-H.; Capini, C.; Ramnoruth, S.; Nel, H.J.; van Gorp, E.; Hyde, C.; Lau, K.; Pahau, H.; et al. T-cell autoreactivity to citrullinated autoantigenic peptides in rheumatoid arthritis patients carrying HLA-DRB1 shared epitope alleles. *Arthritis Res.* **2012**, *14*, R118. [CrossRef] [PubMed]
16. Wu, J.; Li, J.; Li, S.; Zhang, T.P.; Li, L.J.; Lv, T.T.; Pan, H.F.; Ye, D.Q. Association of HLA-DQB1 polymorphisms with rheumatoid arthritis: A meta-analysis. *Postgrad. Med. J.* **2017**, *93*, 618–625. [CrossRef]
17. Traylor, M.; Knevel, R.; Cui, J.; Taylor, J.; Harm-Jan, W.; Conaghan, P.G.; Cope, A.P.; Curtis, C.; Emery, P.; Newhouse, S.; et al. Genetic associations with radiological damage in rheumatoid arthritis: Meta-analysis of seven genome-wide association studies of 2,775 cases. *PLoS ONE* **2019**, *14*, e0223246. [CrossRef] [PubMed]
18. Okada, Y.; Eyre, S.; Suzuki, A.; Kochi, Y.; Yamamoto, K. Genetics of rheumatoid arthritis: 2018 status. *Ann. Rheum. Dis.* **2019**, *78*, 446–453. [CrossRef] [PubMed]
19. Korczowska, I. Rheumatoid arthritis susceptibility genes: An overview. *World J. Orthop.* **2014**, *5*, 544–549. [CrossRef]
20. Magyari, L.; Varszegi, D.; Kovesdi, E.; Sarlos, P.; Farago, B.; Javorhazy, A.; Sumegi, K.; Banfai, Z.; Melegh, B. Interleukins and interleukin receptors in rheumatoid arthritis: Research, diagnostics and clinical implications. *World J. Orthop.* **2014**, *5*, 516–536. [CrossRef]
21. Zhang, C.; Jiao, S.; Li, T.; Zhao, L.; Chen, H. Relationship between polymorphisms in −572G/C interleukin 6 promoter gene polymorphisms (rs1800796) and risk of rheumatoid arthritis: A meta-analysis. *Int. J. Rheum. Dis.* **2020**, *23*, 47–54. [CrossRef] [PubMed]
22. Yu, M.; Hou, J.; Zheng, M.; Cao, Y.; Alike, Y.; Mi, Y.; Zhu, J. IL-21 gene rs6822844 polymorphism and rheumatoid arthritis susceptibility. *Biosci. Rep.* **2020**, *40*. [CrossRef] [PubMed]
23. Mohammadi, F.S.; Aslani, S.; Mostafaei, S.; Jamshidi, A.; Riahi, P.; Mahmoudi, M. Are genetic variations in IL-21–IL-23R–IL-17A cytokine axis involved in a pathogenic pathway of rheumatoid arthritis? Bayesian hierarchical meta-analysis. *J. Cell. Physiol.* **2019**, *234*, 17159–17171. [CrossRef]
24. Cheng, P.; Zhang, Y.; Huang, H.; Zhang, W.; Yang, Q.; Guo, F.; Chen, A. Association between CCR6 and rheumatoid arthritis: A meta-analysis. *Int. J. Clin. Exp. Med.* **2015**, *8*, 5388–5396. [PubMed]
25. Toson, B.; Dos Santos, E.J.; Adelino, J.E.; Sandrin-Garcia, P.; Crovella, S.; Louzada-Júnior, P.; Oliveira, R.D.R.; Pedroza, L.S.R.A.; de Fátima Lobato Cunha Sauma, M.; de Lima, C.P.S.; et al. CCR5Δ32 and the genetic susceptibility to rheumatoid arthritis in admixed populations: A multicentre study. *Rheumatol. (Oxf.)* **2017**, *56*, 495–497.
26. Chen, S.; Deng, C.; Hu, C.; Li, J.; Wen, X.; Wu, Z.; Li, Y.; Zhang, F.; Li, Y. Association of MCP-1-2518A/G polymorphism with susceptibility to autoimmune diseases: A meta-analysis. *Clin. Rheumatol.* **2016**, *35*, 1169–1179. [CrossRef]
27. David, T.; Ling, S.F.; Barton, A. Genetics of immune-mediated inflammatory diseases. *Clin. Exp. Immunol.* **2018**, *193*, 3–12. [CrossRef]
28. Zhang, L.; Yuan, X.; Zhou, Q.; Shi, J.; Song, Z.; Quan, R.; Zhang, D. Associations Between TNFAIP3 Gene Polymorphisms and Rheumatoid Arthritis Risk: A Meta-analysis. *Arch. Med. Res.* **2017**, *48*, 386–392. [CrossRef]
29. Gao, W.; Dong, X.; Yang, Z.; Mao, G.; Xing, W. Association between rs7574865 polymorphism in STAT4 gene and rheumatoid arthritis: An updated meta-analysis. *Eur. J. Intern. Med.* **2020**, *71*, 101–103. [CrossRef]

30. Mustelin, T.; Bottini, N.; Stanford, S.M. The Contribution of PTPN22 to Rheumatic Disease. *Arthritis Rheumatol.* **2019**, *71*, 486–495. [CrossRef]
31. Abbasifard, M.; Imani, D.; Bagheri-Hosseinabadi, Z. PTPN22 gene polymorphism and susceptibility to rheumatoid arthritis (RA): Updated systematic review and meta-analysis. *J. Gene Med.* **2020**, e3204. [CrossRef]
32. Wu, X.; Yang, H.J.; Jung Kim, M.; Zhang, T.; Qiu, J.Y.; Park, S. Association between PTPN22 -1123G/C and susceptibility to rheumatoid arthritis: A systematic review and meta-analysis. *Int. J. Rheum. Dis.* **2019**, *22*, 769–780. [CrossRef] [PubMed]
33. Yamamoto, K.; Okada, Y.; Suzuki, A.; Kochi, Y. Genetic studies of rheumatoid arthritis. *Proc. Jpn. Acad. Ser. B Phys. Biol. Sci.* **2015**, *91*, 410–422. [CrossRef] [PubMed]
34. Yang, X.; Liu, J.; Liu, J.; Liang, Y.; Xu, W.; Leng, R.; Pan, H.; Ye, D. Associations Between PADI4 Gene Polymorphisms and Rheumatoid Arthritis: An Updated Meta-analysis. *Arch. Med. Res.* **2015**, *46*, 317–325. [CrossRef]
35. Bérczi, B.; Gerencsér, G.; Farkas, N.; Hegyi, P.; Veres, G.; Bajor, J.; Czopf, L.; Alizadeh, H.; Rakonczay, Z.; Vigh, É.; et al. Association between AIRE gene polymorphism and rheumatoid arthritis: A systematic review and meta-analysis of case-control studies. *Sci. Rep.* **2017**, *7*, 14096. [CrossRef]
36. Tizaoui, K.; Kim, S.; Jeong, G.; Kronbichler, A.; Lee, K.; Lee, K.; Shin, J. Association of PTPN22 1858C/T Polymorphism with Autoimmune Diseases: A Systematic Review and Bayesian Approach. *J. Clin. Med.* **2019**, *8*, 347. [CrossRef]
37. Lee, Y.H.; Bae, S.-C. Association between susceptibility to rheumatoid arthritis and PADI4 polymorphisms: A meta-analysis. *Clin. Rheumatol.* **2016**, *35*, 961–971. [CrossRef]
38. Li, G.; Shi, F.; Liu, J.; Li, Y. The effect of CTLA-4 A49G polymorphism on rheumatoid arthritis risk: A meta-analysis. *Diagn. Pathol.* **2014**, *9*, 157. [CrossRef]
39. Lee, Y.H.; Bae, S.-C. Monocyte chemoattractant protein-1 promoter -2518 polymorphism and susceptibility to vasculitis, rheumatoid arthritis, and multiple sclerosis: A meta-analysis. *Cell. Mol. Biol. (Noisy-Le-Grand)* **2016**, *62*, 65–71.
40. Yuan, Y.; Shao, W.; Li, Y. Associations between C677T and A1298C polymorphisms of MTHFR and susceptibility to rheumatoid arthritis: A systematic review and meta-analysis. *Rheumatol. Int.* **2017**, *37*, 557–569. [CrossRef]
41. Bagheri-Hosseinabadi, Z.; Imani, D.; Yousefi, H.; Abbasifard, M. MTHFR gene polymorphisms and susceptibility to rheumatoid arthritis: A meta-analysis based on 16 studies. *Clin. Rheumatol.* **2020**, *3*, 1–13. [CrossRef] [PubMed]
42. Liu, Q.; Yang, J.; He, H.; Yu, Y.; Lyu, J. Associations between interleukin-10 polymorphisms and susceptibility to rheumatoid arthritis: A meta-analysis and meta-regression. *Clin. Rheumatol.* **2018**, *37*, 3229–3237. [CrossRef]
43. Du, J.; Wang, X.; Tan, G.; Liang, Z.; Zhang, Z.; Yu, H. The association between genetic polymorphisms of interleukin 23 receptor gene and the risk of rheumatoid arthritis: An updated meta-analysis. *Clin. Immunol.* **2020**, *210*, 108250. [CrossRef]
44. Agonia, I.; Couras, J.; Cunha, A.; Andrade, A.J.; Macedo, J.; Sousa-Pinto, B. IL-17, IL-21 and IL-22 polymorphisms in rheumatoid arthritis: A systematic review and meta-analysis. *Cytokine* **2020**, *125*, 154813. [CrossRef] [PubMed]
45. Song, G.G.; Bae, S.-C.; Lee, Y.H. Associations between functional TNFR2 196 M/R polymorphisms and susceptibility to rheumatoid arthritis: A meta-analysis. *Rheumatol. Int.* **2014**, *34*, 1529–1537. [CrossRef]
46. Zhou, T.-B.; Zhao, H.-L.; Fang, S.-L.; Drummen, G.P.C. Association of transforming growth factor-β1 T869C, G915C, and C509T gene polymorphisms with rheumatoid arthritis risk. *J. Recept. Signal Transduct.* **2014**, *34*, 469–475. [CrossRef]
47. Julià, A.; González, I.; Fernández-Nebro, A.; Blanco, F.; Rodriguez, L.; González, A.; Cañete, J.D.; Maymó, J.; Alperi-López, M.; Olivé, A.; et al. A genome-wide association study identifies SLC8A3 as a susceptibility locus for ACPA-positive rheumatoid arthritis. *Rheumatology* **2016**, *55*, 1106–1111. [CrossRef]
48. Razi, B.; Reykandeh, S.E.; Alizadeh, S.; Amirzargar, A.; Saghazadeh, A.; Rezaei, N. TIM family gene polymorphism and susceptibility to rheumatoid arthritis: Systematic review and meta-analysis. *PLoS ONE* **2019**, *14*, e0211146. [CrossRef]

49. Zheng, W.; Rao, S. Knowledge-based analysis of genetic associations of rheumatoid arthritis to inform studies searching for pleiotropic genes: A literature review and network analysis. *Arthritis Res.* **2015**, *17*, 202. [CrossRef] [PubMed]
50. Freudenberg, J.; Gregersen, P.; Li, W. Enrichment of Genetic Variants for Rheumatoid Arthritis within T-Cell and NK-Cell Enhancer Regions. *Mol. Med.* **2015**, *21*, 180–184. [CrossRef]
51. Fodil, M.; Teixeira, V.H.; Chaudru, V.; Hilliquin, P.; Bombardieri, S.; Balsa, A.; Westhovens, R.; Barrera, P.; Alves, H.; Migliorin, P.; et al. Relationship between SNPs and expression level for candidate genes in rheumatoid arthritis. *Scand. J. Rheumatol.* **2015**, *44*, 2–7. [CrossRef] [PubMed]
52. Zhu, N.; Hou, J.; Wu, Y.; Li, G.; Liu, J.; Ma, G.; Chen, B.; Song, Y. Identification of key genes in rheumatoid arthritis and osteoarthritis based on bioinformatics analysis. *Medicine (USA)* **2018**, *97*, 22. [CrossRef] [PubMed]
53. Liu, T.; Lin, X.; Yu, H. Identifying genes related with rheumatoid arthritis via system biology analysis. *Gene* **2015**, *571*, 97–106. [CrossRef] [PubMed]
54. Gang, X.; Sun, Y.; Li, F.; Yu, T.; Jiang, Z.; Zhu, X.; Jiang, Q.; Wang, Y. Identification of key genes associated with rheumatoid arthritis with bioinformatics approach. *Medicine (USA)* **2017**, *96*, e7673. [CrossRef] [PubMed]
55. Shchetynsky, K.; Diaz-Gallo, L.-M.; Folkersen, L.; Hensvold, A.H.; Catrina, A.I.; Berg, L.; Klareskog, L.; Padyukov, L. Discovery of new candidate genes for rheumatoid arthritis through integration of genetic association data with expression pathway analysis. *Arthritis Res.* **2017**, *19*, 19. [CrossRef] [PubMed]
56. Li, Y.; Lai-Han Leung, E.; Pan, H.; Yao, X.; Huang, Q.; Wu, M.; Xu, T.; Wang, Y.; Cai, J.; Li, R.; et al. Identification of potential genetic causal variants for rheumatoid arthritis by whole-exome sequencing. *Oncotarget* **2017**, *8*, 111119–111129. [CrossRef]
57. Viatte, S.; Plant, D.; Han, B.; Fu, B.; Yarwood, A.; Thomson, W.; Symmons, D.P.M.; Worthington, J.; Young, A.; Hyrich, K.L.; et al. Association of HLA-DRB1 Haplotypes With Rheumatoid Arthritis Severity, Mortality, and Treatment Response. *JAMA* **2015**, *313*, 1645. [CrossRef]
58. Ling, S.F.; Viatte, S.; Lunt, M.; Van Sijl, A.M.; Silva-Fernandez, L.; Symmons, D.P.M.; Young, A.; Macgregor, A.J.; Barton, A. HLA-DRB1 Amino Acid Positions 11/13, 71, and 74 Are Associated With Inflammation Level, Disease Activity, and the Health Assessment Questionnaire Score in Patients With Inflammatory Polyarthritis. *Arthritis Rheumatol.* **2016**, *68*, 2618–2628. [CrossRef]
59. Lopez-Lasanta, M.; Julià, A.; Maymó, J.; Fernández-Gutierrez, B.; Ureña-Garnica, I.; Blanco, F.J.; Cañete, J.D.; Alperi-López, M.; Olivè, A.; Corominas, H.; et al. Variation at interleukin-6 receptor gene is associated to joint damage in rheumatoid arthritis. *Arthritis Res.* **2015**, *17*, 242. [CrossRef]
60. El-Sayed, E.H.; Saleh, M.H.; Al-Shahaly, M.H.; Toraih, E.A.; Fathy, A. IL-37 gene variant (rs3811047): A marker of disease activity in rheumatoid arthritis: A pilot study. *Autoimmunity* **2018**, *51*, 378–385. [CrossRef]
61. Zhi, L.; Yao, S.; Ma, W.; Zhang, W.; Chen, H.; Li, M.; Ma, J. Polymorphisms of RAD51B are associated with rheumatoid arthritis and erosion in rheumatoid arthritis patients. *Sci. Rep.* **2017**, *7*, 1–7. [CrossRef]
62. Kim, K.; Bang, S.-Y.; Lee, H.-S.; Cho, S.-K.; Choi, C.-B.; Sung, Y.-K.; Kim, T.-H.; Jun, J.-B.; Yoo, D.H.; Kang, Y.M.; et al. High-density genotyping of immune loci in Koreans and Europeans identifies eight new rheumatoid arthritis risk loci. *Ann. Rheum. Dis.* **2015**, *74*, e13. [CrossRef] [PubMed]
63. Liu, D.; Liu, J.; Cui, G.; Yang, H.; Cao, T.; Wang, L. Evaluation of the association of UBASH3A and SYNGR1 with rheumatoid arthritis and disease activity and severity in Han Chinese. *Oncotarget* **2017**, *8*, 103385–103392. [CrossRef] [PubMed]
64. Giannini, D.; Antonucci, M.; Petrelli, F.; Bilia, S.; Alunno, A.; Puxeddu, I. One year in review 2020: Pathogenesis of rheumatoid arthritis. *Clin. Exp. Rheumatol.* **2020**, *38*, 387–397. [PubMed]
65. Smolen, J.S.; Landewé, R.B.M.; Bijlsma, J.W.J.; Burmester, G.R.; Dougados, M.; Kerschbaumer, A.; McInnes, I.B.; Sepriano, A.; van Vollenhoven, R.F.; de Wit, M.; et al. EULAR recommendations for the management of rheumatoid arthritis with synthetic and biological disease-modifying antirheumatic drugs: 2019 update. *Ann. Rheum. Dis.* **2020**. [CrossRef] [PubMed]
66. Singh, J.A.; Saag, K.G.; Bridges, S.L.; Akl, E.A.; Bannuru, R.R.; Sullivan, M.C.; Vaysbrot, E.; McNaughton, C.; Osani, M.; Shmerling, R.H.; et al. 2015 American College of Rheumatology Guideline for the Treatment of Rheumatoid Arthritis. *Arthritis Care Res. (Hoboken)* **2016**, *68*, 1–25. [CrossRef]
67. Castañeda, S.; López-Mejías, R.; González-Gay, M.A. Gene polymorphisms and therapy in rheumatoid arthritis. *Expert Opin. Drug Metab. Toxicol.* **2016**, *12*, 225–229. [CrossRef]

68. Chen, Y.; Zou, K.; Sun, J.; Yang, Y.; Liu, G. Are gene polymorphisms related to treatment outcomes of methotrexate in patients with rheumatoid arthritis? A systematic review and meta-analysis. *Pharmacogenomics* **2017**, *18*, 175–195. [CrossRef]
69. Soukup, T.; Dosedel, M.; Pavek, P.; Nekvindova, J.; Barvik, I.; Bubancova, I.; Bradna, P.; Kubena, A.A.; Carazo, A.F.; Veleta, T.; et al. The impact of C677T and A1298C MTHFR polymorphisms on methotrexate therapeutic response in East Bohemian region rheumatoid arthritis patients. *Rheumatol. Int.* **2015**, *35*, 1149–1161. [CrossRef]
70. Qiu, Q.; Huang, J.; Shu, X.; Fan, H.; Zhou, Y.; Xiao, C. Polymorphisms and Pharmacogenomics for the Clinical Efficacy of Methotrexate in Patients with Rheumatoid Arthritis: A Systematic Review and Meta-analysis. *Sci. Rep.* **2017**, *7*, 44015. [CrossRef]
71. Moya, P.; Salazar, J.; Arranz, M.J.; Díaz-Torné, C.; Del Río, E.; Casademont, J.; Corominas, H.; Baiget, M. Methotrexate pharmacokinetic genetic variants are associated with outcome in rheumatoid arthritis patients. *Pharmacogenomics* **2016**, *17*, 11–25. [CrossRef] [PubMed]
72. Lima, A.; Bernardes, M.; Azevedo, R.; Medeiros, R.; Seabra, V. Pharmacogenomics of Methotrexate Membrane Transport Pathway: Can Clinical Response to Methotrexate in Rheumatoid Arthritis Be Predicted? *Int. J. Mol. Sci.* **2015**, *16*, 13760–13780. [CrossRef]
73. Lima, A.; Bernardes, M.; Azevedo, R.; Monteiro, J.; Sousa, H.; Medeiros, R.; Seabra, V. SLC19A1, SLC46A1 and SLCO1B1 Polymorphisms as Predictors of Methotrexate-Related Toxicity in Portuguese Rheumatoid Arthritis Patients. *Toxicol. Sci.* **2014**, *142*, 196–209. [CrossRef]
74. Qiu, Q.; Huang, J.; Lin, Y.; Shu, X.; Fan, H.; Tu, Z.; Zhou, Y.; Xiao, C. Polymorphisms and pharmacogenomics for the toxicity of methotrexate monotherapy in patients with rheumatoid arthritis: A systematic review and meta-analysis. *Medicine. (Baltim.)* **2017**, *96*, e6337. [CrossRef] [PubMed]
75. Shao, W.; Yuan, Y.; Li, Y. Association Between MTHFR C677T Polymorphism and Methotrexate Treatment Outcome in Rheumatoid Arthritis Patients: A Systematic Review and Meta-Analysis. *Genet. Test. Mol. Biomark.* **2017**, *21*, 275–285. [CrossRef]
76. Jekic, B.; Maksimovic, N.; Damnjanovic, T. Methotrexate pharmacogenetics in the treatment of rheumatoid arthritis. *Pharmacogenomics* **2019**, *20*, 1235–1245. [CrossRef] [PubMed]
77. Lee, Y.H.; Bae, S.-C. Association of the ATIC 347 C/G polymorphism with responsiveness to and toxicity of methotrexate in rheumatoid arthritis: A meta-analysis. *Rheumatol. Int.* **2016**, *36*, 1591–1599. [CrossRef] [PubMed]
78. Eektimmerman, F.; Swen, J.J.; Madhar, M.B.; Allaart, C.F.; Guchelaar, H.-J. Predictive genetic biomarkers for the efficacy of methotrexate in rheumatoid arthritis: A systematic review. *Pharm. J.* **2020**, *20*, 159–168. [CrossRef] [PubMed]
79. He, X.; Sun, M.; Liang, S.; Li, M.; Li, L.; Yang, Y. Association between ABCB1 C3435T polymorphism and methotrexate treatment outcomes in rheumatoid arthritis patients: A meta-analysis. *Pharmacogenomics* **2019**, *20*, 381–392. [CrossRef]
80. Maldonado-Montoro, M.; Cañadas-Garre, M.; González-Utrilla, A.; Ángel Calleja-Hernández, M. Influence of IL6R gene polymorphisms in the effectiveness to treatment with tocilizumab in rheumatoid arthritis. *Pharm. J.* **2018**, *18*, 167–172. [CrossRef]
81. Luxembourger, C.; Ruyssen-Witrand, A.; Ladhari, C.; Rittore, C.; Degboe, Y.; Maillefert, J.-F.; Gaudin, P.; Marotte, H.; Wendling, D.; Jorgensen, C.; et al. A single nucleotide polymorphism of IL6-receptor is associated with response to tocilizumab in rheumatoid arthritis patients. *Pharm. J.* **2019**, *19*, 368–374. [CrossRef] [PubMed]
82. Quax, R.A.M.; Koper, J.W.; Huisman, A.M.; Weel, A.; Hazes, J.M.W.; Lamberts, S.W.J.; Feelders, R.A. Polymorphisms in the glucocorticoid receptor gene and in the glucocorticoid-induced transcript 1 gene are associated with disease activity and response to glucocorticoid bridging therapy in rheumatoid arthritis. *Rheumatol. Int.* **2015**, *35*, 1325–1333. [CrossRef] [PubMed]
83. Wu, X.; Sheng, X.; Sheng, R.; Lu, H.; Xu, H. Genetic and clinical markers for predicting treatment responsiveness in rheumatoid arthritis. *Front. Med.* **2019**, *13*, 411–419. [CrossRef]
84. Avila-Pedretti, G.; Tornero, J.; Fernández-Nebro, A.; Blanco, F.; González-Alvaro, I.; Cañete, J.D.; Maymó, J.; Alperiz, M.; Fernández-Gutiérrez, B.; Olivé, A.; et al. Variation at FCGR2A and functionally related genes is

associated with the response to anti-TNF therapy in rheumatoid arthritis. *PLoS ONE* **2015**, *10*, e0122088. [CrossRef] [PubMed]
85. Bek, S.; Bojesen, A.B.; Nielsen, J.V.; Sode, J.; Bank, S.; Vogel, U.; Andersen, V. Systematic review and meta-Analysis: Pharmacogenetics of anti-TNF treatment response in rheumatoid arthritis. *Pharm. J.* **2017**, *17*, 403–411. [CrossRef] [PubMed]
86. Ferreiro-Iglesias, A.; Montes, A.; Perez-Pampin, E.; Cañete, J.D.; Raya, E.; Magro-Checa, C.; Vasilopoulos, Y.; Caliz, R.; Ferrer, M.A.; Joven, B.; et al. Evaluation of 12 GWAS-drawn SNPs as biomarkers of rheumatoid arthritis response to TNF inhibitors. A potential SNP association with response to etanercept. *PLoS ONE* **2019**, *14*, e0213073. [CrossRef]
87. Cuppen, B.V.J.; Pardali, K.; Kraan, M.C.; Marijnissen, A.C.A.; Yrlid, L.; Olsson, M.; Bijlsma, J.W.J.; Lafeber, F.P.J.G.; Fritsch-Stork, R.D.E. Polymorphisms in the multidrug-resistance 1 gene related to glucocorticoid response in rheumatoid arthritis treatment. *Rheumatol. Int.* **2017**, *37*, 531–536. [CrossRef]
88. Yarwood, A.; Eyre, S.; Worthington, J. Genetic susceptibility to rheumatoid arthritis and its implications for novel drug discovery. *Expert Opin. Drug Discov.* **2016**, *11*, 805–813. [CrossRef]
89. Oliver, J.; Plant, D.; Webster, A.P.; Barton, A. Genetic and genomic markers of anti-TNF treatment response in rheumatoid arthritis. *Biomark. Med.* **2015**, *9*, 499–512. [CrossRef]
90. Burmester, G.R.; Durez, P.; Shestakova, G.; Genovese, M.C.; Schulze-Koops, H.; Li, Y.; Wang, Y.A.; Lewitzky, S.; Koroleva, I.; Berneis, A.A.; et al. Association of HLA-DRB1 alleles with clinical responses to the anti-interleukin-17A monoclonal antibody secukinumab in active rheumatoid arthritis. *Rheumatology* **2016**, *55*, 49–55. [CrossRef]
91. Swierkot, J.; Bogunia-Kubik, K.; Nowak, B.; Bialowas, K.; Korman, L.; Gebura, K.; Kolossa, K.; Jeka, S.; Wiland, P. Analysis of associations between polymorphisms within genes coding for tumour necrosis factor (TNF)-alpha and TNF receptors and responsiveness to TNF-alpha blockers in patients with rheumatoid arthritis. *Jt. Bone Spine* **2015**, *82*, 94–99. [CrossRef] [PubMed]
92. Iwaszko, M.; Świerkot, J.; Kolossa, K.; Jeka, S.; Wiland, P.; Bogunia-Kubik, K. Polymorphisms within the human leucocyte antigen-E gene and their associations with susceptibility to rheumatoid arthritis as well as clinical outcome of anti-tumour necrosis factor therapy. *Clin. Exp. Immunol.* **2015**, *182*, 270–277. [CrossRef] [PubMed]
93. Juli, A.; Fernandez-Nebro, A.; Blanco, F.; Ortiz, A.; Cañete, J.D.; Maymó, J.; Alperi-López, M.; Fernández-Gutierrez, B.; Oliv, A.; Corominas, H.; et al. A genome-wide association study identifies a new locus associated with the response to anti-TNF therapy in rheumatoid arthritis. *Pharm. J.* **2016**, *16*, 147–150. [CrossRef]
94. Lee, Y.H.; Bae, S.-C. Associations between PTPRC rs10919563 A/G and FCGR2A R131H polymorphisms and responsiveness to TNF blockers in rheumatoid arthritis: A meta-analysis. *Rheumatol. Int.* **2016**, *36*, 837–844. [CrossRef] [PubMed]
95. Sode, J.; Vogel, U.; Bank, S.; Andersen, P.S.; Hetland, M.L.; Locht, H.; Heegaard, N.H.H.; Andersen, V. Genetic Variations in Pattern Recognition Receptor Loci Are Associated with Anti-TNF Response in Patients with Rheumatoid Arthritis. *PLoS ONE* **2015**, *10*, e0139781. [CrossRef]
96. Nemtsova, M.V.; Zaletaev, D.V.; Bure, I.V.; Mikhaylenko, D.S.; Kuznetsova, E.B.; Alekseeva, E.A.; Zamyatnin, A.A. Epigenetic Changes in the Pathogenesis of Rheumatoid Arthritis. *Front. Genet.* **2019**, *10*, 1–25. [CrossRef]
97. Xiao, Y.; Liu, H.; Chen, L.; Wang, Y.; Yao, X.; Jiang, X. Association of microRNAs genes polymorphisms with arthritis: A systematic review and meta-analysis. *Biosci. Rep.* **2019**, *39*. [CrossRef]

International Journal of
Molecular Sciences

MDPI

Review

Reconsidering the Role of Melatonin in Rheumatoid Arthritis

Iona J. MacDonald [1], Chien-Chung Huang [1,2], Shan-Chi Liu [3] and Chih-Hsin Tang [1,4,5,6,*]

1 School of Medicine, China Medical University, Taichung 40402, Taiwan; ionamac@gmail.com (I.J.M.); u104054003@cmu.edu.tw (C.-C.H.)
2 Division of Immunology and Rheumatology, Department of Internal Medicine, China Medical University Hospital, Taichung 40447, Taiwan
3 Department of Medical Education and Research, China Medical University Beigang Hospital, Yunlin 65152, Taiwan; sdsaw.tw@yahoo.com.tw
4 Graduate Institute of Biomedical Sciences, China Medical University, Taichung 40402, Taiwan
5 Chinese Medicine Research Center, China Medical University, Taichung 40402, Taiwan
6 Department of Biotechnology, College of Health Science, Asia University, Taichung 41354, Taiwan
* Correspondence: chtang@mail.cmu.edu.tw; Tel.: +(886)-2205-2121 (ext. 7726)

Received: 17 March 2020; Accepted: 18 April 2020; Published: 20 April 2020

Abstract: Rheumatoid arthritis (RA) is an inflammatory joint disorder characterized by synovial proliferation and inflammation, with eventual joint destruction if inadequately treated. Modern therapies approved for RA target the proinflammatory cytokines or Janus kinases that mediate the initiation and progression of the disease. However, these agents fail to benefit all patients with RA, and many lose therapeutic responsiveness over time. More effective or adjuvant treatments are needed. Melatonin has shown beneficial activity in several animal models and clinical trials of inflammatory autoimmune diseases, but the role of melatonin is controversial in RA. Some research suggests that melatonin enhances proinflammatory activities and thus promotes disease activity in RA, while other work has documented substantial anti-inflammatory and immunoregulatory properties of melatonin in preclinical models of arthritis. In addition, disturbance of the circadian rhythm is associated with RA development and melatonin has been found to affect clock gene expression in joints of RA. This review summarizes current understanding about the immunopathogenic characteristics of melatonin in RA disease. Comprehensive consideration is required by clinical rheumatologists to balance the contradictory effects.

Keywords: melatonin; rheumatoid arthritis

1. Introduction

Rheumatoid arthritis (RA) is an autoimmune disease that is characterized by synovial proliferation and inflammatory responses, the presence of autoantibodies including rheumatoid factor and anti-citrullinated protein antibodies (ACPA) in sera, cartilage, and bone erosion with deformity, and co-occurring health conditions such as cardiovascular disease events, pulmonary, psychological, and metabolic bone disorders [1]. Proinflammatory cytokines that mediate the progression of RA disease include tumor necrosis factor alpha (TNF-α), interleukin 1 beta (IL-1β), and IL-6. Current international guidelines for patients with early RA recommend starting disease-modifying antirheumatic drugs (DMARDs) as soon as possible, with methotrexate being the preferred choice [2]. Methotrexate is usually supplemented with short-term, low-dose oral or intra-articular glucocorticoids (GCs) for fast relief of pain and swelling and for arresting the inflammatory process. GCs must be carefully managed to prevent their inappropriate use and tapered as soon as possible to avoid long-term adverse effects [2]. The highly efficacious biologic DMARDs targeting the proinflammatory cytokines and Janus kinase inhibitors are intended for patients with persistently active disease after initial methotrexate failure and, in some cases, another conventional DMARD [2]. However, although these novel medications help to control RA disease activity, they are not universally effective in all RA patients [3,4] and many will lose therapeutic responsiveness after a period of time [5]. More potent or complementary treatments are needed.

The anti-inflammatory and antioxidant effects of melatonin have proven beneficial in several inflammatory autoimmune diseases [6]. Melatonin is also capable of regulating responses of T cell subsets, such as $CD4^+$ T helper (Th)1, Th17, and regulatory T cells (Tregs) [7]. However, numerous studies indicate that melatonin, instead of being beneficial, could exacerbate RA disease-related activities. Nevertheless, in recent years, some conflicting results show that melatonin is capable of alleviating RA through anti-inflammatory and immunoregulatory mechanisms. The aim of this review is to elucidate the complex reactions of melatonin in RA and determine whether melatonin could serve as a potential therapeutic agent.

2. Mechanisms of Melatonin

Endocrine circadian rhythms are regulated by the endogenous hormone melatonin (*N*-acetyl-5-methoxytryptamine), which activates specific high-affinity melatonin receptors expressed on several different types of cells, including immunocompetent cells [8]. The pineal gland is the primary source of melatonin, which is also synthesized by tissues and organs of multicellular organisms including the retina, gastrointestinal tract, skin, and leukoctyes (in peripheral blood and in bone marrow) [9]. In the skin, melatonin can regulate cutaneous pigmentation and perform photoprotective and anticancer activities [10,11]. *N*-acetylserotonin, a precursor to melatonin, enters the systemic circulation from different peripheral organs for transformation to melatonin [12]. Furthermore, the effects of melatonin can be mediated by its metabolites because of the rapid metabolism of melatonin at the peripheral sites [13,14]. As the production of melatonin by the non-endocrine organs responds to signals other than circadian cycles, the endocrine, autocrine, and paracrine effects of melatonin mean that this substance is extensively involved in the regulation of the human immune system [9].

The biological effects of melatonin involve three pathways: (i) G-protein-coupled membrane receptor signaling; (ii) nuclear signaling; and (iii) receptor-independent signaling that accounts for radical scavenging activities of melatonin [7,15]. The binding of melatonin to the G protein-coupled melatonin receptors (MT_1 and MT_2) on the plasma membrane of the target cells enables melatonin to stimulate signaling pathways and reduce cell proliferation [16]. MT_1 receptors are expressed throughout the body but mainly in the central nervous system, in the thymus and the spleen, B cells, CD4, and CD8 cells [7]. Neuroanatomical mapping of melatonin receptors has revealed marked differences in distribution patterns of MT_1 and MT_2 proteins in the adult rat brain, with for instance MT_2 receptors identified in the reticular thalamic nucleus, mediating neuronal firing and burst activity related to nonrapid eye movement (NREM) sleep, whereas no MT_1 receptors are found in this area, confirming the highly specific functioning of melatonin receptors in sleep neurophysiology [17]. MT_1 and MT_2 affect gene transcription activities through extracellular signal-regulated kinase (ERK) pathways and CREP phosphorylation [7]. Melatonin receptors have also been identified in RA synovial macrophages [18]. A positive correlation has been observed between the polymorphism of the melatonin receptor type 1B (*MTNR1B*) and levels of rheumatoid factor in Korean patients with RA [19]. Other researchers have reported significantly lower levels of MT_1 expression in RA synovial tissue compared with normal healthy tissue, and the finding that siRNAs against MT_1 reverse melatonin-mediated inhibition of TNF-α and IL-1β production, confirming that melatonin suppresses TNF-α and IL-1β via the MT_1 receptor [20]. Thus, the activity of membrane melatonin receptors and their specific agonists is implicated in circadian rhythmicity [7]. Retinoic acid-related orphan receptor alpha (RORα) is an important member of the ROR subfamily of nuclear receptors, which mediate several physiological functions, such as metabolic, immunologic, and circadian actions [21]. The identified endogenous ligands for RORα consist of sterols and their derivatives [22]. It appears that RORα mediates the indirect effects of melatonin in the periphery, such as immunomodulation, cellular growth, and bone differentiation [23]. Moreover, while RORα is not a receptor for melatonin or its metabolites, the constitutive activity of RORα may be modulated by membrane melatonin receptors [21,23].

Melatonin also displays antioxidant and anti-inflammatory activity, depending on the cellular state [24,25]. Evidence suggests that melatonin serves as a link between circadian rhythms and joint diseases, including RA and osteoarthritis (OA) [26,27]. For instance, oxidative stress induced by RA is reduced by melatonin and/or its metabolites, which not only neutralize the reactive oxygen (ROS) and reactive nitrogen species (RNS), but also upregulate levels of glutathione and antioxidant enzyme expression and activity [28,29]. In RA and OA, melatonin and its metabolites modulate several molecular signaling pathways including those governing inflammation, proliferation, and apoptosis [28,29].

3. A Role for Melatonin in Rheumatoid Arthritis Therapy?

In investigations involving melatonin in animal models of inflammatory autoimmune diseases (multiple sclerosis, systemic lupus erythematosus, inflammatory bowel disease, and type 1 diabetes), melatonin has demonstrated beneficial effects in these diseases, including prophylactic and therapeutic effects in rats with adjuvant-induced arthritis (AA), in which melatonin dose-dependently repressed the inflammatory response and enhanced proliferation of thymocytes and secretion of IL-2 [30]. In addition, melatonin decreased the elevated level of cyclic 3′,5′-AMP (cAMP) induced by forskolin. The drop in thymocyte proliferation induced by injection of Freund's complete adjuvant was highly correlated with a decrease in the levels of Met-enkephalin (Met-Enk) in the thymocytes, which were strikingly augmented by melatonin; this effect was blocked by the Ca^{2+} channel antagonist, nifedipine. The anti-inflammatory and immunoregulatory actions of melatonin involved a G protein-adenyl cyclase-cAMP transmembrane signal and Met-Enk release by thymocytes [30].

3.1. Modulation of the Circadian Clock by Melatonin in RA

Importantly, circadian rhythms exist in almost all cells of the body, and are regulated by circadian clock gene expression [7,15]. Any disruption in these circadian clocks is associated with the onset of inflammatory-related disease states and joint diseases, including RA [7,15]. Patients with RA exhibit abnormal clock gene expression, with disturbances in the hypothalamic-pituitary-adrenal axis influencing changes in circadian rhythms of circulating serum levels of melatonin, IL-6, cortisol and in chronic fatigue [15]. Melatonin exerts its effects in RA by modulating clock gene expression, including the *Cry1* gene [7,15]. By attenuating the expression of the *Cry1* gene, melatonin upregulates levels of cAMP production and increases activation of protein kinase A (PKA) and nuclear factor kappa B (NF-κB), which increases CIA severity in rats [31,32]. As detailed earlier, the diurnal secretion of melatonin is also closely related to the production of IL-12 and NO among RA synovial macrophages and human monocytic myeloid THP-1 cells [33].

A positive correlation has been reported between elevated early morning serum melatonin concentrations and disease activity scores as well as erythrocyte sedimentation rate (ESR) levels in patients with juvenile rheumatoid arthritis, although higher melatonin concentrations did not correlate with disease severity [34], echoing the findings of Forrest and colleagues reported earlier, who noted that elevated ESR and neopterin concentrations following melatonin treatment did not worsen the severity of RA disease [35]. El-Awady and colleagues suggested that melatonin may promote the activity of RA disease, rather than its severity [34]. However, as reported above, Akfhamizadeh and colleagues found no link between elevated morning serum melatonin concentrations and RA disease activity or other disease characteristics, despite also observing significantly higher melatonin values in newly diagnosed RA patients compared with those who had established RA disease [36].

There also appears to be a relationship between melatonin and the *Bmal1* and *ROR* clock genes [15]. It is speculated that high melatonin concentrations in RA patients may modulate *ROR* activation [15]. *ROR* acts as a negative regulator of inflammation via the NF-κB signaling pathway and is essential in the activity of both melatonin and the clock gene *Bmal1*, which helps to maintain 24-h rhythms and regulate immune responses [15,37]. Moreover, ROR proteins bind into the promoter region and drive *Bmal1* gene expression [38]. This activity at the binding site is inhibited by reverse-eritroblastosis viruses (REV-ERBs), which may contribute to *Bmal1* suppression and exacerbation of RA [15].

3.2. Adverse Effects of Melatonin in RA

Evidence suggests that melatonin is not beneficial in RA. For instance, the development of collagen-induced arthritis (CIA) in DBA/1 mice is exacerbated by constant darkness [39] and by daily exogenous administration of melatonin 1 mg/kg [40]. Hansson and colleagues then investigated the effects of surgical pinealectomy in DBA/1 and NFR/N mice with collagen-induced arthritis (CIA) [41]. Serum melatonin levels were reduced in the pinealectomized mice to around 30% of levels in normal or sham-operated controls [41]. In both mouse strains, pinealectomy was associated with a delay in onset of arthritic disease, less severe arthritis (lower clinical scores), and lower serum anti-CII levels compared with sham-operated animals [41]. The researchers interpreted these findings as showing that high physiological levels of melatonin stimulate the immune system and worsen CIA, while inhibiting the release of melatonin is beneficial [41]. Their speculation was supported by observations from mice subjected to 30 days of Bacillus Calmette-Guérin (BCG) inoculations into the left hind paw, inducing chronic granulomatous inflammation [42]. Higher vascular permeability was seen around the granulomatous lesions at midnight than at midday; this rhythmic variation was eliminated by pinealectomy and restored by nocturnal replacement of melatonin [42].

This ability of melatonin to modulate immune response was further illustrated by experiments in which the production of IL-12 and nitric oxide (NO) was significantly increased in the media of melatonin-stimulated RA synovial macrophages and cultured THP-1 cells compared with RPMI-treated synovial macrophage controls [33]. Unexpectedly, the opposite effects in IL-12 and NO levels were seen when RA synovial macrophages were pretreated with lipopolysaccharide (LPS) prior to melatonin, as compared with synovial macrophages treated with LPS alone [33]. This study explained the possible mechanism of joint morning stiffness in relation to diurnal rhythmicity of neuroendocrine pathways [33].

These conclusions are supported by later evidence from in vitro and in vivo studies, as well as clinical investigations, showing how melatonin stimulates the production of NO, T helper type 1 (Th1)-type and other inflammatory cytokines besides IL-12 (IL-1, IL-2, IL-4, IL-5, IL-6, TNF-α, granulocyte-macrophage colony-stimulating factor [GM-CSF], and transforming growth factor [TGF]-β, interferon [IFN]-γ), and enhances both cell-mediated and humoral responses [43–45]. In the early morning, patients with RA exhibit high serum levels of proinflammatory cytokines, especially TNF-α and IL-6, when melatonin serum concentrations are also higher [6,43]. The effects of these circadian rhythms are thought to promote the joint pain and morning stiffness that characterizes RA [6]. Animal studies have shown that melatonin treatment (10 mg/kg) dysregulates circadian clock genes, which may promote the progression of RA [31]. Intriguingly, a dual effect of melatonin as a proinflammatory agent and antioxidant has been observed in CIA rats [32]. In that study, a lower dosage of melatonin (30 μg/kg) increased anti-collagen antibodies, IL-1β, and IL-6 levels in the serum and joints of arthritic rats, worsening the severity of joint damage, while simultaneously lowering oxidative markers nitrite/nitrate and lipid peroxidation in serum, but not in joints [32].

3.3. Neutral or Beneficial Effects of Melatonin in RA

Notably, a cross-sectional study from Iran has reported finding significantly higher morning serum levels of melatonin in patients with RA compared with healthy controls, but no correlation between melatonin and RA disease activity score or other disease characteristics, including age, disease duration, medications, gender, or season of sampling [36]. The study also reported finding higher serum melatonin values in newly diagnosed patients compared with patients with established RA, which needs further investigation [36].

Matrix metalloproteinases (MMPs) are a family of endopeptidases primarily responsible for catalyzing the degradation of the extracellular matrix (ECM) [46]. MMPs play important roles in RA. Elevated levels of circulating MMP-3, MMP-8 and MMP-9 are associated with disease progression in

RA [47]. In particular, MMP-2 and MMP-9 are expressed in synoviocytes, CD34$^+$ endothelial cells, monocytes and macrophages of rheumatoid synovium, indicating that both molecules are critical to pannus formation and invasion in RA progression [47]. Interestingly, melatonin reportedly directly inhibits secreted MMP-9 by binding to the active site and significantly reducing the catalytic activity of MMP-9 in both in vitro and cultured cells, in a dose- and time-dependent manner [46]. Thus, melatonin could have an important role in the prevention of joint destruction in RA.

Research demonstrating that melatonin dose-dependently inhibits the proliferation of RA fibroblast-like synoviocytes (FLS) through the activation of the ERK/P21/P27 pathway suggests that inhibiting the invasion of RA FLS through cartilage and into bone may have important implications in the treatment of RA [48]. Blocking NF-κB signaling appears to be the way in which melatonin protects cells from oxidative stress [28] and largely explains how melatonin suppresses proinflammatory cytokines such as IL-1β and TNF-α [20]. Other pathways and molecules associated with inflammation that are modulated by melatonin include the mitogen-activated protein kinase (MAPK) and nuclear erythroid 2-related factor 2 (Nrf2) pathways, as well as Toll-like receptors [15].

In a clinical trial involving RA patients, six months of melatonin treatment (10 mg/day) was associated with a general decrease from baseline in concentrations of peroxidation markers [35]. Conversely, ESR and neopterin concentrations were increased from baseline with melatonin and significantly higher at six months than concentrations in the placebo-treated cohort, which experienced a significant downward trend in these inflammatory indicators during the trial [35]. Paradoxically, neither the elevations in ESR and neopterin concentrations nor the decrease in tissue peroxidation associated with melatonin translated into significant differences from the placebo group in terms of patients' symptoms, or in the concentrations of proinflammatory cytokines (TNF-α, IL-1β, and IL-6) [35]. The study researchers concluded that melatonin does not appear to be beneficial in RA [35].

The findings of Forrest et al. are discussed by Maestroni et al., who argue that because melatonin enhances the production of Th1-type and inflammatory cytokines in RA, upregulates cell-mediated and humoral responses, and also exacerbates CIA in mice, melatonin likely promotes RA disease and is inappropriate for therapeutic use [49]. Maestroni et al. also emphasized the high blood melatonin concentrations (280 pg/mL) observed 12 h after dosing in the RA cohort [49], in relation to the notion that higher blood melatonin concentrations, especially in the early morning, may be responsible for morning stiffness and joint swelling experienced by patients with arthritis [6,43]. Maestroni et al. conjecture that autoreactive T cells in RA patients synthesize and release melatonin, thereby worsening the disease process [49].

Nevertheless, Korkmaz [50] has defended Forrest et al., pointing out that melatonin has shown strong anti-inflammatory activity in studies using known inflammatory agents, such as zymosan [51], lipopolysaccharide [52,53], and carrageenan [54]. Korkmaz speculated that the high blood melatonin concentrations in the RA cohort may have been a compensatory response to RA inflammation and were comparable to the high levels of melatonin in cerebrospinal fluid and its metabolites in meningitis populations and in pediatric patients with epilepsy [50]. Korkmaz maintained that melatonin is an appropriate adjunctive therapy for RA [50].

Melatonin appears to play an important role in microRNA (miRNA) expression in RA. miRNAs are small, non-coding RNAs that post-transcriptionally mediate protein expression by targeting protein-coding genes implicated in cancer cell proliferation, differentiation, apoptosis, and migration [55]. A recent study found that melatonin appears to inhibit miR-590-3p expression and induce apoptosis in human osteoblasts [55]. In another study, melatonin treatment effectively downregulated TNF-α and IL-1β production in human RA synovial fibroblasts (the MH7A cell line) by suppressing PI3K/AKT, ERK, and NF-κB signaling and upregulating miR-3150a-3p expression [20]. Those investigations confirmed that the MT_1 receptor mediates the anti-inflammatory effects of melatonin and that melatonin not only inhibits inflammatory cytokine release in mice with CIA-induced arthritis, but also attenuates CIA-induced cartilage degradation and bone erosion [20]. This evidence suggests that melatonin targets miRNAs, which could be explored in clinical trials examining the efficacy of melatonin in the treatment of RA. The following figure (Figure 1) and table (Table 1) illustrate the processes through which melatonin exerts its therapeutic effects.

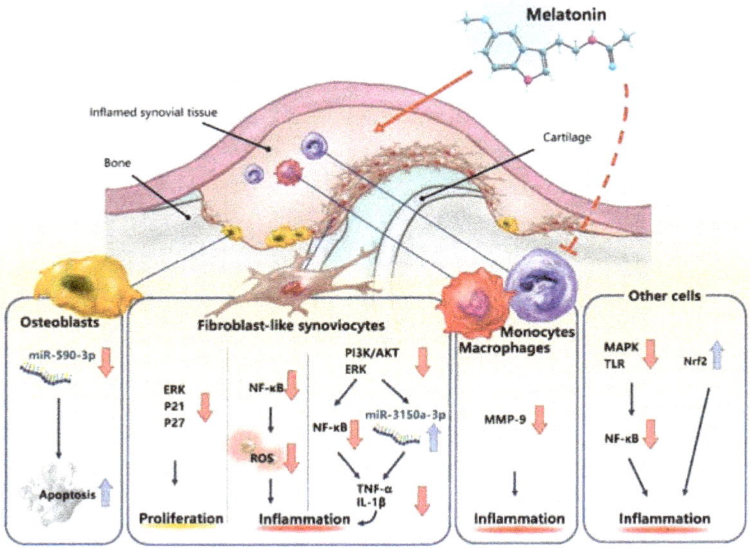

Figure 1. Neutral or beneficial effects of melatonin in rheumatoid arthritis (RA). The dotted line represents the uncertainty over the effects of melatonin upon macrophages and monocytes.

Table 1. Summary of the adverse, neutral, and beneficial effects of melatonin in rheumatoid arthritis.

Adverse/ Neutral/Beneficial	Sample/Animal Model/ Cell Line	Melatonin Level	Effects		References
Adverse	CIA mice	↑	RA	↑	[40]
Adverse	CIA mice (pinealectomy)	↓	Serum anti-CII RA	↓	[41]
Adverse	RA synovial macrophages/ myeloid monocytic cells (THP-1)	↑	IL-12 NO	↑	[33]
Adverse	CIA rats	↑	Anti-collagen antibodies IL-1β and IL-6	↑	[32]
Neutral		Treatment with melatonin	Erythrocyte sedimentation rate (ESR) and neopterin	↑	[35]
Neutral	RA patients' plasma levels	↑			[36]
Beneficial		Treatment with melatonin	MMP-9	↓	[46]
Beneficial	Fibroblast-like synoviocytes (FLS)	Treatment with melatonin	P21/P27 FLS proliferation	↓↓	[48]
Beneficial	Synovial fibroblasts	Treatment with melatonin	miR-3150a-3p IL-1β and TNF-α	↑↓	[20]
Beneficial		Treatment with melatonin	TLR/MAPK Nrf2	↓↑	[15]
Beneficial		Treatment with melatonin	ROS and RNS glutathione and antioxidant enzymes	↓↑	[28]
Beneficial	Osteoblast cells	Treatment with melatonin	miR-590-3p Apoptosis	↓↑	[55]

4. Summary

Various research suggests that melatonin has disease-promoting effects in RA and that it could increase the severity of RA, in contradiction to the beneficial effects of melatonin in other autoimmune inflammatory diseases. However, in the past decade, some studies have demonstrated that melatonin can alleviate RA through the inhibition of RA synovial fibroblast proliferation, TNF-α and IL-1β expression, as well as MMP-9 activity. The anti-inflammatory character of melatonin in RA is associated with regulation of microRNAs (such as miR-3150a-3p). More investigations are therefore warranted to explore the possible double-edged effects of melatonin in RA. The use of melatonin in patients with RA needs thorough consideration by clinical physicians.

Author Contributions: Conceptualization, C.-H.T.; literature collection and preparation, I.J.M., C.-C.H.; writing—original draft preparation, I.J.M., S.-C.L.; writing—review and editing, I.J.M., C.-C.H.; supervision, C.-H.T. All authors have read and agreed to the published version of the manuscript.

Funding: This research was funded by grants from the National Science Council of Taiwan (MOST108-2320-B-039-065; MOST 108-2320-B-039-064-); China Medical University Hospital (DMR-109-208); and China Medical University, Taichung, Taiwan (CMU108-MF-114).

Conflicts of Interest: The authors declare no conflict of interest.

Abbreviations

AA	Adjuvant-induced arthritis
ACPA	Anti-citrullinated protein antibodies
BCG	Bacillus Calmette-Guérin
Ca^{2+}	Calcium
cAMP	Cyclic 3′,5′-AMP
CIA	Collagen-induced arthritis
DMARD	Disease-modifying antirheumaticdrug
ECM	Extracellular matrix
ERK	Extracellular signal-regulated kinase
ESR	Erythrocyte sedimentation rate
FLS	Fibroblast-like synoviocytes
GM-CSF	Granulocyte-macrophage colony-stimulating factor
IFN	Interferon
IL	Interleukin
Met-Enk	Met-enkephalin
MMP	Matrix metalloproteinase
$MT_{1/2}$	High-affinity G protein-coupled melatonin receptors
NF-κB	Nuclear factor kappa B
NO	Nitric oxide
Nrf2	Nuclear erythroid 2-related factor 2
OA	Osteoarthritis
PI3K	Phosphatidylinositol 3-kinase
RA	Rheumatoid arthritis
ROS	Reactive oxygen species
TGF	Transforming growth factor
Th1	Human T helper type 1
TNF	Tumor necrosis factor

References

1. McInnes, I.B.; Schett, G. The pathogenesis of rheumatoid arthritis. *N Engl. J. Med.* **2011**, *365*, 2205–2219. [CrossRef]
2. Mian, A.; Ibrahim, F.; Scott, D.L. A systematic review of guidelines for managing rheumatoid arthritis. *BMC Rheumatol.* **2019**, *3*, 42. [CrossRef] [PubMed]
3. Singh, J.A.; Saag, K.G.; Bridges, S.L. Jr.; Akl, E.A.; Bannuru, R.R.; Sullivan, M.C.; Vaysbrot, E.; McNaughton, C.; Osani, M.; Shmerling, R.H.; et al. 2015 American College of Rheumatology Guideline for the Treatment of Rheumatoid Arthritis. *Arthritis Rheumatol. (Hoboken, N.J.)* **2016**, *68*, 1–26. [CrossRef]

4. Smolen, J.S.; Landewe, R.; Bijlsma, J.; Burmester, G.; Chatzidionysiou, K.; Dougados, M.; Nam, J.; Ramiro, S.; Voshaar, M.; van Vollenhoven, R.; et al. EULAR recommendations for the management of rheumatoid arthritis with synthetic and biological disease-modifying antirheumatic drugs: 2016 update. *Ann. Rheum Dis.* **2017**, *76*, 960–977. [CrossRef] [PubMed]
5. Smolen, J.S.; Aletaha, D.; McInnes, I.B. Rheumatoid arthritis. *Lancet* **2016**, *388*, 2023–2038. [CrossRef]
6. Lin, G.J.; Huang, S.H.; Chen, S.J.; Wang, C.H.; Chang, D.M.; Sytwu, H.K. Modulation by melatonin of the pathogenesis of inflammatory autoimmune diseases. *Int. J. Mol. Sci.* **2013**, *14*, 11742–11766. [CrossRef]
7. Zhao, C.N.; Wang, P.; Mao, Y.M.; Dan, Y.L.; Wu, Q.; Li, X.M.; Wang, D.G.; Davis, C.; Hu, W.; Pan, H.F. Potential role of melatonin in autoimmune diseases. *Cytokine Growth Factor Rev.* **2019**, *48*, 1–10. [CrossRef]
8. Miller, S.C.; Pandi-Perumal, S.R.; Esquifino, A.I.; Cardinali, D.P.; Maestroni, G.J. The role of melatonin in immuno-enhancement: Potential application in cancer. *Int. J. Exp. Pathol.* **2006**, *87*, 81–87. [CrossRef]
9. Cipolla-Neto, J.; Amaral, F.G.D. Melatonin as a Hormone: New Physiological and Clinical Insights. *Endocr. Rev.* **2018**, *39*, 990–1028. [CrossRef]
10. Slominski, A.T.; Zmijewski, M.A.; Semak, I.; Kim, T.K.; Janjetovic, Z.; Slominski, R.M.; Zmijewski, J.W. Melatonin, mitochondria, and the skin. *Cell Mol. Life Sci.* **2017**, *74*, 3913–3925. [CrossRef]
11. Slominski, A.T.; Hardeland, R.; Zmijewski, M.A.; Slominski, R.M.; Reiter, R.J.; Paus, R. Melatonin: A Cutaneous Perspective on its Production, Metabolism, and Functions. *J. Investig. Dermatol.* **2018**, *138*, 490–499. [CrossRef] [PubMed]
12. Slominski, A.T.; Kim, T.K.; Kleszczynski, K.; Semak, I.; Janjetovic, Z.; Sweatman, T.; Skobowiat, C.; Steketee, J.D.; Lin, Z.; Postlethwaite, A.; et al. Characterization of serotonin and N-acetylserotonin systems in the human epidermis and skin cells. *J. Pineal Res.* **2020**, *68*, e12626. [CrossRef] [PubMed]
13. Kim, T.K.; Kleszczynski, K.; Janjetovic, Z.; Sweatman, T.; Lin, Z.; Li, W.; Reiter, R.J.; Fischer, T.W.; Slominski, A.T. Metabolism of melatonin and biological activity of intermediates of melatoninergic pathway in human skin cells. *FASEB J.* **2013**, *27*, 2742–2755. [CrossRef]
14. Slominski, A.T.; Semak, I.; Fischer, T.W.; Kim, T.K.; Kleszczynski, K.; Hardeland, R.; Reiter, R.J. Metabolism of melatonin in the skin: Why is it important? *Exp. Dermatol.* **2017**, *26*, 563–568. [CrossRef] [PubMed]
15. Jahanban-Esfahlan, R.; Mehrzadi, S.; Reiter, R.J.; Seidi, K.; Majidinia, M.; Baghi, H.B.; Khatami, N.; Yousefi, B.; Sadeghpour, A. Melatonin in regulation of inflammatory pathways in rheumatoid arthritis and osteoarthritis: Involvement of circadian clock genes. *Br. J. Pharmacol.* **2018**, *175*, 3230–3238. [CrossRef]
16. Majidinia, M.; Sadeghpour, A.; Mehrzadi, S.; Reiter, R.J.; Khatami, N.; Yousefi, B. Melatonin: A pleiotropic molecule that modulates DNA damage response and repair pathways. *J. Pineal. Res.* **2017**, *63*, e12416. [CrossRef]
17. Lacoste, B.; Angeloni, D.; Dominguez-Lopez, S.; Calderoni, S.; Mauro, A.; Fraschini, F.; Descarries, L.; Gobbi, G. Anatomical and cellular localization of melatonin MT1 and MT2 receptors in the adult rat brain. *J. Pineal. Res.* **2015**, *58*, 397–417. [CrossRef]
18. Maestroni, G.J.; Sulli, A.; Pizzorni, C.; Villaggio, B.; Cutolo, M. Melatonin in rheumatoid arthritis: Synovial macrophages show melatonin receptors. *Ann. N. Y. Acad. Sci.* **2002**, *966*, 271–275. [CrossRef]
19. Ha, E.; Choe, B.K.; Jung, K.H.; Yoon, S.H.; Park, H.J.; Park, H.K.; Yim, S.V.; Chung, J.H.; Bae, H.S.; Nam, M.; et al. Positive relationship between melatonin receptor type 1B polymorphism and rheumatoid factor in rheumatoid arthritis patients in the Korean population. *J. Pineal. Res.* **2005**, *39*, 201–205. [CrossRef]
20. Huang, C.C.; Chiou, C.H.; Liu, S.C.; Hu, S.L.; Su, C.M.; Tsai, C.H.; Tang, C.H. Melatonin attenuates TNF-alpha and IL-1beta expression in synovial fibroblasts and diminishes cartilage degradation: Implications for the treatment of rheumatoid arthritis. *J. Pineal. Res.* **2019**, *66*, e12560. [CrossRef]
21. Slominski, A.T.; Zmijewski, M.A.; Jetten, A.M. RORalpha is not a receptor for melatonin (response to DOI 10.1002/bies.201600018). *Bioessays* **2016**, *38*, 1193–1194. [CrossRef] [PubMed]
22. Slominski, A.T.; Kim, T.K.; Takeda, Y.; Janjetovic, Z.; Brozyna, A.A.; Skobowiat, C.; Wang, J.; Postlethwaite, A.; Li, W.; Tuckey, R.C.; et al. RORalpha and ROR gamma are expressed in human skin and serve as receptors for endogenously produced noncalcemic 20-hydroxy- and 20,23-dihydroxyvitamin D. *FASEB J.* **2014**, *28*, 2775–2789. [CrossRef] [PubMed]
23. Carlberg, C. Gene regulation by melatonin. *Ann. N. Y. Acad. Sci.* **2000**, *917*, 387–396. [CrossRef] [PubMed]
24. Reiter, R.J. The melatonin rhythm: Both a clock and a calendar. *Experientia* **1993**, *49*, 654–664. [CrossRef] [PubMed]

25. Carrillo-Vico, A.; Lardone, P.J.; Naji, L.; Fernandez-Santos, J.M.; Martin-Lacave, I.; Guerrero, J.M.; Calvo, J.R. Beneficial pleiotropic actions of melatonin in an experimental model of septic shock in mice: Regulation of pro-/anti-inflammatory cytokine network, protection against oxidative damage and anti-apoptotic effects. *J. Pineal Res.* **2005**, *39*, 400–408. [CrossRef] [PubMed]
26. Yoshida, K.; Hashimoto, T.; Sakai, Y.; Hashiramoto, A. Involvement of the circadian rhythm and inflammatory cytokines in the pathogenesis of rheumatoid arthritis. *J. Immunol. Res.* **2014**, *2014*, 282495. [CrossRef]
27. Berenbaum, F.; Meng, Q.J. The brain-joint axis in osteoarthritis: Nerves, circadian clocks and beyond. *Nat. Rev. Rheumatol.* **2016**, *12*, 508–516. [CrossRef]
28. Reiter, R.J.; Mayo, J.C.; Tan, D.X.; Sainz, R.M.; Alatorre-Jimenez, M.; Qin, L. Melatonin as an antioxidant: Under promises but over delivers. *J. Pineal. Res.* **2016**, *61*, 253–278. [CrossRef]
29. Hosseinzadeh, A.; Kamrava, S.K.; Joghataei, M.T.; Darabi, R.; Shakeri-Zadeh, A.; Shahriari, M.; Reiter, R.J.; Ghaznavi, H.; Mehrzadi, S. Apoptosis signaling pathways in osteoarthritis and possible protective role of melatonin. *J. Pineal. Res.* **2016**, *61*, 411–425. [CrossRef]
30. Chen, Q.; Wei, W. Effects and mechanisms of melatonin on inflammatory and immune responses of adjuvant arthritis rat. *Int. Immunopharmacol.* **2002**, *2*, 1443–1449. [CrossRef]
31. Bang, J.; Chang, H.W.; Jung, H.R.; Cho, C.H.; Hur, J.A.; Lee, S.I.; Choi, T.H.; Kim, S.H.; Ha, E. Melatonin attenuates clock gene cryptochrome1, which may aggravate mouse anti-type II collagen antibody-induced arthritis. *Rheumatol. Int.* **2012**, *32*, 379–385. [CrossRef] [PubMed]
32. Jimenez-Caliani, A.J.; Jimenez-Jorge, S.; Molinero, P.; Guerrero, J.M.; Fernandez-Santos, J.M.; Martin-Lacave, I.; Osuna, C. Dual effect of melatonin as proinflammatory and antioxidant in collagen-induced arthritis in rats. *J. Pineal. Res.* **2005**, *38*, 93–99. [CrossRef] [PubMed]
33. Cutolo, M.; Villaggio, B.; Candido, F.; Valenti, S.; Giusti, M.; Felli, L.; Sulli, A.; Accardo, S. Melatonin influences interleukin-12 and nitric oxide production by primary cultures of rheumatoid synovial macrophages and THP-1 cells. *Ann. N.Y. Acad. Sci.* **1999**, *876*, 246–254. [CrossRef] [PubMed]
34. El-Awady, H.M.; El-Wakkad, A.S.; Saleh, M.T.; Muhammad, S.I.; Ghaniema, E.M. Serum melatonin in juvenile rheumatoid arthritis: Correlation with disease activity. *Pak. J. Biol. Sci.* **2007**, *10*, 1471–1476. [CrossRef]
35. Forrest, C.M.; Mackay, G.M.; Stoy, N.; Stone, T.W.; Darlington, L.G. Inflammatory status and kynurenine metabolism in rheumatoid arthritis treated with melatonin. *Br. J. Clin. Pharmacol.* **2007**, *64*, 517–526. [CrossRef]
36. Afkhamizadeh, M.; Sahebari, M.; Seyyed-Hoseini, S.R. Morning melatonin serum values do not correlate with disease activity in rheumatoid arthritis: A cross-sectional study. *Rheumatol. Int.* **2014**, *34*, 1145–1151. [CrossRef]
37. Hand, L.E.; Dickson, S.H.; Freemont, A.J.; Ray, D.W.; Gibbs, J.E. The circadian regulator Bmal1 in joint mesenchymal cells regulates both joint development and inflammatory arthritis. *Arthritis. Res. Ther.* **2019**, *21*, 5. [CrossRef]
38. Kouri, V.P.; Olkkonen, J.; Kaivosoja, E.; Ainola, M.; Juhila, J.; Hovatta, I.; Konttinen, Y.T.; Mandelin, J. Circadian timekeeping is disturbed in rheumatoid arthritis at molecular level. *PLoS ONE* **2013**, *8*, e54049. [CrossRef]
39. Hansson, I.; Holmdahl, R.; Mattsson, R. Constant darkness enhances autoimmunity to type II collagen and exaggerates development of collagen-induced arthritis in DBA/1 mice. *J. Neuroimmunol.* **1990**, *27*, 79–84. [CrossRef]
40. Hansson, I.; Holmdahl, R.; Mattsson, R. The pineal hormone melatonin exaggerates development of collagen-induced arthritis in mice. *J. Neuroimmunol.* **1992**, *39*, 23–30. [CrossRef]
41. Hansson, I.; Holmdahl, R.; Mattsson, R. Pinealectomy ameliorates collagen II-induced arthritis in mice. *Clin Exp. Immunol.* **1993**, *92*, 432–436. [CrossRef] [PubMed]
42. Lopes, C.; deLyra, J.L.; Markus, R.P.; Mariano, M. Circadian rhythm in experimental granulomatous inflammation is modulated by melatonin. *J. Pineal. Res.* **1997**, *23*, 72–78. [CrossRef] [PubMed]
43. Sulli, A.; Maestroni, G.J.; Villaggio, B.; Hertens, E.; Craviotto, C.; Pizzorni, C.; Briata, M.; Seriolo, B.; Cutolo, M. Melatonin serum levels in rheumatoid arthritis. *Ann. N. Y. Acad. Sci.* **2002**, *966*, 276–283. [CrossRef] [PubMed]
44. Cutolo, M.; Maestroni, G.J. The melatonin-cytokine connection in rheumatoid arthritis. *Ann. Rheum. Dis.* **2005**, *64*, 1109–1111. [CrossRef] [PubMed]

45. Cutolo, M.; Sulli, A.; Pizzorni, C.; Secchi, M.E.; Soldano, S.; Seriolo, B.; Straub, R.H.; Otsa, K.; Maestroni, G.J. Circadian rhythms: Glucocorticoids and arthritis. *Ann. N. Y. Acad. Sci.* **2006**, *1069*, 289–299. [CrossRef] [PubMed]
46. Rudra, D.S.; Pal, U.; Maiti, N.C.; Reiter, R.J.; Swarnakar, S. Melatonin inhibits matrix metalloproteinase-9 activity by binding to its active site. *J. Pineal. Res.* **2013**, *54*, 398–405. [CrossRef]
47. Zhou, M.; Qin, S.; Chu, Y.; Wang, F.; Chen, L.; Lu, Y. Immunolocalization of MMP-2 and MMP-9 in human rheumatoid synovium. *Int. J. Clin. Exp. Pathol.* **2014**, *7*, 3048–3056.
48. Nah, S.S.; Won, H.J.; Park, H.J.; Ha, E.; Chung, J.H.; Cho, H.Y.; Baik, H.H. Melatonin inhibits human fibroblast-like synoviocyte proliferation via extracellular signal-regulated protein kinase/P21(CIP1)/P27(KIP1) pathways. *J. Pineal. Res.* **2009**, *47*, 70–74. [CrossRef]
49. Maestroni, G.J.; Otsa, K.; Cutolo, M. Melatonin treatment does not improve rheumatoid arthritis. *Br. J. Clin. Pharmacol.* **2008**, *65*, 797–798. [CrossRef]
50. Korkmaz, A. Melatonin as an adjuvant therapy in patients with rheumatoid arthritis. *Br. J. Clin. Pharmacol.* **2008**, *66*, 316–317. [CrossRef]
51. Cuzzocrea, S.; Caputi, A.P. Protective effect of melatonin on zymosan-induced cellular damage. *Biol. Signals Recept.* **1999**, *8*, 136–142. [CrossRef] [PubMed]
52. Mayo, J.C.; Sainz, R.M.; Tan, D.X.; Hardeland, R.; Leon, J.; Rodriguez, C.; Reiter, R.J. Anti-inflammatory actions of melatonin and its metabolites, N1-acetyl-N2-formyl-5-methoxykynuramine (AFMK) and N1-acetyl-5-methoxykynuramine (AMK), in macrophages. *J. Neuroimmunol.* **2005**, *165*, 139–149. [CrossRef] [PubMed]
53. Yu, G.M.; Kubota, H.; Okita, M.; Maeda, T. The anti-inflammatory and antioxidant effects of melatonin on LPS-stimulated bovine mammary epithelial cells. *PLoS ONE* **2017**, *12*, e0178525. [CrossRef] [PubMed]
54. Cuzzocrea, S.; Zingarelli, B.; Gilad, E.; Hake, P.; Salzman, A.L.; Szabo, C. Protective effect of melatonin in carrageenan-induced models of local inflammation: Relationship to its inhibitory effect on nitric oxide production and its peroxynitrite scavenging activity. *J. Pineal. Res.* **1997**, *23*, 106–116. [CrossRef] [PubMed]
55. Meng, X.; Zhu, Y.; Tao, L.; Zhao, S.; Qiu, S. miR-590-3p mediates melatonin-induced cell apoptosis by targeting septin 7 in the human osteoblast cell line hFOB 1.19. *Mol. Med. Rep.* **2018**, *17*, 7202–7208. [CrossRef] [PubMed]

International Journal of
Molecular Sciences

MDPI

Review

Understanding the Molecular Mechanisms Underlying the Pathogenesis of Arthritis Pain Using Animal Models

Jeong-Im Hong [1,2,†], In Young Park [1,2,†] and Hyun Ah Kim [1,2,*]

1 Division of Rheumatology, Department of Internal Medicine, Hallym University Sacred Heart Hospital, Gyeonggi 14068, Korea; jhi1126@naver.com (J.-I.H.); hoyo012@hanmail.net (I.Y.P.)
2 Institute for Skeletal Aging, Hallym University, Chuncheon 24252, Korea
* Correspondence: kimha@hallym.ac.kr; Tel.: +82-31-380-1826
† These authors contributed equally to this work.

Received: 20 November 2019; Accepted: 9 January 2020; Published: 14 January 2020

Abstract: Arthritis, including osteoarthritis (OA) and rheumatoid arthritis (RA), is the leading cause of years lived with disability (YLD) worldwide. Although pain is the cardinal symptom of arthritis, which is directly related to function and quality of life, the elucidation of the mechanism underlying the pathogenesis of pain in arthritis has lagged behind other areas, such as inflammation control and regulation of autoimmunity. The lack of therapeutics for optimal pain management is partially responsible for the current epidemic of opioid and narcotic abuse. Recent advances in animal experimentation and molecular biology have led to significant progress in our understanding of arthritis pain. Despite the inherent problems in the extrapolation of data gained from animal pain studies to arthritis in human patients, the critical assessment of molecular mediators and translational studies would help to define the relevance of novel therapeutic targets for the treatment of arthritis pain. This review discusses biological and molecular mechanisms underlying the pathogenesis of arthritis pain determined in animal models of OA and RA, along with the methodologies used.

Keywords: osteoarthritis; rheumatoid arthritis; animal model; pain

---

1. Introduction

Musculoskeletal diseases, including osteoarthritis (OA) and rheumatoid arthritis (RA), are the leading causes of years lived with disability (YLD) worldwide. Furthermore, YLD due to OA increased by 31.5% from 2006 to 2016, in association with the aging of the population [1]. Pain is the cardinal symptom of both OA and RA, which directly affects the decision to seek medical care. In addition, pain is closely related to function and quality of life, such that knee pain is a better predictor of disability than radiographic changes in OA [2,3] The development of effective therapeutics for optimal pain management has lagged behind other areas, such as inflammation control and the regulation of autoimmunity, which is partially responsible for the current epidemic of opioid and narcotic abuse. A recent report showed that nearly 10% of all opioids prescribed in Australian general practice are prescribed for OA [4]. Similarly, in a survey of Swedish residents aged ≥35 years, 12% of incident opioid dispensations were attributable to OA and/or its related comorbidities [5]. Although there is inconclusive evidence for the benefits of opioids for arthritides and increasing awareness of the risks, opioid prescription rates for OA in the USA remained stable between 2007 and 2014 [6]. On the other hand, despite recent advances in the treatment of RA utilizing effective immunosuppressive therapies based on a better understanding of its underlying mechanism, remaining pain affected almost one third of early RA patients with a good clinical response [4]. By 2014, 41% of patients with RA in the USA were regular users of opioids [7]. Therefore, to optimize the care of patients with OA and RA, the elucidation of the mechanisms underlying the pathogenesis of pain in these diseases is of great importance. Intuitively, pain from arthritis arises from direct nociceptive mechanisms, such as inflammation and structural joint damage. However, in addition to nociception, arthritis pain involves diverse mechanisms, including the processing of pain in the nervous system, as well as psychological distress [8]. Several well-established animal models of OA and RA are available to study the mechanisms underlying the pathogenesis of joint damage and immune/inflammatory regulation. A range of behavioral and neurophysiological approaches have been used for the delineation of pain in animal models of arthritis. Due to the inherent technological challenges in the quantitative assessment of pain in animal models, however, caution is required when attempting to extrapolate discoveries made in animal models to human patients. This review discusses biological and molecular mechanisms underlying the pathogenesis of arthritis pain obtained in animal models of OA and RA along with the methodologies used.

2. Osteoarthritis

2.1. Pain in Clinical OA

Radiographic changes in OA are poorly correlated with pain and physical function, and the risk factors for radiographic OA are not the same as those for OA pain [9–11]. As pain is strongly correlated with person-level psychological, social, and cultural factors aside from joint damage, studies involving human OA subjects have a high risk of being influenced by confounding effects between individual subjects. Studies using a within-person, knee-matched, case-control design minimize such risks by including patients with knees discordant for the presence of pain or pain severity, and have shown that the severity of radiographic knee OA is indeed strongly associated with both the presence of frequent knee pain and severity of pain in diverse ethnic groups [12,13]. On the other hand, a community study showed that a significant number of subjects with Kellgren and Lawrence (KL) grade 4 OA, which is characterized by a marked loss of articular cartilage and profound subchondral bone changes, did not report pain [14]. As hyaline cartilage, the main focus of interest in both clinical and laboratory research on OA, is an aneural tissue, it is unable to generate nociceptive input and is an unlikely source of pain. In an arthroscopic study that probed the human knee without intra-articular anesthesia, a conscious subject reported remarkable sensitivity to the mechanical loading stimulus in anterior synovial tissues, fat pad, and capsule, but not the cartilage [15]. These findings were corroborated by the results of magnetic resonance imaging (MRI) studies correlating pain with synovitis/effusion in OA subjects [16]. It is notable that the sensation experienced with similar probing of the cruciate ligaments and menisci results in variable degrees of pain depending on the location of the probe, while among OA subjects, meniscus degeneration detected in knee MRI is not correlated with pain [17,18]. This discrepancy may be related to differences between study subjects, such as healthy volunteers vs. OA patients. Bone marrow lesions (BMLs), which in MRI scans appear as regions of hyperintense marrow signals, are associated with knee pain as well as the progression of cartilage damage [19,20]. They often occur before joint degeneration is established, and resolution of knee pain is associated with reduced BML size, suggesting that BMLs may serve as a biomarker for OA structural damage as well as pain [16,21]. In a study of two groups of subjects matched by macroscopic cartilage damage score, the expression of nerve growth factor (NGF) in osteochondral channels and osteoclast densities in subchondral bone were higher in a symptomatic than in an asymptomatic group [22]. These observations suggest that subchondral pathology is associated with symptomatic knee OA, independent of cartilage lesions.

In addition to nociceptive mechanisms arising from structural changes, recent evidence indicates that neurophysiological pathways contribute to OA pain, such that persistent tissue damage and inflammation in the joint induce mechanisms of peripheral and central sensitization [23]. In a study involving 2126 subjects with or at risk of knee OA, mechanical temporal summation (an augmented response to repetitive mechanical stimulation and a measure of central sensitization) and pressure pain thresholds (a measure of sensitivity to pain evoked by mechanical stimulation of nociceptors and a reflection of activity-dependent peripheral sensitization) were associated with pain severity but not radiographic OA [24]. Interestingly, the duration of knee OA was not associated with these markers of pain sensitivity, suggesting that individual predisposition to sensitization rather than induction by peripheral nociceptive input from OA pathology may play a role in pain [24]. A study of patients with hand OA revealed that central sensitization was common, and lower local and widespread pressure pain thresholds and the presence of temporal summation were associated with higher hand pain intensity [25]. These results suggest that the sensitization-associated pain phenotype is common to OA in different locations. In a study of 216 patients with different degrees of knee pain, although all subjects showed high physical impairment, low quality of life, and high pain catastrophizing compared to controls, four distinct knee pain profiles with unique combinations of biochemical markers, pain biomarkers, physical impairments, and psychological factors were apparent [26]. These observations suggest that mechanism-based diagnosis and individualized treatment may be possible for the treatment of knee OA pain. In the early stages of OA, pain occurs intermittently in response to specific activities and movement, which is characteristic of nociceptive pain [27]. As OA progresses, however, pain increases, such that it becomes constant and occurs even at rest [28]. There is debate regarding whether the aggravation of pain is indicative of the development of neuropathy arising from damage to the neurons innervating the joint. In two histological studies that used samples of tissue from patients with end-stage OA, relevant changes in joint innervation for the generation of pain, such as tidemark breaching by vascular channels containing sympathetic and sensory nerves, the presence of free nerve fibers within the subchondral bone marrow, and decreased nerve fibers in synovium with inflammation, were demonstrated [29,30]. Clinical trials examining the efficacy of neuromodulating agents, such as serotonin-norepinephrine reuptake inhibitors (SNRIs) and anticonvulsants, showed inconsistent results in pain reduction, however, and none of these agents reached a high level of recommendation in recent OA treatment guidelines [31,32]. NGF induces sensitization of peripheral nociceptive terminals as well as the development of the nervous system, and plays a key role in acute and chronic pain [33]. Biologic agents that specifically block NGF revealed dramatic pain relief among OA patients, and despite their unique side effect profile, such as alterations in peripheral sensation and development of arthropathies, they are in active clinical development [34,35].

2.2. Animal Models for Studying the Pathogenesis of OA Pain

2.2.1. Animal Models

Although a variety of OA animal models have been developed, there is no single model that can replicate all aspects of human OA. The most commonly used animal models employ surgical or chemical induction [36]. Surgically induced OA models reflect posttraumatic human OA and include destabilization of the medial meniscus (DMM), anterior cruciate ligament transection (ACLT), and medial meniscal transection (MNX) models. These models are characterized by a rapid onset of the disease, consistency in the development of pathology, and less dependence on genetic background [37–39]. The monosodium iodoacetate (MIA)-induced arthritis model, which involves cartilage degeneration by suppression of chondrocyte metabolism, is the most widely used chemical model [40]. Although easy and reproducible, a transcriptome study reported that there were large discrepancies in the transcriptome profile between MIA-induced arthritis and human OA [41]. In addition, initiating events, such as the inflammation and inhibition of the glycolytic pathway, and pathological changes, such as subchondral bone necrosis and collapse, in MIA are not typical of human OA [36,42,43]. To produce animal OA models that represent human pathology more closely, noninvasive models have been developed, including bipedal walking and mechanical joint loading models. The bipedal walking model is induced by obligatory bipedal exercise, and pathogenic changes in this model are consistent with the pathology observed in humans [22]. The mechanical joint loading model is induced through vertically compressive loading on the knee and ankle joints, which shows a pathogenesis similar to human OA [44]. The STR/ort mouse develops spontaneous OA at a young age [45], whereas other mouse strains are relatively resistant to the spontaneous development of OA [46]. The selection of a suitable animal model is required to investigate the mechanism underlying the progression of the disease and pain and to evaluate the efficacy of therapeutics [47].

2.2.2. Behavioral Tests to Assess Pain in OA Animal Models

There are many approaches for assessing the behaviors associated with OA pain in animal models [48]. The most common behavioral assays are the von Frey, weight bearing, hot plate, rotarod, and spontaneous pain-related behavior tests. The von Frey test is used to evaluate mechanical allodynia in mice and rats [49]. Briefly, the rodents are placed individually on a mesh grid and calibrated von Frey filaments are applied to the hind paw in ascending order of size, until the fiber bends by force. The animal response, including withdrawal and shaking or licking the paw, is considered a positive pain response [50]. Static weight bearing is assessed using an incapacitance meter, and the average weight bearing applied to the hind paw between the injured limb and contralateral limb is measured [50]. A recent study showed that the positioning of the animal in the incapacitance test may affect its weight distribution, so care should be taken to minimize the influence of positioning [51]. Catwalk automated gait analyses measure changes in spontaneous gait due to joint pain. Animals pass an illuminated glass platform while gait is recorded with a video camera connected to a computer, and the changes in gait pattern, such as swing speed and stride length, are analyzed [52]. Thermal hyperalgesia is assessed using the hot plate test, where the rodent is placed on a metal surface maintained at a constant temperature. The response time (latency) is measured until licking or shaking of the ipsilateral hind paw and jumping on a hot plate occur [53]. Testing latency should be performed without incurring tissue damage and each trial should be separated by an interval of at least 10 min [54]. The rotarod test is used to evaluate changes in motor skill. The rodent is placed on a rotarod machine with automatic timers and falling sensors, and the rod speed is accelerated gradually from 0 to 40 rpm/min [55]. The moving time until falling off is measured. The number of trials in hot plate and rotarod tests should be minimized to exclude learning effects [48,55]. Finally, the Laboratory Animal Behavior Observation Registration and Analysis System (LABORAS) test measures the spontaneous pain-related behavior of rodents, including ambulation, and exploratory behavior. Animals are housed in the LABORAS cage and their behaviors are recorded for 2–12 h [56,57]. For all pain measurement tests, the influence of stress, such as laboratory environment and testing duration, on the pain response should be taken into consideration.

It is notable that, until recently, the most commonly used induction methods to study OA pain were distinct from those most often used to investigate the pathophysiology and regulation of structural joint damage [36]. DMM and MIA models are the most commonly used models in pain research and show mechanical, thermal, and spontaneous pain behavior occurring at the onset of OA [58,59]. In general, chemically induced models exhibit pain responses evoked with von Frey, incapacitance, and hot plate tests more quickly than surgically induced models. Therefore, pain responses in the MIA model appear rapidly within 1 week post-injection [50,60–64], while more insidious responses are observed in the DMM model. In one study, STR/ort mice, which develop spontaneous OA, did not show any signs of pain, such as mechanical allodynia, cold sensitivity, or joint compression-related vocalization, with the development of OA [65]. This is reminiscent of human OA, in which pain does not develop, despite advanced joint damage. On the other hand, mechanical joint loading-induced OA animals develop a robust pain phenotype, except for thermal hyperalgesia [44]. Table 1 briefly summarizes the pathology and pain behaviors reported in OA models [38,65–90].

Table 1. Common OA models and reported pain behaviors.

Type	Model (Onset of Pathology)	Pros/Cons	Pathological Findings	Behavioral Assay (Pain Response Onset)	Findings	Molecular Pathogenesis Identified
Surgical	DMM (4 wk)	Mimics human post-traumatic OA, slow disease progression and mild cartilage damage, useful in assessing therapies. Need specially trained surgeon, risk of infection.	-Cartilage degradation -Synovial hyperplasia -Bone sclerosis -Osteophyte formation	von Frey (4 wk), incapacitance (4 wk), hot plate (8 wk), LABORAS (8 wk), gait abnormality (10 wk)	Pain response is progressively induced in early phase. Most representative method: von Frey	Loss of PKCδ exacerbates pain in DMM. ADAMTS-5 inhibition attenuates pain in DMM. Knockout of RANKL inhibits pain in ACLT mice. Knockout of Netrin-1 inhibits pain in ACLT mice.
	MNX (2 wk)	More rapid disease onset and higher damage in the joint compared with human disease, useful in assessing therapies. Need specially trained surgeon, risk of infection.		von Frey (1 wk), incapacitance (3 d), cold plate (5 wk)		
	ACLT (2 wk)			von Frey (1 wk), incapacitance (1 wk), hot plate (4 wk), rotarod (4 wk), LABORAS (1 wk), gait (8 w)		
Chemical	MIA (3–7 d)	Easy local injection method, rapid induction of severe joint degeneration, useful for studies in pain behavior. More difficult to translate to human setting.	-Inhibition of glycolysis and disruption of chondrocyte metabolism -Cartilage degradation -Synovial hyperplasia -Osteophyte formation	von Frey (1 wk), incapacitance (3 d), hot plate (6 d), rotarod (15 d), gait (6 d), LABORAS (14 d)	Pain response is induced rapidly within a week post-injection. Most representative methods: von Frey and incapacitance	Neutralization of CCL-17 ameliorates pain in CIOA. Increase of IRF-4, CCL-17 in CIOA.
	CIOA (1–4 wk)	Most rapid progression, useful in assessing therapies. More difficult to translate to human setting.	-Cartilage degradation -Osteophyte formation	von Frey (1 wk), incapacitance (1 wk), hot plate (1 wk)		
Spontaneous/ noninvasive	STR/ort (8–16 wk)	Might mimic primary human OA, no specially trained personnel required. Long period for the development of OA, high variability of the disease phenotype and incidence.	-Cartilage degradation -Osteophyte formation	von Frey (no difference), gait (20 w), cold plate (no difference)	Pain response does not show significant variation with age.	STR/ort mice do not show any signs of pain even when treated with the opioid antagonist naloxone.
	Mechanical joint loading (1 wk)	Noninvasive, suitable to study the effects of mechanical loading and intra-articular fracture, rapid induction of severe joint degeneration. Need specialized equipment.	-Cartilage degradation -Bone sclerosis -Osteophyte formation	von Frey (2 wk), incapacitance (4 wk), hot plate (no difference), rotarod (5 wk)	Pain response is progressively induced in early phase.	Anti-NGF alleviates pain in mechanical joint loading model.

DMM, destabilization of medial meniscus; MNX, medial meniscal transection; ACLT, anterior cruciate ligament transection; MIA, monosodium iodoacetate; CIOA, collagenase-induced arthritis; OA, osteoarthritis; LABORAS, laboratory animal behavior observation registration and analysis system; d, day; wk, week(s); PKCδ, protein kinase C delta; ADAMTS-5, a disintegrin and metalloproteinase with thrombospondin motifs 5; RANKL, receptor activator of nuclear factor kappa-B ligand; CCL-17, chemokine (c-c motif) ligand 17; IRF-4, of interferon regulatory factor 4; NGF, nerve growth factor.

2.2.3. Understanding the Molecular Mechanism Underlying the Pathogenesis of OA Pain via Experiments in Animal Models

In animal models, as in humans, the extent of joint damage and pain are not always correlated [36]. For example, in one study that used a rat model of partial MNX- and MIA-induced OA, the majority of pain responses were apparent within 1 week of surgery or iodoacetate injection, whereas gross joint damage was not evident until around day 21, mirroring the clinical situation where the extent of joint damage is not always correlated with pain [91]. In a recent study that used CRISPR/Cas9 technology to ablate OA-associated genes, although ablation of matrix metalloproteinase 13 (MMP-13) or interleukin 1beta (IL-1β) markedly attenuated structural deterioration, the extent of pain relief was modest compared to the ablation of NGF, which significantly increased joint damage, despite its profound analgesic effect [92]. In MNX- and MIA-induced OA of rats, it was shown that pain responses to NGF locally administered into the knee cavity were increased in OA compared to non-OA joints, indicating that local production of NGF may be crucial for the generation of pain [62,93]. In a DMM model, the loss of protein kinase C delta (PKCδ) expression prevented cartilage degeneration but exacerbated OA-associated hyperalgesia [94]. Increases in sensory neuron distribution in knee OA synovium and activation of the NGF-tropomyosin receptor kinase (TrkA) axis in innervating dorsal root ganglia were highly correlated with knee OA hyperalgesia, indicating the role of NGF/TrkA signaling in OA pain, independent of cartilage preservation [94]. On the other hand, cartilage degradation products generated during joint damage may directly induce pain. A disintegrin and metalloproteinase with thrombospondin motifs 5 (ADAMTS-5), a critical mediator of cartilage degeneration during the development of OA, was found to mediate pain, because both ADAMTS-5 knockout (KO) mice and anti-ADAMTS-5 antibody in wild-type (WT) mice showed inhibition of pain as well as joint degeneration induced with DMM [95,96]. Hyalectan fragments generated by ADAMTS-5 have been suggested to directly stimulate nociceptive neurons as well as glial activation, promoting increased pain perception [97,98]. Intra-articular injection of the 32-amino-acid (32-mer) aggrecan fragment provoked knee hyperalgesia in a Toll-like receptor 2 (TLR-2)-dependent way, and induced the expression of the proalgesic chemokine (c-c motif) ligand 2 (CCL-2) in dorsal root ganglion (DRG) nociceptive neurons [99]. On the other hand, the release of the proalgesic chemokine monocyte chemoattractant protein 1 (MCP-1) in DRG cultures by S100 calcium-binding protein A8 (S100A8) and alpha-2 -macroglobulin (α2M) was mediated by TLR-4, while TLR-4 KO mice were not protected from mechanical allodynia or from joint damage induced with DMM [100]. Further research is needed to elucidate the biological effects of damage-associated molecular patterns (DAMPs), which act as TLR ligands on pain-sensing neurons, as well as the complex balance between pro- and anti-inflammatory signaling pathways activated by OA DAMPs [101].

OA animal models differ in terms of the inflammatory response evoked in the synovium. In general, chemical-induced models tend to exhibit more inflammation in the synovium compared to surgical models. As synovitis is observed before the thinning of the articular cartilage or subchondral bone changes in the MIA model, the abovementioned augmentation of pain behavior in the MIA model may reflect the influence of inflammation on pain [102]. The collagenase-induced OA (CIOA) model, which is induced by chemical instability resulting from intra-articular injection of collagenase, also exhibits pronounced synovitis and early exhibition of thermal hyperalgesia, manifesting as early as 1 week after injection [61], while DMM mice do not exhibit thermal hyperalgesia until the late phase of the disease [95]. Persistent inflammation with fibrosis in the synovial tissue of MIA model was accompanied by pain avoidance behavior before articular cartilage degeneration and by an increase in calcitonin gene-related peptide (CGRP)-positive fibers in the DRG and synovium [103]. CIOA induced an increase in interferon regulatory factor 4 (IRF-4), CCL-17 and chemokine (c-c motif) receptor 4 (CCR-4), the CCL-17 receptor; gene-deficient mice were protected from pain as well as joint destruction, indicating that these molecules are required for the development of OA pain [104]. The therapeutic neutralization of CCL-17 ameliorated both pain and joint damage, whereas the cyclooxygenase 2 (COX-2) inhibitor only ameliorated pain [104].

Subchondral changes in bone are common in most OA animal models. A recent study showed that osteoclast-initiated subchondral bone remodeling plays an important role in the generation of pain in ACLT-induced animal OA [84]. Netrin-1 secreted by osteoclasts led to sensory nerve axonal growth in subchondral bone, and reduced osteoclast formation, induced by the knockout of receptor activator of nuclear factor kappa-B ligand (RANKL) in osteocytes, inhibited pain behavior in OA mice, suggesting that the modulation of subchondral bone remodeling may have therapeutic potential for OA pain [77]. This result is consistent with findings of clinical trials of drugs that modify subchondral bone. Strontium ranelate, an osteoporosis drug that simultaneously enhances osteoprotegerin (OPG) expression and downregulates RANKL expression in primary human osteoblastic cells, leading to decreased osteoclastogenesis and bone resorption, has been shown to ameliorate pain as well as cartilage volume loss and bone marrow lesions in OA patients [105–107]. Bisphosphonates, which inhibit osteoclast activity, are effective for reducing pain and BML size in OA patients [108]. These results demonstrate the potential of finding novel therapeutic molecules for pain by reciprocal use of data derived from both clinical and animal studies.

Obesity has been identified as a key risk factor for the development and progression of OA in numerous epidemiological studies in different ethnic populations. Three studies evaluated the relationship between obesity and OA development via the inhibition of transient receptor potential cation channel, subfamily V, member 4 (TRPV-4), lecithin-cholesterol acyltransferase (Lcat), apolipoprotein A1 (Apoa1), and low-density lipoprotein receptor (Ldlr) in mice fed with a high-fat diet (60% kcal), Western-type diet (4.5 Kcal/g) or cholesterol-rich diet [109–111]. OA was spontaneous or collagenase-induced and, overall, these genes were OA-preventing. On the other hand, how obesity affects pain has not been studied in sufficient detail. It is notable that obese leptin-deficient (ob/ob) and leptin receptor-deficient (db/db) mice with leptin signaling impairment do not show increased incidence of knee OA [112]. However, diet-induced obesity significantly increases the severity of OA following intra-articular fracture, with increases in synovitis and inflammatory cytokine IL-12p70 level [113]. On the other hand, in one study, pain behavior measured with thermal hyperalgesia and spontaneous activity tests were not significantly correlated with either weight gain or OA induced by DMM in obese mice fed a high-fat diet [114]. Adenoviral overexpression of the genes encoding the cholesterol hydroxylases cholesterol 25-hydroxylase (CH25H) and 25-hydroxycholesterol 7α-hydroxylase (CYP7B1) in mouse joint tissues caused OA, whereas knockout or knockdown of these hydroxylases abrogated it. In addition, pain induced with DMM in CH25H KO mice was attenuated, suggesting a role of cholesterol metabolism in OA pain [67].

Age is another strong risk factor for OA in human patients. Although it varies by strain and sex, some inbred strains of mice, such as STR/ort and C57BL/6, spontaneously develop OA with age, and spontaneous joint damage does develop in the majority of mouse strains >12 months of age [115]. Although pain is common among elderly people due to a variety of causes, such as age-related musculoskeletal diseases, comorbid illness, and psychological changes, unlike the structural changes in OA, aging has not been shown to be associated with pain in OA subjects. This is in contrast to reports showing age-related peripheral and central nociceptive changes, such as a decreased density of unmyelinated fibers [116], widespread degenerative changes in spinal dorsal horn sensory neurons [117], and declines in the neural opioid and non-opioid analgesic mechanisms mediating endogenous pain inhibitory systems [118]. Systemic inflammation was shown to correlate with pain in older adults with knee OA, such that an increase in serum tumor necrosis factor alpha (TNF-α) and high sensitivity C-reactive protein (hs-CRP) corresponded to increased knee pain and high levels of the soluble receptors for TNF-α correlated with decreased physical function [119–121]. On the other hand, mice with a deletion of the IL-6 gene were found to have more severe age-related OA compared to age-matched WT controls, reflecting the complicated relationship between inflammation and OA according to species [122]. Molecular features of cellular aging include genomic instability, dysregulated nutrient sensing, loss of proteostasis, and mitochondrial dysfunction [123]. Senescent cells (SnCs) exhibit proinflammatory secretome, known as the senescence-associated secretory phenotype (SASP) that indices degenerative changes in cells and tissues [124]. Chondrocytes respond to oxidative stress by upregulating p53 and p21 expression and activating p38 mitogen-activated protein kinases (MAPK) and phosphorylation of phosphatidylinositol 3-kinase (PI3K)/Akt signaling pathways, which in turn stimulates a SASP [125,126]. ACLT in mice led to the accumulation of SnCs in the articular cartilage and synovium, and selective elimination of these cells attenuated the development of post-traumatic OA [127]. Remarkably, pain was relieved in the joints soon after SnC clearance, before any tissue structural changes occurred, which implies that cellular senescence drives pain of OA, independent of joint damage.

Although female sex is a risk factor for both OA and OA-associated pain, female mice have been infrequently used for the study of OA [128], with only 20% to 30% of studies using female mice and many studies using only male mice. The reasons for this sex imbalance in OA animal models are speculative. A study that used DMM mice showed that male mice develop more severe OA than female mice, suggesting that sex is a key factor in the progression of OA [129]. In addition, OA models using STR/ort and IL-6 KO mice have shown a higher prevalence of OA in male than female mice [122,130]. A study that used the CIOA mouse model showed sex-related differences in the prevalence of cartilage damage in addition to differences between mouse strains [131]. On the other hand, we have shown that joint damage and pain behavior develop similarly after DMM in both male and female C57/BL6 mice [132]. However, TRPV-1 antagonist capsazepine significantly reduced DMM-induced pain and the expression of TRPV-1 in DRG only in male mice [103]. In another study that used DMM in C57BL/6 mice, although OA changes were evident in 12-month-old females, the extents of cartilage degradation, subchondral bone plate sclerosis, and osteophytes were milder than in males [78]. The development of OA changes after DMM surgery depends on the activity level of the animals, which may explain this discrepancy. As pain is such a prominent feature that shows sex-related differences, not only in OA, but also in other illnesses, it is important to study the mechanisms underlying the sex differences in pain [133]. Proper use and representation of female mice in OA pain research is urgently needed to be able to elucidate sex differences in this debilitating disease (Figure 1).

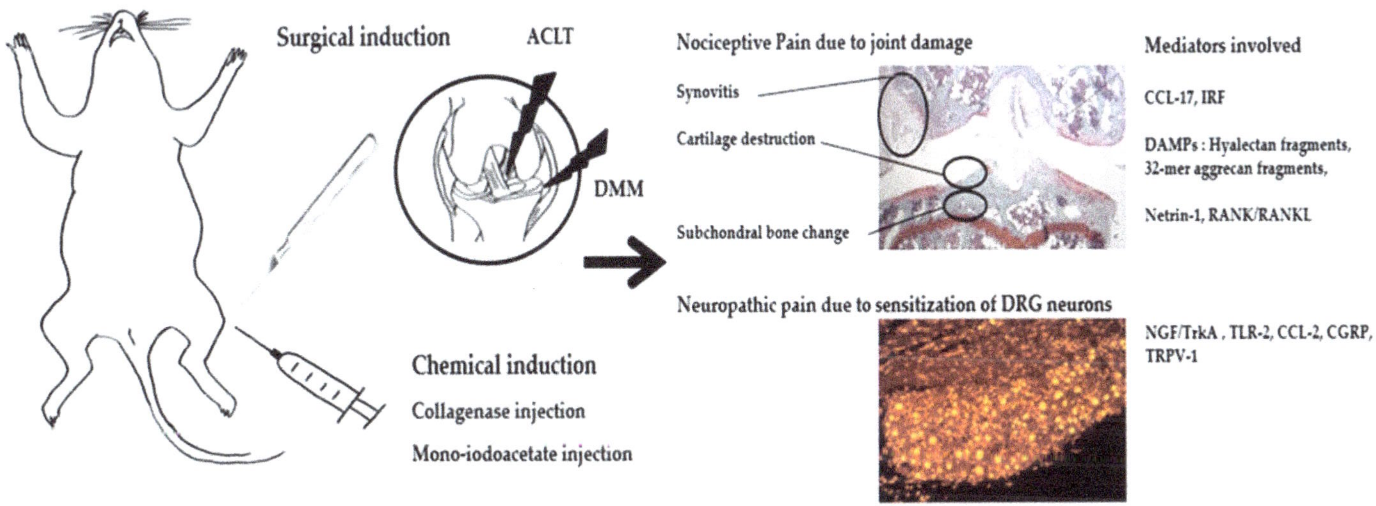

Figure 1. Summary of molecular mediators of pain in OA animal model. ACLT, anterior cruciate ligament transection; DMM, destabilization of the ligament transection; DRG, dorsal root ganglion; CCL-17, chemokine (c-c motif) ligand 17; IRF, interferon regulatory factor; DAMPs, damage associated molecular patterns; 32-mer, 32-animo-acid; RANK/RANKL, receptor activator of nuclear factor kappa-B/RANK ligand; NGF/TrkA, nerve growth factor/tropomyosin receptor kinase; TLR-2, toll-like receptor 2; CCL-2, chemokine (c-c motif) ligand 2; CGRP, calcitonin gene related peptide; TRPV-1, transient receptor potential cation channel subfamily V member 1.

3. Rheumatoid Arthritis

3.1. Pain in Clinical RA

Compared to OA, which is considered a type of noninflammatory arthritis, research endeavors in RA have focused on the regulation of abnormal immune responses and inflammation, with pain considered a byproduct of inflammation that would be controlled by reducing disease activity. Although biological disease-modifying anti-rheumatic drugs (DMARDs) have revolutionized disease control and long-term outcomes of RA, substantial numbers of patients still suffer from pain despite low disease activity. The use of biological DMARDs has provided new insights into the unique qualities of pain manifestations independent of inflammation in RA [134]. The blockade of TNF-α improves pain faster than the resolution of inflammation or tissue damage, indicating a direct role for TNF-α in nociceptor sensitization pathways [135]. This direct analgesic effect is not shared by all cytokine blockers, as neutralization of IL-1β has a less pronounced influence on pain despite its profound role in attenuating inflammation and structural damage [136]. In a study of nociceptive central nervous system (CNS) activity using functional MRI in RA patients treated with a monoclonal antibody to TNF-α, neuronal activity in the thalamus and the somatosensory cortex, areas typically involved in pain perception, was significantly reduced as early as 24 h after the infusion [137]. This indicates that pain in RA is mediated by a mechanism independent of inflammation or joint damage. Pain is an important contributor to the patient global assessment of RA disease activity and discordance between patients and physicians [138].

There has been some speculation on the mechanism underlying persistent pain despite the absence of inflammation. It may result from irreversible joint damage and from changes in the CNS processing signals from the joint [139]. Central sensitization is present in people with RA, such that the prevalence of patients fulfilling fibromyalgia classification increases throughout the course of the disease [140].

Conditioned pain modulation, a measure of inhibitory pathways leading to a diffuse decrease in pain in response to acutely painful stimuli, is impaired in RA patients, and this association is mediated by sleep problems [141]. Patients with established RA also show increased sensitivity to pressure-induced pain at non-joint sites, such as the sternum and anterior tibia, as well as over joints, further indicating that central mechanisms contribute to pain in RA [142]. In a study of 108 RA patients, electrophysiological evidence of neuropathy, including pure sensory or sensory motor axonal neuropathy and demyelinating neuropathy, was present in 57.4% of cases [139]. Local inflammatory responses arising from synovitis as well as systemic inflammation caused by circulating proinflammatory cytokines may augment central pain processing in RA. The potentiation of anti-rheumatic medication is indicated mostly to control inflammation, and a high disease activity score driven by pain should be distinguished to avoid over-treatment. A better understanding of the mechanism of such pain is thus of paramount importance.

3.2. Animal Models for Studying the Pathogenesis of RA Pain

3.2.1. Animal Models

Animal models of RA are divided into immunization and transfer models [143]. The former is induced by active immunization with normal joint constituents, such as type II collagen (CII) or proteoglycan, and encompass both innate and adaptive immune responses. The collagen-induced arthritis (CIA) model, the most commonly used animal model of RA, is induced by intradermal injection of heterologous CII in complete Freund's adjuvant (CFA) into the tail [144], leading to an autoimmune response in the joint, such as increased infiltration of circulating immune cells, chronic inflammation, and tissue damage, mimicking human RA [145]. Inflammatory polyarthritis is induced in specific mouse strains, such as DBA1 and C57BL/6. In antigen-induced arthritis (AIA), injection of methylated bovine serum albumin (mBSA) mixed with CFA into the base of the tail or knee joint of mice or rats leads to monoarticular arthritis. The subsequent pathology includes immune complex-mediated inflammation followed by articular T cell-mediated responses [146]. On the other hand, the transfer model is induced by injection of pathogenic autoantibodies or serum, and recapitulates the effector phase of RA. The collagen antibody-induced arthritis (CAIA) model is induced by injecting a cocktail of anti-CII antibodies and lipopolysaccharide (LPS), and is applicable independent of mouse strain or genotype [147]. The K/BxN serum-transfer arthritis model is induced by injecting anti-glucose-6-phosphate isomerase (anti-GPI)-positive serum from K/BxN mice into commonly used mouse strains, leading to pathological changes resembling human RA. Both models circumvent the induction phase of RA, and lead to joint inflammation and destruction of articular cartilage as well as elevated inflammatory markers in serum. In addition, a variety of genetically modified knockout or transgenic mice, such as IL-1 receptor antagonist knockout (IL-1RA-KO), IL-6 receptor (IL-6R) knock-in, and TNF-α transgenic (Tg) mice, were used to study the influence of molecular mediators in inflammation and to test the efficacy of novel therapeutics [143,144,148–151].

3.2.2. Behavioral Tests to Assess Pain in RA Animal Models

Experimental methods for assessing pain behaviors in RA models are largely similar to those used for OA models, although there are discrepancies in response patterns. In addition, because RA models generally exhibit polyarthritis, modalities useful for measuring asymmetric joint pathology sometimes cannot be used for RA models. Compared to OA, RA models exhibit a greater degree of joint inflammation, which is reflected in their pain behaviors. Mechanical allodynia measured with von Frey fiber and thermal hypersensitivity measured with hot plate response time tend to appear earlier in RA models compared to OA models. While static weight bearing is useful for pain assessment in OA models, because of its polyarticular nature, it is not appropriate for assessment of many RA models. It is notable that in human TNF-Tg (hTNF-Tg) mice, gait parameters measured using catwalk analyses have revealed the association between gait abnormalities and the extent of cartilage damage and bone erosions, but not with the extent of synovitis [152]. These observations indicate that functional impairment in animal models of RA is dependent more on joint destruction than on inflammation.

Both the CIA and CAIA models clearly exhibit mechanical allodynia and thermal hypersensitivity in the early phase of arthritis [153]. While mechanical hypersensitivity persists until the late phase, thermal hyperalgesia tends to decrease to the basal level in the late phase [153]. Moreover, the CIA and CAIA models also display changes in spontaneous behavior, such as reduced climbing, locomotion, and grooming activities [153]. The AIA model displays pathological changes in a single joint, as in OA models, while pain behaviors measured using von Frey or incapacitance tests occur earlier compared to OA models [154]. In this model, mechanical allodynia, thermal hypersensitivity, and abnormal incapacitance tests are normalized in the later phase [154]. The K/BxN model exhibits persistent pain with mechanical hypersensitivity, which does not return to baseline levels during disease progression and outlasts inflammation [155]. Table 2 briefly summarizes the pathology and pain behaviors reported in RA models [134,137,153–167].

Table 2. Common RA models and reported behaviors.

Type	Model (Trigger, Onset of Pathology)	Pros/Cons	Pathological Findings	Behavioral Assay (Pain Response Onset)	Findings	Molecular Pathogenesis Identified
Induced (onset after first immunization)	CIA (CII/adjuvant)	Most common induced model, RA-like pathogenesis. Restricted strains in mice, severe progressive disease.	-Adaptive immune system activation against endogenous joint epitopes. -Inflammation -Immune cell infiltration -Joint destruction and synovial hyperplasia	von Frey (30 d), rotarod (5 d), locomotion (25 d), tail flick (1 wk), Hargreaves (24 d)	Pain response is induced rapidly after induction. Pain response increases in early phase and persists. Most representative methods: von Frey and Hargreaves	Anti-Cat S and FKN attenuate pain in CIA. Gabapentin and buprenorphine attenuate pain in CAIA. Knockout of TLR-4 inhibits pain in K/BxN.
	CAIA (Anti-CII Ab)	Efficient and robust to study the effector phase of RA, diverse susceptible strains. Does not involve full spectrum of immune activation.	-Inflammation -Immune cell infiltration -Joint destruction	von Frey (6 d), hot plate (15 d), locomotion (5 d)		
	K/BxN (Serum/Anti-GPI Ab)			von Frey (2 d), Hargreaves (3 d), locomotion (3 d)		
	AIA (mBSA/adjuvant)	Local RA-like pathogenesis, localized inflammation. Damage to cartilage less severe than in RA.	-Adaptive immune system activation against exogenous epitopes -Inflammation -Immune cell infiltration -Joint destruction and synovial hyperplasia	von Frey (22 d), Hargreaves (7 d), gait (15 d), incapacitance (17 d)	Pain response is induced rapidly after induction. Pain response increases in early phase and restores in late phase. Most representative methods: von Frey and incapacitance	Anti-IL-17 alleviates pain in AIA. Increase of IL-1RI and pCREB in AIA.
Spontaneous	TNF-Tg (hTNF overexpression)	Useful for studies in effect of excess TNF in RA. Only been identified in mice, does not involve full spectrum of immune activation.	-Inflammation -Immune cell infiltration -Joint destruction and synovial hyperplasia -Pannus formation	von Frey (6 wk), tail flick (10 wk), Hargreaves (6 wk)	Pain response increases in early phase and persists. Most representative methods: von Frey and Hargreaves	Increase of the nociceptive brain activity in TNF-Tg mice.
	IL-1RA−/− (Genetic deficiency of 1L-1Ra)	Useful for studies in effect of IL-1 signaling in RA. Only been identified in mice.		No behavioral data available to date.		

CIA, collagen-induced arthritis; CAIA, collagen antibody-induced arthritis; AIA, antigen-induced arthritis; TNF-Tg, tumor necrosis factor transgene; IL-1RA−/−, interleukin-1 receptor antagonist knockout; CII, collagen type II; Ab, antibody; mBSA, methylated bovine serum albumin; GPI, glucose-6-phosphateisomerase; hTNF, human tumor necrosis factor; RA, rheumatoid arthritis; d, day; wk, week(s); Cat S, cathepsin S; FKN, fractalkine; TLR-4, toll-like receptor 4; IL-1RI, interleukin-1 receptor type I; pCREB, phospho-CREB.

3.2.3. Understanding the Molecular Mechanism Underlying the Pathogenesis of RA Pain via Experiments in Animal Models

Compared to research on the pathogenesis of aberrant immunity and inflammation, the mechanism of pain in RA animal models has been explored only recently (Figure 2).

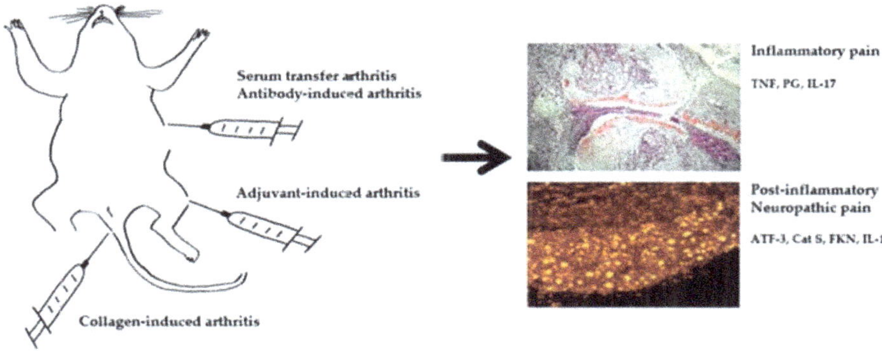

Figure 2. Summary of molecular mediators of pain RA animal model. TNF, tumor necrosis factor; PG, prostaglandin; IL-17, interleukin 17; ATF-3, activating transcription factor 3; Cat S, cathepsin S; FKN, fractalkine; IL-1, interleukin 1.

Although pain behavior largely parallels the development of inflammation, as in human patients, it is not always concordant with the degree of inflammation. As in humans, pain outlasts inflammation in monophasic RA models induced with antibodies. In the K/BxN serum transfer arthritis model, mechanical allodynia develops congruent with joint swelling and persists after the resolution of inflammation [155]. A transition from an inflammatory to a neuropathic pain state is indicated because TNF and prostaglandin inhibitors alleviate allodynia at the peak of joint inflammation, while only gabapentin relieves allodynia following its resolution [126]. Activating transcription factor 3 (ATF-3), a marker of nerve injury, is significantly increased in the lumbar dorsal root ganglia during the late phase, further corroborating the development of neuropathic pain [126]. TLR-4, a receptor mediating innate immunity and response to DAMPs, has been implicated as a mediator of pain, such that TLR-4 KO mice display a significant reversal of mechanical hypersensitivity and diminished appearance of glial activation markers after the resolution of peripheral inflammation induced by K/BxN serum transfer [168]. In the CAIA model, pain exists prior to, and outlasts, the visual signs of inflammation [169]. As in KBxN serum transfer arthritis, a lack of antinociceptive effects of diclofenac in the post-inflammatory phase of arthritis, and time-dependent activation of spinal astrocytes and microglia, are observed. In a study on a mouse model of CIA, significant reductions in both mechanical and thermal pain thresholds were detected on the day of onset of clinical arthritis [170]. While mechanical pain thresholds remained significantly reduced compared to naive mice for up to 28 days after the onset of arthritis, thermal thresholds returned more quickly to the levels observed in naive mice. In a study on a rat model of CIA, significant mechanical hypersensitivity developed before the onset of clinical signs of arthritis, consistent with observations in patients with RA, who often develop pain ahead of overt inflammatory signs [171]. In that study, significant microglial and astrocytic responses, alongside T cell infiltration, were observed in the spinal cord, and intrathecal delivery of a cathepsin S (Cat S) inhibitor and a fractalkine neutralizing antibody, microglial inhibitors, attenuated mechanical hypersensitivity. In another study, the role of proinflammatory cytokines in the generation of pain was investigated in AIA model induced by mBSA. Immunized mice showed mechanical hypernociception, which was abrogated by an antibody against IL-17 [172]. In another study, IL-1R type I (IL-1RI) expression in lumbar DRGs was significantly upregulated in AIA rats, and although treatment with anakinra did not significantly reduce the severity of arthritis or mechanical hyperalgesia, it reduced thermal hyperalgesia [173]. Anakinra treatment downregulated the expression of TRPV-1, which was accompanied by a pronounced reduction in thermal hyperalgesia. Mechanical hyperalgesia in an AIA model was paralleled by the upregulation of phospho-CREB (pCREB) in the lumbar DRG neurons [174]. This was prevented by IL-1 inhibitor, but not by TNF neutralization, suggesting again the importance of IL-1β in neuroplastic changes in sensory neurons in inflammatory arthritis. In a study on a mono-arthritic multi flare rat streptococcal cell wall (SCW) model, in which a local injection of SCW caused the rapid onset of inflammation and pain, prophylactic administration of etanercept inhibited paw swelling and pain [175]. However, the extent of inhibition of pain was less than that of inflammation. The mechanism underlying the dissociation between inflammation and pain has been explored in Fc gamma receptor 1 (FcγR1) KO mice [176]. In a study that employed AIA and CFA models, FcγR1 signaling was upregulated in joint sensory neurons, while the blockade or global genetic deletion of FcγR1 significantly attenuated arthritis pain and hyperactivity of joint sensory neurons without changes in joint inflammation [176]. Antibodies specific for CII or cartilage oligomeric matrix protein (COMP) were found to elicit mechanical hypersensitivity in mice independent of inflammation [160]. Interestingly, CII-immune complex and CII antibodies did not induce mechanical hypersensitivity or pain-like behavior in FcγR chain-deficient mice, suggesting functional coupling between autoantibodies and pain transmission. In murine glucose-6-phosphate isomerase (G6PI)–induced arthritis, nonremitting arthritis induced by depletion of regulatory T cells led to more severe bone destruction and more persistent thermal hyperalgesia [177]. Up-regulation of the neuronal injury marker ATF-3 in sensory neurons ahead of clinical inflammation indicated an early and persisting affection of sensory neurons by G6PI-induced arthritis [177]. These results indicate that the mechanism underlying pain in RA animal models precedes inflammation.

Inflammation and suppression of pain-related spontaneous behaviors, such as locomotor activity, operant responses, and place avoidance, are strongly correlated in rapid-onset models of arthritis [134]. However, the more slowly progressing K/BxN mouse strain shows a significant delay between peak clinical progression and decreased mobility [178]. This finding is suggestive of a psychoaffective component to pain-suppressed behaviors, which is commonly observed in human RA.

4. Conclusions

Recent advances in animal experimentation and molecular biology have led to significant progress in our understanding of the mechanisms underlying the pathogenesis of arthritis pain. The concept that pain is a mere byproduct of joint damage and nociceptive response has become outdated. Aside from DAMPs produced from joint destruction, various nociceptive players, such as NGF- TrkA axis, CGRP, TRPV-1, and SASP, have been proposed as molecular mediators of OA pain. For RA, pain independent of inflammation has been correlated with ATF-3, TLR-4, and FcγR1. With the advances in cutting edge molecular techniques such as single cell polymerase chain reaction (PCR) and CRISPR/Cas9 mediated gene regulation, the knowledge base for pain pathogenesis would be significantly and rapidly expanded. Despite the inherent difficulty in extrapolating data gained in animal pain behavior studies to human arthritis, the critical assessment of various molecular mediators and translational studies would help to define the biological relevance of novel therapeutic targets for the treatment of arthritis pain.

Author Contributions: Acquisition and interpretation of data for the work, J.-I.H.; drafting the work, I.Y.P., J.-I.H. and H.A.K.; conception or design of the work, acquisition and interpretation of data for the work, H.A.K. All authors have read and agreed to the published version of the manuscript.

Funding: This research was supported by a grant of the Basic Science Research Program through the National Research Foundation (NRF) of Korea funded by the Ministry of Education (2017R1A2B2001881), and by the Hallym University Research Fund.

Conflicts of Interest: The authors declare no conflict of interest.

References

1. GBD 2016 Disease and Injury Incidence and Prevalence Collaborators. Global, regional, and national incidence, prevalence, and years lived with disability for 328 diseases and injuries for 195 countries, 1990–2016: A systematic analysis for the Global Burden of Disease Study 2016. *Lancet* **2017**, *390*, 1211–1259. [CrossRef]
2. Hadler, N. Knee pain is the malady—Not osteoarthritis. *Ann. Intern. Med.* **1992**, *116*, 598–599. [CrossRef] [PubMed]
3. Kim, I.; Kim, H.A.; Seo, Y.I.; Song, Y.W.; Jeong, J.Y.; Kim, D.H. The prevalence of knee osteoarthritis in elderly community residents in Korea. *J. Korean Med. Sci.* **2010**, *25*, 293–298. [CrossRef] [PubMed]
4. Ackerman, I.N.; Zomer, E.; Gilmartin-Thomas, J.F.; Liew, D. Forecasting the future burden of opioids for osteoarthritis. *Osteoarthr. Cartil.* **2018**, *26*, 350–355. [CrossRef] [PubMed]
5. Thorlund, J.B.; Turkiewicz, A.; Prieto-Alhambra, D.; Englund, M. Opioid use in knee or hip osteoarthritis: A region-wide population-based cohort study. *Osteoarthr. Cartil.* **2019**, *27*, 871–877. [CrossRef] [PubMed]
6. DeMik, D.E.; Bedard, N.A.; Dowdle, S.B.; Burnett, R.A.; McHugh, M.A.; Callaghan, J.J. Are We Still Prescribing Opioids for Osteoarthritis? *J. Arthroplast.* **2017**, *32*, 3578–3582. [CrossRef] [PubMed]
7. Curtis, J.R.; Xie, F.; Smith, C.; Saag, K.G.; Chen, L.; Beukelman, T.; Mannion, M.; Yun, H.; Kertesz, S. Changing Trends in Opioid Use Among Patients with Rheumatoid Arthritis in the United States. *Arthritis Rheumatol.* **2017**, *69*, 1733–1740. [CrossRef]
8. Rifbjerg-Madsen, S.; Christensen, A.W.; Christensen, R.; Hetland, M.L.; Bliddal, H.; Kristensen, L.E.; Danneskiold-Samsoe, B.; Amris, K. Pain and pain mechanisms in patients with inflammatory arthritis: A Danish nationwide cross-sectional DANBIO registry survey. *PLoS ONE* **2017**, *12*, e0180014. [CrossRef]
9. Davis, M.A.; Ettinger, W.H.; Neuhaus, J.M.; Barclay, J.D.; Segal, M.R. Correlates of knee pain among US adults with and without radiographic knee osteoarthritis. *J. Rheumatol.* **1992**, *19*, 1943–1949.
10. Creamer, P.; Lethbridge-Cejku, M.; Hochberg, M.C. Factors associated with functional impairment in symptomatic knee osteoarthritis. *Rheumatology* **2000**, *39*, 490–496. [CrossRef]
11. Bedson, J.; Croft, P.R. The discordance between clinical and radiographic knee osteoarthritis: A systematic search and summary of the literature. *BMC Musculoskelet. Disord.* **2008**, *9*, 116. [CrossRef] [PubMed]
12. Neogi, T.; Felson, D.; Niu, J.; Nevitt, M.; Lewis, C.E.; Aliabadi, P.; Sack, B.; Torner, J.; Bradely, L.; Zhang, Y. Association between radiographic features of knee osteoarthritis and pain: Results from two cohort studies. *BMJ* **2009**, *339*, b2844. [CrossRef] [PubMed]
13. Wang, K.; Kim, H.A.; Felson, D.T.; Xu, L.; Kim, D.H.; Nevitt, M.C.; Yoshimura, N.; Kawaguchi, H.; Lin, J.; Kang, X.; et al. Radiographic Knee Osteoarthritis and Knee Pain: Cross-sectional study from Five Different Racial/Ethnic Populations. *Sci. Rep.* **2018**, *8*, 1364. [CrossRef] [PubMed]
14. Son, K.M.; Lee, H.S.; Kim, D.H.; Paik, M.C.; Jang, D.G.; Lee, S.Y.; Kim, H.A. The Absence of Symptom in Subjects with Advanced Knee OA. *Rheum. Dis.* **2016**, *75*, 825–826. [CrossRef]
15. Dye, S.F.; Vaupel, G.L.; Dye, C.C. Conscious neurosensory mapping of the internal structures of the human knee without intraarticular anesthesia. *Am. J. Sports Med.* **1998**, *26*, 773–777. [CrossRef]
16. Zhang, Y.; Nevitt, M.; Niu, J.; Lewis, C.; Torner, J.; Guermazi, A.; Roemer, F.; McCulloch, C.; Felson, D.T. Fluctuation of knee pain and changes in bone marrow lesions, effusions, and synovitis on magnetic resonance imaging. *Arthritis Rheum.* **2011**, *63*, 692–699. [CrossRef]
17. Englund, M.; Guermazi, A.; Gale, D.; Hunter, D.J.; Aliabadi, P.; Clancy, M.; Felson, D.T. Incidental meniscal findings on knee MRI in middle-aged and elderly persons. *N. Engl. J. Med.* **2008**, *359*, 1108–1115. [CrossRef]
18. Kim, H.A.; Kim, I.; Song, Y.W.; Kim, D.H.; Niu, J.; Guermazi, A.; Crema, M.D.; Hunter, D.J.; Zhang, Y. The association between meniscal and cruciate ligament damage and knee pain in community residents. *Osteoarthr. Cartil.* **2011**, *19*, 1422–1428. [CrossRef]
19. Felson, D.T.; Chaisson, C.E.; Hill, C.L.; Totterman, S.M.; Gale, M.E.; Skinner, K.M.; Kazis, L.; Gale, D.R. The association of bone marrow lesions with pain in knee osteoarthritis. *Ann. Intern. Med.* **2001**, *134*, 541–549. [CrossRef]
20. Yusuf, E.; Kortekaas, M.C.; Watt, I.; Huizinga, T.W.; Kloppenburg, M. Do knee abnormalities visualised on MRI explain knee pain in knee osteoarthritis? A systematic review. *Ann. Rheum. Dis.* **2011**, *70*, 60–67. [CrossRef]

21. Alliston, T.; Hernandez, C.J.; Findlay, D.M.; Felson, D.T.; Kennedy, O.D. Bone marrow lesions in osteoarthritis: What lies beneath. *J. Orthop. Res.* **2018**, *36*, 1818–1825. [CrossRef] [PubMed]
22. Aso, K.; Shahtaheri, S.M.; Hill, R.; Wilson, D.; McWilliams, D.F.; Walsh, D.A. Associations of Symptomatic Knee Osteoarthritis with Histopathologic Features in Subchondral Bone. *Arthritis Rheumatol.* **2019**, *71*, 916–924. [CrossRef] [PubMed]
23. Arendt-Nielsen, L. Pain sensitisation in osteoarthritis. *Clin. Exp. Rheumatol.* **2017**, *35* (Suppl. 107), 68–74. [PubMed]
24. Neogi, T.; Frey-Law, L.; Scholz, J.; Niu, J.; Arendt-Nielsen, L.; Woolf, C.; Nevitt, M.; Bradley, L.; Felson, D.T.; Multicenter Osteoarthritis, S. Sensitivity and sensitisation in relation to pain severity in knee osteoarthritis: Trait or state? *Ann. Rheum. Dis.* **2015**, *74*, 682–688. [CrossRef]
25. Steen Pettersen, P.; Neogi, T.; Magnusson, K.; Berner Hammer, H.; Uhlig, T.; Kvien, T.K.; Haugen, I.K. Peripheral and Central Sensitization of Pain in Individuals with Hand Osteoarthritis and Associations with Self-Reported Pain Severity. *Arthritis Rheumatol.* **2019**, *71*, 1070–1077. [CrossRef]
26. Egsgaard, L.L.; Eskehave, T.N.; Bay-Jensen, A.C.; Hoeck, H.C.; Arendt-Nielsen, L. Identifying specific profiles in patients with different degrees of painful knee osteoarthritis based on serological biochemical and mechanistic pain biomarkers: A diagnostic approach based on cluster analysis. *Pain* **2015**, *156*, 96–107. [CrossRef]
27. Eitner, A.; Hofmann, G.O.; Schaible, H.G. Mechanisms of Osteoarthritic Pain. Studies in Humans and Experimental Models. *Front. Mol. Neurosci.* **2017**, *10*, 349. [CrossRef]
28. Felson, D.T. Developments in the clinical understanding of osteoarthritis. *Arthritis Res. Ther.* **2009**, *11*, 203. [CrossRef]
29. Eitner, A.; Pester, J.; Nietzsche, S.; Hofmann, G.O.; Schaible, H.G. The innervation of synovium of human osteoarthritic joints in comparison with normal rat and sheep synovium. *Osteoarthr. Cartil.* **2013**, *21*, 1383–1391. [CrossRef]
30. Suri, S.; Gill, S.E.; de Massena, C.S.; Wilson, D.; McWilliams, D.F.; Walsh, D.A. Neurovascular invasion at the osteochondral junction and in osteophytes in osteoarthritis. *Ann. Rheum. Dis.* **2007**, *66*, 1423–1428. [CrossRef]
31. Pergolizzi, J.V., Jr.; Raffa, R.B.; Taylor, R., Jr.; Rodriguez, G.; Nalamachu, S.; Langley, P. A review of duloxetine 60 mg once-daily dosing for the management of diabetic peripheral neuropathic pain, fibromyalgia, and chronic musculoskeletal pain due to chronic osteoarthritis pain and low back pain. *Pain Pract.* **2013**, *13*, 239–252. [CrossRef] [PubMed]
32. Bannuru, R.R.; Osani, M.C.; Vaysbrot, E.E.; Arden, N.K.; Bennell, K.; Bierma-Zeinstra, S.M.A.; Kraus, V.B.; Lohmander, L.S.; Abbott, J.H.; Bhandari, M.; et al. OARSI guidelines for the non-surgical management of knee, hip, and polyarticular osteoarthritis. *Osteoarthr. Cartil.* **2019**, *27*, 1578–1589. [CrossRef] [PubMed]
33. Miller, R.E.; Malfait, A.M.; Block, J.A. Current status of nerve growth factor antibodies for the treatment of osteoarthritis pain. *Clin. Exp. Rheumatol.* **2017**, *35* (Suppl. 107), 85–87. [PubMed]
34. Dakin, P.; DiMartino, S.J.; Gao, H.; Maloney, J.; Kivitz, A.J.; Schnitzer, T.J.; Stahl, N.; Yancopoulos, G.D.; Geba, G.P. The Efficacy, Tolerability, and Joint Safety of Fasinumab in Osteoarthritis Pain: A Phase IIb/III Double-Blind, Placebo-Controlled, Randomized Clinical Trial. *Arthritis Rheumatol.* **2019**, *71*, 1824–1834. [CrossRef] [PubMed]
35. Lane, N.E.; Schnitzer, T.J.; Birbara, C.A.; Mokhtarani, M.; Shelton, D.L.; Smith, M.D.; Brown, M.T. Tanezumab for the treatment of pain from osteoarthritis of the knee. *N. Engl. J. Med.* **2010**, *363*, 1521–1531. [CrossRef] [PubMed]
36. Little, C.B.; Zaki, S. What constitutes an "animal model of osteoarthritis"—The need for consensus? *Osteoarthr. Cartil.* **2012**, *20*, 261–267. [CrossRef]
37. Glasson, S.S.; Blanchet, T.J.; Morris, E.A. The surgical destabilization of the medial meniscus (DMM) model of osteoarthritis in the 129/SvEv mouse. *Osteoarthr. Cartil.* **2007**, *15*, 1061–1069. [CrossRef]
38. Zhou, S.; Lu, W.; Chen, L.; Ge, Q.; Chen, D.; Xu, Z.; Shi, D.; Dai, J.; Li, J.; Ju, H.; et al. AMPK deficiency in chondrocytes accelerated the progression of instability-induced and ageing-associated osteoarthritis in adult mice. *Sci. Rep.* **2017**, *7*, 43245. [CrossRef]
39. Wondimu, E.B.; Culley, K.L.; Quinn, J.; Chang, J.; Dragomir, C.L.; Plumb, D.A.; Goldring, M.B.; Otero, M. Elf3 Contributes to Cartilage Degradation in vivo in a Surgical Model of Post-Traumatic Osteoarthritis. *Sci. Rep.* **2018**, *8*, 6438. [CrossRef]

40. Maumus, M.; Roussignol, G.; Toupet, K.; Penarier, G.; Bentz, I.; Teixeira, S.; Oustric, D.; Jung, M.; Lepage, O.; Steinberg, R.; et al. Utility of a Mouse Model of Osteoarthritis to Demonstrate Cartilage Protection by IFNgamma-Primed Equine Mesenchymal Stem Cells. *Front. Immunol.* **2016**, *7*, 392. [CrossRef]
41. Barve, R.A.; Minnerly, J.C.; Weiss, D.J.; Meyer, D.M.; Aguiar, D.J.; Sullivan, P.M.; Weinrich, S.L.; Head, R.D. Transcriptional profiling and pathway analysis of monosodium iodoacetate-induced experimental osteoarthritis in rats: Relevance to human disease. *Osteoarthr. Cartil.* **2007**, *15*, 1190–1198. [CrossRef] [PubMed]
42. Clements, K.M.; Ball, A.D.; Jones, H.B.; Brinckmann, S.; Read, S.J.; Murray, F. Cellular and histopathological changes in the infrapatellar fat pad in the monoiodoacetate model of osteoarthritis pain. *Osteoarthr. Cartil.* **2009**, *17*, 805–812. [CrossRef] [PubMed]
43. Guzman, R.E.; Evans, M.G.; Bove, S.; Morenko, B.; Kilgore, K. Mono-iodoacetate-induced histologic changes in subchondral bone and articular cartilage of rat femorotibial joints: An animal model of osteoarthritis. *Toxicol. Pathol.* **2003**, *31*, 619–624. [CrossRef] [PubMed]
44. Ter, H.F.; Luiz, A.P.; Santana-Varela, S.; Chessell, I.P.; Welsh, F.; Wood, J.N.; Chenu, C. Noninvasive Mechanical Joint Loading as an Alternative Model for Osteoarthritic Pain. *Arthritis Rheumatol.* **2019**, *71*, 1078–1088. [CrossRef]
45. Sokoloff, L.; Crittenden, L.B.; Yamamoto, R.S.; Jay, G.E., Jr. The genetics of degenerative joint disease in mice. *Arthritis Rheum.* **1962**, *5*, 531–546. [CrossRef] [PubMed]
46. Kim, H.A.; Cheon, E.J. Animal Model of Osteoarthritis. *J. Rheum. Dis.* **2012**, *19*. [CrossRef]
47. Zhang, R.X.; Ren, K.; Dubner, R. Osteoarthritis pain mechanisms: Basic studies in animal models. *Osteoarthr. Cartil.* **2013**, *21*, 1308–1315. [CrossRef]
48. Deuis, J.R.; Dvorakova, L.S.; Vetter, I. Methods Used to Evaluate Pain Behaviors in Rodents. *Front. Mol. Neurosci.* **2017**, *10*, 284. [CrossRef]
49. Chaplan, S.R.; Bach, F.W.; Pogrel, J.W.; Chung, J.M.; Yaksh, T.L. Quantitative assessment of tactile allodynia in the rat paw. *J. Neurosci. Methods* **1994**, *53*, 55–63. [CrossRef]
50. Pitcher, T.; Sousa-Valente, J.; Malcangio, M. The Monoiodoacetate Model of Osteoarthritis Pain in the Mouse. *J. Vis. Exp.* **2016**. [CrossRef]
51. Jacobs, B.Y.; Allen, K.D. Factors affecting the reliability of behavioral assessments for rodent osteoarthritis models. *Lab. Anim.* **2019**. [CrossRef] [PubMed]
52. Herold, S.; Kumar, P.; Jung, K.; Graf, I.; Menkhoff, H.; Schulz, X.; Bahr, M.; Hein, K. CatWalk gait analysis in a rat model of multiple sclerosis. *BMC Neurosci.* **2016**, *17*, 78. [CrossRef] [PubMed]
53. Gholami, M.; Saboory, E.; Mehraban, S.; Niakani, A.; Banihabib, N.; Azad, M.R.; Fereidoni, J. Time dependent antinociceptive effects of morphine and tramadol in the hot plate test: Using different methods of drug administration in female rats. *Iran. J. Pharm. Res.* **2015**, *14*, 303–311. [PubMed]
54. O'Callaghan, J.P.; Holtzman, S.G. Quantification of the analgesic activity of narcotic antagonists by a modified hot-plate procedure. *J. Pharmacol. Exp. Ther.* **1975**, *192*, 497–505. [PubMed]
55. Shiotsuki, H.; Yoshimi, K.; Shimo, Y.; Funayama, M.; Takamatsu, Y.; Ikeda, K.; Takahashi, R.; Kitazawa, S.; Hattori, N. A rotarod test for evaluation of motor skill learning. *J. Neurosci. Methods* **2010**, *189*, 180–185. [CrossRef]
56. Lynch, J.J.; Castagne, V.; Moser, P.C.; Mittelstadt, S.W. Comparison of methods for the assessment of locomotor activity in rodent safety pharmacology studies. *J. Pharmacol. Toxicol. Methods* **2011**, *64*, 74–80. [CrossRef]
57. Quinn, L.P.; Stean, T.O.; Trail, B.; Duxon, M.S.; Stratton, S.C.; Billinton, A.; Upton, N. LABORAS: Initial pharmacological validation of a system allowing continuous monitoring of laboratory rodent behaviour. *J. Neurosci. Methods* **2003**, *130*, 83–92. [CrossRef]
58. Miller, R.E.; Tran, P.B.; Das, R.; Ghoreishi-Haack, N.; Ren, D.; Miller, R.J.; Malfait, A.M. CCR2 chemokine receptor signaling mediates pain in experimental osteoarthritis. *Proc. Natl. Acad. Sci. USA* **2012**, *109*, 20602–20607. [CrossRef]
59. Nwosu, L.N.; Mapp, P.I.; Chapman, V.; Walsh, D.A. Blocking the tropomyosin receptor kinase A (TrkA) receptor inhibits pain behaviour in two rat models of osteoarthritis. *Ann. Rheum. Dis.* **2016**, *75*, 1246–1254. [CrossRef]
60. Harvey, V.L.; Dickenson, A.H. Behavioural and electrophysiological characterisation of experimentally induced osteoarthritis and neuropathy in C57Bl/6 mice. *Mol. Pain* **2009**, *5*, 18. [CrossRef]

61. Lee, C.H.; Wen, Z.H.; Chang, Y.C.; Huang, S.Y.; Tang, C.C.; Chen, W.F.; Hsieh, S.P.; Hsieh, C.S.; Jean, Y.H. Intra-articular magnesium sulfate (MgSO4) reduces experimental osteoarthritis and nociception: Association with attenuation of N-methyl-D-aspartate (NMDA) receptor subunit 1 phosphorylation and apoptosis in rat chondrocytes. *Osteoarthr. Cartil.* **2009**, *17*, 1485–1493. [CrossRef] [PubMed]
62. Ashraf, S.; Mapp, P.I.; Burston, J.; Bennett, A.J.; Chapman, V.; Walsh, D.A. Augmented pain behavioural responses to intra-articular injection of nerve growth factor in two animal models of osteoarthritis. *Ann. Rheum. Dis.* **2014**, *73*, 1710–1718. [CrossRef] [PubMed]
63. Yuan, X.C.; Zhu, B.; Jing, X.H.; Xiong, L.Z.; Wu, C.H.; Gao, F.; Li, H.P.; Xiang, H.C.; Zhu, H.; Zhou, B.; et al. Electroacupuncture Potentiates Cannabinoid Receptor-Mediated Descending Inhibitory Control in a Mouse Model of Knee Osteoarthritis. *Front. Mol. Neurosci.* **2018**, *11*, 112. [CrossRef] [PubMed]
64. Comi, E.; Lanza, M.; Ferrari, F.; Mauri, V.; Caselli, G.; Rovati, L.C. Efficacy of CR4056, a first-in-class imidazoline-2 analgesic drug, in comparison with naproxen in two rat models of osteoarthritis. *J. Pain Res.* **2017**, *10*, 1033–1043. [CrossRef] [PubMed]
65. Poulet, B.; de Souza, R.; Knights, C.B.; Gentry, C.; Wilson, A.M.; Bevan, S.; Chang, Y.M.; Pitsillides, A.A. Modifications of gait as predictors of natural osteoarthritis progression in STR/Ort mice. *Arthritis Rheumatol.* **2014**, *66*, 1832–1842. [CrossRef] [PubMed]
66. Van der Kraan, P.M.; Vitters, E.L.; van Beuningen, H.M.; van de Putte, L.B.; van den Berg, W.B. Degenerative knee joint lesions in mice after a single intra-articular collagenase injection. A new model of osteoarthritis. *J. Exp. Pathol.* **1990**, *71*, 19–31.
67. Choi, W.S.; Lee, G.; Song, W.H.; Koh, J.T.; Yang, J.; Kwak, J.S.; Kim, H.E.; Kim, S.K.; Son, Y.O.; Nam, H.; et al. The CH25H-CYP7B1-RORalpha axis of cholesterol metabolism regulates osteoarthritis. *Nature* **2019**, *566*, 254–258. [CrossRef]
68. Suter, E.; Herzog, W.; Leonard, T.R.; Nguyen, H. One-year changes in hind limb kinematics, ground reaction forces and knee stability in an experimental model of osteoarthritis. *J. Biomech.* **1998**, *31*, 511–517. [CrossRef]
69. Janusz, M.J.; Hookfin, E.B.; Heitmeyer, S.A.; Woessner, J.F.; Freemont, A.J.; Hoyland, J.A.; Brown, K.K.; Hsieh, L.C.; Almstead, N.G.; De, B.; et al. Moderation of iodoacetate-induced experimental osteoarthritis in rats by matrix metalloproteinase inhibitors. *Osteoarthr. Cartil.* **2001**, *9*, 751–760. [CrossRef]
70. Mason, R.M.; Chambers, M.G.; Flannelly, J.; Gaffen, J.D.; Dudhia, J.; Bayliss, M.T. The STR/ort mouse and its use as a model of osteoarthritis. *Osteoarthr. Cartil.* **2001**, *9*, 85–91. [CrossRef]
71. Fang, H.; Huang, L.; Welch, I.; Norley, C.; Holdsworth, D.W.; Beier, F.; Cai, D. Early Changes of Articular Cartilage and Subchondral Bone in The DMM Mouse Model of Osteoarthritis. *Sci. Rep.* **2018**, *8*, 2855. [CrossRef] [PubMed]
72. Knights, C.B.; Gentry, C.; Bevan, S. Partial medial meniscectomy produces osteoarthritis pain-related behaviour in female C57BL/6 mice. *Pain* **2012**, *153*, 281–292. [CrossRef] [PubMed]
73. Yu, D.G.; Yu, B.; Mao, Y.Q.; Zhao, X.; Wang, X.Q.; Ding, H.F.; Cao, L.; Liu, G.W.; Nie, S.B.; Liu, S.; et al. Efficacy of zoledronic acid in treatment of teoarthritis is dependent on the disease progression stage in rat medial meniscal tear model. *Acta Pharmacol. Sin.* **2012**, *33*, 924–934. [CrossRef] [PubMed]
74. Di Cesare Mannelli, L.; Micheli, L.; Zanardelli, M.; Ghelardini, C. Low dose native type II collagen prevents pain in a rat osteoarthritis model. *BMC Musculoskelet. Disord.* **2013**, *14*, 228. [CrossRef]
75. Ko, F.C.; Dragomir, C.; Plumb, D.A.; Goldring, S.R.; Wright, T.M.; Goldring, M.B.; van der Meulen, M.C. In vivo cyclic compression causes cartilage degeneration and subchondral bone changes in mouse tibiae. *Arthritis Rheum.* **2013**, *65*, 1569–1578. [CrossRef]
76. Ruan, M.Z.; Patel, R.M.; Dawson, B.C.; Jiang, M.M.; Lee, B.H. Pain, motor and gait assessment of murine osteoarthritis in a cruciate ligament transection model. *Osteoarthr. Cartil.* **2013**, *21*, 1355–1364. [CrossRef]
77. Naik, S.R.; Wala, S.M. Arthritis, a complex connective and synovial joint destructive autoimmune disease: Animal models of arthritis with varied etiopathology and their significance. *J. Postgrad. Med.* **2014**, *60*, 309–317. [CrossRef]
78. Huang, H.; Skelly, J.D.; Ayers, D.C.; Song, J. Age-dependent Changes in the Articular Cartilage and Subchondral Bone of C57BL/6 Mice after Surgical Destabilization of Medial Meniscus. *Sci. Rep.* **2017**, *7*, 42294. [CrossRef]
79. Kung, L.H.W.; Ravi, V.; Rowley, L.; Bell, K.M.; Little, C.B.; Bateman, J.F. Comprehensive Expression Analysis of microRNAs and mRNAs in Synovial Tissue from a Mouse Model of Early Post-Traumatic Osteoarthritis. *Sci. Rep.* **2017**, *7*, 17701. [CrossRef]

80. Van Dalen, S.C.; Blom, A.B.; Slöetjes, A.W.; Helsen, M.M.; Roth, J.; Vogl, T.; van de Loo, F.A.; Koenders, M.I.; van der Kraan, P.M.; van den Berg, W.B.; et al. Interleukin-1 is not involved in synovial inflammation and cartilage destruction in collagenase-induced osteoarthritis. *Osteoarthr. Cartil.* **2017**, *25*, 385–396. [CrossRef]
81. Kim, J.E.; Song, D.H.; Kim, S.H.; Jung, Y.; Kim, S.J. Development and characterization of various osteoarthritis models for tissue engineering. *PLoS ONE* **2018**, *13*, e0194288. [CrossRef] [PubMed]
82. Tawonsawatruk, T.; Sriwatananukulkit, O.; Himakhun, W.; Hemstapat, W. Comparison of pain behaviour and osteoarthritis progression between anterior cruciate ligament transection and osteochondral injury in rat models. *Bone Joint Res.* **2018**, *7*, 244–251. [CrossRef]
83. Xie, J.; Zhang, D.; Lin, Y.; Yuan, Q.; Zhou, X. Anterior Cruciate Ligament Transection-Induced Cellular and Extracellular Events in Menisci: Implications for Osteoarthritis. *Am. J. Sports Med.* **2018**, *46*, 1185–1198. [CrossRef] [PubMed]
84. Zhu, S.; Zhu, J.; Zhen, G.; Hu, Y.; An, S.; Li, Y.; Zheng, Q.; Chen, Z.; Yang, Y.; Wan, M.; et al. Subchondral bone osteoclasts induce sensory innervation and osteoarthritis pain. *J. Clin. Invest.* **2019**, *129*, 1076–1093. [CrossRef] [PubMed]
85. Tu, M.; Yang, M.; Yu, N.; Zhen, G.; Wan, M.; Liu, W.; Ji, B.; Ma, H.; Guo, Q.; Tong, P.; et al. Inhibition of cyclooxygenase-2 activity in subchondral bone modifies a subtype of osteoarthritis. *Bone Res.* **2019**, *7*, 1–10. [CrossRef] [PubMed]
86. Carcole, M.; Zamanillo, D.; Merlos, M.; Fernandez-Pastor, B.; Cabanero, D.; Maldonado, R. Blockade of the Sigma-1 Receptor Relieves Cognitive and Emotional Impairments Associated to Chronic Osteoarthritis Pain. *Front. Pharmacol.* **2019**, *10*, 468. [CrossRef]
87. Jacobs, H.N.; Rathod, S.; Wolf, M.T.; Elisseeff, J.H Intra-articular Injection of Urinary Bladder Matrix Reduces Osteoarthritis Development. *AAPS J.* **2017**, *19*, 141–149. [CrossRef]
88. Fang, H.; Beier, F. Mouse models of osteoarthritis: Modelling risk factors and assessing outcomes. *Nat. Rev. Rheumatol.* **2014**, *10*, 413–421. [CrossRef]
89. Bapat, S.; Hubbard, D.; Munjal, A.; Hunter, M.; Fulzele, S. Pros and cons of mouse models for studying osteoarthritis. *Clin. Transl. Med.* **2018**, *7*, 36. [CrossRef]
90. Thysen, S.; Luyten, F.P.; Lories, R.J. Targets, models and challenges in osteoarthritis research. *Dis. Model Mech.* **2015**, *8*, 17–30. [CrossRef]
91. Fernihough, J.; Gentry, C.; Malcangio, M.; Fox, A.; Rediske, J.; Pellas, T.; Kidd, B.; Bevan, S.; Winter, J. Pain related behaviour in two models of osteoarthritis in the rat knee. *Pain* **2004**, *112*, 83–93. [CrossRef] [PubMed]
92. Zhao, L.; Huang, J.; Fan, Y.; Li, J.; You, T.; He, S.; Xiao, G.; Chen, D. Exploration of CRISPR/Cas9-based gene editing as therapy for osteoarthritis. *Ann. Rheum. Dis.* **2019**, *78*, 676–682. [CrossRef] [PubMed]
93. Malfait, A.M.; Miller, R.J. Emerging Targets for the Management of Osteoarthritis Pain. *Curr. Osteoporos. Rep.* **2016**, *14*, 260–268. [CrossRef] [PubMed]
94. Kc, R.; Li, X.; Kroin, J.S.; Liu, Z.; Chen, D.; Xiao, G.; Levine, B.; Li, J.; Hamilton, J.L.; van Wijnen, A.J.; et al PKCdelta null mutations in a mouse model of osteoarthritis alter osteoarthritic pain independently of joint pathology by augmenting NGF/TrkA-induced axonal outgrowth. *Ann. Rheum. Dis.* **2016**, *75*, 2133–2141. [CrossRef]
95. Malfait, A.M.; Ritchie, J.; Gil, A.S.; Austin, J.S.; Hartke, J.; Qin, W.; Tortorella, M.D.; Mogil, J.S. ADAMTS-5 deficient mice do not develop mechanical allodynia associated with osteoarthritis following medial meniscal destabilization. *Osteoarthr. Cartil.* **2010**, *18*, 572–580. [CrossRef] [PubMed]
96. Miller, R.E.; Tran, P.B.; Ishihara, S.; Larkin, J.; Malfait, A.M. Therapeutic effects of an anti-ADAMTS-5 antibody on joint damage and mechanical allodynia in a murine model of osteoarthritis. *Osteoarthr. Cartil.* **2016**, *24*, 299–306. [CrossRef]
97. Chan, C.C.; Roberts, C.R.; Steeves, J.D.; Tetzlaff, W. Aggrecan components differentially modulate nerve growth factor-responsive and neurotrophin-3-responsive dorsal root ganglion neurite growth. *J. Neurosci. Res.* **2008**, *86*, 581–592. [CrossRef]
98. Chen, D.; Shen, J.; Zhao, W.; Wang, T.; Han, L.; Hamilton, J.L.; Im, H.J. Osteoarthritis: Toward a comprehensive understanding of pathological mechanism. *Bone Res.* **2017**, *5*, 16044. [CrossRef]
99. Miller, R.E.; Ishihara, S.; Tran, P.B.; Golub, S.B.; Last, K.; Miller, R.J.; Fosang, A.J.; Malfait, A.M. An aggrecan fragment drives osteoarthritis pain through Toll-like receptor 2. *JCI Insight* **2018**, *3*. [CrossRef]

100. Miller, R.E.; Belmadani, A.; Ishihara, S.; Tran, P.B.; Ren, D.; Miller, R.J.; Malfait, A.M. Damage-associated molecular patterns generated in osteoarthritis directly excite murine nociceptive neurons through Toll-like receptor 4. *Arthritis Rheumatol.* **2015**, *67*, 2933–2943. [CrossRef]
101. Miller, R.E.; Scanzello, C.R.; Malfait, A.M. An emerging role for Toll-like receptors at the neuroimmune interface in osteoarthritis. *Semin. Immunopathol.* **2019**, *41*, 583–594. [CrossRef] [PubMed]
102. Ivanavicius, S.P.; Ball, A.D.; Heapy, C.G.; Westwood, F.R.; Murray, F.; Read, S.J. Structural pathology in a rodent model of osteoarthritis is associated with neuropathic pain: Increased expression of ATF-3 and pharmacological characterisation. *Pain* **2007**, *128*, 272–282. [CrossRef] [PubMed]
103. Hoshino, T.; Tsuji, K.; Onuma, H.; Udo, M.; Ueki, H.; Akiyama, M.; Abula, K.; Katagiri, H.; Miyatake, K.; Watanabe, T.; et al. Persistent synovial inflammation plays important roles in persistent pain development in the rat knee before cartilage degradation reaches the subchondral bone. *BMC Musculoskelet. Disord.* **2018**, *19*, 291. [CrossRef] [PubMed]
104. Lee, M.C.; Saleh, R.; Achuthan, A.; Fleetwood, A.J.; Forster, I.; Hamilton, J.A.; Cook, A.D. CCL17 blockade as a therapy for osteoarthritis pain and disease. *Arthritis Res. Ther.* **2018**, *20*, 62. [CrossRef] [PubMed]
105. Atkins, G.J.; Welldon, K.J.; Halbout, P.; Findlay, D.M. Strontium ranelate treatment of human primary osteoblasts promotes an osteocyte-like phenotype while eliciting an osteoprotegerin response. *Osteoporos. Int.* **2009**, *20*, 653–664. [CrossRef] [PubMed]
106. Reginster, J.Y.; Badurski, J.; Bellamy, N.; Bensen, W.; Chapurlat, R.; Chevalier, X.; Christiansen, C.; Genant, H.; Navarro, F.; Nasonov, E.; et al. Efficacy and safety of strontium ranelate in the treatment of knee osteoarthritis: Results of a double-blind, randomised placebo-controlled trial. *Ann. Rheum. Dis.* **2013**, *72*, 179–186. [CrossRef]
107. Pelletier, J.P.; Roubille, C.; Raynauld, J.P.; Abram, F.; Dorais, M.; Delorme, P.; Martel-Pelletier, J. Disease-modifying effect of strontium ranelate in a subset of patients from the Phase III knee osteoarthritis study SEKOIA using quantitative MRI: Reduction in bone marrow lesions protects against cartilage loss. *Ann. Rheum. Dis.* **2015**, *74*, 422–429. [CrossRef]
108. Laslett, L.L.; Dore, D.A.; Quinn, S.J.; Boon, P.; Ryan, E.; Winzenberg, T.M.; Jones, G. Zoledronic acid reduces knee pain and bone marrow lesions over 1 year: A randomised controlled trial. *Ann. Rheum. Dis.* **2012**, *71*, 1322–1328. [CrossRef]
109. O'Conor, C.J.; Griffin, T.M.; Liedtke, W.; Guilak, F. Increased susceptibility of Trpv4-deficient mice to obesity and obesity-induced osteoarthritis with very high-fat diet. *Ann. Rheum. Dis.* **2013**, *72*, 300–304. [CrossRef]
110. Triantaphyllidou, I.E.; Kalyvioti, E.; Karavia, E.; Lilis, I.; Kypreos, K.E.; Papachristou, D.J. Perturbations in the HDL metabolic pathway predispose to the development of osteoarthritis in mice following long-term exposure to western-type diet. *Osteoarthr. Cartil.* **2013**, *21*, 322–330. [CrossRef]
111. De Munter, W.; Blom, A.B.; Helsen, M.M.; Walgreen, B.; van der Kraan, P.M.; Joosten, L.A.; van den Berg, W.B.; van Lent, P.L. Cholesterol accumulation caused by low density lipoprotein receptor deficiency or a cholesterol-rich diet results in ectopic bone formation during experimental osteoarthritis. *Arthritis Res. Ther.* **2013**, *15*, R178. [CrossRef] [PubMed]
112. Griffin, T.M.; Huebner, J.L.; Kraus, V.B.; Guilak, F. Extreme obesity due to impaired leptin signaling in mice does not cause knee osteoarthritis. *Arthritis Rheum.* **2009**, *60*, 2935–2944. [CrossRef] [PubMed]
113. Louer, C.R.; Furman, B.D.; Huebner, J.L.; Kraus, V.B.; Olson, S.A.; Guilak, F. Diet-induced obesity significantly increases the severity of posttraumatic arthritis in mice. *Arthritis Rheum.* **2012**, *64*, 3220–3230. [CrossRef] [PubMed]
114. Wu, C.L.; Jain, D.; McNeill, J.N.; Little, D.; Anderson, J.A.; Huebner, J.L.; Kraus, V.B.; Rodriguiz, R.M.; Wetsel, W.C.; Guilak, F. Dietary fatty acid content regulates wound repair and the pathogenesis of osteoarthritis following joint injury. *Ann. Rheum. Dis.* **2015**, *74*, 2076–2083. [CrossRef]
115. Jay, G.E., Jr.; Sokoloff, L. Natural history of degenerative joint disease in small laboratory animals. II. Epiphyseal maturation and osteoarthritis of the knee of mice of inbred strains. *Ann. Arch. Pathol.* **1956**, *62*, 129–135.
116. Ochoa, J.; Mair, W.G. The normal sural nerve in man. II. Changes in the axons and Schwann cells due to ageing. *Acta Neuropathol.* **1969**, *13*, 217–239. [CrossRef]
117. Ko, M.L.; King, M.A.; Gordon, T.L.; Crisp, T. The effects of aging on spinal neurochemistry in the rat. *Brain Res. Bull.* **1997**, *42*, 95–98. [CrossRef]
118. Hamm, R.J.; Knisely, J.S. Environmentally induced analgesia: Age-related decline in a neurally mediated, nonopioid system. *Psychol. Aging* **1986**, *1*, 195–201. [CrossRef]

119. Stannus, O.P.; Jones, G.; Blizzard, L.; Cicuttini, F.M.; Ding, C. Associations between serum levels of inflammatory markers and change in knee pain over 5 years in older adults: A prospective cohort study. *Ann. Rheum. Dis.* **2013**, *72*, 535–540. [CrossRef]
120. Greene, M.A.; Loeser, R.F. Aging-related inflammation in osteoarthritis. *Osteoarthr. Cartil.* **2015**, *23*, 1966–1971. [CrossRef]
121. Penninx, B.W.; Abbas, H.; Ambrosius, W.; Nicklas, B.J.; Davis, C.; Messier, S.P.; Pahor, M. Inflammatory markers and physical function among older adults with knee osteoarthritis. *J. Rheumatol.* **2004**, *31*, 2027–2031. [PubMed]
122. De Hooge, A.S.; van de Loo, F.A.; Bennink, M.B.; Arntz, O.J.; de Hooge, P.; van den Berg, W.B. Male IL-6 gene knock out mice developed more advanced osteoarthritis upon aging. *Osteoarthr. Cartil.* **2005**, *13*, 66–73. [CrossRef] [PubMed]
123. Jeon, O.H.; David, N.; Campisi, J.; Elisseeff, J.H. Senescent cells and osteoarthritis: A painful connection. *J. Clin. Investig.* **2018**, *128*, 1229–1237. [CrossRef] [PubMed]
124. Campisi, J. Aging, cellular senescence, and cancer. *Ann. Rev. Physiol.* **2013**, *75*, 685–705. [CrossRef] [PubMed]
125. Yu, S.M.; Kim, S.J. Thymoquinone-induced reactive oxygen species causes apoptosis of chondrocytes via PI3K/Akt and p38kinase pathway. *Exp. Biol. Med.* **2013**, *238*, 811–820. [CrossRef]
126. Freund, A.; Patil, C.K.; Campisi, J. p38MAPK is a novel DNA damage response-independent regulator of the senescence-associated secretory phenotype. *EMBO J.* **2011**, *30*, 1536–1548. [CrossRef]
127. Jeon, O.H.; Kim, C.; Laberge, R.M.; Demaria, M.; Rathod, S.; Vasserot, A.P.; Chung, J.W.; Kim, D.H.; Poon, Y.; David, N.; et al. Local clearance of senescent cells attenuates the development of post-traumatic osteoarthritis and creates a pro-regenerative environment. *Nat. Med.* **2017**, *23*, 775–781. [CrossRef]
128. Lorenz, J.; Grassel, S. Experimental osteoarthritis models in mice. *Methods Mol. Biol.* **2014**, *1194*, 401–419. [CrossRef]
129. Ma, H.L.; Blanchet, T.J.; Peluso, D.; Hopkins, B.; Morris, E.A.; Glasson, S.S. Osteoarthritis severity is sex dependent in a surgical mouse model. *Osteoarthr. Cartil.* **2007**, *15*, 695–700. [CrossRef]
130. Mahr, S.; Menard, J.; Krenn, V.; Muller, B. Sexual dimorphism in the osteoarthritis of STR/ort mice may be linked to articular cytokines. *Ann. Rheum. Dis.* **2003**, *62*, 1234–1237. [CrossRef]
131. Van Osch, G.J.; van der Kraan, P.M.; Vitters, E.L.; Blankevoort, L.; van den Berg, W.B. Induction of osteoarthritis by intra-articular injection of collagenase in mice. Strain and sex related differences. *Osteoarthr. Cartil.* **1993**, *1*, 171–177. [CrossRef]
132. Park, I.Y.; Hong, J.I.; Hwang, H.S.; Kim, H.A. Evaluation of cartilage degeneration and osteoarthritis pain on female and male mouse model of osteoarthritis. *Osteoarthr. Cartil.* **2018**, *26*, S360. [CrossRef]
133. Sorge, R.E.; Totsch, S.K. Sex Differences in Pain. *J. Neurosci. Res.* **2017**, *95*, 1271–1281. [CrossRef] [PubMed]
134. Fischer, B.D.; Adeyemo, A.; O'Leary, M.E.; Bottaro, A. Animal models of rheumatoid pain: Experimental systems and insights. *Arthritis Res. Ther.* **2017**, *19*, 146. [CrossRef] [PubMed]
135. Maini, R.; St Clair, E.W.; Breedveld, F.; Furst, D.; Kalden, J.; Weisman, M.; Smolen, J.; Emery, P.; Harriman, G.; Feldmann, M.; et al. Infliximab (chimeric anti-tumour necrosis factor alpha monoclonal antibody) versus placebo in rheumatoid arthritis patients receiving concomitant methotrexate: A randomised phase III trial. ATTRACT Study Group. *Lancet* **1999**, *354*, 1932–1939. [CrossRef]
136. Singh, J.A.; Christensen, R.; Wells, G.A.; Suarez-Almazor, M.E.; Buchbinder, R.; Lopez-Olivo, M.A.; Tanjong Ghogomu, E.; Tugwell, P. Biologics for rheumatoid arthritis: An overview of Cochrane reviews. *Cochrane Database Syst. Rev.* **2009**. [CrossRef]
137. Hess, A.; Axmann, R.; Rech, J.; Finzel, S.; Heindl, C.; Kreitz, S.; Sergeeva, M.; Saake, M.; Garcia, M.; Kollias, G.; et al. Blockade of TNF-alpha rapidly inhibits pain responses in the central nervous system *Proc. Natl. Acad. Sci. USA* **2011**, *108*, 3731–3736. [CrossRef]
138. Smolen, J.S.; Strand, V.; Koenig, A.S.; Szumski, A.; Kotak, S.; Jones, T.V. Discordance between patient and physician assessments of global disease activity in rheumatoid arthritis and association with work productivity. *Arthritis Res. Ther.* **2016**, *18*, 114. [CrossRef]
139. McWilliams, D.F.; Walsh, D.A. Pain mechanisms in rheumatoid arthritis. *Clin. Exp. Rheumatol.* **2017**, *35* (Suppl. 107), 94–101.
140. Wolfe, F.; Hauser, W.; Hassett, A.L.; Katz, R.S.; Walitt, B.T. The development of fibromyalgia–I: Examination of rates and predictors in patients with rheumatoid arthritis (RA). *Pain* **2011**, *152*, 291–299. [CrossRef]

141. Lee, Y.C.; Lu, B.; Edwards, R.R.; Wasan, A.D.; Nassikas, N.J.; Clauw, D.J.; Solomon, D.H.; Karlson, E.W. The role of sleep problems in central pain processing in rheumatoid arthritis. *Arthritis Rheum.* **2013**, *65*, 59–68. [CrossRef] [PubMed]
142. Joharatnam, N.; McWilliams, D.F.; Wilson, D.; Wheeler, M.; Pande, I.; Walsh, D.A. A cross-sectional study of pain sensitivity, disease-activity assessment, mental health, and fibromyalgia status in rheumatoid arthritis. *Arthritis Res. Ther.* **2015**, *17*, 11. [CrossRef] [PubMed]
143. Krock, E.; Jurczak, A.; Svensson, C.I. Pain pathogenesis in rheumatoid arthritis-what have we learned from animal models? *Pain* **2018**, *159* (Suppl. 1), S98–S109. [CrossRef] [PubMed]
144. Bas, D.B.; Su, J.; Wigerblad, G.; Svensson, C.I. Pain in rheumatoid arthritis: Models and mechanisms. *Pain Manag.* **2016**, *6*, 265–284. [CrossRef]
145. Buckley, B.J.; Ali, U.; Kelso, M.J.; Ranson, M. The Urokinase Plasminogen Activation System in Rheumatoid Arthritis: Pathophysiological Roles and Prospective Therapeutic Targets. *Curr. Drug Targets* **2019**, *20*, 970–981. [CrossRef]
146. Asquith, D.L.; Miller, A.M.; McInnes, I.B.; Liew, F.Y. Animal models of rheumatoid arthritis. *Eur. J. Immunol.* **2009**, *39*, 2040–2044. [CrossRef]
147. Caplazi, P.; Baca, M.; Barck, K.; Carano, R.A.; DeVoss, J.; Lee, W.P.; Bolon, B.; Diehl, L. Mouse Models of Rheumatoid Arthritis. *Vet. Pathol.* **2015**, *52*, 819–826. [CrossRef]
148. Bevaart, L.; Vervoordeldonk, M.J.; Tak, P.P. Evaluation of therapeutic targets in animal models of arthritis: How does it relate to rheumatoid arthritis? *Arthritis Rheum.* **2010**, *62*, 2192–2205. [CrossRef]
149. Moudgil, K.D.; Kim, P.; Brahn, E. Advances in rheumatoid arthritis animal models. *Curr. Rheumatol. Rep.* **2011**, *13*, 456–463. [CrossRef]
150. Roy, T.; Ghosh, S. Animal models of rheumatoid arthritis: Correlation and usefulness with human rheumatoid arthritis. *Indo. Am. J. Pharm. Res.* **2013**, *3*, 6131–6142.
151. Abramson, S.B.; Amin, A. Blocking the effects of IL-1 in rheumatoid arthritis protects bone and cartilage. *Rheumatology* **2002**, *41*, 972–980. [CrossRef] [PubMed]
152. Hayer, S.; Bauer, G.; Willburger, M.; Sinn, K.; Alasti, F.; Plasenzotti, R.; Shvets, T.; Niederreiter, B.; Aschauer, C.; Steiner, G.; et al. Cartilage damage and bone erosion are more prominent determinants of functional impairment in longstanding experimental arthritis than synovial inflammation. *Dis. Model. Mech.* **2016**, *9*, 1329–1338. [CrossRef] [PubMed]
153. Impellizzeri, D.; Esposito, E.; Di Paola, R.; Ahmad, A.; Campolo, M.; Peli, A.; Morittu, V.M.; Britti, D.; Cuzzocrea, S. Palmitoylethanolamide and luteolin ameliorate development of arthritis caused by injection of collagen type II in mice. *Arthritis Res. Ther.* **2013**, *15*, R192. [CrossRef] [PubMed]
154. Jochmann, E.; Boettger, M.K.; Anand, P.; Schaible, H.G. Antigen-induced arthritis in rats is associated with increased growth-associated protein 43-positive intraepidermal nerve fibres remote from the joint. *Arthritis Res. Ther.* **2015**, *17*, 299. [CrossRef]
155. Christianson, C.A.; Corr, M.; Firestein, G.S.; Mobargha, A.; Yaksh, T.L.; Svensson, C.I. Characterization of the acute and persistent pain state present in K/BxN serum transfer arthritis. *Pain* **2010**, *151*, 394–403. [CrossRef]
156. Christianson, C.A.; Corr, M.; Yaksh, T.L.; Svensson, C.I. K/BxN serum transfer arthritis as a model of inflammatory joint pain. *Methods Mol. Biol.* **2012**, *851*, 249–260. [CrossRef]
157. Qu, L.; Caterina, M.J. Enhanced excitability and suppression of A-type K(+) currents in joint sensory neurons in a murine model of antigen-induced arthritis. *Sci. Rep.* **2016**, *6*, 28899. [CrossRef]
158. Zhou, L.L.; Zhu, Y.M.; Qian, F.Y.; Yuan, C.C.; Yuan, D.P.; Zhou, X.P. MicroRNA-143-3p contributes to the regulation of pain responses in collagen-induced arthritis. *Mol. Med. Rep.* **2018**, *18*, 3219–3228. [CrossRef]
159. Balkrishna, A.; Sakat, S.S.; Joshi, K.; Paudel, S.; Joshi, D.; Joshi, K.; Ranjan, R.; Gupta, A.; Bhattacharya, K.; Varshney, A. Anti-Inflammatory and Anti-Arthritic Efficacies of an Indian Traditional Herbo-Mineral Medicine "Divya Amvatari Ras" in Collagen Antibody-Induced Arthritis (CAIA) Mouse Model Through Modulation of IL-6/IL-1beta/TNF-alpha/NFkappaB Signaling. *Front. Pharmacol.* **2019**, *10*, 659. [CrossRef]
160. Bersellini Farinotti, A.; Wigerblad, G.; Nascimento, D.; Bas, D.B.; Morado Urbina, C.; Nandakumar, K.S.; Sandor, K.; Xu, B.; Abdelmoaty, S.; Hunt, M.A.; et al. Cartilage-binding antibodies induce pain through immune complex-mediated activation of neurons. *J. Exp. Med.* **2019**, *216*, 1904–1924. [CrossRef]
161. Fernandez-Zafra, T.; Gao, T.; Jurczak, A.; Sandor, K.; Hore, Z.; Agalave, N.M.; Su, J.; Estelius, J.; Lampa, J.; Hokfelt, T.; et al. Exploring the transcriptome of resident spinal microglia after collagen antibody-induced arthritis. *Pain* **2019**, *160*, 224–236. [CrossRef] [PubMed]

162. Park, D.S.; Seo, B.K.; Baek, Y.H. Analgesic effect of electroacupuncture on inflammatory pain in collagen-induced arthritis rats: Mediation by alpha2- and beta-adrenoceptors. *Rheumatol. Int.* **2013**, *33*, 309–314. [CrossRef] [PubMed]
163. Filippin, L.I.; Teixeira, V.N.; Viacava, P.R.; Lora, F.S.; Xavier, L.L.; Xavier, R.M. Temporal development of muscle atrophy in murine model of arthritis is related to disease severity. *J. Cachexia Sarcopenia Muscle* **2013**, *4*, 231–238. [CrossRef] [PubMed]
164. Bonnet, C.S.; Williams, A.S.; Gilbert, S.J.; Harvey, A.K.; Evans, B.A.; Mason, D.J. AMPA/kainate glutamate receptors contribute to inflammation, degeneration and pain related behaviour in inflammatory stages of arthritis. *Ann. Rheum. Dis.* **2015**, *74*, 242–251. [CrossRef] [PubMed]
165. Fujikado, N.; Saijo, S.; Iwakura, Y. Identification of arthritis-related gene clusters by microarray analysis of two independent mouse models for rheumatoid arthritis. *Arthritis Res. Ther.* **2006**, *8*, R100. [CrossRef]
166. Akitsu, A.; Ishigame, H.; Kakuta, S.; Chung, S.H.; Ikeda, S.; Shimizu, K.; Kubo, S.; Liu, Y.; Umemura, M.; Matsuzaki, G.; et al. IL-1 receptor antagonist-deficient mice develop autoimmune arthritis due to intrinsic activation of IL-17-producing CCR2(+)Vgamma6(+)gammadelta T cells. *Nat. Commun.* **2015**, *6*, 7464. [CrossRef]
167. Schinnerling, K.; Rosas, C.; Soto, L.; Thomas, R.; Aguillon, J.C. Humanized Mouse Models of Rheumatoid Arthritis for Studies on Immunopathogenesis and Preclinical Testing of Cell-Based Therapies. *Front. Immunol.* **2019**, *10*, 203. [CrossRef]
168. Christianson, C.A.; Dumlao, D.S.; Stokes, J.A.; Dennis, E.A.; Svensson, C.I.; Corr, M.; Yaksh, T.L. Spinal TLR4 mediates the transition to a persistent mechanical hypersensitivity after the resolution of inflammation in serum-transferred arthritis. *Pain* **2011**, *152*, 2881–2891. [CrossRef]
169. Bas, D.B.; Su, J.; Sandor, K.; Agalave, N.M.; Lundberg, J.; Codeluppi, S.; Baharpoor, A.; Nandakumar, K.S.; Holmdahl, R.; Svensson, C.I. Collagen antibody-induced arthritis evokes persistent pain with spinal glial involvement and transient prostaglandin dependency. *Arthritis Rheum.* **2012**, *64*, 3886–3896. [CrossRef]
170. Inglis, J.J.; Notley, C.A.; Essex, D.; Wilson, A.W.; Feldmann, M.; Anand, P.; Williams, R. Collagen-induced arthritis as a model of hyperalgesia: Functional and cellular analysis of the analgesic actions of tumor necrosis factor blockade. *Arthritis Rheum.* **2007**, *56*, 4015–4023. [CrossRef]
171. Clark, A.K.; Grist, J.; Al-Kashi, A.; Perretti, M.; Malcangio, M. Spinal cathepsin S and fractalkine contribute to chronic pain in the collagen-induced arthritis model. *Arthritis Rheum.* **2012**, *64*, 2038–2047. [CrossRef] [PubMed]
172. Pinto, L.G.; Cunha, T.M.; Vieira, S.M.; Lemos, H.P.; Verri, W.A., Jr.; Cunha, F.Q.; Ferreira, S.H. IL-17 mediates articular hypernociception in antigen-induced arthritis in mice. *Pain* **2010**, *148*, 247–256. [CrossRef] [PubMed]
173. Ebbinghaus, M.; Uhlig, B.; Richter, F.; von Banchet, G.S.; Gajda, M.; Brauer, R.; Schaible, H.G. The role of interleukin-1beta in arthritic pain: Main involvement in thermal, but not mechanical, hyperalgesia in rat antigen-induced arthritis. *Arthritis Rheum.* **2012**, *64*, 3897–3907. [CrossRef] [PubMed]
174. Segond von Banchet, G.; Konig, C.; Patzer, J.; Eitner, A.; Leuchtweis, J.; Ebbinghaus, M.; Boettger, M.K.; Schaible, H.G. Long-Lasting Activation of the Transcription Factor CREB in Sensory Neurons by Interleukin-1beta During Antigen-Induced Arthritis in Rats: A Mechanism of Persistent Arthritis Pain? *Arthritis Rheumatol.* **2016**, *68*, 532–541. [CrossRef] [PubMed]
175. Chakravarthy, K.; Faltus, R.; Robinson, G.; Sevilla, R.; Shin, J.; Zielstorff, M.; Byford, A.; Leccese, E.; Caniga, M.J.; Hseih, S.; et al. Etanercept ameliorates inflammation and pain in a novel mono-arthritic multi-flare model of streptococcal cell wall induced arthritis. *BMC Musculoskelet. Disord.* **2014**, *15*, 409. [CrossRef] [PubMed]
176. Wang, L.; Jiang, X.; Zheng, Q.; Jeon, S.M.; Chen, T.; Liu, Y.; Kulaga, H.; Reed, R.; Dong, X.; Caterina, M.J.; et al. Neuronal FcgammaRI mediates acute and chronic joint pain. *J. Clin. Invest.* **2019**, *130*, 3754–3769. [CrossRef]
177. Ebbinghaus, M.; Muller, S.; Segond von Banchet, G.; Eitner, A.; Wank, I.; Hess, A.; Hilger, I.; Kamradt, T.; Schaible, H.G. Contribution of Inflammation and Bone Destruction to Pain in Arthritis: A Study in Murine Glucose-6-Phosphate Isomerase-Induced Arthritis. *Arthritis Rheumatol.* **2019**, *71*, 2016–2026. [CrossRef]
178. Frommholz, D.; Illges, H. Maximal locomotor depression follows maximal ankle swelling during the progression of arthritis in K/BxN mice. *Rheumatol. Int.* **2012**, *32*, 3999–4003. [CrossRef]

International Journal of
Molecular Sciences

MDPI

Review

Wnt Signaling and Biological Therapy in Rheumatoid Arthritis and Spondyloarthritis

Daniela Cici *, Addolorata Corrado, Cinzia Rotondo and Francesco P. Cantatore

Rheumatology Clinic, Department of Medical and Surgical Sciences, University of Foggia, 71121 Foggia, Italy; ada.corrado@unifg.it (A.C.); cinzia.rotondo@gmail.com (C.R.); francescopaolo.cantatore@unifg.it (F.P.C.)

* Correspondence: daniela.cici@gmail.com

Received: 9 October 2019; Accepted: 6 November 2019; Published: 7 November 2019

Abstract: The Wnt signaling pathway plays a key role in several biological processes, such as cellular proliferation and tissue regeneration, and its dysregulation is involved in the pathogenesis of many autoimmune diseases. Several evidences support its role especially in bone complications of rheumatic diseases. In Rheumatoid Arthritis (RA), the Wnt signaling is implicated in systemic and localized bone loss, while available data of its role in Spondyloarthritis (SpA) are conflicting. In the last few decades, the quality of life of rheumatic patients has been dramatically improved by biological therapy, targeting cytokines involved in the pathogenesis of these diseases like tumor necrosis factor (TNF)α, interleukin (IL)-1, IL-6, IL-17. In this review, we reviewed the role of Wnt signaling in RA and SpA, focusing on the effect of biological therapy on this pathway and its possible clinical implications.

Keywords: Wnt signaling; Dkk-1; biologics; rheumatoid arthritis; ankylosing spondylitis; axial spondyloarthritis; bone homeostasis

1. Introduction

Wnt signaling is a key pathway involved in several biological processes, such as cellular proliferation, cell migration, tissue homeostasis and regeneration, embryonic development and stem cell maintenance. Furthermore, the dysregulation of Wnt signaling is believed to be involved in the pathogenesis of cancer, vascular disorders and autoimmune diseases [1].

The Wnt family in humans currently includes 19 different glycoproteins [2] that can trigger multiple signaling cascades: the "canonical pathway", also known as the "Wnt/β-catenin pathway", and several "noncanonical pathways" (Figure 1). To trigger the Wnt canonical pathway, Wnt ligands must bind their 7-pass transmembrane Frizzled receptors and the coreceptor low-density lipoprotein receptor-related protein (LRP) 5/6 [3]. In the absence of Wnt ligands, β-catenin is kept at a low level through the ubiquitin-proteasome system. It is located in an intracellular binding complex, composed of glycogen synthase kinase-3β (GSK3β), caseine kinase I (CKI), adenomatous polyposis coli (APC), and Axin [4]: GSK3β and CKI phosphorylate cytosolic β-catenin, Axin acts as a scaffold allowing the aforementioned phosphorylation and APC mediates phosphorylated β-catenin binding to the ubiquitin-mediated proteolysis pathway. The binding of the Wnt proteins to their coreceptor complex leads to the recruitment of the cytosolic disheveled proteins, which block the β-catenin degradation and allow its translocation into the nucleus, where it acts as a transcriptional regulator involved in the expression of several targeted genes [5].

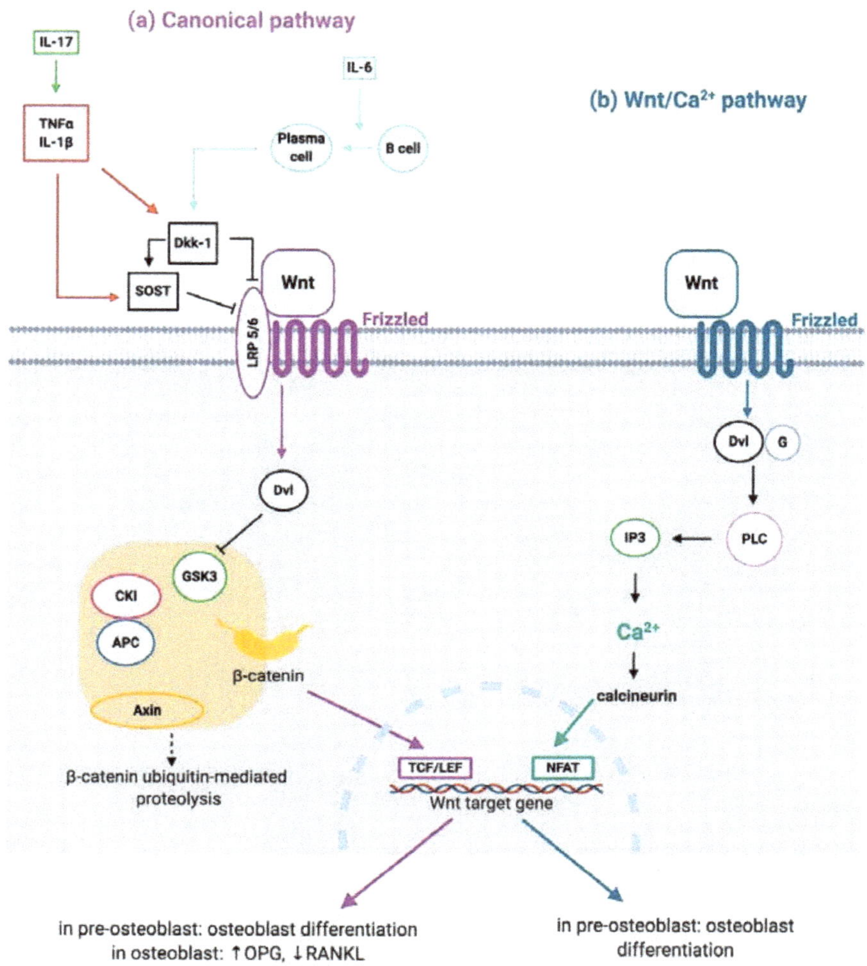

Figure 1. Wnt signaling pathways. (**a**) Canonical Wnt pathway: in the absence of Wnt ligands, β-catenin is degraded by a complex composed of glycogen synthase kinase-3β (GSK3), caseine kinase I (CKI), adenomatous polyposis coli (PCI) and Axin. Wnt proteins binding to their coreptor complex (Frizzled + low-density lipoprotein receptor-related protein (LRP) 5/6) leads to inhibition of GSK3 mediated by disheveled (Dvl) protein. In this condition, β-catenin translocates into the nucleus and together with T-cell factor (TCF)/lymphoid enhancer factor 1 (LEF) induces the expression of Wnt target genes, leading to osteoblast differentiation, up-regulation of osteoprotegerin (OPG) and down-regulation of Receptor activator of nuclear factor-kappa B ligand (RANKL). Dickkopf (Dkk) protein and sclerostin (SOST) inhibit this pathway by binding LRP5/6; moreover, Dkk-1 induces SOST. Pro-inflammatory cytokines tumor necrosis factor (TNF)α and interleukin (IL)-1β induce Dkk-1 and SOST; IL-17 down-regulates Wnt canonical pathway indirectly, enhancing the production of TNFα and IL-1β; furthermore, IL-6 induces differentiation of B cells into plasma cells which express Dkk-1. (**b**) Wnt/Ca^{2+} pathway: Wnt proteins binding to the Frizzled receptor lead to the activation of Dvl via activation of G-proteins (G). Dvl leads to cytoplasmic calcium (Ca^{2+}) release from the endoplasmic reticulum via phospholipase C (PLC) and inositol 1,4,5-trisphosphate (IP3). Intracellular Ca^{2+} in turn activates calcineurin, which activates the nuclear factor of activated T-cells (NFAT), inducing the expression of Wnt target genes, leading to osteoblast differentiation.

The "noncanonical pathways" are numerous β-catenin independent signaling cascades, like planer cell polarity (PCP) and Wnt/calcium (Wnt/Ca^{2+}) pathways. The PCP pathway is involved in cytoskeletal organization and coordinated polarization of cells within the plane of epithelial sheets [6]; the Wnt/Ca^{2+} pathway is involved in cancer, inflammation and neurodegeneration [7].

The Wnt signaling is regulated by different inhibitors, such as the secreted frizzled-related protein, the Wnt inhibitory factor 1, sclerostin and the Dickkopf (Dkk) family of secreted proteins. In particular, sclerostin is a protein encoded by the *SOST* gene primarily expressed by mature osteocytes, which decreases the life span of osteoblasts by stimulating their apoptosis; it inhibits Wnt signaling by binding the Wnt co-receptors LRP5/6 antagonizing downstream signaling; moreover, sclerostin also interacts with LRP4, a protein that specifically facilitates the aforementioned inhibitory action of sclerostin on Wnt/β-catenin signaling [8]. Dkk is a family of proteins comprising at least four different forms (Dkk-1 to Dkk-4); the best studied is Dkk-1, a powerful antagonist of canonical Wnt/β-catenin signaling: it binds with high affinity LRP5 and LRP6 and a single-pass transmembrane receptor, Kremen 1/2, which results in internalization of the complex and the consequent inhibition of Wnt signaling [9]. Moreover, Dkk-1 further inhibits Wnt signaling by inducing the other antagonist sclerostin [10]. Interestingly, it has been reported that $1,25(OH)_2D_3$ plays a role in the regulation of the Wnt signaling pathway: indeed, it is able to induce the expression of LRP5 in osteoblasts targeting the *LRP5* gene [11].

The Wnt signaling is considered to be one of the main regulators of bone metabolism. It is involved in osteoblast differentiation from mesenchymal precursors and osteochondroprogenitor cells, in osteoblast regulation, proliferation and survival [1]. Moreover, it is also involved in osteoclastogenesis regulation: the canonical pathway leads to osteoprotegerin (OPG) expression, which acts as an inhibitor of the receptor activator of nuclear factor-kappa B (RANK)/RANK ligand (RANKL) signal, crucial to osteoclastogenesis [12]. Furthermore, Wnt inhibitor Dkk-1 seems to play a key role in osteoporosis [1,13,14]. In this regard, it is worth mentioning the emerging role of microRNAs (miRNAs) as regulators of the Wnt signaling. miRNAs are small noncoding RNA molecules which transcriptionally regulate gene expression by targeting mRNA with partially complementary sequences. Several miRNAs target key components of Wnt signaling cascade, leading to an attenuation or an enhancing of Wnt signals [15]. For example, the expression of miR-37c, miR-23a, miR-30e determines a decrease of Wnt signal and therefore a decreased osteoblast differentiation by targeting Wnt receptor or co-receptor (Wnt3, LRP5, LRP6). Conversely, miR-27a, miR-142, miR-29a, miR-218, miR-98, miR-335, miR-542 target Wnt inhibitors and negative regulators (such as APC, secreted frizzled-related proteins, Dkk-1, Kremen2, sclerostin), thus inducing Wnt signaling and osteogenic differentiation [15]. Moreover, a dysregulated expression of miRNAs targeting Wnt pathway components may lead to bone homeostasis impairment, such as osteoporosis. For example, an up-regulation of miR-320 could play a role in osteoporosis development through negatively regulating Wnt signal; on the contrary, miR-542 expression seems to prevent osteoporosis in mice models and it was down-regulated in postmenopausal osteoporotic patients [15]. Other non-coding RNAs, such as long non-coding RNAs and circular RNAs, act as regulators of Wnt pathway [16–19].

Inflammatory diseases are often characterized by bone metabolism impairment: local and systemic bone loss in RA, destructive and productive bone lesions in Spondyloarthritis (SpA). Interestingly, the Wnt signaling is believed to be implicated in the pathogenesis of many autoimmune diseases, including systemic lupus erythematosus, systemic sclerosis, rheumatoid arthritis (RA), ankylosing spondylitis (AS), psoriasis [1].

Autoimmune diseases are caused by a defective over activity of the immune system that leads the body to attack "self" components and damage its own tissues. The treatment for autoimmune diseases mainly focuses on relieving symptoms, given the incomplete understanding of their pathogenesis [20]. It has been shown that the Wnt signaling plays a regulatory role in the homeostasis of the immune system, as reviewed by Shi et al. [20]. It plays a key role in the maintenance, proliferation, differentiation, and self-renewal of hematopoietic stem cells, cells able to differentiate into hematopoietic progenitor cells, which can further differentiate into immune cells, such as T cells, B cells, NK cells, and macrophages. Moreover, several evidences support the role played by the Wnt pathway in immune cells differentiation and proliferation: the canonical pathway regulates T cell differentiation both in thymus and in peripheral lymphoid tissues, and its dysregulation could lead to autoimmunity or immune deficiency; the absence of Wnt-responsive transcription factors could lead to a defective development of T and B cells; the expression of a stable form of β-catenin in vitro enhances the survival of regulatory T (Treg) cells, therefore an activation of Wnt canonical pathway in inflammatory conditions could inhibit Treg cells function, thus triggering an immune response and the development of autoimmune responses. Furthermore, the Wnt signaling is also crucial for the differentiation of hematopoietic stem cells into normal functioning B cells; it is involved in the immune homeostasis through its activation in dendritic cells, regulating functions that contribute to the balance between tolerance and inflammation.

Interestingly, the Wnt signaling is down-regulated directly or indirectly by pro-inflammatory cytokines, such as tumor necrosis factor (TNF)α and interleukin (IL)-1 β (through the induction of Dkk-1 and sclerostin), IL-6, IL-17 [10,21,22]. Moreover, B cells differentiate into plasma cells which inhibit the Wnt signaling through the expression of Dkk-1 [23].

In the last few decades, there has been a revolution in the treatment of chronic inflammatory rheumatic diseases. Biological agents able to inhibit molecular targets directly involved in the pathogenesis of these diseases have been developed, dramatically improving the quality of life of patients suffering from inflammatory joint diseases, particularly RA and Spondyloarthritis (SpA). Anti-TNFα agents have been approved for the treatment of various inflammatory diseases, and have proven effective in RA, psoriatic arthritis (PsA), AS; they represent the most used biologic drugs since 2000 and are usually well tolerated. Anakinra is a human IL-1 receptor antagonist that acts by competitively inhibiting the binding of IL-1 with the IL-1 type 1 receptor; currently approved for the treatment of RA, cryopyrin-associated periodic syndromes, and Still's disease [24]. Tocilizumab is an IL-6 receptor antagonist approved for the treatment of adults with moderate to severe active RA. Its safety and short- and long-term efficacy have been demonstrated, in terms of clinical and radiographic outcomes and health-related quality of life [25]. Secukinumab is a monoclonal antibody which selectively binds to and neutralizes IL-17A, effective in the treatment of psoriasis and PsA [26].

The aim of this review is to focus on the relation between the Wnt signaling and the biological therapy for RA and SpA (Table 1). A literature search for reviews and studies in PubMed, Google Scholar and Scopus databases was performed. The search was limited to the last ten years and only articles with abstract in English language were considered. The keywords used were "wnt signaling", "wnt rheumatoid arthritis", "wnt spondyloarthritis", "wnt psoriatic arthritis", "wnt ankylosing spondylitis", "dkk rheumatoid arthritis", "dkk spondyloarthritis", "wnt osteoporosis", "wnt biological therapy", "abatacept wnt", "tnf wnt". We scanned the reference list of the selected articles to identify other relevant papers.

Table 1. Wnt signaling and biological therapy in arthritis.

Study	Disease	Patients	Observation Time	Treatment	Effect on Wnt Signaling	Reference
Adami et al. 2016	RA	54	6 months	TNFi (adalimumab, certolizumab, etanercept, infliximab, golimumab)	↓ Dkk-1 ↔ sclerostin	[27]
Fassio et al. 2019	RA	17	2 months	TNFi (certolizumab)	↓ Dkk-1 ↓ sclerostin	[25]

Table 1. *Cont.*

Study	Disease	Patients	Observation Time	Treatment	Effect on Wnt Signaling	Reference
Wang et al. 2011	RA	100	6 months	TNFi (infliximab); IL-1Ra (anakinra)	↓ Dkk-1	[21]
Briot et al. 2015	RA	103	1 year	Anti-IL-6 (tocilizumab)	↓ Dkk-1 ↔ sclerostin	[28]
Terpos et al. 2011	RA	22	8 weeks	Anti-IL-6 (tocilizumab)	↓ Dkk-1	[29]
Fassio et al. 2019	PsA	28	6 months	Anti-IL-17 (secukinumab)	↑ Dkk-1	[20]
Daoussis et al. 2010	AS	45	3 months	TNFi	↑ Dkk-1	[30]
Kwon et al. 2012	AS	56	3 months	TNFi (etanercept, adalimumab, infliximab)	↔ Dkk-1	[31]
Zhao et al. 2019	SpA	30	6 months	TNFi	↓ Dkk-1	[32]
Saad et al. 2012	AS	30	1 year	TNFi (infliximab, adalimumab, etanercept)	↑ sclerostin	[33]
Korkosz et al. 2014	AS	40	6 months	TNFi (etanercept, adalimumab)	↓ Dkk-1	[34]

RA: rheumatoid arthritis; PsA: psoriatic arthritis; AS: ankylosing spondylitis; SpA: spondyloarthritis; TNFi: tumour necrosis factor inhibitor; Il-1Ra: IL-1 receptor antagonist; ↓: decreased; ↔: unchanged; ↑: increased.

2. Wnt Signaling in RA

RA is a chronic autoimmune inflammatory disease, that primarily attacks synovial joints. It is characterized by symmetric polyarticular inflammation, most commonly involving the small joints of hands and feet, which can lead to progressive joint damage and resulting functional disability with a decreased quality of life.

Several studies support the hypothesis of a potential involvement of Wnt signaling in the etiology of RA, in particular Wnt7b [20]: higher levels of Wnt ligands, Frizzled receptors, and Wnt inducible signaling pathway proteins were observed in the synovium of RA patients, also as pro-inflammatory cytokines TNFα, IL-1β and IL-6. Moreover, it has been demonstrated that Wnt inhibitor Dkk-1 promotes synovial angiogenesis, a critical process in the pathogenesis of RA [35]: vascular proliferation occurs during pannus formation in the affected joints [36,37], during which the synovium becomes locally invasive at the interface with cartilage and bone. The pannus plays a key role in the joint damage observed in RA [37]. Furthermore, also miRNAs have been implicated in the pathogenesis of RA by targeting Wnt signaling pathways. Indeed, a downregulated expression of miR-152 was found in arthritic rat model, whereas upregulation of this miRNA in fibroblast-like synoviocytes indirectly upregulated the expression of secreted frizzled-related protein 4, a Wnt negative regulator, thus leading to canonical Wnt pathway inhibition and to a significant decrease of fibroblast-like synoviocytes proliferation [38]. Consistently, miR-375 was also downregulated in fibroblast-like synoviocytes of arthritic rat model, and its upregulation inhibited the canonical Wnt pathway by targeting Frizzled 8. Interestingly, increased miR-375 also inhibited the pathogenesis of arthritis in the rat model, as indicated by decreases in disease markers, showing a role played by this miRNA in the pathogenesis of the disease through the canonical Wnt signaling pathway [39]. In addition, in synovium from RA patients, miR-663 was found upregulated, whereas APC expression was decreased. It was therefore revealed that this miRNA could active the canonical Wnt pathway by targeting APC [40].

RA is characterized by bone involvement represented by generalized osteoporosis and localized bone loss, which includes erosions and iuxta-articular osteopenia of affected joints [41].

Both bone erosions and systemic bone loss are due to an imbalance of the osteoblast–osteoclast axis. The chronic inflammatory state typical of RA leads to bone loss: pro-inflammatory cytokines TNFα, IL-1β and IL-6 upregulate the RANK/RANKL pathway, leading to increased osteoclast activity, prolonged osteoclast lifespan and bone resorption [42]. OPG acts as a competitive inhibitor of RANKL, reducing osteoclastogenesis and bone resorption. Moreover, several evidences suggest a connection between systemic osteoporosis in RA patients and low 25(OH) vitamin D levels. In numerous studies conducted on RA patients, low levels of 25(OH) vitamin D showed a significant association with disease activity and bone loss. As a matter of fact, vitamin D acts as a wide spectrum immunomodulator, with effect on several cells of the immune system (B and T cells, monocytes/macrophages), promoting an anti-inflammatory immune status [42].

The Wnt signaling plays a central role in bone development and homeostasis: its canonical pathway leads to osteoblast commitment, proliferation, and differentiation, enhances osteoblast and osteocyte survival; furthermore, it has been suggested that *OPG* gene expression is regulated by the Wnt/β-catenin signaling pathway [12]. Indeed, animal studies show that Wnt signaling inhibitor Dkk-1 is able to downregulate OPG and upregulate RANKL expression [43]. In addition, Wnt canonical pathway is downregulated in systemic osteoporosis: several studies found monogenic causes of osteoporosis [44], like mutations in genes encoding for LRP5 [45,46] and different Wnt proteins [47–51]. Moreover, the Wnt inhibitors Dkk-1 and sclerostin play a key role in systemic bone loss. Dkk-1 levels are higher in postmenopausal osteoporosis patients than in age-matched controls [13], and in osteoporosis patients higher Dkk-1 serum levels highly correlated with bone mass variables with inverse associations found between serum Dkk-1 expression and lumbar and femur T-score [52]; Dkk-1 expression in osteoblastic cultures from osteoporotic subjects is higher than in control cells [14]. Further studies suggest that Dkk-1 is a key inhibitor of systemic bone formation, like increased bone mass and osteoblast activity in Dkk-1 deficient mice [27,53] and osteopenia in mice over-expressing Dkk-1 [30]; in naïve normal growing female mice, human monoclonal anti-Dkk-1 antibodies are able to significantly improve both trabecular and cortical bone mineral densities [28].

Overexpression of *SOST* gene in mice leads to low bone mass as a result of reduction in osteoblast activity [29]; on the contrary, loss-of-function mutations of *SOST* gene lead to van Buchem disease and sclerosteosis, diseases distinguished by osteoblast hyperactivity and consequent increased bone density [54]. Interestingly, dual inhibition of sclerostin and Dkk-1 with a bispecific antibody resulted in a greater increased bone formation when compared to neutralization of each of the Wnt antagonists alone. These evidences further prove the synergical action of sclerostin and Dkk-1 in inhibiting the Wnt pathway [8].

Wnt signaling is involved in the bone alterations typical of RA: systemic and localized bone loss. In this regard, in the latest years, Wnt inhibitors Dkk-1 and sclerostin have gained more importance in understanding the physiopathological processes underlying RA. In a recent study by Singh et al., sclerostin serum levels were significantly higher in RA patients than in controls, and showed significant correlation with disease activity scores and inflammation markers, but not with bone destruction [55]. In animal models, Dkk-1 blockade in TNF-transgenic mice prevented the development of bone erosions [10]. Moreover, treatment with sclerostin antibodies in human TNF transgenic mice with late stage inflammatory arthritis, lead to a great improvement in bone complications: in this study, the treatment reversed systemic and periarticular osteopenia, improved articular cartilage damage, blocked progression of bone erosion and, when combined with TNF inhibitors, it was also able to reverse and repair articular cartilage damage and cortical bone erosions [31].

Interestingly, different studies showed that serum level of Dkk-1 is higher in patients with RA than in controls, and correlates with disease activity, elevated acute-phase reactants and more severe bone destruction in patients with RA [35,55–57]. Dkk-1 may be a biomarker of structural damage and a predictor of structural progression; therefore, it could represent a therapeutic target in RA [56]. In this regard, treatment with anti-Dkk-1 antibodies seems promising: in mouse models of RA, anti-Dkk-1 antibodies were able to block inflammatory bone erosions, as demonstrated by radiographic and histopathological examinations, due to a decreased osteoclast formation in the affected joints [22]. More evidences supporting the role of Wnt in bone homeostasis in RA come from studies focused on abatacept (CTLA-4Ig). Abatacept inhibits TNF-mediated osteoclastogenenis in vitro without T cells and inhibits inflammatory bone erosion in vivo in an animal model of RA [58]. CTLA-4Ig is a recombinant fusion protein based on CTLA-4, a protein physiologically produced by activated T cells that functions as a negative regulator of T cell-mediated immune responses. Indeed, full T cell activation requires two signals: the initial recognition of a specific antigen by a T cell receptor, after which T cells are unresponsive to further antigenic presentations (anergy); secondly, a co-stimulatory signal, such as the binding of CD80 or CD86 on the CD28 receptor on T cells. Abatacept and CTL4-a inhibit T cell activation by binding to CD80 and CD86 [59,60].

Roser-Page et al investigated the effect of abatacept on bone turnover in mice and found that its anabolic activity is linked to Wnt signaling [59,61] The authors reported that CTLA-4Ig administration in healthy mice induced bone gain due to an increased osteoblast bone formation and they also found increased expression of Wnt ligand Wnt-10b in purified T cells from the animals. The authors therefore hypothesized that abatacept induces Wnt-10b in anergized T cells, therefore promoting bone formation [59]. These findings were later confirmed by another study from the same research group conducted on mouse genetic models of Wnt-10b and T cell deficiency [8]. The data collected supported the hypothesis that the anabolic activity of abatacept in vivo is indeed mediated by a mechanism involving T cells and Wnt-10b: in the absence of either T cells or Wnt-10b, CTLA-4Ig did not lead to bone formation, on the contrary its effect was a significant loss of bone mass. Moreover, the authors also reported an increased expression of sclerostin following abatacept administration in healthy mice. Therefore, the authors hypothesized that in basal conditions, abatacept-induced Wnt-10b expression from T cells compensates for production of sclerostin and CTLA-4Ig promotes bone formation; however, in the absence of Wnt-10b, the net effect of abatacept is increased sclerostin production and consequent suppression of bone formation. These findings suggest caution in the treatment of RA immunocompromised patients, in whom abatacept administration may lead to unpredictable outcomes on bone formation [61].

These findings indicate that bone complications typical of RA might be the result of both enhanced bone resorption and impaired bone formation, in consequence of increased TNFα-driven osteoclast activity and overproduction of Wnt inhibitor Dkk-1, both locally (erosions) and systemically (RA-associated osteoporosis) [62].

Biological therapy is able to slow down bone destruction and inhibit radiological progression in RA [63]. Several studies show how this effect may be connected with the Wnt signaling. The studies evaluating the effect of biological therapy on Wnt pathway in RA were mainly focused on TNFα inhibitors, IL-1 receptor antagonist (IL-1Ra) anakinra and anti-IL-6 monoclonal antibody tocilizumab.

Most of the studies were conducted with TNFα inhibitors, showing a decrease in serum concentration of Dkk-1 in RA patients undergoing this biological treatment [34,35,43,62]. In particular, Adami et al. found a reduction in Dkk-1 serum levels in RA patients after 6 months of anti-TNFα treatment (most patients were treated with adalimumab and certolizumab, less with etanercept, infliximab and golimumab); they did not observe any changes in sclerostin serum levels, therefore suggesting that the changes of Dkk-1 were not associated with a feedback with sclerostin [62]. Conversely, Fassio et al. recently found a rapid decline in both Dkk-1 and sclerostin serum levels in RA patients after 2 months of treatment with TNFα inhibitor certolizumab-pegol, accompanied by dramatic changes in bone turnover [43]. The rapidity of the reduction in serum Dkk-1 levels observed after initiation of the treatment further proves the TNFα-dependent induction of Dkk-1 in vivo, already demonstrated in vitro [22], as also suggested by Daoussis et al [34]. Wang et al. found that the serum Dkk-1 concentration was significantly increased in RA patients than in healthy controls and patients affected by other rheumatic diseases, moreover, increasing Dkk-1 levels were associated with bone erosion and correlated with levels of inflammatory markers like serum C-reactive protein levels and erythrocyte sedimentation rates. Furthermore, in their study, treatment with anti-TNFα agent infliximab and anti-IL-1 anakinra induced a significant reduction of circulating levels of Dkk-1 [35]. Therefore, Dkk-1 may serve as a new clinical indicator for RA: a biomarker of disease activity and bone erosion, as well as a marker of response to biological therapy with TNFα blockers and IL-1Ra. These evidences suggest the strong connection between the dysregulation of the Wnt signaling pathway, TNFα-dependent inflammation and bone metabolism alterations in RA.

The key role of IL-6 in the pathogenesis of bone changes in RA through the regulation of the Wnt pathway has been suggested by studies evaluating the levels of Dkk-1 in RA patients after treatment with anti-IL-6 monoclonal antibody tocilizumab. In the 1-year prospective open study conducted by Briot et al. [64], a significant decrease in serum level of Dkk-1 was observed following tocilizumab administration, confirming the results from a previous study by Terpos et al. [65]. It has been suggested that tocilizumab does not affect the whole osteocyte functions since no significant change was observed in sclerostin serum levels [64]. These studies suggest a critical role of IL-6 in bone homeostasis in RA and how its dysregulation may be connected with the bone complications of this disease. Indeed, several in vitro and animal studies support this theory [65]: increased osteoclastogenesis and reduced osteoblast activity in IL-6 transgenic mice; decreased levels of RANKL produced by T-lymphocytes in IL-6-deficient mice; furthermore, blockade of IL-6 receptor through neutralizing antibodies blocks TNF- and RANKL-mediated osteoclastogenesis in vitro and in vivo as shown by Axmann et al. [32]. Thus, anti-IL-6 therapy may have a direct effect on bone metabolism impairment in RA patients.

3. Wnt Signaling in SpA

The term SpA refers to a group of inflammatory rheumatic diseases that share genetic background, pathophysiological mechanisms, and clinical features. Depending on the leading manifestation, SpAs can be classified as axial (mainly involving the axial skeleton, i.e. sacroiliac joints and spine) or peripheral (distinguished by arthritis, enthesitis or dactylitis). The latter includes reactive arthritis, arthritis associated with inflammatory bowel disease, PsA and so-called undifferentiated peripheral SpA [66]. Unlike RA bone involvement, SpA is characterized by the co-existence of both destructive and productive bone lesions, which suggests an alteration of a bone remodelling in the affected joints [33,67,68].

In particular, in PsA bone erosions are associated with new bone formation, typically at the edges of the cartilage joint at the insertion of the enthesis [69]. IL-17 is an important cytokine involved in the pathogenesis of bone lesions of PsA, via the inhibition of the Wnt signaling [70]. In a recent study conducted by Fassio et al. [26] serum levels of Dkk-1 in PsA patients were found lower than in healthy subjects and significantly increased after treatment with monoclonal anti-IL-17A antibody secukinumab. The aforementioned treatment appeared to restore normal Dkk-1 serum levels in these patients, resulting in the loss of the significant gap vs the healthy controls after six months of therapy. These findings suggest a drug-induced inhibition of local bone over-proliferation, typical of the bone lesions in PsA.

Axial SpA (axSpA)

Pathologically, axSpA is characterized by a three-stage process, resulting in a paradoxical bone destruction and formation. It has been postulated that the initial inflammation (in which TNFα is the principal cytokine involved [71]) causes erosions in cartilage and bone; these lesions are then filled in by fibrous tissue, that is later ossified leading to abnormal bony outgrowth (syndesmophytes, bone bridges and complete ankyloses) [9,68,72]. The Wnt signaling and its inhibitors, such as Dkk-1 and sclerostin, might play a role in the third phase of axSpA, due to their role in bone homeostasis [9,73].

In AS the primary site of inflammation is located at the enthesis or subchondral bone marrow, with bone marrow edema, lymphocytic infiltrates, increased osteoclast density, and increased microvessel density as typical findings in acute inflammation [35]. TNFα is a primary cytokine in axSpa [73], not only for its pro-inflammatory effect [71,74], but also as a stimulator of osteoclastogenesis [67] and for its effect on the Wnt signaling (enhancing the expression of Wnt inhibitors, Dkk-1 and sclerostin [10,21,23,63,75]).

Treatment with TNFα inhibitors has greatly improved the clinical outcome of axSpA patients, reducing the signs and symptoms improving the health-related quality of life. However, it is still unclear whether they slow the structural damage and radiographic progression or not [63,67,68]. In this context, several studies focused on the role of Dkk-1 in axSpA, in relation to bone formation and treatment with TNFα inhibitors [33,34,76–78].

Studies have shown that Dkk-1 is involved in the pathogenesis of structural damage and in molecular mechanisms of syndesmophyte formation and new bone formation in SpA, but most data are conflicting [33,34]. Various studies showed that Dkk-1 circulating levels respond in a different way to TNFα blockade in patients with AS and in patients with RA. It has been shown that serum levels of Dkk-1 were significantly higher in patients with AS compared to patients with RA and healthy controls and were further increased in AS patient receiving anti-TNFα treatment [34]; the authors hypothesized that the higher levels of Dkk-1 may reflect a counter-balancing mechanism to attenuate Wnt signaling, which is turned on after resolution of inflammation following the treatment. Conversely, another study revealed that circulating levels of Dkk-1 were lower in patient with AS compared to healthy controls and did not change after anti-TNFα treatment [33]. It could be therefore hypothesized that in AS the circulating levels of Dkk-1 are unable to suppress Wnt-mediated bone formation, and thus the inability of TNFα to induce Dkk-1 in SpA may be one explanation why anti-TNFα therapy might not block new bone formation [63].

Levels of functional Dkk-1 are increased in AS patients with no syndesmophyte growth compared to patients with syndesmophyte growth, suggesting that low levels of serum DKK-1 are necessary to develop syndesmophytes. Therefore, inhibition of Wnt signaling could protect from the development of syndesmophytes through an inhibition of bone formation processes [76]. In an animal model of transgenic mice overexpressing TNF, which develops bilateral sacroiliitis, Dkk-1 blockade promotes the expression of type X collagen and the formation of hypertrophic chondrocytes, promoting the ankylosis of sacroiliac joints, without affecting inflammatory processes [77]. Nevertheless, a prospective study on SpA patients showed that treatment with TNFα blockers induced a significant decrease of circulating levels of Dkk-1, which correlated with the reduction of MRI bone marrow edema of sacroiliac joint and spine, suggesting that the reduction of Dkk-1 by anti-TNFα agents could be related to the inhibitory effects of these drugs on new bone formation in SpA [78].

The hypothesis that the Wnt pathway plays an important role in the pathogenesis of AS is supported by studies that focused on another Wnt signaling inhibitor, sclerostin. It was observed that sclerostin expression was nearly absent in osteocytes in the periarticular bone of AS patients, suggesting a specific alteration of osteocyte function in this disease [79]. Moreover, serum sclerostin levels were found lower in AS patients than in healthy controls [79,80]. Interestingly, radiographic progression was associated with significantly lower sclerostin levels, suggesting that a low sclerostin level in AS could increase susceptibility for syndesmophyte formation [79]. Furthermore, although increasing after anti-TNFα treatment, sclerostin levels were still lower than in healthy subjects after 12 months of therapy [80]. Moreover, since AS patients with higher baseline sclerostin levels showed a rapid reduction of inflammatory parameters following the treatment and a concomitantly gradual increase in this Wnt inhibitor, the authors hypothesized that low sclerostin serum levels could be a possible marker of persistent inflammation in AS patients under anti-TNF therapy.

These data confirm the potential role of Wnt signaling in the pathogenesis of structural bone changes in SpA. Several physiopathogenetic hypothesis have been proposed to explain the conflicting available data on Wnt involvement in bone changes observed in SpA patients. There is a difference between the total levels of Dkk-1 and receptor-bound and thus functional Dkk-1, showing a minor capacity of Dkk-1 in axSpA patients to bind the LRP coreceptor [22,34,76]. Another explanation could be that Dkk-1 serum levels in patients with axSpA could be related to disease duration [72], as Dkk-1 serum levels were found higher in patients with early axSpA compared with patients with established disease.

This explanation may also clarify the link between TNFα and Dkk-1, and could contribute to explain the relationship between inflammation and osteoproliferation. The lower levels of Dkk-1 in patients with established axSpA may explain why TNFα blockers in this stage of the disease did not lead to a change in Dkk-1 levels in the study conducted by Kwon et al. [33] and is not able to avoid the development of syndesmophytes [68]. On the contrary, in patients with early axSpA, anti-TNFα treatment could lead to a decrease in Dkk-1 serum levels [75,78] and also to a better radiographic outcome, as shown by a longitudinal cohort study conducted by Haroon et al. [81]. In this study, radiographic progression was slower in AS patients who underwent TNFα-blocker therapy earlier in the course of disease than in patients in whom treatment was delayed. Indeed, in the early stages of the disease, inflammation and osteoproliferation may be coupled. Considering the three-stage pathological process of axSpA (inflammation, erosion, osteoproliferation), targeting the inflammation with TNFα inhibitors in patients at an early stage of the disease, may avoid the development of the next stages and thus the new bone formation processes. In other terms, if early inflammatory lesions resolve without undergoing chronic changes, the sequelae of new bone formation following inflammation might be halted [68,72]. Therefore, anti-TNFα treatment in the early stages of the disease may prevent development of osteogenesis, while at later stages osteogenesis and inflammation appear to be two separate therapeutic targets [63,68,75].

The clinical application of this theory is to establish the therapeutic time window to avoid the new bone formation process and improving the radiographic outcome through TNFα inhibitors, before the disconnection between inflammation and osteoproliferation [75]. This window might be characterized by higher serum levels of Dkk-1 in axSpA patients than in controls.

4. Conclusions

The Wnt signaling is involved in pathological aspects of rheumatic diseases, with several evidences supporting its role especially in bone complications, bone loss and new bone formation.

Higher serum levels of Wnt inhibitor Dkk-1 found in RA patients than in controls and its decrease after biological treatment (TNFα inhibitors, IL-1Ra, anti-IL-6 antibody), suggest the strong connection between the dysregulation of Wnt signaling leading to bone loss—both locally and systemically—in RA and the pro-inflammatory state typical of the disease. Interestingly, Dkk-1 concentration correlates with disease activity, elevated acute-phase reactants and more severe bone damage, suggesting its role as a possible biomarker of structural damage and new therapeutic target in RA. Moreover, in RA patients, higher levels of another Wnt inhibitors, sclerostin, correlates with disease activity scores and inflammation markers; in addition, in RA mice models anti-sclerostin antibodies arrested the bone damage progression and in combination with anti-TNF led to regression of cortical bone erosions.

In axSpA, the role of Wnt signaling has not yet been fully understood. There is evidence of a critical time window in the early stages of the disease when treatment with TNFα inhibitors might lead to two otherwise separate therapeutic targets: reducing signs and symptoms, and slowing the structural damage and radiographic progression. Further exploration of Dkk-1's role and the connection between bone formation and inflammatory response is needed in order to achieve a better knowing of the biologic background of the disease; this would subsequently lead to better management of current therapeutic options.

Author Contributions: Conceptualization, A.C. and F.P.C.; literature collection and preparation, D.C. and A.C.; writing—original draft preparation, D.C. and A.C.; writing—review and editing, D.C., A.C. and C.R.; supervision, F.P.C.

Funding: This work received no external funding.

Conflicts of Interest: The authors declare no conflict of interest.

Abbreviations

AS	Ankylosing spondylitis
axSpA	Axial spondyloarthritis
CKI	Caseine kinase I
DKK	Dickkopf
GSK3β	Glycogen synthase kinase-3β
IL	Interleukin
IL-1Ra	IL-1 receptor antagonist
LRP	Low-density lipoprotein receptor-related protein
OPG	Osteoprotegerin
PCK/Ca^{2+}	Protein kinase C/calcium
PCP	Planer cell polarity
PsA	Psoriatic arthritis
RA	Rheumatoid arthritis
RANK	Receptor activator of nuclear factor-kappa B
RANKL	RANK ligand
SpA	Spondyloarthritis
TNF	Tumor necrosis factor
Treg	Regulatory T

References

1. Maruotti, N.; Corrado, A.; Neve, A.; Cantatore, F.P. Systemic effects of Wnt signaling. *J. Cell. Physiol.* **2013**, *228*, 1428–1432. [CrossRef] [PubMed]
2. Komiya, Y.; Habas, R. Wnt signal transduction pathways. *Organogenesis* **2008**, *4*, 68–75. [CrossRef] [PubMed]
3. Tamai, K.; Semenov, M.; Kato, Y.; Spokony, R.; Liu, C.; Katsuyama, Y.; Hess, F.; Saint-Jeannet, J.P.; He, X. LDL-receptor-related proteins in Wnt signal transduction. *Nature* **2000**, *407*, 530–535. [CrossRef] [PubMed]
4. Moon, R.T.; Bowerman, B.; Boutros, M.; Perrimon, N. The promise and perils of Wnt signaling through beta-catenin. *Science* **2002**, *296*, 1644–1646. [CrossRef] [PubMed]
5. Yu, J.; Virshup, D.M. Updating the Wnt pathways. *Biosci. Rep.* **2014**, *34*, 593–607. [CrossRef]
6. Veeman, M.T.; Axelrod, J.D.; Moon, R.T. A second canon: Functions and mechanisms of β-catenin-independent Wnt signaling. *Dev. Cell* **2003**, *5*, 367–377. [CrossRef]
7. Bengoa-Vergniory, N.; Kypta, R.M. Canonical and noncanonical Wnt signaling in neural stem/progenitor cells. *Cell. Mol. Life Sci.* **2015**, *72*, 4157–4172. [CrossRef]
8. Delgado-Calle, J.; Sato, A.Y.; Bellido, T. Role and mechanism of action of sclerostin in bone. *Bone* **2017**, *96*, 29–37. [CrossRef]
9. Xie, W.; Zhou, L.; Li, S.; Hui, T.; Chen, D. Wnt/β-catenin signaling plays a key role in the development of spondyloarthritis. *Ann. N. Y. Acad. Sci.* **2016**, *1364*, 25–31. [CrossRef]
10. Heiland, G.R.; Zwerina, K.; Baum, W.; Kireva, T.; Distler, J.H.; Grisanti, M.; Asuncion, F.; Li, X.; Ominsky, M.; Richards, W.; et al. Neutralisation of Dkk-1 protects from systemic bone loss during inflammation and reduces sclerostin expression. *Ann. Rheum. Dis.* **2010**, *69*, 2152–2159. [CrossRef]
11. Fretz, J.A.; Zella, L.A.; Kim, S.; Shevde, N.K.; Pike, J.W. 1,25-Dihydroxyvitamin D3 regulates the expression of low-density lipoprotein receptor-related protein 5 via deoxyribonucleic acid sequence elements located downstream of the start site of transcription. *Mol. Endocrinol.* **2006**, *20*, 2215–2230. [CrossRef] [PubMed]
12. Glass, D.A.; Bialek, P.; Ahn, J.D.; Starbuck, M.; Patel, M.S.; Clevers, H.; Taketo, M.M.; Long, F.; McMahon, A.P.; Lang, R.A.; et al. Canonical Wnt signaling in differentiated osteoblast controls osteoclast differentiation. *Dev. Cell* **2005**, *8*, 751–764. [CrossRef] [PubMed]
13. Tian, J.; Xu, X.J.; Shen, L.; Yang, Y.P.; Zhu, R.; Shuai, B.; Zhu, X.W.; Li, C.G.; Ma, C.; Lv, L. Association of serum Dkk-1 levels with β-catenin in patients with postmenopausal osteoporosis. *J. Huazhong Univ. Sci. Technolog. Med. Sci.* **2015**, *35*, 212–218. [CrossRef] [PubMed]
14. Corrado, A.; Neve, A.; Macchiarola, A.; Gaudio, A.; Marucci, A.; Cantatore, F.P. RANKL/OPG ratio and DKK-1 expression in primary osteoblastic cultures from osteoarthritic and osteoporotic subjects. *J. Rheumatol.* **2013**, *40*, 684–694. [CrossRef] [PubMed]

15. Bellavia, D.; De Luca, A.; Carina, V.; Costa, V.; Raimondi, L.; Salamanna, F.; Alessandro, R.; Fini, M.; Giavaresi, G. Deregulated miRNAs in bone health: Epigenetic roles in osteoporosis. *Bone* **2019**, *122*, 52–75. [CrossRef] [PubMed]
16. Yu, C.Y.; Kuo, H.C. The emerging roles and functions of circular RNAs and their generation. *J. Biomed. Sci.* **2019**, *26*, 29. [CrossRef] [PubMed]
17. Yao, C.; Yu, B. Role of Long Noncoding RNAs and Circular RNAs in Nerve Regeneration. *Front. Mol. Neurosci.* **2019**, *12*, 165. [CrossRef]
18. Liang, W.C.; Wong, C.W.; Liang, P.P.; Shi, M.; Cao, Y.; Rao, S.T.; Tsui, S.K.; Waye, M.M.; Zhang, Q.; Fu, W.M.; et al. Translation of the circular RNA circβ-catenin promotes liver cancer cell growth through activation of the Wnt pathway. *Genome Biol.* **2019**, *20*, 84. [CrossRef]
19. Yang, S.; Sun, Z.; Zhou, Q.; Wang, W.; Wang, G.; Song, J.; Li, Z.; Zhang, Z.; Chang, Y.; Xia, K.; et al. MicroRNAs, long noncoding RNAs, and circular RNAs: Potential tumor biomarkers and targets for colorectal cancer. *Cancer Manag. Res.* **2018**, *10*, 2249–2257. [CrossRef]
20. Shi, J.; Chi, S.; Xue, J.; Yang, J.; Li, F.; Liu, X. Emerging Role and Therapeutic Implication of Wnt Signaling Pathways in Autoimmune Diseases. *J. Immunol. Res.* **2016**, *2016*, 9392132. [CrossRef]
21. Di Munno, O.; Ferro, F. The effect of biologic agents on bone homeostasis in chronic inflammatory rheumatic diseases. *Clin. Exp. Rheumatol.* **2019**, *37*, 502–507. [PubMed]
22. Diarra, D.; Stolina, M.; Polzer, K.; Zwerina, J.; Ominsky, M.S.; Dwyer, D.; Korb, A.; Smolen, J.; Hoffmann, M.; Scheinecker, C.; et al. Dickkopf-1 is a master regulator of joint remodeling. *Nat. Med.* **2007**, *13*, 156–163. [CrossRef] [PubMed]
23. Schett, G.; Stach, C.; Zwerina, J.; Voll, R.; Manger, B. How antirheumatic drugs protect joints from damage in rheumatoid arthritis. *Arthritis Rheum.* **2008**, *58*, 2936–2948. [CrossRef] [PubMed]
24. European Medicines Agency. Summary of Product Characteristics—Kineret. Available online: https://www.ema.europa.eu/documents/product-information/kineret-epar-product-information_en.pdf (accessed on 29 September 2019).
25. Sarzi-Puttini, P.; Ceribelli, A.; Marotto, D.; Batticciotto, A.; Atzeni, F. Systemic rheumatic diseases: From biological agents to small molecules. *Autoimmun. Rev.* **2019**, *18*, 583–592. [CrossRef] [PubMed]
26. Fassio, A.; Gatti, D.; Rossini, M.; Idolazzi, L.; Giollo, A.; Adami, G.; Gisondi, P.; Girolomoni, G.; Viapiana, O. Secukinumab produces a quick increase in WNT signalling antagonists in patients with psoriatic arthritis. *Clin. Exp. Rheumatol.* **2019**, *37*, 133–136.
27. Morvan, F.; Boulukos, K.; Clément-Lacroix, P.; Roman Roman, S.; Suc-Royer, I.; Vayssière, B.; Ammann, P.; Martin, P.; Pinho, S.; Pognonec, P.; et al. Deletion of a single allele of the Dkk1 gene leads to an increase in bone formation and bone mass. *J. Bone Miner. Res.* **2006**, *21*, 934–945. [CrossRef]
28. Glantschnig, H.; Hampton, R.A.; Lu, P.; Zhao, J.Z.; Vitelli, S.; Huang, L.; Haytko, P.; Cusick, T.; Ireland, C.; Jarantow, S.W.; et al. Generation and selection of novel fully human monoclonal antibodies that neutralize Dickkopf-1 (DKK1) inhibitory function in vitro and increase bone mass in vivo. *J. Biol. Chem.* **2010**, *285*, 40135–40147. [CrossRef]
29. Winkler, D.G.; Sutherland, M.K.; Geoghegan, J.C.; Yu, C.; Hayes, T.; Skonier, J.E.; Shpektor, D.; Jonas, M.; Kovacevich, B.R.; Staehling-Hampton, K.; et al. Osteocyte control of bone formation via sclerostin, a novel BMP antagonist. *EMBO J.* **2003**, *22*, 6267–6276. [CrossRef]
30. Li, J.; Sarosi, I.; Cattley, R.C.; Pretorius, J.; Asuncion, F.; Grisanti, M.; Morony, S.; Adamu, S.; Geng, Z.; Qiu, W.; et al. Dkk1-mediated inhibition of Wnt signaling in bone results in osteopenia. *Bone* **2006**, *39*, 754–766. [CrossRef]
31. Chen, X.X.; Baum, W.; Dwyer, D.; Stock, M.; Schwabe, K.; Ke, H.Z.; Stolina, M.; Schett, G.; Bozec, A. Sclerostin inhibition reverses systemic, periarticular and local bone loss in arthritis. *Ann. Rheum. Dis.* **2013**, *72*, 1732–1736. [CrossRef]
32. Axmann, R.; Böhm, C.; Krönke, G.; Zwerina, J.; Smolen, J.; Schett, G. Inhibition of interleukin-6 receptor directly blocks osteoclast formation in vitro and in vivo. *Arthritis Rheum.* **2009**, *60*, 2747–2756. [CrossRef] [PubMed]
33. Kwon, S.R.; Lim, M.J.; Suh, C.H.; Park, S.G.; Hong, Y.S.; Yoon, B.Y.; Kim, H.A.; Choi, H.J.; Park, W. Dickkopf-1 level is lower in patients with ankylosing spondylitis than in healthy people and is not influenced by anti-tumor necrosis factor therapy. *Rheumatol. Int.* **2012**, *32*, 2523–2527. [CrossRef] [PubMed]

34. Daoussis, D.; Liossis, S.N.; Solomou, E.E.; Tsanaktsi, A.; Bounia, K.; Karampetsou, M.; Yiannopoulos, G.; Andonopoulos, A.P. Evidence that Dkk-1 is dysfunctional in Ankylosing Spondylitis. *Arthritis Rheum.* **2010**, *62*, 150–158. [CrossRef] [PubMed]
35. Wang, S.Y.; Liu, Y.Y.; Ye, H.; Guo, J.P.; Li, R.; Liu, X.; Li, Z.G. Circulating dickkopf-1 is correlated with bone erosion and inflammation in Rheumatoid Arthritis. *J. Rheumatol.* **2011**, *38*, 821–827. [CrossRef] [PubMed]
36. Strunk, J.; Heinemann, E.; Neeck, G.; Schmidt, K.L.; Lange, U. A new approach to studying angiogenesis in rheumatoid arthritis by means of power Doppler ultrasonography and measurement of serum vascular endothelial growth factor. *Rheumatology* **2004**, *43*, 1480–1483. [CrossRef] [PubMed]
37. Paleolog, E.M. Angiogenesis in rheumatoid arthritis. *Arthritis Res.* **2002**, *4*, S81–S90. [CrossRef] [PubMed]
38. Miao, C.G.; Yang, Y.Y.; He, X.; Huang, C.; Huang, Y.; Qin, D.; Du, C.L.; Li, J. MicroRNA-152 modulates the canonical Wnt pathway activation by targeting DNA methyltransferase 1 in arthritic rat model. *Biochimie.* **2014**, *106*, 149–156. [CrossRef] [PubMed]
39. Miao, C.G.; Shi, W.J.; Xiong, Y.Y.; Yu, H.; Zhang, X.L.; Qin, M.S.; Du, C.L.; Song, T.W.; Li, J. miR-375 regulates the canonical Wnt pathway through FZD8 silencing in arthritis synovial fibroblasts. *Immunol. Lett.* **2015**, *164*, 1–10. [CrossRef]
40. Miao, C.G.; Shi, W.J.; Xiong, Y.Y.; Yu, H.; Zhang, X.L.; Qin, M.S.; Du, C.L.; Song, T.W.; Zhang, B.; Li, J. MicroRNA-663 activates the canonical Wnt signaling through the adenomatous polyposis coli suppression. *Immunol. Lett.* **2015**, *166*, 45–54. [CrossRef]
41. Maruotti, N.; Corrado, A.; Cantatore, F.P. Osteoporosis and rheumatic diseases. *Reumatismo* **2014**, *66*, 125–135. [CrossRef]
42. Bellavia, D.; Costa, V.; De Luca, A.; Maglio, M.; Pagani, S.; Fini, M.; Giavaresi, G. Vitamin D Level Between Calcium-Phosphorus Homeostasis and Immune System: New Perspective in Osteoporosis. *Curr. Osteoporos. Rep.* **2016**. [CrossRef] [PubMed]
43. Fassio, A.; Adami, G.; Gatti, D.; Orsolini, G.; Giollo, A.; Idolazzi, L.; Benini, C.; Vantaggiato, E.; Rossini, M.; Viapiana, O. Inhibition of tumor necrosis factor-alpha (TNF-alpha) in patients with early rheumatoid arthritis results in acute changes of bone modulators. *Int. Immunopharmacol.* **2019**, *67*, 487–489. [CrossRef] [PubMed]
44. Mäkitie, R.E.; Costantini, A.; Kämpe, A.; Alm, J.J.; Mäkitie, O. New insights into monogenic causes of osteoporosis. *Fron. Endocrinol.* **2019**, *10*, 70. [CrossRef] [PubMed]
45. Gong, Y.; Slee, R.B.; Fukai, N.; Rawadi, G.; Roman-Roman, S.; Reginato, A.M.; Wang, H.; Cundy, T.; Glorieux, F.H.; Lev, D.; et al. LDL receptor-related protein 5 (LRP5) affects bone accrual and eye development. *Cell* **2001**, *107*, 513–523. [CrossRef]
46. Levasseur, R.; Lacombe, D.; de Vernejoul, M.C. LRP5 mutations in osteoporosis-pseudoglioma syndrome and high-bone-mass disorders. *Joint Bone Spine* **2005**, *72*, 207–214. [CrossRef] [PubMed]
47. Laine, C.M.; Joeng, K.S.; Campeau, P.M.; Kiviranta, R.; Tarkkonen, K.; Grover, M.; Lu, J.T.; Pekkinen, M.; Wessman, M.; Heino, T.J.; et al. WNT1 mutations in early-onset osteoporosis and osteogenesis imperfecta. *N Engl. J. Med.* **2013**, *369*, 1809–1816. [CrossRef] [PubMed]
48. Mäkitie, R.E.; Haanpää, M.; Valta, H.; Pekkinen, M.; Laine, C.M.; Lehesjoki, A.E.; Schalin-Jäntti, C.; Mäkitie, O. Skeletal characteristics of WNT1 osteoporosis in children and young adults. *J. Bone Miner. Res.* **2016**, *31*, 1734–1742. [CrossRef]
49. Zheng, H.F.; Tobias, J.H.; Duncan, E.; Evans, D.M.; Eriksson, J.; Paternoster, L.; Yerges-Armstrong, L.M.; Lehtimäki, T.; Bergström, U.; Kähönen, M.; et al. WNT16 influences bone mineral density, cortical bone thickness, bone strength, and osteoporotic fracture risk. *PLos Genet.* **2012**, *8*, e1002745. [CrossRef]
50. Gori, F.; Lerner, U.; Ohlsson, C.; Baron, R. A new WNT on the bone: WNT16, cortical bone thickness, porosity and fractures. *Bonekey Rep.* **2015**, *4*, 669. [CrossRef]
51. Ohlsson, C.; Henning, P.; Nilsson, K.H.; Wu, J.; Gustafsson, K.L.; Sjögren, K.; Törnqvist, A.; Koskela, A. Zhang, F.P.; Lagerquist, M.K.; et al. Inducible Wnt16 inactivation: WNT16 regulates cortical bone thickness in adult mice. *J. Endocrinol.* **2018**, *237*, 113–122. [CrossRef]
52. Butler, J.S.; Murray, D.; Hurson, C.J.; O'Brien, J.; Doran, P.P.; O'Byrne, J.M. The role of Dkk1 in bone mass regulation: Correlating serum Dkk1 expression with bone mineral density. *J. Orthop. Res.* **2011**, *29*, 414–418. [CrossRef] [PubMed]
53. McDonald, M.M.; Morse, A.; Schindeler, A.; Mikulec, K.; Peacock, L.; Cheng, T.; Bobyn, J.; Lee, L.; Baldock, P.A.; Croucher, P.I.; et al. Homozygous Dkk1 Knockout Mice Exhibit High Bone Mass Phenotype Due to Increased Bone Formation. *Calcif. Tissue Int.* **2018**, *102*, 105–116. [CrossRef] [PubMed]

54. Sebastian, A.; Loots, G.G. Genetics of Sost/SOST in sclerosteosis and van Buchem disease animal models. *Metabolism.* **2018**, *80*, 38–47. [CrossRef] [PubMed]
55. Singh, A.; Gupta, M.K.; Mishra, S.P. Study of correlation of level of expression of Wnt signaling pathway inhibitors sclerostin and dickkopf-1 with disease activity and severity in rheumatoid arthritis patients. *Drug Discov. Ther.* **2019**, *13*, 22–27. [CrossRef]
56. Seror, R.; Boudaoud, S.; Pavy, S.; Nocturne, G.; Schaeverbeke, T.; Saraux, A.; Chanson, P.; Gottenberg, J.E.; Devauchelle-Pensec, V.; Tobón, G.J.; et al. Increased Dickkopf-1 in Recent-onset Rheumatoid Arthritis is a New Biomarker of Structural Severity. Data from the ESPOIR Cohort. *Sci. Rep.* **2016**, *6*, 18421. [CrossRef]
57. Garnero, P.; Tabassi, N.C.; Voorzanger-Rousselot, N. Circulating Dickkopf-1 and radiological progression in patients with early Rheumatoid Arthritis treated with etanercept. *J. Rheumatol.* **2008**, *35*, 2313–2315. [CrossRef]
58. Axmann, R.; Herman, S.; Zaiss, M.; Franz, S.; Polzer, K.; Zwerina, J.; Herrmann, M.; Smolen, J.; Schett, G. CTLA-4 directly inhibits osteoclast formation. *Ann. Rheum. Dis.* **2008**, *67*, 1603–1609. [CrossRef]
59. Roser-Page, S.; Vikulina, T.; Zayzafoon, M.; Weitzmann, M.N. CTLA-4Ig-induced T cell anergy promotes Wnt-10b production and bone formation in a mouse model. *Arthritis Rheumatol.* **2014**, *66*, 990–999. [CrossRef]
60. Blair, H.A.; Deeks, E.D. Abatacept: A Review in Rheumatoid Arthritis. *Drugs* **2017**, *77*, 1221–1233. [CrossRef]
61. Roser-Page, S.; Vikulina, T.; Weiss, D.; Habib, M.M.; Beck, G.R., Jr.; Pacifici, R.; Lane, T.F.; Weitzmann, M.N. CTLA-4Ig (abatacept) balances bone anabolic effects of T cells and Wnt-10b with antianabolic effects of osteoblastic sclerostin. *Ann. N. Y. Acad. Sci.* **2018**, *1415*, 21–33. [CrossRef]
62. Adami, G.; Orsolini, G.; Adami, S.; Viapiana, O.; Idolazzi, L.; Gatti, D.; Rossini, M. Effects of TNF Inhibitors on Parathyroid Hormone and Wnt Signaling Antagonists in Rheumatoid Arthritis. *Calcif. Tissue Int.* **2016**, *99*, 360–364. [CrossRef] [PubMed]
63. Szentpétery, Á.; Horváth, Á.; Gulyás, K.; Pethö, Z.; Bhattoa, H.P.; Szántó, S.; Szücs, G.; FitzGerald, O.; Schett, G.; Szekanecz, Z. Effects of targeted therapies on the bone in arthritides. *Autoimmun. Rev.* **2017**, *16*, 313–320. [CrossRef] [PubMed]
64. Briot, K.; Rouanet, S.; Schaeverbeke, T.; Etchepare, F.; Gaudin, P.; Perdriger, A.; Vray, M.; Steinberg, G.; Roux, C. The effect of tocilizumab on bone mineral density, serum levels of Dickkopf-1 and bone remodeling markers in patients with Rheumatoid Arthritis. *Joint Bone Spine* **2015**, *82*, 109–115. [CrossRef] [PubMed]
65. Terpos, E.; Fragiadaki, K.; Konsta, M.; Bratengeier, C.; Papatheodorou, A.; Sfikakis, P.P. Early effects of IL-6 receptor inhibition on bone homeostasis: A pilot study in women with rheumatoid arthritis. *Clin. Exp. Rheumatol.* **2011**, *29*, 921–925. [PubMed]
66. Poddubnyy, D.; Sieper, J. Current Unmet Needs in Spondyloarthritis. *Curr. Rheumatol. Rep.* **2019**, *21*, 43. [CrossRef] [PubMed]
67. Osta, B.; Benedetti, G.; Miossec, P. Classical and paradoxical effects of TNF-α on bone homeostasis. *Front. Immunol.* **2014**, *5*, 48. [CrossRef] [PubMed]
68. Magrey, M.N.; Khan, M.A. The Paradox of Bone Formation and Bone Loss in Ankylosing Spondylitis: Evolving New Concepts of Bone Formation and Future Trends in Management. *Curr. Rheumatol. Rep.* **2017**, *19*, 17. [CrossRef] [PubMed]
69. Schett, G. Bone formation in psoriatic arthritis: A report from the GRAPPA 2013 Annual Meeting. *J. Rheumatol.* **2014**, *41*, 1218–1219. [CrossRef] [PubMed]
70. Uluçkan, Ö.; Jimenez, M.; Karbach, S.; Jeschke, A.; Graña, O.; Keller, J.; Busse, B.; Croxford, A.L.; Finzel, S.; Koenders, M.; et al. Chronic skin inflammation leads to bone loss by IL-17-mediated inhibition of Wnt signaling in osteoblasts. *Sci. Transl. Med.* **2016**, *8*, 330ra37. [CrossRef]
71. Tam, L.S.; Gu, J.; Yu, D. Pathogenesis of ankylosing spondylitis. *Nat. Rev. Rheumatol.* **2010**, *6*, 399–405. [CrossRef]
72. Rubio Vargas, R.; Melguizo Madrid, E.; González Rodríguez, C.; Navarro Sarabia, F.; Dominguez Quesada, C.; Ariza Ariza, R.; Navarro Compán, V. Association between serum dickkopf-1 levels and disease duration in axial spondyloarthritis. *Reumatol. Clin.* **2017**, *13*, 197–200. [CrossRef] [PubMed]
73. Sieper, J.; Poddubnyy, D. Axial spondyloarthritis. *Lancet* **2017**, *390*, 73–84. [CrossRef]
74. Biton, J.; Boissier, M.C.; Bessis, N. TNFα: Activator or inhibitor of regulatory T cells? *Joint Bone Spine* **2012**, *79*, 119–123. [CrossRef] [PubMed]
75. Korkosz, M.; Gasowski, J.; Leszczyński, P.; Pawlak-Buś, K.; Jeka, S.; Siedlar, M.; Grodzicki, T. Effect of tumour necrosis factor-α inhibitor on serum level of dickkopf-1 protein and bone morphogenetic protein-7

in ankylosing spondylitis patients with high disease activity. *Scand. J. Rheumatol.* **2014**, *43*, 43–48. [CrossRef] [PubMed]

76. Heiland, G.R.; Appel, H.; Poddubnyy, D.; Zwerina, J.; Hueber, A.; Haibel, H.; Baraliakos, X.; Listing, J.; Rudwaleit, M.; Schett, G.; et al. High level of functional dickkopf-1 predicts protection from syndesmophyte formation in patients with ankylosing spondylitis. *Ann. Rheum. Dis.* **2012**, *71*, 572–574. [CrossRef]
77. Uderhardt, S.; Diarra, D.; Katzenbeisser, J.; David, J.P.; Zwerina, J.; Richards, W.; Kronke, G.; Schett, G. Blockade of Dickkopf (DKK)-1 induces fusion of sacroiliac joints. *Ann. Rheum. Dis.* **2010**, *69*, 592–597. [CrossRef]
78. Zhao, Z.; Wang, G.; Wang, Y.; Yang, J.; Wang, Y.; Zhu, J.; Huang, F. Correlation between magnetic resonance imaging (MRI) findings and the new bone formation factor Dkk-1 in patients with spondyloarthritis. *Clin. Rheumatol.* **2019**, *38*, 465–475. [CrossRef]
79. Appel, H.; Ruiz-Heiland, G.; Listing, J.; Zwerina, J.; Herrmann, M.; Mueller, R.; Haibel, H.; Baraliakos, X.; Hempfing, A.; Rudwaleit, M.; et al. Altered skeletal expression of sclerostin and its link to radiographic progression in ankylosing spondylitis. *Arthritis Rheum.* **2009**, *60*, 3257–3262. [CrossRef]
80. Saad, C.G.; Ribeiro, A.C.; Moraes, J.C.; Takayama, L.; Goncalves, C.R.; Rodrigues, M.B.; de Oliveira, R.M.; Silva, C.A.; Bonfa, E.; Pereira, R.M. Low sclerostin levels: A predictive marker of persistent inflammation in ankylosing spondylitis during anti-tumor necrosis factor therapy? *Arthritis Res. Ther.* **2012**, *14*, R216. [CrossRef]
81. Haroon, N.; Inman, R.D.; Learch, T.J.; Weisman, M.H.; Lee, M.; Rahbar, M.H.; Ward, M.M.; Reveille, J.D.; Gensler, L.S. The impact of tumor necrosis factor alpha inhibitors on radiographic progression in ankylosing spondylitis. *Arthritis Rheum.* **2013**, *65*, 2645–2654. [CrossRef]

International Journal of *Molecular Sciences*

MDPI

Review

Role of Microparticles in the Pathogenesis of Inflammatory Joint Diseases

Magdalena Krajewska-Włodarczyk [1,2,*], Agnieszka Owczarczyk-Saczonek [3], Zbigniew Żuber [4], Maja Wojtkiewicz [5] and Joanna Wojtkiewicz [6]

1 Department of Rheumatology, Municipal Hospital in Olsztyn, 10-900 Olsztyn, Poland
2 Department of Internal Medicine, School of Medicine, Collegium Medicum, University of Warmia and Mazury, 10-900 Olsztyn, Poland
3 Department of Dermatology, Sexually Transmitted Diseases and Clinical Immunology, School of Medicine, Collegium Medicum, University of Warmia and Mazury, 10-900 Olsztyn, Poland; aganek@wp.pl
4 Department of Pediatrics, Faculty of Medicine and Health Sciences, Andrzej Frycz Modrzewski Kraków University, 30-705 Kraków, Poland; zbyszekzuber@interia.pl
5 Faculty of Earth Sciences, Department of Geomatics and Cartography Nicolaus Copernicus University, 87-100 Torun, Poland; maja.wojtkiewicz@umk.pl
6 Department of Pathophysiology, School of Medicine, Collegium Medicum, University of Warmia and Mazury, 10-900 Olsztyn, Poland; joanna.wojtkiewicz@uwm.edu.pl
* Correspondence: magdalenakw@op.pl

Received: 4 September 2019; Accepted: 30 October 2019; Published: 1 November 2019

Abstract: Rheumatoid arthritis (RA), juvenile idiopathic arthritis (JIA), ankylosing spondylitis (AS), and psoriatic arthritis (PsA) make up a group of chronic immune-mediated inflammatory diseases (IMIDs). The course of these diseases involves chronic inflammation of joints and enthesopathies, which can result in joint damage and disability. Microparticles (MPs) are a group of small spherical membranous vesicles. The structure and cellular origin of MPs, mechanisms that stimulate their secretion and the place of their production, determine their biological properties, which could become manifest in the pathogenesis of immune-mediated inflammatory diseases. Microparticles can stimulate synovitis with proinflammatory cytokines and chemokines. MPs may also contribute to the pathogenesis of rheumatic diseases by the formation of immune complexes and complement activation, pro-coagulation activity, activation of vascular endothelium cells, and stimulation of metalloproteinase production. It seems that in the future, microparticles can become a modern marker of disease activity, a response to treatment, and, possibly, they can be used in the prognosis of the course of arthritis. The knowledge of the complexity of MPs biology remains incomplete and it requires further comprehensive studies to explain how they affect the development of rheumatic diseases. This review focuses on the immunopathogenic and therapeutic role of MPs in chronic immune-mediated inflammatory joint diseases.

Keywords: microparticles; joint inflammatory diseases

1. Introduction

Cell membrane microparticles (MPs), or microvesicles, are fragments of surface membranes of activated eukaryotic cells. Their size, which determines their diameter as lying within the interval of 0.1 to 1 μm, is their main defining criterion. Therefore, the diameter of MPs is greater than that of exosomes and smaller than that of apoptotic bodies or small platelets. In physiological conditions, when cells mature, age, and undergo apoptosis, microparticles are released by exfoliation or by shedding to body fluids from cell membranes of all morphotic elements of blood and vascular endothelium [1,2]. MPs can be found in plasma, in whole blood, in umbilical blood, in cerebrospinal fluid, in urine, in milk, and in saliva. Microparticles do not have a cell nucleus, but they contain cytoplasmic material and surface antigens of their parent cells, owing to which their origin can be determined [2–4] (Table 1). Increased secretion of MPs in physiological conditions takes place in pregnant women, after intensive physical effort, in obese people, and in smokers [5]. Increased secretion of microparticles from activated platelets, leukocytes, erythrocytes, smooth muscle cells, and vascular endothelium cells takes place in immune-mediated diseases. An increased number of microparticles have been found in immune thrombocytopenia [6], in systemic lupus erythematosus [7], in rheumatoid arthritis [8], and in psoriasis [9,10]. The presence in MPs membrane of intercellular adhesion molecule 1 (ICAM-1) and vascular cell adhesion molecule 1 (VCAM-1) enables microparticles to join other cells and to take part in intermembrane transport of enzymes and receptor proteins, cytokines, growth factors, and nucleic acids: Micro RNA (miRNA), messenger RNA (mRNA), and deoxyribonucleic acid (DNA) [11,12].

Table 1. Cells of origin of microparticles and their clusters of differentiation.

Parent Cells	Surface Membrane Antigens of MPs Reflecting Their Cell of Origin
Platelets	CD41, CD41a, CD42a, CD42b, CD61, CD62p, PS, TF
Endothelium cells	CD31, CD51, CD62e, CD105, CD144, CD146, PS, TF
Erythrocytes	CD235a
Leukocytes	CD45
Monocytes	CD14, PS, TF
Neutrophils	CD66b
Th-cells	CD4
Ts-cells	CD8
B-cells	CD20

CD—cluster of differentiation, MPs—microparticles, PS—phosphatidylserine, TF—tissue factor.

As many as 90% of all circulating microparticles are MPs derived from platelets and megakaryocytes (PMPs) [13]. PMPs have a number of receptors on their membrane surface, including adhesive proteins. For PMPs, the most frequent surface markers are: Glycoprotein IIb (CD41), Ib (CD42b), IIb/IIIa (CD41a), IIIa (CD61), selectin P (CD62P) [3], and sphingolysine, arachidonic acid (AA), and bioactive lipids [5,14,15]. Contact of platelet-derived microparticles with target cells can result in monocyte chemotaxis, stimulation of cytokine secretion, activation of endothelial cells, and increased tissue factor expression on endothelial cell surface [16]. Platelet microparticles stimulate phagocytic activity of granulocytes by increasing the expression of the adhesive molecule CD11b on them [17]. An increased number of platelet-derived microparticles have been observed in atherosclerosis [18], diabetes [19], coronary artery disease [20], thrombotic thrombocytopenic purpura [21], aplastic anaemia, and paroxysmal nocturnal haemoglobinuria [22]. However, it is very likely that the activation of monocytes/macrophages, B-cells, T-cells, and endothelial cells observed in patients with inflammatory diseases may result in an increased release of MPs from these cells, raising their levels in plasma.

It has been proposed that excessive production of MPs may predispose to autoimmune diseases such as rheumatoid arthritis and systemic lupus erythematosus [23] but their role in the pathogenesis of these autoimmune diseases may differ. In patients with SLE, a prototypic autoimmune disease characterized by the production of antibodies to components of the cell nucleus and the formation of immune complexes, circulating MPs differ in their amount and composition compared to from those in patients with RA or healthy controls. MPs from SLE patients contain more immunoglobulins (IgG, IgA, and IgM) and complement components (C1q, C1s, C3, C4b, and C9) on their surface indicating the role of MPs as a source of immune complexes [24]. MPs containing DNA and RNA in SLE can behave as self-adjuvants for the production of autoantibodies. They can also increase tolerance of immature B-lymphocytes and break the tolerance of mature B-cells. MPs endocytosed by plasmacytoid dendritic cells are able to contact intracellular TLR7 (toll-like receptor-7) and TLR9, leading to the production of proinflammatory cytokines including type 1 interferon (IFN-1) and IL-6 (interleukin-6) [25].

2. The Mechanism of Microparticle Formation

The primary settings for MPs release are cellular activation and death. An increase in the intracellular concentration of calcium ions secreted by cytoplasmic reticulum is a response to multiple factors, including: An increase in the number of free radicals, increased shear force, adenosine diphosphate (ADP) secreted by activated platelets, expression of CD40 ligand (CD40L) on T-cells [26]. In these conditions, activation of calcium concentration-dependent enzymes takes place; these include gelsolin, which facilitates the separation of actin fibers from platelet cytoskeleton [27]; aminophospholipid translocase, which transports aminophospholipids from the outer membrane into the cell interior [28]; floppase, which transports phospholipids from the inner lipid bilayer outwards [29]; calpain, which destroys cytoskeleton actin fibers [30]; and scramblase, which affects transmembrane phospholipid transport [31] (Figure 1). The activated enzymes contribute to the loss of asymmetric distribution of phospholipids in the cell membrane in which phosphatidylserine (PS) and phosphatidylethanolamine (PE) are present mainly in the inner cytoplasmic layer, and phosphatidylcholine (PC) and sphingomyelin (SM) are present in the outer layer of the lipid bilayer. The asymmetry loss process resulting from transferring phosphatidylserine and phosphatidylethanolamine to the outer layer of the cell membrane and simultaneous cytoskeleton destabilization allow the formation and secretion of microparticles [26,32].

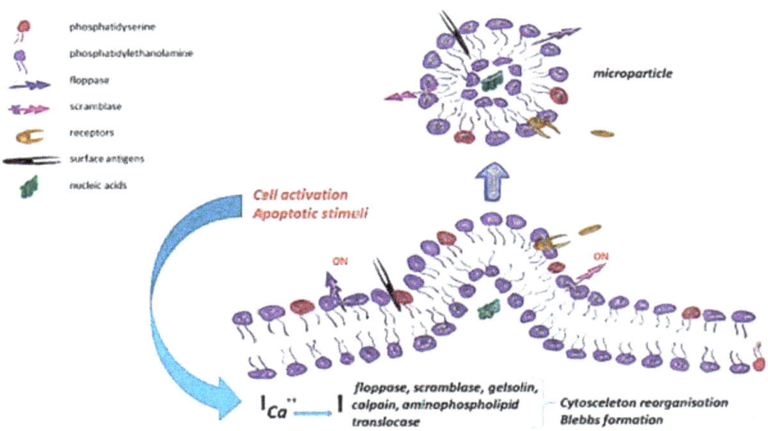

Figure 1. Microparicle formation following cellular activation and cytoskeletal.

An increase in the intracellular concentration of calcium, as a response to cell activation or apoptotic stimuli, results in the activation of calcium concentration-dependent enzymes: Gelsolin, aminophospholipid translocase, floppase, calpain, and scramblase. During this process, membrane asymmetry is lost, leading to the exposure of phosphatidylserine and phosphatidylethanolamine normally present in the inner leaflet of the membrane bilayer. Destabilization of the cytoskeleton results in cellular contraction and membrane blebbing.

3. Methods of Microparticle Detection

There are no standardized microparticle testing techniques and each laboratory conducting such testing develops its own MPs detection methods and standards. However, common protocol among researchers is to start collecting MPs from blood with a centrifugation to collect platelet-free plasma to avoid the activation and subsequent release of microparticles from platelets. Microparticle identification is a technical challenge because they are much smaller than cells of origin (diameters of 10–100× less). Microparticles can be isolated from blood, other biological fluids, or from cell cultures. Since MPs are cell-derived structures, a cytometric test is the "gold standard" and is the most widely used method of microparticle detection on the basis of light scattering as well as binding of marker antibodies to identify the cell of origin [33]. The MPs population to the flow cytometry settings is defined by using size calibration beads. However, MPs smaller than approximately 0.5 μm in diameter are not efficiently resolved by conventional flow cytometers. Available digital flow cytometers do not count all MPs because of their limited forward scatter (FS) sensitivity [34]. Recently, high-sensitivity flow cytometers with significantly improved light scatter detection became available and provide sufficient size resolution for the identification of MPs subtypes [35]. Microparticles generally expose phosphatidylserine and membrane antigens of their parent cells. MPs as cell-derived membrane structures in the cytometry test are commonly determined with annexin V, usually stained with phycoerythrin and antibodies against specific cell antigens, stained with fluorescein isothiocyanate. Labeled annexin V binds mainly to phosphatidylserine, which is typical of all types of microparticles and which is present on the MPs membranous surface and less frequently in membrane permeability disorders; it can also connect to phosphatidylserine located inside microparticles [36]. Annexin V is often used to identify microparticles, but some MPs may not show a tendency to bind to this protein [37]. The use of antibodies against different membranous antigens enables identification of the cellular origin of microparticles.

Another method of microparticle determination is based on ELISA (enzyme-linked immunosorbent assay), which makes use of test plates coated with annexin V or antibodies specific to cell membrane antigens [38]. When total phosphorus or phospholipid activity is determined, ELISA enables quantitative determination of microparticles [39].

4. Role of Microparticles in Inflammatory Joint Diseases

Rheumatoid arthritis (RA), juvenile idiopathic arthritis (JIA), ankylosing spondylitis (AS), and psoriatic arthritis (PsA) are chronic immune-mediated inflammations, leading to chronic joint inflammations and/or enthesopathies and to many extra-articular complications. Increasing numbers of circulating microparticles in immune-mediated diseases have been reported; the increase is particularly manifested if vessels are also affected; it usually concerns microparticles of platelet origin and—less frequently—those of endothelial origin [40–46]. The few studies conducted to date have suggested, or even confirmed, a pathogenic link between microparticles and immune-dependent diseases [6–10,47,48]. MPs can be detected in inflammatory joint diseases in blood and other biological fluids (Table 2).

Table 2. Microparticles in blood and other biological fluids in inflammatory joint diseases.

Disease	Microparticles	References
RA	Increased number of PMPs in peripheral blood and synovial fluid in RA	[8,49–51]
RA	Increased number of circulating MPs exposing complement components in early RA	[51]
RA	Increased number of monocyte-, B-cell-, T-cell-, platelet-derived MPs in high disease activity in RA	[51,52]
RA	Monocyte-derived MPs present in a much larger amount in synovial fluid than in plasma in RA	[53]
RA	Significantly increased number of granulocyte-derived MPs in synovial fluid in the RA patients with aCCP antibodies	[54]
RA	Increased number of MPs with CD3, CD14, and CD19 antigens in the urine of RA patients with high disease activity	[52]
JIA	Increased number of PMPs in synovial fluid in JIA compared to osteoarthritis	[8]
JIA	Much higher number of PMPs in synovial fluid in active JIA than in serum	[55]
PsA	Increased number of circulating PMPs and EMPs in PsA	[47]
PsA	Increased number of PMPs in synovial fluid in PsA	[8]
AS	Decrease in the number of MPMs and EMPs during the anti-TNFα treatment in AS	[56]
AS	No differences in the number of MPs between AS patients and healthy control, but significantly higher expression of CD4, CD62, CD14 and lower expression of CD41 in the MPs surface in AS	[57]

aCCP—anti cyclic citrullinated peptide antibodies; AS—ankylosing spondylitis; CD—cluster of differentiation; MPMs—monocyte-derived microparticles; PMPs—platelet-derived microparticles; PsA—psoriatic arthritis; RA—rheumatoid arthritis; JIA—juvenile idiopathic arthritis.

4.1. Rheumatoid Arthritis

An increase in circulating MPs secretion is closely linked to an increase in cytokine production and appears to be a significant factor which affects inflammation development within the synovial membrane in rheumatoid arthritis [46]. In one of the first studies assessing the relationship between MPs and rheumatoid arthritis in a group of 19 patients, Knifjj-Dutmer et al. observed an increased number of circulating PMPs compared to a group of healthy individuals, and a significant relationship between the number of circulating microparticles of platelet origin and the disease activity assessed by the DAS28 score [49]. Moreover, researchers suggested a possible effect of PMPs on the development of cardiovascular diseases in patients with RA, leading to increased mortality linked to vascular complications, compared to the general population [49]. Viñuela-Berni et al. observed an increased number of MPs with CD3, CD14, CD19, CD41, and CD63E antigens in plasma of RA patients with high disease activity (DAS 28 > 5.1) [52]. The link between the intensity of inflammation in RA and the number and activity of released microparticles of endothelial origin was confirmed by Barbati et al. The total pool of circulating MPs and endothelial MPs (EMPs) initially increased, then decreased after four months of anti-TNFα therapy [58]. The microparticles with CD3, CD14, CD19, CD41, and CD63E antigens also stimulated secretion of TNFα and IL-1, IL-17 by monocytes in vitro [52]. The potential role of microparticles in the pathogenesis of rheumatoid arthritis appears to be very complex (Table 3).

Table 3. Potential role of microparticles in the development of rheumatoid arthritis.

MPs as a Potential Pathogenetic Factor of RA	References
Activation of Immunocompetent Cells	
Activation of B-cells by macrophage/monocyte-derived MPs from synovial fluid	Messer et al. [59]
Participation in Formation of Immune Complexes	
Increased number of C1q, C4, C3-binding MPs in synovial fluid and in peripheral blood	Biro et al. [60]
mpIC present in synovial fluid	Cloutier et al. [61]
Increased Secretion of Matrix Metalloproteinases	
Monocyte- and B-cell-derived MPs can induce the release of MMP3, MMP9, MMP13 in FLS	Distler et al. [62]
Modulation of Chemokine and Cytokine Release	
Monocyte- and granulocyte-derived MPs from synovial fluid modulate MCP-1, IL-6, IL-8, and CCL5 release by synoviocytes	Berckmans et al. [63]
Increased secretion of TNFα and IL-1, IL-17 by monocytes stimulated by monocyte-, B-cell-, T-cell-, platelet-derived MPs from peripheral blood	Viñuela-Berni et al. [52]
Pro-Coagulation Activity	
Monocyte- and granulocyte-derived MPs from synovial fluid are strongly coagulant via the factor VII-dependent pathway	Berckmans et al. [64]
Activation of Vascular Endothelium Cells	
MPs from articular fluid stimulate FLS production and release of VEGF	Berckmans et al. [63]
Stimulating effect of leukocyte-derived MPs on production and release by rheumatoid synoviocytes of proangiogenic CXC	Reich et al. [65]

C—complement component; CCL—C-C motif chemokine ligand; CXC—CXC chemokines; FLS—fibroblast-like synoviocyte; IL—interleukin; MCP—monocyte chemoattractant protein; MMP—metalloproteinase; MPs—microparticles; RA—rheumatoid factor; TNF—tumor necrosis factor; VEGF—vascular endothelium growth factor.

Apart from serum, microparticles have been detected in other body fluids of the patients. Viñuela-Berni et al. observed an increased number of MPs with CD3, CD14, and CD19 antigens in the urine of RA patients with high disease activity [52]. Boilard et al. [8] analyzed samples of synovial fluid in RA patients and found it to contain large numbers of PMPs (slightly less than 2 × 105 CD41+ MPs/μL). Synovial fluid of RA patients contained (much less than PMPs) MPs with surface antigens of neutrophils, monocytes, and T-cells. It was an interesting observation to determine a group of neutrophils present in rheumatoid synovial fluid, with simultaneously present leukocyte CD45 antigen and a platelet CD41 antigen. The immunofluorescence signal was a result of attaching to neutrophils of the bodies corresponding to PMPs rather than whole platelets [8]. Interestingly, the number of PMPs determined in rheumatoid fluid in this study was much higher than in serum of RA patients in the study by Knijff et al. [49], where it was 600 per μL. Michael et al. [54] determined the number of MPs in synovial fluid in RA patients and found a considerably larger number of MPs derived from granulocytes, monocytes, and T-cells than in patients with degenerative joint disease and in the control group. Moreover, the number of granulocyte-derived MPs in RA patients was significantly larger in the patients with aCCP antibodies.

It is not completely clear how platelets infiltrate synovial fluid, although undamaged platelets, platelet aggregates, and platelets attached to leukocytes have been found in studies with RA patients for many years [66–68]. It is probable that collagen, fibrinogen, proteolytic enzymes, inflammatory cytokines, and shear forces in a joint could stimulate the production of platelet-derived MPs. It is also possible that, owing to their size, microparticles can penetrate synovial fluid and synovial membranes because the number of platelet microparticles in synovial fluid in RA patients is considerably larger than the number of PMPs in peripheral blood, which may suggest locally increased microparticle release from activated platelets in vessels near joints. Platelets can be activated locally by stimulation through collagen, a specific platelet receptor containing glycoprotein VI (GPVI) [69]. In a study by Boilard et al., platelet activation mediated by the GPVI, conducted in vivo on an animal model with transgenic K/BxN mice, induced release of microparticles containing both forms of interleukin 1 (IL-1): IL-1α and IL-β, stimulating production and secretion of IL-6 and IL-8 by fibroblast-like synoviocytes (FLS). The findings of the study suggest the pro-inflammatory potential of PMPs and their active participation in pathogenesis of rheumatoid arthritis [8]. Activation of platelet receptor, GPVI, leads to activation of spleen tyrosine kinase (SYK) in platelets and B-cells, further activating Bruton's tyrosine kinase (BTK), which plays a key role in the activation of B-cells, which is essential in their proper function and development. Bruton's kinase inhibition with the BTK selective inhibitor was examined by Hsu et al. and found to reduce collagen-induced production of PMPs [70]. In another study, BTK blockade in activated platelet culture also resulted in a decrease in production of microparticles and inhibition of production and release of IL-6 and IL-8 [71,72].

Apart from platelet-derived microparticles, synovial fluid in RA patients was found to contain MPs from monocytes, granulocytes, T- and B-cells, and erythrocytes [50,73,74]. Monocyte-derived MPs, as determined by Headland et al., were present in a much larger amount in synovial fluid than in plasma of RA patients. Researchers obtained some interesting findings on an animal model, where they observed a protective effect of monocyte-derived microparticles on articular cartilage, which is associated with decreasing secretion of IL-8 and prostaglandin E2 [53].

Microparticles exhibit high pro-coagulation activity mediated by the TF/VII factor, thereby stimulating thrombin production. They can also contribute to developing proatherogenic vasculitis and to the formation of "rice bodies" within joints as a manifestation of local coagulation processes [64]. In their study with RA patients, concerning non-differentiated arthritis, Berckmans et al. found incubation of MPs obtained from synovial fluid in the presence of FLS obtained by the biopsy of the synovial membrane to result in an increase in production and release by synoviocytes of IL-6, IL-8, monocyte chemoattractant protein 1 (MPC-1), RANTES (regulation on activation normal T-cells expressed and secreted) chemokine, and vascular endothelium growth factor (VEGF) [63]. A local increase in VEGF secretion can stimulate angiogenesis within articular tissues in RA, especially at its early stages [74]. Stimulation of angiogenesis in joints affected by RA can also be mediated by chemokines. Reich et al. observed a stimulating effect of leukocyte-derived MPs on production and release by rheumatoid synoviocytes of proangiogenic CXC chemokine with an ELR motive—a sequence of three amino acids: Glutamic acid-leucine-arginine (Glu-Leu-Arg). In their study, the authors observed increasing mRNA expression for ligands of chemokine CXC ELR+: CXCL1, CXCL2, CXCL3, CXCL5, and CXCL6 [65].

Matrix metalloproteinases (MMP) are responsible for processes of extracellular matrix component transformation and degradation. Distler et al. demonstrated that MPs derived from B-cells and monocytes can stimulate rheumatoid FLS additionally to synthesis of metalloproteinases 1, 3, 9, and 13, which participate in the destruction of the extracellular matrix of cartilaginous and bone tissue in RA. In this study, the microparticles under study stimulated the production of IL-6, IL-8, MCP-1, and MCP-2 by fibroblasts [62].

The complement system, comprising approximately 40 proteins, plays an important role in the regulation of innate immune response by stimulating phagocytosis and intensification of an inflammatory reaction. The system is activated in a cascade manner. Removing apoptotic and necrotic cells is one of the functions of the complement system [75]. These cells activate the complement system mainly through a conventional pathway, as a result of a reaction of the C1q component with the CH2 domain of the antibody Fc fragment [76–78]. Microparticles with membranous features of apoptotic and necrotic cells (with exposed phosphatidylserine, phosphatidylethynolamine, oxidated phospholipids) can participate in the development of inflammation in RA by activating the complement cascade. It has been shown that MPs formed from apoptotic Jurkat leukemia cell [79] and stimulated neutrophils [80,81] can bind the C1q and, thereby, activate the complement in vitro through a conventional activation pathway. Biro et al. found C1q, C4, and/or C3 components on microparticles isolated from synovial fluid and—to a lesser extent—on microparticles obtained from serum [60]. It seems that microparticles, especially those derived from platelets, exposing the CD41 antigen, can also take part in the formation of immune complexes (IC), usually described as structures containing antibodies, antigens, and complement components. Cloutier et al. used high resolution flow cytometry and transmission electron microscopy and detected MPs in IC present in synovial fluid in RA patients, forming specific mpIC [61].

Microparticles in rheumatoid synovial fluid can undergo the process of protein citrullination—posttranslational deimination of arginine residues catalyzed by peptidylarginine deiminase (PAD), which results in the production of antibodies against cyclic citrullinated peptides (aCCP). For platelet microparticles described in the study by Cloutier et al., with expression of the FcγRIIa receptor, mpIC were formed not by connecting antibodies to this receptor, but by binding MPs to citrullinated proteins, such as fibrinogen and vimentin. The researchers confirmed that platelet MPs can react with aCCP antibodies in a mechanism which follows citrullination of PMPs surface proteins and by binding microparticles and citrullinated proteins. The paper also describes a stimulating effect of platelet mpIC on the production of leukotrienes by neutrophils. The researchers made an interesting observation by comparing the amount of mpIC in synovial fluid collected from RA and PsA patients. Despite the presence of MPs and immunoglobulins in synovial fluid of PsA patients, the amount of detected mpIC was nearly twenty times smaller than in RA patients (2000 ± 900 mpICs/μL vs 39,400 ± 9400 mpICs/μL) [82]. Unlike the previous study, two other studies found no proof of any relationship between the amount of circulating microparticles and immune complexes containing MPs in RA patients and the indices conventionally used to assess the disease activity [49,82]. This may indicate a highly effective vascular and reticular-endothelial mechanism of IC elimination or local formation of mpIC in joints affected by inflammation.

A very important role in pathogenesis of RA is played by activated B-cells. Data from the study by Messer et al. suggest the role of microparticles in synovial fluid in inducing the release of B-cell activating factor (BAFF), thymic stromal lymphopoietin (TSLP), and antileukoprotease (SLPI) by fibroblast-like synoviocytes. MPs present in synovial fluid stimulated the secretion of BAFF to the same extent as IFN-γ used as a control. The effect was observed both among the RA patients—study participants—and in patients with degenerative joint disease, which indicated the activity of MPs in stimulating B-cells, regardless of the disease type. The main difference in this study was quantitative.

The number of MPs in synovial fluid in RA patients was considerably larger than in individuals with no joint inflammation. The study assessed the ability of MPs from THP-1 monocytic–macrophagic cell line and from the CEM lymphocyte line to synthesize and release BAFF, TLSP, and SLPI by activated FLS. Microparticles of monocytic–macrophagic origin had high inflammatory activity, which indicates the important participation of monocytes in initiation of an inflammatory response. MPs from activated T-cells which, in turn, stimulate the secretion of IL-6 and IL-8, did not stimulate the release of BAFF, but of TLSP and SLPI by synoviocytes. Those same MPs, did not affect the release of BAFF, TLSP, or SLPI after being treated with actinomycin D, which suggested no effect of MPs from apoptotic T-cells on activation of B-cells [59].

4.2. Juvenile Idiopathic Arthritis

There are only a few papers on circulating MPs in other joint inflammations. In a recent study with 26 children with JIA, Kumar et al. found a greater number of PMPs in plasma of patients with the active disease compared to the patients with disease remission [55] despite the absence of a difference in the number of platelets. Additionally the number of PMPs in synovial fluid in JIA was close to the number of PMPs in serum of individuals with active disease. The researchers suggested the potential usability of PMPs determination as a sensitive indicator of JIA activity. As in the study by Knifjj-Dutmer et al. [49], the number of PMPs in patients with the active disease did not correlate with the number of circulating platelets, ESR and CRP. Boilard et al. [8] analyzed samples of synovial fluid in JIA patients and found an increased number of PMPs in synovial fluid of patients with JIA, whereas the number of PMPs was not determinable in synovial fluid of 95% of patients with osteoarthritis.

4.3. Ankylosing Spondylitis

In a study with 82 male AS patients and a group of healthy individuals, Sari et al. did not find any difference in the number of PMPs or EMPs in plasma between the groups under study. No differences were also found between the number of PMPs and EMPs in patients with high disease activity as defined by BASDAI > 4 (Bath Ankylosing Spondylitis Disease Activity Index) and its low activity [56]. This notwithstanding, a significant decrease in the number of MPMs and EMPs was observed during the anti-TNFα treatment (etanercept, infliximab, adalimumab) compared with a conventional therapy. This may indirectly indicate the role of MPs in AS pathogenesis and, because both the number of PMPs and EMPs increases in vascular endothelium disorders, a positive vascular effect of anti-TNFα treatment. In a study with AS patients, Bradley did not observe any differences in the number of MPs between them and the control group; in contrast, significantly higher expression of CD4, CD62, CD14, VCam1 and lower expression of CD41 and CD54 was observed in the MPs surface in the patients compared with healthy individuals as well as significantly more frequent positive immunofluorescence of AV-labeled MPs in the patients [57], which implies a relationship between different cellular origin and a mechanism leading to MPs formation (in this case—apoptosis) and AS development.

4.4. Psoriatic Arthritis

An increase in the number of circulating endothelial, platelet, and monocyte-derived MPs in psoriatic patients was also observed in a study conducted by Takeshita et al. [9]. In another paper, Papadavid et al. described a considerable increase in the number of PMPs correlating with an increase in the concentration of interleukin 12 (IL-12) and an increase in the disease activity as assessed by the PASI (Psoriasis Area Severity Index) [83]. In another study with patients with severe psoriasis (with or without psoriatic arthritis), Ho et al. observed a larger number of circulating PMPs and EMPs in patients compared with the control group [47]. The researchers did not observe any differences in the number of MPs between patients with psoriasis and those with psoriatic arthritis. Contrary to expectations, no difference was observed in the number of PMPs or EMPs before and after a three-month treatment with IL12/23 p40 subunit inhibitor, despite a significant clinical improvement measured with PASI. Increased number of PMPs in synovial fluid of patients with PsA compared to osteoarthritis was described by Boilard et al. [8].

5. Microparticles as an Indicator of Disease Activity

Microparticles have been attracting increasing attention as potential indicators of eukaryotic cell activation. They could provide valuable information on inflammatory processes in progress, disease activity, and the response to treatment as well as prognosis as a disease assessment indicator.

Hsu et al. demonstrated that release of MPs from platelets activated with collagen decreased considerably after the activity of kinase BTK was inhibited [70]. Reduction of PMPs numbers in other studies with BTK inhibitor in platelet cultures was associated with a decrease in production and the release of inflammatory cytokines IL-6 and IL-8 [71,72]. A considerable increase in the number of platelet, monocyte, and lymphocyte-derived microparticles (CD3, CD19) has been observed in RA patients with high disease activity [52]. Rodrigez-Cario et al. examined the amount of circulating microparticles and their origin in 114 RA patients. The total number of MPs in platelet poor plasma was much higher in individuals with arthritis compared to a group of healthy individuals. The occurrence of different MPs subtypes in this study differed considerably in the RA group and was associated with the clinical course of joint inflammation: The amount of endothelial MPs was associated with the disease duration, the amount of granulocyte MPs was associated with the disease activity as assessed by DAS28, whereas the amount of monocyte-derived MPs was associated with the presence of the rheumatoid factor. The amount of MPs was also associated with the presence of traditional cardiovascular risk factors [59]. The findings of Cloutier et al. could indicate the possibility of using the studies of circulating mpICs to assess RA activity [60]. However, different conclusions were presented by van Eijk et al. based on a study with 24 patients with an early form of RA [51]. The disease activity was assessed based on the ESR, C-reactive protein (CRP) level, and DAS28 score. Moreover, the level of serum amyloid-P (SAP) and the amount of circulating MPs and MPs presenting the C1q complement component was determined in the patients. Nine patients were reassessed after an eight-week intensive treatment according to the COBRA (COmBination therapy in Rheumatoid Arthritis) regimen, which included a combined treatment with methotrexate, sulfasalazine, and prednisolone. As expected, ESR, CRP, and DAS28 improved as a result of the treatment; however, contrary to expectations, neither the amount of circulating MPs, nor MPs with the attached C1q component decreased, which suggests the absence of any connection between the activity of inflammation and MPs release and mpIC production [51]. In a recent paper, Chen demonstrated that inhibition of PMPs formation in an animal model of CIA (collagen-induced arthritis) and reduction of circulating PMPs was associated with a clinical decrease in the disease activity assessed as joint swelling and stiffness [84].

6. The Potential Role of Mesenchymal Stem Cells-Derived Microparticles in Inflammatory Joint Disease Therapy

Immunomodulating properties of mesenchymal stem cells (MSC) are used in current studies of new therapeutic options in inflammatory joint diseases [85,86]. Cosenza et al. studied the delayed-T hypersensitivity model (DTH) and CIA and found MSCs-derived MPs administered parenterally to have an immunosuppressive effect by inhibiting T- and B-cell proliferation and inducing Treg cells [87]. Compared to MSC, MSCs-derived MPs were more effective in stimulating CD4+CD25+Foxp3+ Treg and CD4+IL-10+ Tr1 in vitro. In the DTH model, MSCs-derived MPs proved to be more effective in inhibiting the inflammation than MSC, and they significantly inhibited the formation of erosions in the CIA model. In another paper, Cosenza et al. described the anti-inflammatory effect on macrophage maturation of MSCs-derived MPs with lower membranous expression of TNFα and higher expression of IL-10 [88]. Microparticles formed from adipose-derived MSCs (ASCs) can inhibit in vitro the expression of inflammatory cytokines and chemokines secreted by fibroblast-like synoviocytes [89] and also increase the production of anti-inflammatory IL-10 and collagen II in chondrocyte cultures [90].

7. Summary

Microparticles have special biological properties which allow them to play a role in pathogenesis of chronic inflammation. They can also be used as a sensitive indicator of an inflammation in progress. Most studies with patients with joint inflammations have reported an increase in circulating MPs and MPs in synovial fluid in joints affected by the inflammation. Participation of microparticles in the pathogenesis of RA, JIA, AS, and PsA is complex. Microparticles can stimulate the production and release of inflammatory factors, take part in their transport, in the formation of immune complexes, and induce formation of autoantibodies. In future, MPs determination can be used as one of the elements of disease activity assessment, of monitoring the response to treatment, or forecasting the course of a joint inflammation. Microparticles derived from stem cells can also become a cell-free biological therapeutic option in joint inflammations. It is necessary to continue the study of MPs in the context of inflammatory joint diseases to determine their value as biomarkers for diagnostic, prognostic, and therapeutic purposes.

Funding: This research received no external funding.

Acknowledgments: This study is supported by the statutory grant School of Medicine, Collegium Medicum, University of Warmia and Mazury in Olsztyn, Poland.

Conflicts of Interest: The authors declare no conflict of interest.

Abbreviations

aCCP	Anti-cyclic citrullinated peptide autoantibodies
AS	Ankylosing spondylitis
BAFF	B-cell-activating factor
BTK	Bruton's tyrosine kinase
CRP	C reactive protein
DAS 28	Disease activity score 28
EMPs	Endothelial microparticles
FLS	Fibroblast-like synoviocytes
IC	Immune complexes
ICAM-1	Intercellular adhesion molecule 1
IFN-γ	Interferon γ
IMIDs	Immune-mediated inflammatory diseases
JIA	Juvenile idiopathic arthritis
MPC-1	Monocyte chemoattractant protein-1
mpIC	Microparticles in immune complexes
mRNA	Messenger RNA
miRNA	Micro-ribonucleic acid
MMP	Matrix metalloproteinases
MPs	Microparticles
PMPs	Platelet-derived microparticles
PsA	Psoriatic arthritis
RA	Rheumatoid arthritis
SLPI	Secretory leukocyte protease inhibitor
SYK	Spleen tyrosine kinase
TF	Tissue factor
TLR	Toll-like receptor
TSLP	Thymic stromal lymphopoetin
VCAM-1	Vascular cell adhesion molecule 1
VEGF	Vascular endothelial growth factor

References

1. Gelderman, M.P.; Simak, J. Flow cytmometric analysis of cell membrane microparticles. *Methods Mol. Biol.* **2008**, *484*, 79–93. [CrossRef] [PubMed]
2. Piccin, A.; Murphy, W.G.; Smith, O.P. Circulating microparticles: Pathophysiology and clinical implications. *Blood Rev.* **2007**, *21*, 157–171. [CrossRef] [PubMed]
3. Maślanka, K.; Michur, H.; Smoleńska-Sym, G. Mikrocząstki błon komórkowych. *Acta Haemat. Pol.* **2009**, *40*, 481–491.
4. Simak, J.; Gelderman, M.P. Cell membrane microparticles in blood and blood products: Potentially pathogenic agents and diagnostic markers. *Trans. Med. Rev.* **2006**, *20*, 1–26. [CrossRef]
5. Barry, O.P.; Pratico, D.; Lawson, J.A.; FitzGerald, G.A. Transcellular activation of platelets and endothelial cells by bioactive lipids in platelet microparticles. *J. Clin. Investig.* **1997**, *99*, 2118–2127. [CrossRef]
6. Semple, J.W.; Provan, D.; Garvey, M.B.; Freedman, J. Recent progress in understanding the pathogenesis of immune thrombocytopenia (ITP). *Curr. Opin. Haematol.* **2010**, *17*, 590–595. [CrossRef]
7. Burbano, C.; Villar-Vesga, J.; Orejuela, J.; Muñoz, C.; Vanegas, A.; Vásquez, G.; Rojas, M.; Castaño, D. Potential Involvement of Platelet-Derived Microparticles and Microparticles Forming Immune Complexes during Monocyte Activation in Patients with Systemic Lupus Erythematosus. *Front. Immunol.* **2018**, *9*, 322. [CrossRef]
8. Boilard, E.; Nigrovic, P.A.; Larabee, K.; Watts, G.F.; Coblyn, J.S.; Weinblatt, M.E.; Massarotti, E.M.; Remold-O'Donnell, E.; Farndale, R.W.; Ware, J.; et al. Platelets amplify inflammation in arthritis via collagen-dependent microparticle production. *Science* **2010**, *327*, 580–583. [CrossRef]
9. Takeshita, J.; Mohler, E.R.; Krishnamoorthy, P.; Moore, J.; Rogers, W.T.; Zhang, L.; Gelfand, J.M.; Mehta, N.N. Endothelial Cell-, Platelet-, and Monocyte/Macrophage-Derived Microparticles are Elevated in Psoriasis Beyond Cardiometabolic Risk Factors. *J. Am. Heart Assoc.* **2014**, *3*, e000507. [CrossRef]
10. Martínez-Sales, V.; Vila, V.; Ricart, J.M.; Vayá, A.; Todolí, J.; Nńñez, C.; Contreras, T.; Ballester, C.; Reganon, E. Increased circulating endothelial cells and microparticles in patients with psoriasis. *Clin. Hemorheol. Microcirc.* **2015**, *60*, 283–290. [CrossRef]
11. Hunter, M.P.; Ismail, N.; Zhang, X.; Aguda. B.D.; Lee, E.J.; Yu, L.; Xiao, T.; Schafer, J.; Lee, M.L.; Schmittgen, T.D.; et al. Detection of microRNA expression in human peripheral blood microvesicles. *PLoS ONE* **2008**, *3*, e3694. [CrossRef] [PubMed]
12. Risitano, A.; Beaulieu, L.M.; Vitseva, O.; Freedman, J.E. Platelets and platelet-like particles mediate intercellular RNA transfer. *Blood* **2012**, *119*, 6288–6295. [CrossRef] [PubMed]
13. Siljander, P.R. Platelet-derived microparticles—An updated perspective. *Thromb. Res.* **2011**, *127*, 30–33. [CrossRef]
14. Baj-Krzyworzeka, M.; Majka, M.; Pratico, D.; Ratajczak, J.; Vilaire, G.; Kijowski, J.; Reca, R.; Janowska-Wieczorek, A.; Ratajczak, M.Z. Platelet-derived microparticles stimulate proliferation, survival, adhesion and chemotaxis of hematopoietic cells. *Exp. Hematol.* **2002**, *30*, 450–459. [CrossRef]
15. Barry, O.P.; Kazanietz, M.G.; Pratico, D.; FitzGerald, G.A. Arachidonic acid in platelet microparticles up-regulates cyclooxygenase-2-dependent prostaglandin formation via a protein kinase C/mitogen-activated protein kinase-dependent pathway. *J. Biol. Chem.* **1999**, *274*, 7545–7556. [CrossRef] [PubMed]
16. Barry, O.P.; Pratico, D.; Savani, R.C.; FitzGerald, G.A. Modulation of monocyte-endothelial cell interactions by platelet microparticles. *J. Clin. Investig.* **1998**, *102*, 136–144. [CrossRef]
17. Merten, M.; Pakala, P.; Thiagarajan, P.; Benedict, C.R. Platelet microparticles promote platelet interactions with subendothelial matrix in a glycoprotein IIb/IIIa-dependent mechanism. *Circulation* **1999**, *99*, 2577–2582. [CrossRef]
18. Tan, K.T.; Lip, G.Y. The potential role of platelet microparticles in atherosclerosis. *Thromb. Haemost.* **2005**, *94*, 488–492. [CrossRef]
19. Koga, H.; Sugiyama, S.; Kugiyama, K.; Watanabe, K.; Fukushima, H.; Tanaka, T.; Sakamoto, T.; Yoshimura, M.; Jinnouchi, H.; Ogawa, H. Elevated levels of VE-cadherin-positive endothelial microparticles in patients with type 2 diabetes mellitus and coronary artery disease. *J. Am. Coll. Cardiol.* **2005**, *45*, 1622–1630. [CrossRef]
20. Vidal, C.; Spaulding, C.; Picard, F.; Schaison, F.; Melle, J.; Weber, S.; Fontenay-Roupie, M. Flow cytometry detection of platelet procoagulation activity and microparticles in patients with unstable angina treated by percutaneous coronary angioplasty and stent implantation. *Thromb. Haemost.* **2001**, *86*, 784–790. [CrossRef]

21. Joseph, J.E.; Harrison, P.; Mackie, I.J.; Isenberg, D.A.; Machin, S.J. Increased circulating platelet-leucocyte complexes and platelet activation in patients with antiphospholipid syndrome, systemic lupus erythematosus and rheumatoid arthritis. *Br. J. Haematol.* **2001**, *115*, 451–459. [CrossRef] [PubMed]
22. Hugel, B.; Socie, G.; Vu, T.; Toti, F.; Gluckman, E.; Freyssinet, J.M.; Scrobohaci, M.L. Elevated levels of circulating procoagulant microparticles in patients with paroxysmal nocturnal hemoglobinuria and aplastic anemia. *Blood* **1999**, *93*, 3451–3456. [CrossRef] [PubMed]
23. Dye, J.R.; Ullal, A.J.; Pisetsky, D.S. The role of microparticles in the pathogenesis of rheumatoid arthritis and systemic lupus erythematosus. *Scand. J. Immunol.* **2013**, *78*, 140–148. [CrossRef] [PubMed]
24. Østergaard, O.; Nielsen, C.T.; Iversen, L.V.; Tanassi, J.T.; Knudsen, S.; Jacobsen, S.; Heegaard, N.H. Unique protein signature of circulating microparticles in systemic lupus erythematosus. *Arthritis Rheum.* **2013**, *65*, 2680–2690. [CrossRef] [PubMed]
25. Pisetsky, D.S.; Lipsky, P.E. Microparticles as autoadjuvants in the pathogenesis of SLE. *Nat. Rev. Rheumatol.* **2010**, *6*, 368–372. [CrossRef]
26. Morel, O.; Morel, N.; Freyssinet, J.M.; Toti, F. Platelet microparticles and vascular cells interactions: A checkpoint between the haemostatic and thrombotic responses. *Platelets* **2008**, *19*, 9–23. [CrossRef]
27. McLaughlin, P.J.; Gooch, J.T.; Mannherz, H.G.; Weeds, A.G. Structure of gelsolin segment 1-actin complex and the mechanism of filament serving. *Nature* **1993**, *364*, 685–692. [CrossRef]
28. Beleznay, Z.; Zachowski, A.; Devaux, P.F.; Navazo, M.P.; Ott, P. ATP-dependent aminophospholipid translocation in erythrocyte vesicles: Stoichiometry of transport. *Biochemistry* **1993**, *32*, 3146–3152. [CrossRef]
29. Connor, J.; Pak, C.H.; Zwaal, R.F.; Schroit, A.J. Bidirectional transbilayer movement of phospholipid analogs in human red blood cells. Evidence for an ATP-dependent and protein-mediated process. *J. Biol. Chem.* **1992**, *267*, 19412–19417.
30. Kelton, J.G.; Warkentin, T.E.; Hayward, C.P.; Murphy, W.G.; Moore, J.C. Calpain activity in patients with thrombotic thrombocytopenic purpura is associated with platelet microparticles. *Blood* **1992**, *80*, 2246–2251. [CrossRef]
31. Zwaal, R.F.; Comfurius, P.; Bevers, E.M. Mechanism and function of change in membrane-phospholipid asymetry in platelets and erythrocytes. *Biochim. Soc. Trans.* **1993**, *21*, 248–253. [CrossRef] [PubMed]
32. Schroit, A.J.; Tanaka, Y.; Madsen, J.; Fidler, I.J. The recognition of red blood cells by macrofages: Role of phosphatidyl-serine and possible implication of membrane phospholipid asymetry. *Biol. Cell* **1984**, *51*, 227–238. [CrossRef] [PubMed]
33. Thiagarajan, P.; Tait, J.F. Collagen-induced exposure of anionic phospholipid in platelet and platelet derived microparticles. *J. Biol. Chem.* **1991**, *266*, 24302–24307. [PubMed]
34. Van der Pol, E.; van Gemert, M.J.; Sturk, A.; Nieuwland, R.; van Leeuwen, T.G. Single vs. swarm detection of microparticles and exosomes by flow cytometry. *J. Thromb. Haemost.* **2012**, *10*, 919–930. [CrossRef] [PubMed]
35. Lacroix, R.; Robert, S.; Poncelet, P.; Dignat-George, F. Overcoming limitations of microparticle measurement by flow cytometry. *Semin. Thromb Hemost.* **2010**, *36*, 807–818. [CrossRef] [PubMed]
36. Dachary-Prigent, J.; Freyssinet, J.M.; Pasquet, J.M.; Carron, J.C.; Nurden, A.T. Annexin-V as a probe of aminophospholipid exposure and platelet membrane vesiculation—A flow-cytometry study showing a role for free sulfhydryl-groups. *Blood* **1993**, *81*, 2554–2565. [CrossRef]
37. Connor, D.E.; Exner, T.; Ma, D.D.; Joseph, J.E. The majority of circulating platelet-derived microparticles fail to bind annexin V, lack phospholipid-dependent procoagulant activity and demonstrate greater expression of glycoprotein lb. *Thromb. Haemost.* **2010**, *103*, 1044–1052. [CrossRef]
38. Miyamoto, S.; Marcinkiewicz, C.; Edmunds, L.H.; Niewiarowski, S. Measurement of platelet microparticles during cardiopulmonary bypass by means of captured ELISA for GpIIb/IIIa. *Thromb. Haemost.* **1998**, *80*, 225–230. [CrossRef]
39. Nomura, S. Measuring circulating cell derived microparticles. *J. Thromb. Haemost.* **2004**, *2*, 1847–1848. [CrossRef]
40. Baka, Z.; Senolt, L.; Vencovsky, J.; Mann, H.; Simon, P.S.; Kittel, A.; Buzás, E.; Nagy, G. Increased serum concentration of immune cell derived microparticles in polymyositis/dermatomyositis. *Immunol. Lett.* **2010**, *128*, 124–130. [CrossRef]
41. Brogan, P.A.; Shah, V.; Brachet, C.; Harnden, A.; Mant, D.; Klein, N.; Dillon, M.J. Endothelial and platelet microparticles in vasculitis of the young. *Arthritis Rheum.* **2004**, *50*, 927–936. [CrossRef] [PubMed]

42. Dignat-George, F.; Camoin-Jau, L.; Sabatier, F.; Arnoux, D.; Anfosso, F.; Bardin, N.; Veit, V.; Combes, V.; Gentile, S.; Moal, V. Endothelial microparticles: A potential contribution to the thrombotic complications of the antiphospholipid syndrome. *Thromb. Haemost.* **2004**, *91*, 667–673. [CrossRef] [PubMed]
43. Erdbruegger, U.; Grossheim, M.; Hertel, B.; Wyss, K.; Kirsch, T.; Woywodt, A.; Haller, H.; Haubitz, M. Diagnostic role of endothelial microparticles in vasculitis. *Rheumatology* **2008**, *47*, 18205. [CrossRef] [PubMed]
44. Nagahama, M.; Nomura, S.; Ozaki, Y.; Yoshimura, C.; Kagawa, H.; Fukuhara, S. Platelet activation markers and soluble adhesion molecules in patients with systemic lupus erythematosus. *Autoimmunity* **2001**, *33*, 85–94. [CrossRef]
45. Oyabu, C.; Morinobu, A.; Sugiyama, D.; Saegusa, J.; Tanaka, S.; Morinobu, S.; Tsuji, G.; Kasagi, S.; Kawano, S.; Kumagai, S. Plasma platelet-derived microparticles in patients with connective tissue diseases. *J. Rheumatol.* **2011**, *38*, 680–684. [CrossRef]
46. Sellam, J.; Proulle, V.; Jungel, A.; Ittah, M.; Miceli, R.C.; Gottenberg, J.E.; Toti, F.; Benessiano, J.; Gay, S.; Freyssinet, J.M. Increased levels of circulating microparticles in primary Sjögren's syndrome, systemic lupus erythematosus and rheumatoid arthritis and relation with disease activity. *Arthritis Res. Ther.* **2008**, *11*, R156. [CrossRef]
47. Ho, J.C.; Lee, C.H.; Lin, S.H. No Significant Reduction of Circulating Endothelial-Derived and Platelet-Derived Microparticles in Patients with Psoriasis Successfully Treated with Anti-IL12/23. *Biomed. Res. Int.* **2016**, *2016*, 3242143. [CrossRef]
48. Pelletier, F.; Garnache-Ottou, F.; Angelot, F.; Biichlé, S.; Vidal, C.; Humbert, P.; Saas, P.; Seillès, E.; Aubin, F. Increased levels of circulating endothelial-derived microparticles and small-size platelet-derived microparticles in psoriasis. *J. Investig. Dermatol.* **2011**, *131*, 1573–1576. [CrossRef]
49. Knijff-Dutmer, E.A.; Koerts, J.; Nieuwland, R.; Kalsbeek-Batenburg, E.M.; van de Laar, M.A. Elevated levels of platelet microparticles are associated with disease activity in rheumatoid arthritis. *Arthritis Rheum.* **2002**, *46*, 1498–1503. [CrossRef]
50. Beyer, C.; Pisetsky, D.S. The role of microparticles in the pathogenesis of rheumatic diseases. *Nat. Rev. Rheumatol.* **2010**, *6*, 21–29. [CrossRef]
51. Van Eijk, I.C.; Tushuizen, M.E.; Sturk, A.; Dijkmans, B.A.; Boers, M.; Voskuyl, A.E.; Diamant, M.; Wolbink, G.J.; Nieuwland, R.; Nurmohamed, M.T. Circulating microparticles remain associated with complement activation despite intensive anti-inflammatory therapy in early rheumatoid arthritis. *Ann. Rheum. Dis.* **2010**, *69*, 1378–1382. [CrossRef] [PubMed]
52. Viñuela-Berni, V.; Doníz-Padilla, L.; Figueroa-Vega, N.; Portillo-Salazar, H.; Abud-Mendoza, C.; Baranda, L.; González-Amaro, R. Proportions of several types of plasma and urine microparticles are increased in patients with rheumatoid arthritis with active disease. *Clin. Exp. Immunol.* **2015**, *180*, 442–451. [CrossRef] [PubMed]
53. Headland, S.E.; Jones, H.R.; Norling, L.V.; Kim, A.; Souza, P.R.; Corsiero, E.; Gil, C.D.; Nerviani, A.; Dell'Accio, F.; Pitzalis, C.; et al. Neutrophil-derived microvesicles enter cartilage and protect the joint in inflammatory arthritis. *Sci. Transl. Med.* **2015**, *7*. [CrossRef] [PubMed]
54. Michael, B.N.R.; Kommoju, V.; Kavadichanda Ganapathy, C.; Negi, V.S. Characterization of cell-derived microparticles in synovial fluid and plasma of patients with rheumatoid arthritis. *Rheumatol. Int.* **2019**, *39*, 1377–1387. [CrossRef] [PubMed]
55. Kumar, N.; Punnen, K.A.; Nair, S.C.; Jayaseelan, V.; Kumar, T.S. Platelet microparticles level in juvenile idiopathic arthritis: A pediatric population-based cross-sectional study in a tertiary care center. *Indian J. Rheumatol.* **2019**, *14*, 182–186. [CrossRef]
56. Sari, I.; Bozkaya, G.; Kirbiyik, H.; Alacacioglu, A.; Ates, H.; Sop, G.; Can, G.; Taylan, A.; Piskin, O.; Yildiz, Y.; et al. Evaluation of circulating endothelial and platelet microparticles in men with ankylosing spondylitis. *J. Rheumatol.* **2012**, *39*, 594–599. [CrossRef] [PubMed]
57. Bradley, N. Plasma Microparticle Levels are not Raised in Patients with Ankylosing Spondylitis. *Rheumatology* **2014**, *53*, i137. [CrossRef]
58. Barbati, C.; Vomero, M.; Colasanti, T.; Diociaiuti, M.; Ceccarelli, F.; Ferrigno, S.; Finucci, A.; Miranda, F.; Novelli, L.; Perricone, C.; et al. TNFα expressed on the surface of microparticles modulates endothelial cell fate in rheumatoid arthritis. *Arthritis Res. Ther.* **2018**, *20*, 273. [CrossRef]
59. Messer, L.; Alsaleh, G.; Freyssinet, J.M.; Zobairi, F.; Leray, I.; Gottenberg, J.E.; Sibilia, J.; Toti-Orfanoudakis, F.; Wachsmann, D. Microparticle-induced release of B-lymphocyte regulators by rheumatoid synoviocytes. *Arthritis Res. Ther.* **2009**, *11*, R40. [CrossRef]

60. Biro, E.; Nieuwland, R.; Tak, P.P.; Pronk, L.M.; Schaap, M.C.; Sturk, A.; Hack, C.E. Activated complement components and complement activator molecules on the surface of cell-derived microparticles in patients with rheumatoid arthritis and healthy individuals. *Ann. Rheum. Dis.* **2007**, *66*, 1085–1092. [CrossRef]
61. Cloutier, N.; Tan, S.; Boudreau, L.H.; Cramb, C.; Subbaiah, R.; Lahey, L.; Albert, A.; Shnayder, R.; Gobezie, R.; Nigrovic, P.A.; et al. The exposure of autoantigens by microparticles underlies the formation of potent inflammatory components: The microparticle-associated immune complexes. *EMBO Mol. Med.* **2013**, *5*, 235–249. [CrossRef] [PubMed]
62. Distler, J.H.; Jungel, A.; Huber, L.C.; Seemayer, C.A.; Reich, C.F., 3rd; Gay, R.E.; Michel, B.A.; Fontana, A.; Gay, S.; Pisetsky, D.S.; et al. The induction of matrix metalloproteinase and cytokine expression in synovial fibroblasts stimulated with immune cell microparticles. *Proc. Natl. Acad. Sci. USA* **2005**, *102*, 2892–2897. [CrossRef] [PubMed]
63. Berckmans, R.J.; Nieuwland, R.; Kraan, M.C.; Schaap, M.C.; Pots, D.; Smeets, T.J.; Sturk, A.; Tak, P.P. Synovial microparticles from arthritic patients modulate chemokine and cytokine release by synoviocytes. *Arthritis Res. Ther.* **2005**, *7*, 536–544. [CrossRef] [PubMed]
64. Berckmans, R.J.; Nieuwland, R.; Tak, P.P.; Böing, A.N.; Romijn, F.P.; Kraan, M.C.; Breedveld, F.C.; Hack, C.E.; Sturk, A. Cell-derived microparticles in synovial fluid from inflamed arthritic joints support coagulation exclusively via a factor VII-dependent mechanism. *Arthritis Rheum.* **2002**, *46*, 2857–2866. [CrossRef]
65. Reich, N.; Beyer, C.; Gelse, K.; Akhmetshina, A.; Dees, C.; Zwerina, J.; Schett, G.; Distler, O.; Distler, J.H. Microparticles stimulate angiogenesis by inducing ELR(+) CXC-chemokines in synovial fibroblasts. *J. Cell Mol. Med.* **2011**, *15*, 756–762. [CrossRef]
66. Endresen, G.K. Investigation of blood platelets in synovial fluid from patients with rheumatoid arthritis. *Scand. J. Rheumatol.* **1981**, *10*, 204–208. [CrossRef]
67. Endresen, G.K.; Forre, O. Human platelets in synovial fluid. A focus on the effects of growth factors on the inflammatory responses in rheumatoid arthritis. *Clin. Exp. Rheumatol.* **1992**, *10*, 181–187.
68. Farr, M.; Wainwright, A.; Salmon, M.; Hollywell, C.A.; Bacon, P.A. Platelets in the synovial fluid of patients with rheumatoid arthritis. *Rheumatol. Int.* **1984**, *4*, 13–17. [CrossRef]
69. Moroi, M.; Jung, S.M. Platelet glycoprotein VI: Its structure and function. *Thromb. Res.* **2004**, *114*, 221–233. [CrossRef]
70. Hsu, J.; Gu, Y.; Tan, S.L.; Narula, S.; Demartino, J.A.; Liao, C. Bruton's Tyrosine Kinase mediates platelet receptor-induced generation of microparticles: A potential mechanism for amplification of inflammatory responses in rheumatoid arthritis synovial joints. *Immunol. Lett.* **2012**, *150*, 97–104. [CrossRef]
71. Tan, S.L.; Liao, C.; Lucas, M.C.; Stevenson, C.; Demartino, J.A. Targeting the SYK-BTK axis for the treatment of immunological and hematological disorders: Recent progress and therapeutic perspectives. *Pharmacol. Ther.* **2013**, *138*, 294–309. [CrossRef] [PubMed]
72. Uckun, F.M.; Qazi, S. Bruton's tyrosine kinase as a molecular target in treatment of leukemias and lymphomas as well as inflammatory disorders and autoimmunity. *Expert Opin. Ther. Pat.* **2010**, *20*, 1457–1470. [CrossRef] [PubMed]
73. Ardoin, S.P.; Shanahan, J.C.; Pisetsky, D.S. The role of microparticles in inflammation and thrombosis. *Scand. J. Immunol.* **2007**, *66*, 159–165. [CrossRef] [PubMed]
74. Distler, J.H.; Distler, O. Inflammation: Microparticles and their roles in inflammatory arthritides. *Nat. Rev. Rheumatol.* **2010**, *6*, 385–386. [CrossRef]
75. Gaipl, U.S.; Kuenkele, S.; Voll, R.E.; Beyer, T.D.; Kolowos, W.; Heyder, P.; Kalden, J.R.; Herrmann, M. Complement binding is an early feature of necrotic and a rather late event during apoptotic cell death. *Cell Death Differ.* **2001**, *8*, 327–334. [CrossRef]
76. Ciurana, C.L.; Zwart, B.; van Mierlo, G.; Hack, C.E. Complement activation by necrotic cells in normal plasma environment compares to that by late apoptotic cells and involves predominantly IgM. *Eur. J. Immunol.* **2004**, *34*, 2609–2619. [CrossRef]
77. Taylor, P.R.; Carugati, A.; Fadok, V.A.; Cook, H.T.; Andrews, M.; Carroll, M.C.; Savill, J.S.; Henson, P.M.; Botto, M.; Walport, M.J. A hierarchical role for classical pathway complement proteins in the clearance of apoptotic cells in vivo. *J. Exp. Med.* **2000**, *192*, 359–366. [CrossRef]
78. Zwart, B.; Ciurana, C.; Rensink, I.; Manoe, R.; Hack, C.E.; Aarden, L.A. Complement activation by apoptotic cells occurs predominantly via IgM and is limited to late apoptotic (secondary necrotic) cells. *Autoimmunity* **2004**, *37*, 95–102. [CrossRef]

79. Nauta, A.J.; Trouw, L.A.; Daha, M.R.; Tijsma, O.; Nieuwland, R.; Schwaeble, W.J.; Gingras, A.R.; Mantovani, A.; Hack, E.C.; Roos, A. Direct binding of C1q to apoptotic cells and cell blebs induces complement activation. *Eur. J. Immunol.* **2002**, *32*, 1726–1736. [CrossRef]
80. Gasser, O.; Hess, C.; Miot, S.; Deon, C.; Sanchez, J.C.; Schifferli, J.A. Characterisation and properties of ectosomes released by human polymorphonuclear neutrophils. *Exp. Cell Res.* **2003**, *285*, 243–257. [CrossRef]
81. Gasser, O.; Schifferli, J.A. Microparticles released by human neutrophils adhere to erythrocytes in the presence of complement. *Exp. Cell Res.* **2005**, *307*, 381–387. [CrossRef] [PubMed]
82. Nielsen, C.T.; Ostergaard, O.; Stener, L.; Iversen, L.V.; Truedsson, L.; Gullstrand, B.; Jacobsen, S.; Heegaard, N.H. Increased IgG on cell-derived plasma microparticles in systemic lupus erythematosus is associated with autoantibodies and complement activation. *Arthritis Rheum.* **2012**, *64*, 1227–1236. [CrossRef] [PubMed]
83. Papadavid, E.; Diamanti, K.; Spathis, A.; Varoudi, M.; Andreadou, I.; Gravanis, K.; Theodoropoulos, K.; Karakitsos, P.; Lekakis, J.; Rigopoulos, D.; et al. Increased levels of circulating platelet-derived microparticles in psoriasis: Possible implications for the associated cardiovascular risk. *World J. Cardiol.* **2016**, *8*, 667–675. [CrossRef] [PubMed]
84. Chen, X. Rac1 regulates platelet microparticles formation and rheumatoid arthritis deterioration. *Platelets* **2019**, 1–8. [CrossRef] [PubMed]
85. Krajewska-Włodarczyk, M.; Owczarczyk-Saczonek, A.; Placek, W.; Osowski, A.; Engelgardt, P.; Wojtkiewicz, J. Role of Stem Cells in Pathophysiology and Therapy of Spondyloarthropathies-New Therapeutic Possibilities? *Int. J. Mol. Sci.* **2017**, *19*, 80. [CrossRef] [PubMed]
86. Tang, C.H. Research of Pathogenesis and Novel Therapeutics in Arthritis. *Int. J. Mol. Sci.* **2019**, *20*, 1646. [CrossRef] [PubMed]
87. Cosenza, S.; Toupet, K.; Maumus, M.; Luz-Crawford, P.; Blanc-Brude, O.; Jorgensen, C.; Noël, D. Mesenchymal stem cells-derived exosomes are more immunosuppressive than microparticles in inflammatory arthritis. *Theranostics* **2018**, *8*, 1399–1410. [CrossRef]
88. Cosenza, S.; Ruiz, M.; Toupet, K.; Jorgensen, C.; Noël, D. Mesenchymal stem cells derived exosomes and microparticles protect cartilage and bone from degradation in osteoarthritis. *Sci. Rep.* **2017**, *7*, 16214. [CrossRef]
89. Ragni, E.; Perucca Orfei, C.; De Luca, P.; Lugano, G.; Viganò, M.; Colombini, A.; Valli, F.; Zacchetti, D.; Bollati, V.; de Girolamo, L. Interaction with hyaluronan matrix and miRNA cargo as contributors for in vitro potential of mesenchymal stem cell-derived extracellular vesicles in a model of human osteoarthritic synoviocytes. *Stem Cell Res. Ther.* **2019**, *10*, 109. [CrossRef]
90. Tofiño-Vian, M.; Guillén, M.I.; Pérez Del Caz, M.D.; Silvestre, A.; Alcaraz, M.J. Microvesicles from Human Adipose Tissue-Derived Mesenchymal Stem Cells as a New Protective Strategy in Osteoarthritic Chondrocytes. *Cell Physiol. Biochem.* **2018**, *47*, 11–25. [CrossRef]

MDPI
St. Alban-Anlage 66
4052 Basel
Switzerland
Tel. +41 61 683 77 34
Fax +41 61 302 89 18
www.mdpi.com

International Journal of Molecular Sciences Editorial Office
E-mail: ijms@mdpi.com
www.mdpi.com/journal/ijms

www.ingramcontent.com/pod-product-compliance
Lightning Source LLC
Chambersburg PA
CBHW041934260926
51850CB00018B/157
9783036575926